CLINICAL GASTROENTEROLOGY
A COMPREHENSIVE GUIDE

Dr. Ahmed Mohamed Helmy

ALLIED HEALTH PRESS

Clinical Gastroenterology: A Comprehensive Guide

Author: **Dr. Ahmed Mohamed Helmy**

Allied Health Press
4164 Lakeshore Road
Burlington ON L7L 1A4
Canada
www.alliedhealthpress.com
Email: orders@arclereducation.com

ISBN: 978-1-77956-832-8

ABOUT THE AUTHOR

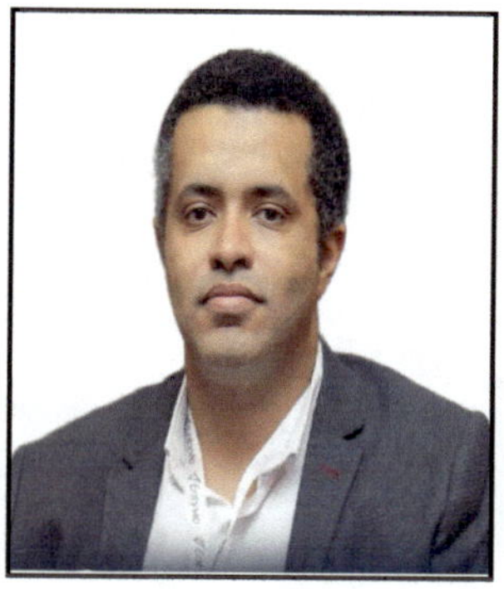

Dr. Ahmed Helmy is a physician with over 15 years of extensive experience in internal medicine, gastroenterology, hepatology, and gastrointestinal (GI) endoscopy. His clinical acumen is rooted in a solid academic foundation and years of dedicated practice in both hospital and academic settings.He began his medical career at Raghi GIT and Hepatology Hospital, Assiut University, where he completed a rigorous residency program. Building on that, he earned a master's degree in gastroenterology, hepatology, and infectious diseases from the same esteemed institution. To further refine his technical skills, Dr. Helmy pursued advanced training and received a GI endoscopy diploma from Ain Shams University, one of Egypt's leading medical universities.

Dr. Helmy currently serves as a consultant of gastroenterology and endoscopy at Assiut P.Staff Hospital, where he specializes in the diagnosis, treatment, and procedural management of a broad spectrum of gastrointestinal conditions. His clinical focus includes chronic liver disease, inflammatory bowel disease, gastrointestinal bleeding, and advanced endoscopic techniques.

In addition to his clinical role, Dr. Helmy is a recognized leader in gastroenterology research. His scholarly interests center around improving diagnostic accuracy and therapeutic strategies in hepatogastroenterology. He has contributed to academic forums, with particular emphasis on liver disease epidemiology, novel endoscopic technologies, and the intersection of infectious diseases with GI disorders. His work has informed evidence-based practices and has been instrumental in shaping regional treatment protocols. Dr. Helmy remains committed to advancing the field through a combination of patient-centered care, academic collaboration, and continuous research innovation.

Brief Table of Contents

Detailed Table of Contents

CHAPTER 10

Gallbladder and Biliary Tract Disorders 299

CHAPTER 11

Gastrointestinal Bleeding 331

CHAPTER 12

Nutritional Aspects in Gastroenterology 365

CHAPTER 13

Pediatric Gastroenterology 399

CHAPTER 14

GI Oncology 433

LIST OF FIGURES

PREFACE

The human digestive system goes through a process of phenomenal changes that transform the food we consume into the compounds our bodies require. The moment one bites an apple, a process of mechanical and chemical conversion begins, breaking down complex molecules into a usable form that can be absorbed and utilized. Not only does the system enable the retrieval of energy and essential compounds, but it also protects our health from the onset of harmful pathogens and toxins entering the body. Malfunctions in the processes can result in discomfort, disease, or fatal diseases, hence the need for practitioners and students to comprehend digestive health.

To understand how the gastrointestinal tract functions, one has to grasp the dynamic interplay between the nervous system, microbes, fluids, and tissues. Each part of the tract—mouth to anus—serves unique functions: secretion, digestion, absorption, and elimination. New imaging modalities, endoscopy, and molecular diagnostics have provided clinicians with a degree of insight into these functions heretofore unobtainable, allowing them to diagnose disorders early and provide directed treatments. The greater our understanding, the better we can enhance patient outcomes with directed interventions and prevention.

Clinical Gastroenterology: A Comprehensive Guide synthesizes novel knowledge, practice, and research to present a wide-ranging overview of gastrointestinal well-being. It seeks to meet educational and reference needs as far as possible, striking a balance between clear explanations and evidence-based recommendations. Practitioners will be able to consult whatever is appropriate, whether they are dealing with common problems or managing complex cases, according to prevailing standards of clinical care.

Chapter 1 introduces the basic principles of gastrointestinal anatomy and physiology. It outlines the structure of the tract's layers, the functions of digestive secretions, and the control of motility. It is through an understanding of these fundamentals that clinicians can make sense of signs and symptoms found in practice.

Chapter 2 describes the diagnostic procedures used in contemporary gastroenterology. Laboratory diagnostics, imaging techniques like ultrasound and CT, and endoscopic methods like capsule endoscopy and high-end endoscope systems are discussed. The readers will know how to choose and apply each technique in the proper way.

Chapter 3 discusses several esophageal conditions, including motility diseases like achalasia and inflammatory diseases like eosinophilic esophagitis. The chapter discusses issues of management in depth, including drug treatment and dilation methods.

Chapter 4 discusses gastric diseases, including peptic ulcer disease, gastritis, and dyspepsia.

The chapter discusses *Helicobacter pylori*'s role, acid suppression therapy, and surgery for refractory conditions.

Chapter 5 discusses disorders of the small intestine, including celiac disease, other malabsorption syndromes, and neoplasms. It emphasizes approaches to nutritional support and interpretation of results of small bowel biopsies.

Chapter 6 covers disorders of the colon like irritable bowel syndrome, diverticular disease, and chronic constipation. Dietary management is highlighted, as is the employment of motility agents and when colonoscopic evaluation should be obtained.

Chapter 7 outlines the spectrum of inflammatory bowel disease (IBD) and includes ulcerative colitis and Crohn's disease. The management includes the use of biological therapies, immunomodulatory drugs, and surgery.

Chapter 8 discusses liver disease, including hepatitis, cirrhosis, and metabolic liver disease. The chapter discusses diagnostic scoring, antiviral treatment, and transplantation criteria.

Chapter 9 discusses pancreatic disease, focusing on acute pancreatitis and chronic pancreatitis, exocrine deficiency, and the diagnosis of pancreatic masses. Principles of nutritional and endoscopic management are outlined.

Chapter 10 addresses gallbladder and biliary tract disease, such as cholelithiasis, cholangitis, and strictures of the biliary tract. ERCP and modern surgical techniques are discussed.

Chapter 11 addresses gastrointestinal bleeding, both upper and lower, in pathogenesis. Stabilization recommendations, endoscopic hemostasis, and radiologic procedures are covered.

Chapter 12 considers nutritional issues in gastroenterology, such as enteral and parenteral nutrition, the management of micronutrient deficiency, and weight control strategies in gastrointestinal disease.

Chapter 13 presents an overview of pediatric gastroenterology, emphasizing prevalent disorders affecting infants and children, including gastroesophageal reflux, developmental motility disorders, and congenital abnormalities. Considerations regarding growth and development are integrated throughout the discussion.

Chapter 14 covers gastrointestinal oncology, which comprises screening guidelines, staging criteria, and multidisciplinary management of esophageal, stomach, colon, and pancreatic cancer.

Chapter 15 discusses new innovations and the future of gastroenterology. Subtopics are microbiome therapies, next-generation endoscopic platforms, and precision medicine strategies.

This text is intended for gastroenterology fellows, practicing physicians, and allied health professionals who need a complete, integrated reference. Medical students and residents will also find useful the clear explanation of basic principles, while experienced practitioners will appreciate the up-to-date discussion of diagnostic and therapeutic advances.

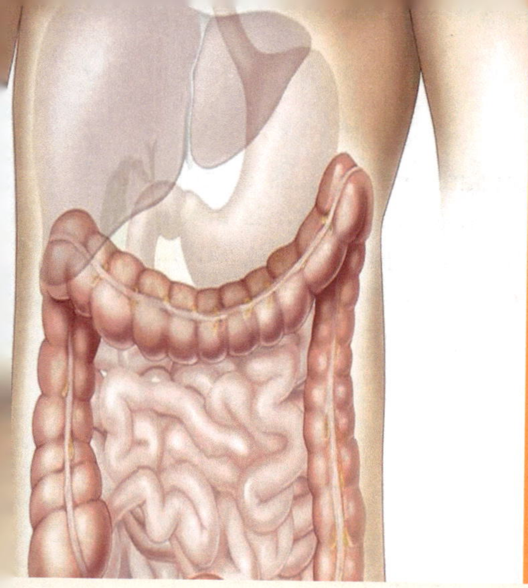

Chapter 1

FUNDAMENTALS OF GASTROINTESTINAL PHYSIOLOGY AND ANATOMY

Contents

Introduction

The gastrointestinal (GI) system is the center of human health with its complex and interdependent functionalities. The digestive tract and organs constitute the system responsible predominantly for the ingestion, breakdown, and assimilation of nutrients. It transforms food into essential sources of energy while, at the same time, eliminating waste products, thereby performing dual functions in nutrient assimilation and management of metabolic waste. The complex GI tract architecture from the oral cavity to the anus consists of specialized areas, each serving a particular function, e.g., enzymatic digestion of food in the stomach and nutrient absorption in the small intestine. An in-depth study of these anatomical structures adds to a better understanding of their physiological functions as well as the probable complications arising from their malfunctioning, thereby setting the stage for the subsequent research into gastrointestinal health and treatment of related diseases. Each part of the gastrointestinal tract is particularly designed to optimize the digestion process, beginning with the mechanical and enzymatic digestion of food. The salivary glands initiate the process of digestion in the oral cavity by secreting enzymes that start carbohydrate breakdown, which is continued in the stomach, where secretions of the stomach play an important role in protein digestion. The small intestine is the major site of the absorption of nutrients, aided by its extensive surface area made up of villi and microvilli.

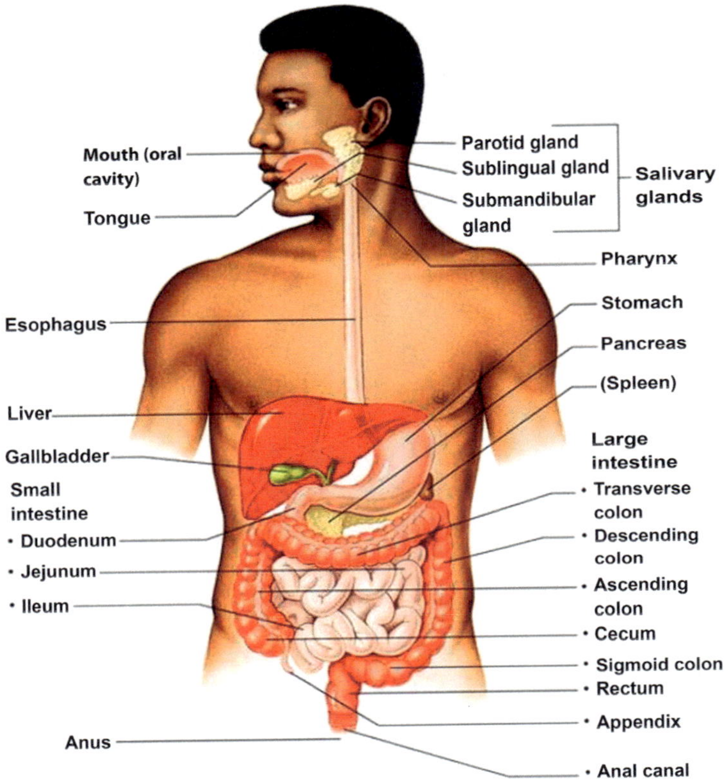

Figure 1.1. Gastrointestinal physiology and anatomy.

Source: https://i.pinimg.com/736x/65/81/d0/6581d0ab629f12c17a0190abae2fa664--anatomy-and-physiology.jpg.

The role of the pancreas and liver is equally important as they supply digestive enzymes and bile that emulsify fat, an important step towards nutrient uptake. Understanding of these processes highlights the importance of intact GI physiology towards the maintenance of health; any deviation within this system may result in the creation of conditions such as malabsorption or gastrointestinal reflux, emphasizing the importance of subsequent research and intervention. Pathophysiologic conditions within the gastrointestinal tract have a tendency to be the result of, or the cause of, disruption of normal physiological function. For example, constipation can represent interruption of normal gut motility, with significant clinical implications for general health and well-being. It can manifest as straining, reduced frequency of bowel action, and the perception of incomplete bowel evacuation, indicative of possible underlying pathologies that affect colonic transit and mechanisms of defecation. A closer examination of constipation reveals several classifications and treatment strategies aimed at these presentations. Knowledge of the pharmacological agents used in treatment, especially in the presence of underlying disease, highlights the requirement for evidence-based practice within gastrointestinal medicine. This illustrates the interaction between gastrointestinal anatomy and physiology, with the way in which detailed anatomical knowledge allows the effective management of functional disorders (Focal Spot, Fall/Winter 2010/2011; Gardiner & Hilton, 2016) (Figure 1.1).

Definition and Importance of the Gastrointestinal System

The gastrointestinal (GI) system, identified as an intricate organ system essential for human health, consists of a series of hollow organs forming a continuous tube extending from the mouth to the anus. The main function is to provide the ability to digest and assimilate nutrients in the food ingested and, at the same time, manage the excretion of waste products. The system consists of the mouth, esophagus, stomach, intestines, liver, pancreas, and gallbladder, each with a distinct function in the digestion process. The GI tract processes the food ingested into necessary nutrients for energy, cellular growth, and cellular repair. For this reason, it is important to know the anatomy and physiology of the GI system to learn about how our bodies function, thus enabling us to have crucial knowledge of both health and the pathological consequences of its malfunction or structural defects. The GI system's function is more than mundane digestion; it is connected to the body's overall homeostasis. The regulation of the absorption of necessary substances by the GI system influences various physiological processes, such as metabolism and immunity. It is also responsible for maintaining the acid-base balance of the body. The synergistic functions of several organs and systems, as indicated by the research work of White indicate the interdependence of digestion on other bodily processes. Without an effectively functioning GI system, the body is susceptible to deficiencies in nutrients, gastrointestinal diseases, and a host of systemic complications that endanger overall health. For this reason, knowledge of its definition and significance is crucial to understanding the larger aspects of human physiology and health. In addition, the role of the gastrointestinal (GI) system involves more than the absorption of nutrients; it also has a role in advanced cognitive functions, as described by the distributed cognition model of Christensen (2006). Control of GI functions involves not only mechanical and biochemical processes but also neural and hormonal signaling that coordinates a wide range of physiological responses. This system of interaction emphasizes the importance of voluntary and involuntary control of digestive processes so that the organism may effectively manage meals of diverse composition and duration. A comprehensive appreciation of the anatomy and physiological processes of the GI system is thus essential to any human physiology study, emphasizing its role as a structural and functional basis of health that enables many physiological processes, along with cognitive processes, to optimize nutrition and digestion.

Overview of Gastrointestinal Functions

The gastrointestinal (GI) tract is a highly developed system for macronutrient breakdown, nutrient absorption, and elimination of waste. It is designed to carry out several functions efficiently, from the mechanical and chemical breakdown of food in the oral cavity to the esophagus, stomach, and intestines. This process entails a series of coordinated muscular contractions known as peristalsis, which advances the food bolus through the digestive tract. The secretions of the digestive system, such as saliva, gastric juice, and bile, also take part in the breakdown of macronutrients into their absorbable forms: amino acids, fatty acids, and monosaccharides. The GI tract is therefore not only central to nutrition but also acts as a disease barrier, which highlights its vital role in maintaining the general state of health. The gastrointestinal system's functions are also inextricably linked with its multifaceted neural and hormonal regulation. The enteric nervous system, which is also known as the second brain, autonomously regulates digestive functions and also maintains considerable communication with the central nervous system. Hormonal regulators such as gastrin, cholecystokinin, and secretin are released upon food intake and trigger digestive functions. The hormones are also responsible for coordinating the timing of gastric emptying, the release of enzymes, and the release of bile to ensure the digestive process is finely attuned to the availability of food substances. According to research, age-related changes may affect these neuromuscular functions, particularly in the ascending colon, where cholinergic responses are affected, which may be responsible for decreased efficiency in gastrointestinal motility and nutrient absorption (Broad et al., 2018). Additionally, gastrointestinal functions are not only affected by mechanical and chemical processes but are also significantly affected by various physiological factors, such as changes in hormones. Conditions like Irritable Bowel Syndrome (IBS) and Inflammatory Bowel Disease (IBD) show the impact of interactions among hormones that lead to severe alterations in intestinal function and then manifest symptoms like pain and changes in bowel habits. It has also been discovered through research that hormonal changes, particularly in the company of progesterone, exacerbate such symptoms, indicating the need for therapeutic interventions that target hormonal pathways to alleviate discomfort yet treat the underlying causes of the disorders (Linson, 2013). Such discoveries make it important to have an interdisciplinary approach to the understanding of gastrointestinal physiology that unites anatomy, neurology, and endocrinology levels of understanding to contribute to better health outcomes.

Relevance to Health and Disease

The gastrointestinal system is of fundamental importance in maintaining overall health through the digestion and absorption of nutrients. These nutrients are required for cellular function, growth, and repair, thus influencing a range of physiological mechanisms. In the case of the gastrointestinal system functioning optimally, it can thus modulate the absorption of vitamins, minerals, and macronutrients, all of which are required for metabolic well-being. Abnormalities in digestive function, however, can lead to malabsorption syndromes and gastrointestinal disease, such as celiac disease or Crohn's disease. These syndromes are examples of the influence an impaired gastrointestinal tract can have on health, further supporting the relationship between gastrointestinal physiology and general well-being. Awareness of these mechanisms is also integral in the development of therapeutic algorithms for optimizing health outcomes in patients with chronic gastrointestinal disease. The influence of dietary components on impacting gastrointestinal health also includes that of environmental contaminants, further supporting concerns regarding the influence of toxins and their resulting health consequences. An example is that of cadmium (Cd), identified as a prominent nephrotoxin and with adverse effects on the developing nervous system, particularly in infants. Evidence indicates that gastrointestinal absorption of Cd is greater in neonates than in adults, giving rise to concern regarding dietary exposure. An example of Cd presence in infant foods and cereal-based foods reflects differences in absorption that can have a decisive influence on health outcomes in this vulnerable population. The adverse effects of Cd highlight the role of the decisive relationship between gastrointestinal physiology and environmental health, making dietary intake a cause of significant health risk and thus requiring strict controls in food safety and surveillance. In addition, differences in gastrointestinal absorption mechanisms between age groups require a precise comprehension of nutrient bioavailability and toxicity. Infant digestion physiology, for example, reflects typical patterns with profound effects on dietary cadmium retention and bioavailability. The evidence suggests that the decreased solubility of cadmium during infant digestion, compared to adult digestion, leads to decreased absorption; the risk, however, arises from the enhanced uptake in this age group. The impact clearly demonstrates how factors such as age-related enzyme function and gut microbiome maturation can affect dietary constituents' health effects. More importantly, the complexity of these interactions has significant implications for pediatric nutrition, underscoring the importance of the role of expert dietary counseling in minimizing toxic exposure while maintaining adequate intake of essential nutrients. This body of research highlights the strong rationale for the integration of an understanding of public health campaigns to safeguard the health of susceptible populations, including infants and young children.

1.1. Anatomy of the Gastrointestinal Tract

The gastrointestinal (GI) tract anatomy is a complex organization of structures that function in harmony to promote digestion and absorption of nutrients. It starts in the oral cavity, where the food is mechanically fragmented and mixed with saliva, the start of the process of digestion. As the food moves through the pharynx and esophagus, it enters the stomach, a muscular organ that plays a basic role in the resumption of the digestive process. The stomach is subdivided into regions, including the fundus, body, and antrum, which play crucial roles in the mixing with gastric secretions and the regulation of its passage into the duodenum. The mention of respective anatomical structures along the GI tract highlights their functional significance in the process of digestion, with each section playing a specific role in ensuring effective breakdown and nutrient absorption. The small intestine is another demonstration of the complexity of structure in the GI tract. Subdivided into three parts, duodenum, jejunum, and ileum, the small intestine is the primary site of nutrient absorption. The villi and microvilli present enhance the surface area immensely, thereby enhancing its absorptive capability. In this context, the structure and function of intestinal walls become of paramount importance. Recent studies using computational fluid dynamics have demonstrated the dynamics of the gastric functions of trituration and mixing and gained greater insight into the role of various components, including the pyloric canal and the proximal duodenal cap, in the overall process of digestion (Vijay, 2020). Admitting these anatomical subtleties serves to reinforce the harmony of structure and function in the GI tract. Also, the transition into the large intestine represents a critical phase in the GI tract functions, with reabsorption of excess water and preparation of the waste for expulsion. The large intestine, comprising the cecum, colon, rectum, and anal canal, is responsible for maintaining electrolyte homeostasis and storing a diverse microbiome that is crucial to fermentation and vitamin synthesis. Anatomical organization in the large intestine is such that it accommodates progressive compaction of waste and also sustains the microbial populations key to health. Synthesis of anatomical and physiological findings reveals that the structural organization of each segment dictates the digestive processes performed throughout the complete gastrointestinal tract (Dunton, 1963). Such findings highlight the need for extensive anatomical knowledge of the gastrointestinal tract as key to understanding its complex physiological processes (Figure 1.2).

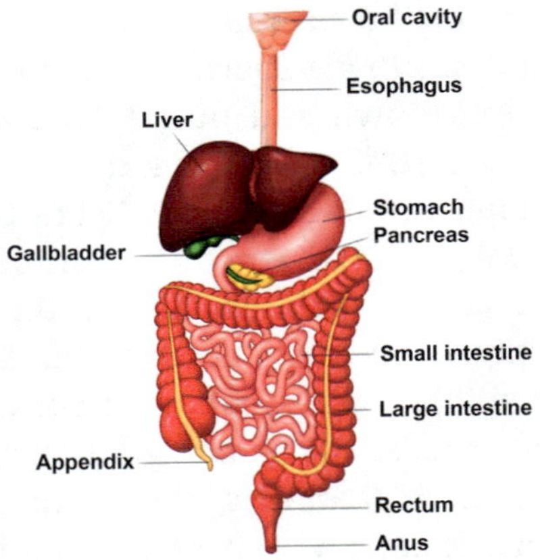

Figure 1.2. Anatomy of the gastrointestinal tract.

Source: https://cdn1.byjus.com/wp-content/uploads/2017/12/Gastrointestinal-Tract.png.

1.1.1. Structure of the Digestive Organs

The anatomy of the digestive organs is precisely designed to allow for the intricate functions of digestion, absorption, and elimination of wastes. From the oral cavity, food is mechanically fragmented by the teeth and mixed with saliva, which is a secretion containing enzymes that begin the digestion of carbohydrates. The esophagus is then a muscular tube that propels food to the stomach through the action of peristalsis, which is rhythmic contractions of the esophageal muscles. Gastric secretions within the stomach further fragment food into a semi-fluid substance known as chyme. The structural composition of the stomach, comprising a number of layers of muscle and mucosal tissue, plays a central role in allowing these functions to occur, suggesting the importance of effective coordination of various anatomical structures to accomplish their overall functions within the process of digestion. As food enters the small intestine, its structural alterations become more central. The small intestine comprises three compartments: the duodenum, jejunum, and ileum, each playing specific roles in digestion and nutrient absorption. Of note, the presence of villi and microvilli in the lining of the intestine greatly increases the surface area, and consequently, the efficiency of nutrient absorption. The cooperation of pancreatic digestive enzymes and bile from the liver also aids in fat emulsification and the digestion of proteins and carbohydrates.

The highly specialized architecture of the small intestine not only assists in digestion but also permits variability in the absorption of drugs, as changes in motility and the chemical makeup of intestinal fluid can affect the bioavailability of orally ingested drugs, suggesting the importance of an in-depth understanding of gastrointestinal anatomy within pharmacology (Vinarov et al., 2021).

The structure of the large intestine, or colon, is the central aspect of the digestive process, particularly that of water absorption and the creation of feces. It is comprised of several segments, including the cecum, colon, and rectum, and is larger in diameter than the small intestine, as well as having a specific organization of muscular tissue that facilitates the efficient transit and storage of waste material. Of special interest is the existence of a dense microbiome in the large intestine, which not only affects digestive processes but also the general state of health. The interaction of the gut microbiome with the structural properties of the large intestine has implications for a wide range of physiological processes, such as immune function and inflammatory processes, but also exhibits significant variability based on dietary habits and disease status (Rodrigues et al., 2019). Therefore, a thorough understanding of the structural properties of digestive organs is the foundation of an understanding of their functional processes and possible dysfunctions in the general context of gastrointestinal physiology (Figure 1.3).

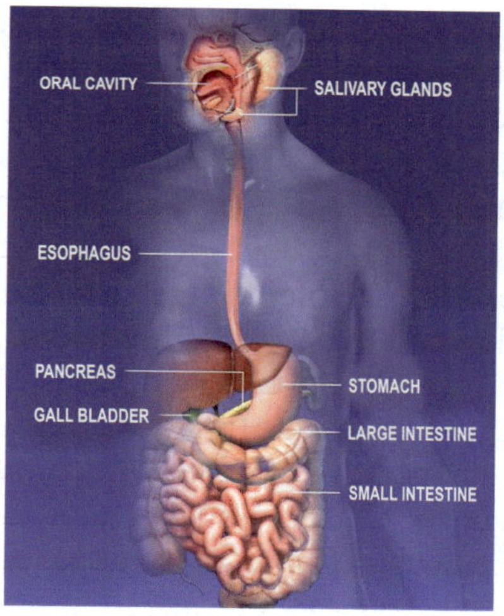

Figure 1.3. Structure of the digestive organs.

Source: https://www.visiblebody.com/hs-fs/hubfs/Learn_Articles/Digestive_System/2B_Digestive_System_Structures.jpg?width=957&height=1355&name=2B_Digestive_System_Structures.jpg.

1.1.2. Organization of the Gastrointestinal System

The organization of the gastrointestinal system is a complex interaction between structural elements and functional processes that collectively facilitate the digestion and absorption of nutrients. The system comprises various anatomical structures, including the oral cavity, esophagus, stomach, small intestine, large intestine, and accessory organs like the liver and pancreas. Each structure is uniquely designed to perform specific functions in the digestion process, varying from mechanical breakdown in the oral cavity to nutrient absorption in the small intestine. The coordinated flow of food through the gastrointestinal tract, propelled by peristaltic contractions, is an example of the dynamic nature of the system. The interaction of anatomical structures and coordinated movements exemplifies the importance of organization in the efficient functioning of the gastrointestinal system, where food ingested is efficiently processed, leading to the absorption of essential nutrients necessary for overall health and energy homeostasis. In addition, the organization of the gastrointestinal system goes beyond mere anatomical structures, incorporating a complex set of biochemical processes involving numerous secretions. Specialized digestive lining cells secrete enzymes, acids, and hormones that are vital in the breakdown of food. For example, gastric glands in the stomach secrete hydrochloric acid, which helps to digest proteins and generates an acidic environment necessary for the activation of digestive enzymes. Similarly, the pancreas secretes digestive enzymes into the small intestine, which degrade carbohydrates, proteins, and fats. These secretions are of critical importance in the process of digestion and are accurately regulated by neural and hormonal stimuli, thereby ensuring the efficacy of digestion. The complex interaction between cellular structure and biochemical function is a prime example of the gastrointestinal system's complexity, highlighting its basic function in the absorption of nutrients and overall physiological processes. Additionally, the physiological organization of the gastrointestinal system is deeply dependent upon its vascular and neural endowments, which play a vital role in regulating and maintaining homeostasis. The circulatory supply to the gastrointestinal system is specially organized to ensure that nutrients absorbed are effectively distributed to the liver and other systemic vascular pathways. The mesenteric arteries, which are branches of the abdominal aorta, supply essential blood to the intestines. The autonomic nervous system, including the enteric nervous system, is also essential in modulating digestive processes, such as the coordination of peristalsis and the release of digestive enzymes. This complex system of vascular and neural connections not only facilitates the mechanical and biochemical functioning of the gastrointestinal system but also ensures that the organism responds appropriately to the varied demands of digestion and nutrient absorption under different physiological conditions.

The structure of the gastrointestinal system thus represents an integrated interaction of anatomical, biochemical, vascular, and neural components required to ensure health and well-being.

1.1.3. Role of Accessory Organs in Digestion

The human digestive system is an intricate system of organs, each with a specific function carried out with astounding efficiency. Of all organs, the accessory organs, the liver, pancreas, and gallbladder, are integral to the digestive process, significantly aiding the absorption and use of nutrients. The liver, the largest internal organ, secretes bile, a required fluid needed for the emulsification of fats. Emulsification allows for the effective degradation of lipids by pancreatic enzymes, maximizing nutrient degradation and absorption in the small intestine. As such, the diverse functions of the liver go beyond digestion to metabolic control, an achievement of the interrelatedness of digestive and metabolic functions in the human body. The pancreas complements the functions of the liver by playing a dual role in endocrine and exocrine functions. In terms of digestion, the pancreas releases digestive enzymes, such as amylase, lipase, and proteases, into the small intestine.

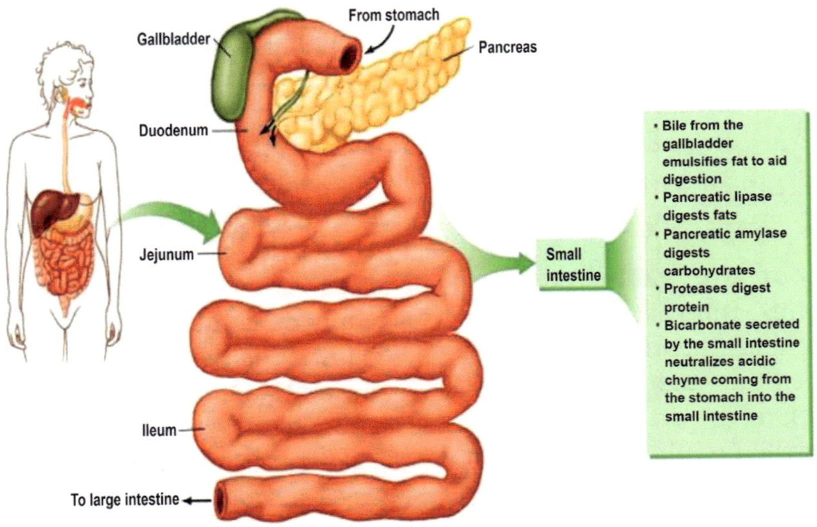

Figure 1.4. Role of accessory organs in digestion.

Source: https://image.slideserve.com/247868/digestion-accessory-organs-l.jpg.

These enzymes have a central role in the degradation of carbohydrates, fats, and proteins, respectively, to facilitate the effective absorption of essential nutrients. Additionally, the pancreas has a central role in glucose regulation in the blood by releasing insulin and glucagon, a hormone that is a testament to its role as an accessory organ, showing interrelatedness of digestion and metabolic control. This dual function is a testament to the unique function of accessory organs in enabling homeostasis, an achievement of a sophisticated physiological network that is inherent to nutrient processing and general health. Even though smaller in size than other organs, the gallbladder is equally important in acting as a reservoir for bile. In response to food, more so fatty foods, the gallbladder contracts to secrete stored bile into the duodenum, thereby enabling fat absorption and digestion. This process is necessary, as normal secretion of bile guarantees that fats are emulsified to enable them to be broken down effectively by lipases. Coordination of gallbladder contraction and the release of pancreatic enzymes and intestinal peristalsis is a classic demonstration of a well-coordinated digestive response. All these accessory organs not only optimize and amplify macronutrient digestion but also participate in larger physiological processes, including detoxification and hormonal homeostasis (Bulletin of the University of Nebraska: Annual catalog of the College of Medicine, 1966; Coaten, 2024). Their functions illustrate the interconnectedness of the gastrointestinal system and the significance of the system in general well-being and nutrient absorption (Figure 1.4).

1.2. Physiology of Digestion

The physiology of digestion is a delicate interplay between anatomical structures and physiological processes that transform food ingested into nutrients required by the body. The gastrointestinal (GI) tract is at the center of the process and consists of a chain of organs, like the stomach, intestines, and accessory organs, like the liver and pancreas. All the organs play a specific role in mechanical and chemical digestion, beginning from the chewing of food in the oral cavity and ending at nutrient absorption in the small intestine. The mucous membranes of the GI tract, particularly the mucosa, are designed to enable the absorption and translocation of nutrients across the epithelial barrier, thus demonstrating the delicate interplay between structure and function in the GI tract. The delicate interplay is facilitated by the dynamic changes that occur in the mucosal folds during peristalsis, a vital mechanism for effective movement of nutrients (Keet, 1974). The movement of digestive material is facilitated by coordinated muscular contraction known as peristalsis and segmentation, which have varied functions in the process of moving digestive material. Peristalsis is a wave-like muscular contraction that propels food through the digestive tract, permitting one-way movement that is vital for effective digestion and absorption. Segmentation is characterized by the intermittent constriction of circular muscles in the intestine, which blends intestinal content and improves nutrient absorption by increasing the contact between the digested food and the intestinal lining. The elaborate pattern of contraction permits the gastrointestinal tract to maximize the extraction of nutrients while maximizing the time food spends in the digestive tract. The normal physiological movements of the mucosa are indicative of the success of these mechanisms, as the curvature of the folds of the mucosa is in agreement with the contractions of the intestinal walls (Keet, 1974). The role of different hormones and enzymes involved in the process of digestion cannot be overlooked either. Gastrin, secretin, and cholecystokinin are the hormones responsible for coordinating the process of digestion by regulating the secretion of enzymes, gastric motility, and bile secretion, and thereby controlling the complex digestion and absorption of nutrients. The role of enzymes begins in the mouth with salivary amylase, continues in the stomach with pepsin and gastric lipase, and concludes in the small intestine, where pancreatic enzymes and bile salts further break down the food material. This well-coordinated interaction of enzymatic and hormonal functions ensures that digestion not only efficiently fragments food into pieces but also pre-empts nutrients for absorption into the body. A clear understanding of these physiological principles is mandatory for understanding the integrated nature of the gastrointestinal system and moving forward with progress in the fields of medical and nutritional science (Figure 1.5).

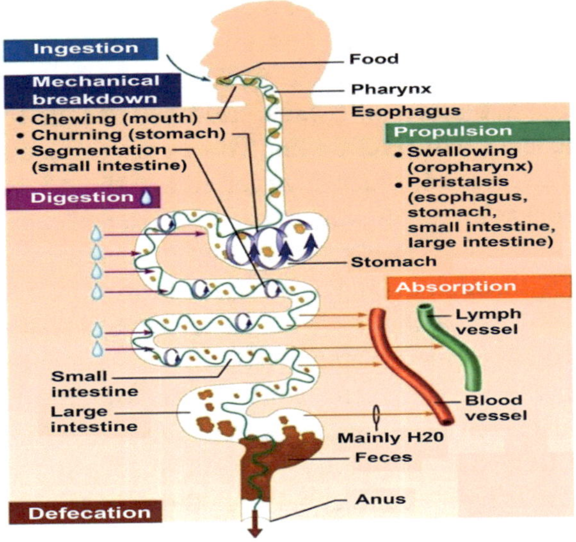

Figure 1.5. Physiology of digestion.

Source: https://1.bp.blogspot.com/-2qcpMFshcYA/XS9i1UuBi5I/AAAAAAAAE-s/xh5V2sM4XHIJCEmv KOJQT6M3Gbin VzhfwCLcBGAs/s1600/The-Physiology-Of-Digestion.jpg.

1.2.1. Mechanical Digestion Processes

The mechanical digestion process is integral to the function of the gastrointestinal (GI) system, as it prepares food for enzymatic digestion. The process occurs within the oral cavity, where food is chewed and masticated. The first mechanical process is to increase the surface area of food particles, thus optimizing the following enzymatic processes. Saliva serves a dual function, as it not only aids in the lubrication of food for swallowing but also contains enzymes like amylase that begin carbohydrate digestion. Effective mechanical digestion is important, as large food particles can confound the action of digestive enzymes, resulting in reduced nutrient absorption. The process is also closely coupled with sensory mechanisms that respond to food texture and composition, ultimately influencing appetite as well as the efficiency of digestion. Understanding these initial steps in mechanical digestion increases our understanding of how the body prepares food for subsequent breakdown and absorption later in digestion. Once food leaves the oral cavity, it travels to the stomach, where mechanical digestion continues through a combination of gastric secretions and muscular contractions. The three layers of stomach muscle produce a churning action that thoroughly mixes food with gastric juices, thus optimizing the breakdown process. Recent research has shown that these digestive mechanics allow for complete mixing of chyme, which is integral to effective enzymatic action and the continuation of chemical digestion under acidic pH (Liu et al., 2023). The contractions not only mechanically break up larger food particles but also function to push food toward the pyloric sphincter, which controls the rate at which chyme moves into the small intestine. The intricate interaction between chemical and mechanical digestion emphasizes the sheer importance of muscular function and gastric dynamics in the effective processing of ingested nutrients. As the process continues in the next phase, food moves to the small intestine, where mechanical and chemical digestive processes cooperate to optimize the absorption of nutrients and maximise their uptake. Peristaltic activity and segmentation contractions in the small intestine allow effective mixing of the chyme with digestive enzymes and bile, thus enhancing the emulsification of fats and the hydrolysis of proteins and carbohydrates. In this regard, mechanical digestion not only entails the tearing of food into infinitesimal pieces but also optimising its interaction with intestinal epithelial absorptive surfaces. The evidence points towards such optimal mixing in the maximisation of the use of the chemical processes initiated in the gut, which in turn determines nutritional absorption (Balters et al., 2017). As these chemical and mechanical phases coexist, they form a well-established network that is part and parcel of the digestive and absorptive processes that are integral to human physiology (Figure 1.6).

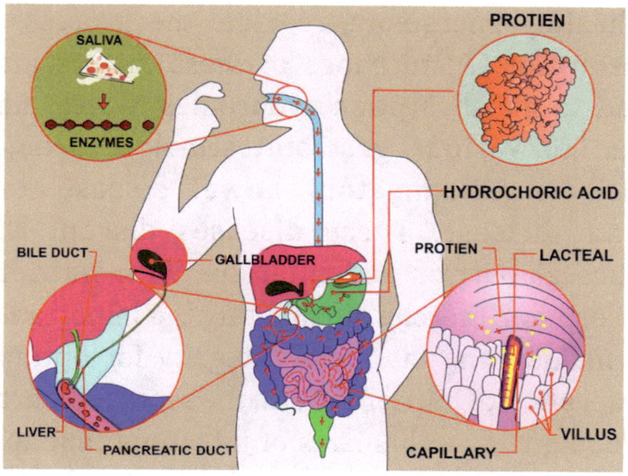

Figure 1.6. Mechanical digestion processes.

Source: https://www.wikihow.com/images/8/8a/Study-the-Physiology-of-Digestion-in-the-Human-Body-Step-9-Version-3.jpg.

1.2.2. Chemical Digestion and Enzymatic Action

The process of chemical digestion is a crucial part of the gastrointestinal system, where complex food molecules are broken down to units that may be absorbed. The complex process is sustained by enzymatic action, which allows the body to use macronutrients efficiently. Digestive enzymes, produced by various glands such as the salivary glands, pancreas, and mucosa of the intestine, specifically act on biomolecules such as carbohydrates, proteins, and fats. For instance, amylase is the first enzyme to break down the carbohydrates in the mouth, while proteases and lipases degrade the proteins and fats further in the stomach and small intestine. The enzyme breakdown allows for the absorption of nutrients as well as prepares food structures for further metabolic processes. Knowledge of the enzymatic processes provides information on the overall mechanisms of gastrointestinal physiology and provides possibilities for exploring possible therapeutic modalities of digestive diseases. The process of interaction between enzymes and substrates is critical in maximizing digestive efficiency since the specificity of the enzyme activity plays an important role in preventing barriers to digestion. For instance, treatments of carbohydrate-degrading enzymes (MEP) modify the structural properties of dietary fibers, which significantly enhance the bioavailability of nutrients. Research shows that the enzyme treatments make the arabinoxylans more soluble and yield shorter chains that enhance fermentation processes in the gastrointestinal tract. The enhancement of microbial fermentation leads to the production of short-chain fatty acids (SCFA), which play an essential role in maintaining gut integrity and health. By stimulating the growth of probiotic bacteria such as those in the Lachnospiraceae and Ruminococcaceae families, enzymatic activity protects the healthy microbiome and reduces inflammation, thus demonstrating the possible interplay of enzymatic function, digestion, and overall gastrointestinal function (Yacoubi, 2016). Furthermore, the role of enzymatic activity transcends simple digestion, for it plays a significant role in overall systemic well-being and health. An appreciation of the manner in which enzymatic modulation influences the diversity of gut microbiota is critical to the design of maximized dietary protocols and therapeutic interventions. For instance, increased production of short-chain fatty acids (SCFAs), such as butyrate, illustrates an interconnection between enzymatic activity and anti-inflammatory mechanisms that support a harmonious intestinal ecology. Such an awareness conforms to the guiding principles of holistic health, in which digestive function is interconnected with general physiological processes. The reconciliation of ancient wisdom and modern biochemical paradigms facilitates a more sophisticated appreciation of human health, thereby bridging mechanistic disease models and holistic healing philosophies. Such is the situation with the recent discovery of chemical digestion and enzymatic activity, in which one discovers layers of profundity that illustrate the sophistication of human health (Balick et al., 1997) (Figure 1.7).

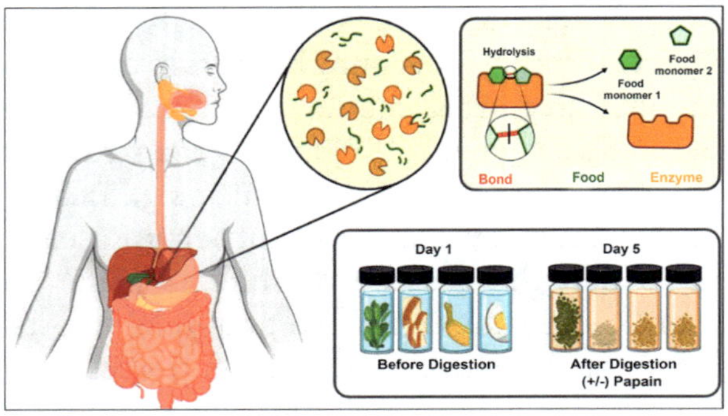

Figure 1.7. Chemical digestion and enzymatic action.

Source: https://pubs.acs.org/cms/10.1021/acs.jchemed.2c00992/asset/images/acs.jchemed.2c00992.social.jpeg_v03

1.2.3. Absorption of Nutrients

The mechanism of nutrient absorption is an essential part of gastrointestinal physiology, predominantly taking place in the small intestine, where the surface area is amplified through specialized structures called villi and microvilli. These structural specializations enhance the effective absorption of essential nutrients such as carbohydrates, proteins, fats, vitamins, and minerals. The mechanism begins through the delivery of the chyme to the duodenum, where enzymes and bile salts help break down food into smaller molecules.

The carbohydrates are hydrolyzed to monosaccharides, proteins are hydrolyzed to amino acids, and lipids are hydrolyzed to fatty acids and glycerol. Enzymatic digestion is essential as it prepares the macromolecules for absorption across the intestinal epithelium. The coordination of digestive enzymes and epithelial transport mechanisms ensures effective absorption of nutrients into the blood, highlighting the relationship between anatomy and physiology in the mechanism of nutrient assimilation. Additionally, several physiological factors, including the integrity of the intestinal mucosa and the existence of a healthy microbiota, regulate the process of absorption. Disturbance of these factors may lead to malabsorption syndromes, which may lead to various gastrointestinal disorders, such as inflammatory bowel disease and celiac disease. These diseases disrupt the mucosal barrier and interfere with nutrient absorption, thereby highlighting the importance of maintaining intestinal integrity for optimal absorption of nutrients. With the recent research probing the mechanisms of intestinal function, models such as human intestinal organoids have been recognized as essential tools to explore the pathophysiology of nutrient absorption. These organoids reproduce the primary characteristics of human intestinal tissue and enable researchers to explore the complexity of nutrient transport and the mechanisms of gastrointestinal diseases, thereby providing insights into potential therapeutic implications (Flood et al., 2023).

In nutrient absorption research, it is important to investigate the role of antioxidants in maintaining intestinal health, especially under the risk of oxidative stress. Current evidence suggests that reactive oxygen species (ROS) can impair nutrient absorption through damage to the intestinal epithelium. For example, chilling stress research in peanut seedlings has reported ROS accumulation to be linked to compromised photosynthesis and nutrient transport, showing that plants also face nutrient absorption problems under stress conditions (Dong et al., 2024). This observation not only emphasizes the transferability of nutrient absorption problems across different biological systems but also calls for further efficient ROS-scavenging processes in maintaining epithelial integrity. Such understanding of plant and human physiological dynamics can inform strategies toward optimizing nutrient absorption in different settings, thus yielding improved health and agricultural outcomes (Figure 1.8).

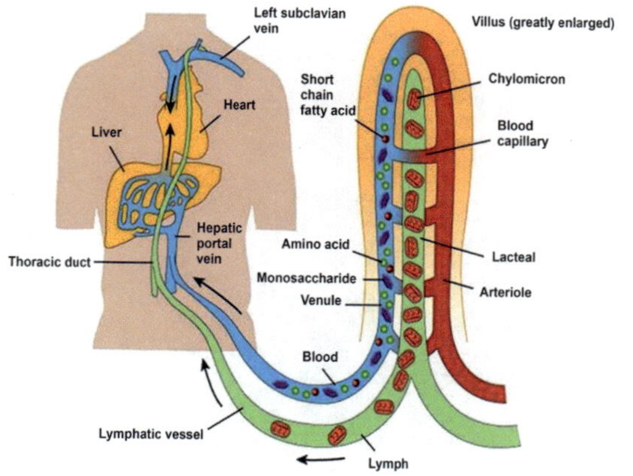

Figure 1.8. Absorption of nutrients.

Source: https://genefitletics.com/wp-content/uploads/2020/01/nutrient-absorption-hair-copy.jpg.

1.3. Regulation of Gastrointestinal Function

Regulation of gastrointestinal (GI) function is a subtle balance of neural, hormonal, and local mechanisms that, working together, provide effective digestion and nutrient absorption. Neural control is mainly through the autonomic nervous system, regulating involuntary functions such as peristalsis, rhythmic contraction of the smooth muscles of the GI tract. The enteric nervous system, or second brain, is a complex network of neurons capable of controlling gut functions independently and reacting to changes in the local environment rapidly. On food intake into the gut, mechanoreceptors and chemoreceptors trigger reflexes that coordinate muscle function and secretory processes, thus illustrating the sophisticated responsiveness of the GI system to external and internal stimuli, ensuring homeostasis and aiding effective digestion (Cornell University, 2000). Hormonal control is equally important in the GI tract, allowing organs to communicate with one another to optimize digestive processes. Primary hormones such as gastrin, secretin, and cholecystokinin (CCK) are released from specialist cells within the stomach and intestines in response to diverse stimuli, such as food intake.

Gastrin, for instance, is released on food intake, stimulating gastric acid secretion and increasing motility, while secretin and CCK increase the secretion of pancreatic enzymes and bile secretion, respectively. Coordination of hormonal function not only supports digestion but also assists appetite regulation and energy balance regulation, thus illustrating the dynamic relationship between the digestive system and metabolic health. Such sophisticated interactions illustrate the importance of hormonal signals in driving digestive efficiency (Cornell University, 2000). Along with neural and hormonal systems, local regulatory mechanisms are integral to the accuracy of gastrointestinal function. The intestinal wall is made up of different cell types that are responsible for the production of local modulators that influence smooth muscle contraction and secretory function. For instance, the release of nitric oxide (NO) by enteric neurons leads to relaxation of smooth muscles, thereby influencing peristalsis and enhancing blood flow for absorption. In addition to this, local factors like pH and nutrient concentration are able to trigger localized responses that modify digestive processes based on the gastrointestinal tract content. This particular control is significant as it enables the gastrointestinal system to adjust to different types and amounts of food, ensuring optimal nutrient absorption under differing physiological conditions. In conclusion, both local and systemic control of gastrointestinal function highlights its significance to health maintenance and disease management (Cornell University, 2000) (Figure 1.9).

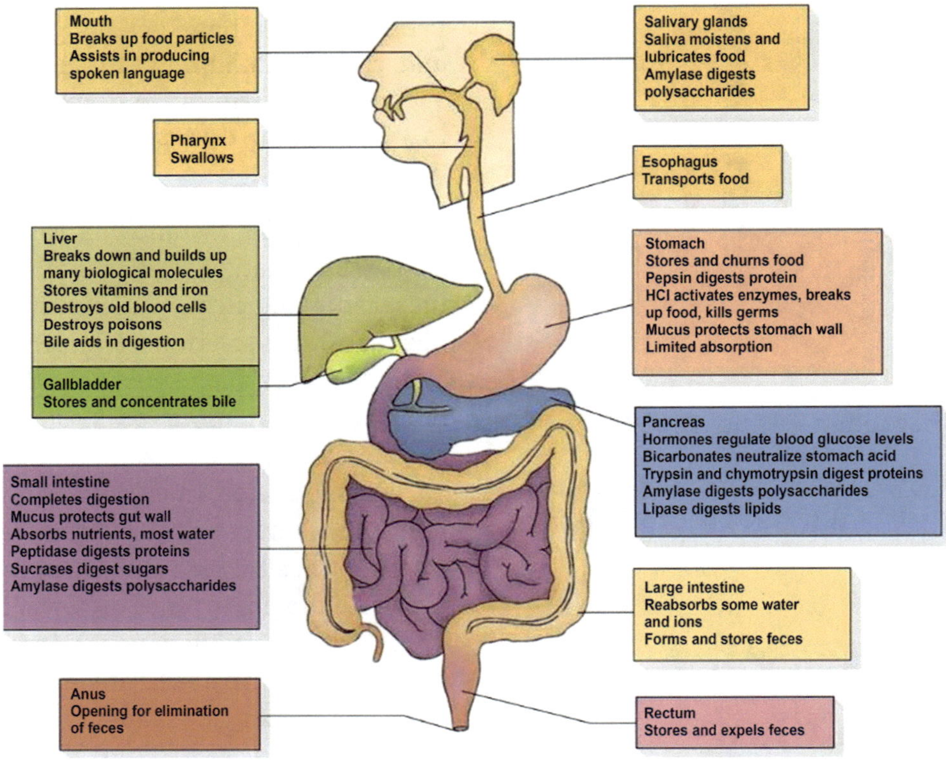

Figure 1.9. Regulation of gastrointestinal function.

Source: https://i0.wp.com/basicmedicalkey.com/wp-content/uploads/2016/09/F000358f35-19-9781455726509.jpg?fit=1026%2C837&ssl=1.

1.3.1. Neural Control Mechanisms

The neural control mechanisms of the gastrointestinal (GI) tract play an important role in organizing digestive activity. These functions are primarily carried out by the enteric nervous system (ENS), or second brain, due to its high degree of autonomy and complexity. The ENS is composed of over 100 million neurons in the walls of the GI tract, making it strong enough to function independently as well as in coordination with the central nervous system (CNS). This dual capability enhances the regulation of gastrointestinal activities such as motility, secretion, and blood supply. In addition, the ENS employs a wide array of neurotransmitters and neuropeptides, such as acetylcholine and nitric oxide, to regulate smooth muscle contractions and coordinate reflex activity that enhances digestive efficiency. The intricate interactions between these neural elements emphasize the role of the ENS in persistent gastrointestinal homeostasis and adaptation to physiological demands. One of the features essential to the neural control mechanisms of the GI tract is their capacity to adapt with time, especially in response to changes related to aging. The evidence indicates that the efficiency of colonic neuromuscular response decreases with age, with far-reaching implications for digestive health. For instance, a study documented that in elderly individuals, electrically induced contractions mediated by cholinergic pathways were significantly weaker compared to those in young individuals, a sign of a reduction in cholinergic activity (Broad et al., 2018). Furthermore, although there were no significant changes in the populations of myenteric neurons in ascending and descending colon segments, differences in neurotransmitter release and receptor sensitivity could be the reasons behind these age differences.

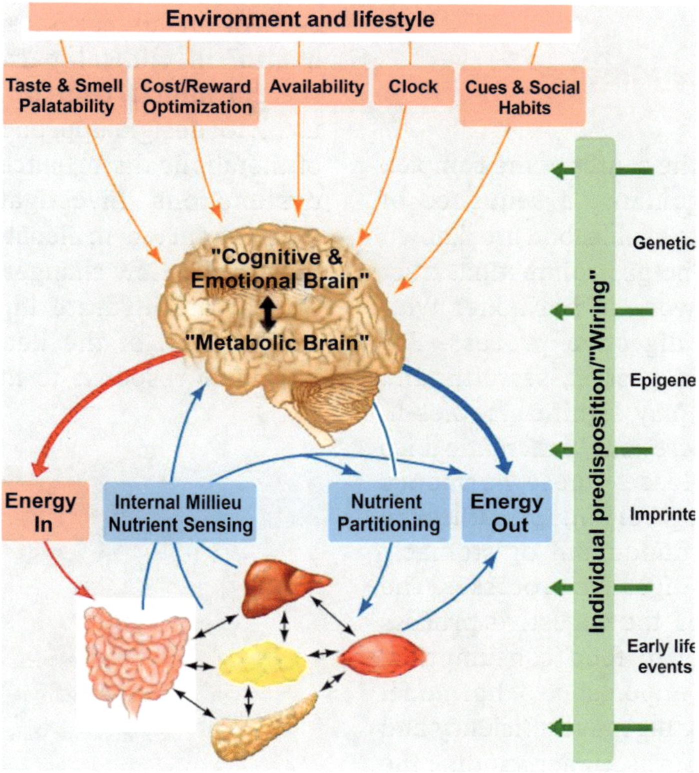

Figure 1.10. Neural control mechanisms.

Source: https://www.researchgate.net/profile/Huiyuan-Zheng-2/publication/5451434/figure/fig1/AS:341282137362435@1458379410242/Schematic-diagram-showing-the-major-factors-determining-neural-control-of-appetite-and.png.

Such observations underscore the significance of knowledge of neuromuscular dynamics in the aging population, opening the door to better clinical management of gastrointestinal abnormalities prevalent in elderly populations. In addition, interaction between the enteric nervous system (ENS) and autonomic nervous system (ANS) adds to the complexity of neural regulatory mechanisms of the gastrointestinal tract. The ANS, with sympathetic and parasympathetic components, regulates activity of the ENS and, in turn, modifies motility and secretory functions. The parasympathetic component largely facilitates digestive functions by stimulating enhanced peristalsis and the release of digestive enzymes, while sympathetic stimulation suppresses these activities in times of stress or the fight-or-flight response. Bidirectional communication allows a highly specific response to the immediate physiological needs of the body. Awareness of such neural control mechanisms is essential in the understanding of many gastrointestinal diseases, which may emerge due to disturbance in neural transmission or deranged interaction between ENS and ANS. Hence, an exploration of the therapeutic potential directed towards these mechanisms can provide new directions towards the treatment of digestive disorders across different age groups (Burnstock, 2011) (Figure 1.10).

1.3.2. Hormonal Regulation of Digestion

Hormonal control is at the center of the complex digestive process, organizing a sequence of physiological reactions to enable food breakdown and nutrient uptake. The gastrointestinal tract houses a complex network of hormones with specific roles in the digestive process. For instance, hormones like gastrin, secretin, and cholecystokinin (CCK) play significant roles in the control of gastric secretions, pancreatic juice secretion, and bile release. These hormones are released following certain stimuli, like food presence in the duodenum or stomach, triggering a cascade of digestive processes. The control system ensures the digestive process responds appropriately to food consumption, and thus highlights the importance of hormonal signaling in maintaining digestive efficiency and gastrointestinal homeostasis. Understanding the dynamic process is the basis of exploring the bigger picture of hormonal control's implications on digestion. The release of particular hormones in the gastrointestinal tract is strongly correlated with the diet content. For instance, carbohydrates are significantly implicated in the activation of hormonal signals and the efficiency of the digestive process. The diversity of types and amounts of carbohydrates that reach the colon can be strongly influenced by hormonal control, as shown by the microbial fermentation processes in digestion. Recent research has been focused on the role of short-chain fatty acids (SCFA) generated by the process of carbohydrate fermentation, which can further influence hormonal responses and overall gut health. This relationship explains how hormones not only enable digestion but are also implicated in the complex interactions between diet, microbiota, and metabolic processes, referring to a multifaceted approach to gastrointestinal physiology and anatomy. From an understanding of these interactions, a greater appreciation is developed for the importance of hormonal control of digestion and its relevance to health. In clinical paradigms, awareness of the hormonal control of digestion can be used to design approaches to the treatment of metabolic disturbances and gastrointestinal dysfunctions. Investigational work, such as that conducted in ileostomy models, provides insight into how changes in diet and the nature of the carbohydrate ingested may affect the composition of the ileal microbiota and the hormonal response to nutrient absorption.

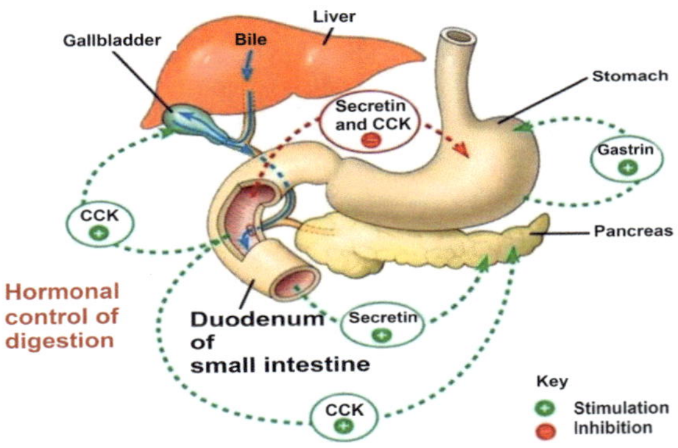

Figure 1.11. Hormonal regulation of digestion.

Source: https://image.slidesharecdn.com/digestivesystemashok-170322140625/95/digestive-system-ashok-19-638.jpg?cb=1490192145.

The results derived from such studies demonstrate that intestinal health and hormonal secretion can be substantially altered by adapting dietary approaches. Research concerned with the hormonal climate under varying dietary conditions identifies potential for the use of hormonal mechanisms to enhance digestive function and prevent disease. In this way, appreciation of the crucial role of hormones in the regulation of digestion not only contributes to our basic knowledge of the gastrointestinal physiology and anatomy but also identifies promising directions for therapeutic intervention to facilitate digestive health and restore metabolic balance in a wide range of populations (Figure 1.11).

1.3.3. Feedback Mechanisms in Gastrointestinal Physiology

The gastrointestinal (GI) tract is a complex system that is controlled by many feedback mechanisms that regulate and optimize digestion processes. Feedback mechanisms are classified broadly as hormonal or neural. Hormonal feedback involves the release of certain peptides that transmit information regarding the body's state of digestion to other organs. For example, the release of gastrin from the stomach triggers acid production, while other hormones, such as secretin and cholecystokinin (CCK), control the pancreas and gallbladder activities and ensure homeostasis. On the other hand, neural feedback involves the utilization of short and long reflex arcs that are initiated with the arrival of food in the GI tract, which trigger motility and secretion for the activation of digestion. The intricate balance of these hormonal and neural stimuli ensures that digestion is executed optimally while adjusting to various kinds of food and varying physiological needs. The control of gastric acid secretion illustrates how feedback mechanisms harmonize with one another. With the arrival of food in the stomach, stretch receptors detect distention, which leads to the release of gastrin, which triggers the secretion of gastric acid needed for the digestion of food. With the decrease in the pH of the stomach content, the feedback response is the release of somatostatin, which suppresses the synthesis of gastrin in order to prevent hyperacidity. This cycle illustrates the delicate balance achieved in the gastrointestinal system, where various variables such as pH, nutrient content, and hormone activity interact with each other. Further, such coordination is not solely reactive in nature; predictive feedback mechanisms are present, and the body can anticipate food intake based on sensory stimuli. Anticipatory responses are also essential to successful digestion, and they underscore the significance of feedback mechanisms that not only control ongoing processes but also anticipate and prepare the gastrointestinal tract for upcoming challenges. Acid-base balance regulation is another essential process controlled by feedback mechanisms in gastrointestinal physiology. Digestion is a process that can significantly impact the body's acid-base status and, therefore, requires a coordinated response from multiple systems, including the lungs and kidneys. Food ingestion into the stomach can initiate the creation of acidic content that must be neutralized in order to maximize digestion and avoid damaging the lining of the intestines. Pancreas bicarbonate secretion and the buffering actions of varied bodily fluids are, therefore, initiated, working collectively to sustain acid-base homeostasis. This regulatory process illustrates the dependence of physiological systems on each other; the gastrointestinal tract does not work in isolation but is dependent on integrated feedback mechanisms that allow the coordination of its activities with overall systemic needs, such as those described in reference to acid-base regulation, manifesting in vivo as a coordinated phenomenon involving bodily fluids and regulatory systems other than the gastrointestinal system (White, 2025).

1.4. Gastrointestinal Motility

The multifaceted process of gastrointestinal motility lies at the center of the digestive system's operation, allowing for the passage of food through specific areas of the gastrointestinal tract. The process of this type is controlled by a multifaceted coordination of muscular contractions, neural patterns, and hormonal control. These contractions are required for the mixing of food with digestive enzymes, the digestion of nutrients, and the passage of chyme through the digestive tract. One of the primary characteristics of gastrointestinal motility is the ability to synchronize, which is largely dependent on the enteric nervous system. This intrinsic nervous system controls reflexes governing peristalsis, rhythmic contraction allowing for the transport of food undergoing digestion. In addition, the digestive system's motility is sensitive to the presence of food, modulating the strength and frequency of contraction with regard to the body's physiological state, ensuring proper digestion and nutrient absorption. In addition, the operation of the vagus nerve, a part of the autonomic nervous system, is important to the consideration of gastrointestinal motility. As a primary interface between the gastrointestinal tract and the central nervous system, it transmits sensory and motor signals important to the digestive process. Activation of the vagus nerve increases peristalsis and overall motility, as well as its function in regulating gastric secretions and enzyme release. The effects of vagal activation have implications beyond bodily digestion; they are intimately linked to emotional and psychological health. By suppressing stress responses and optimizing digestive efficiency, vagal function not only aids digestion but is involved in psychosomatic interactions influencing appetite and nutrient assimilation. The convergence of gastrointestinal function and neural controls highlights their importance as a unifying theme of study. Besides neural controls, gastrointestinal motility is also strongly modulated by a variety of mechanical and hormonal factors that regulate digestive functions. Gastrin, secretin, and cholecystokinin (CCK) are examples of hormones that get released on the ingestion of food and, in turn, modulate gastric motility and gastric compartmental emptying rates. CCK, for instance, not only provokes the release of bile from the gallbladder but also inhibits gastric motility, thus facilitating fat digestion. Moreover, the complexity of gastrointestinal motility is also apparent in clinical practice, where irritable bowel syndrome (IBS) and gastroparesis disrupt normal motility patterns. These also highlight the tenuous balance achieved by heterogeneous physiological mechanisms and illustrate how their disruption that produces significant gastrointestinal distress and impaired nutrient absorption. A comprehension of the basics of gastrointestinal motility is therefore important in states of health and disease, uncovering avenues of therapy and optimization of patients' outcomes (Figure 1.12).

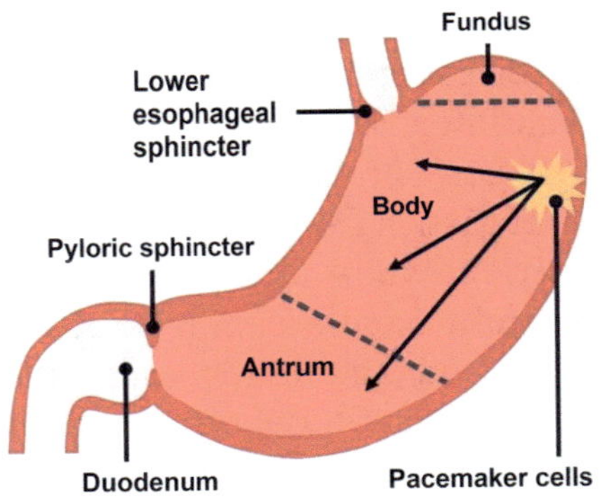

Figure 1.12. Gastrointestinal motility.

Source: https://cdn.lecturio.com/assets/Regions-of-the-stomach-and-their-functions.jpg.

1.4.1. Types of Motility: Peristalsis and Segmentation

Understanding the different types of gastrointestinal motility is important in understanding the complex mechanisms that enable digestion and absorption of nutrients. The two major types of motility, peristalsis and segmentation, perform different yet integrated functions in the gastrointestinal tract. Peristalsis involves synchronous, smooth wave-like muscle contractions that propel food along the digestive tract and are effective in transporting chyme from the esophagus to the rectum. The unidirectional movement depends on a series of contractions and relaxations ahead of and behind the bolus, thereby ensuring effective progression along the gastrointestinal tract. Segmentation involves rhythmic contractions intended to churn and mix intestinal contents, allowing for increased contact with the mucosal surface. The bidirectional movement significantly enhances the ability of the body to absorb nutrients through extensive contact with the intestinal wall. The function of peristalsis and segmentation goes beyond mechanical transport; these mechanisms have a significant role in maintaining homeostasis within the gastrointestinal tract. With peristalsis, an increase in the pressure gradient increases effective propulsion, while segmentation increases the contact area, thereby increasing the absorption of nutrients. Empirical evidence has shown that the maintenance of these patterns of motility is important in ensuring functional gastrointestinal wellness. For instance, interference of peristaltic function may lead to diseases such as gastroesophageal reflux disease or constipation, while interference of segmentation may prevent nutrient absorption and lead to malnutrition. Further, recent studies have shown fascinating dynamics regarding the motility of mucosal folds, wherein contraction of the intestinal wall alters the orientation of these folds, allowing transit during peristaltic and segmental activity (Keet , 1974). In addition, extensive research has investigated the role of genetic determinants in motility with a focus on disease conditions like cystic fibrosis (CF). Evidence has indicated that mutations of the CF transmembrane conductance regulator can lead to reduced peristaltic contractions in the intestines, as demonstrated by CFTR knockout models (Liu et al., 2022). Such evidence is indicative of the complex interdependence of genetic determinants and gastrointestinal motility, with a lot of information being gained about how systemic disease can cause disruption in normal digestive function. Knowledge of the mechanisms controlling peristalsis and segmentation and their relationship to genetic variables highlights the key role of these processes in the maintenance of gastrointestinal well-being and the prevention of associated disorders. Such investigations improve the understanding of how motility is involved in normal and disease conditions in the gastrointestinal tract and, hence, the development of future therapeutic interventions (Figure 1.13).

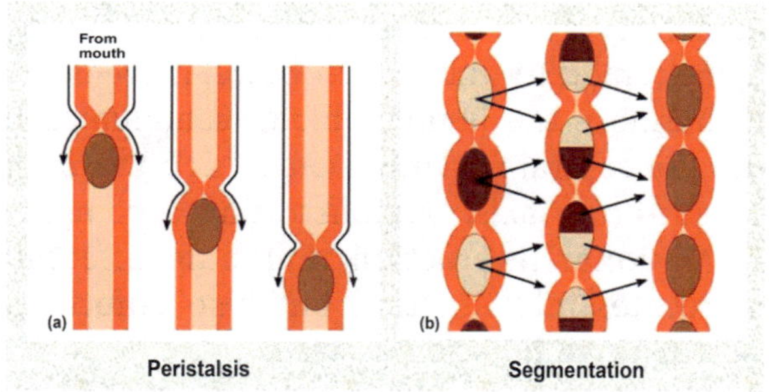

Figure 1.13. Types of motility: peristalsis and segmentation.

Source: https://image.slideserve.com/1418318/peristalsis-versus-segmentation-l.jpg.

1.4.2. Factors Influencing Motility

Gastrointestinal motility is influenced by an entire range of variables, all of which act in concert to optimize digestion and nutrient absorption. Synchronization of the muscular contractions of the gastrointestinal tract is controlled by intrinsic neural circuits, with additional modulation by the autonomic nervous system. Of particular importance, the enteric nervous system (ENS) controls these movements, responding to a variety of stimuli, including the presence of food, hormonal, and local chemical changes. For instance, distension of the intestines and stomach results in reflexive responses augmenting peristalsis to enable food passage through the digestive apparatus. External factors, such as rates of exercise and stress, can significantly modify motility patterns and result in conditions like irritable bowel syndrome or constipation, and demonstrating the fine balance necessary for normal gastrointestinal function. The composition of the gut microbiota has been recognized as a key determinant of gastrointestinal motility and digestive health. With a diverse range of beneficial microbes colonizing the gut, the microbiome is dynamically involved in a variety of physiological processes, including the regulation of motility. Research indicates that such gut bacteria are able to produce short-chain fatty acids and other metabolites that augment motility and regular bowel movements. Furthermore, the gut microbiome communicates with the central nervous system (CNS) through the gut-brain axis, demonstrating a complex, bidirectional interaction, not only affecting gastrointestinal function but also emotional and cognitive function as well.

Alteration of this microbiota by diet, disease, or pharmacological intervention may result in altered motility and worsen gastrointestinal disease, and highlighting the significance of a healthy microbiome for optimal digestive function (Kanmani et al., 2020). Pharmaceutical considerations are central to the modulation of gastrointestinal motility, especially in terms of drug absorption and efficacy. Alterations in motility have significant effects on the pharmacokinetics of drugs administered orally, leading to varying rates of absorption among individuals based on differences in gastrointestinal transit time, pH, and luminal environment. For example, factors such as gastric emptying time, diet, and patient-related physiological factors all cumulatively modify the efficacy of drug absorption. Recent studies have indicated that variability in the formulation and delivery of drugs might mitigate the effect of variability on oral drug exposure, suggesting that drug development might maximize therapeutic responses (Vinarov et al., 2021). This interaction highlights the fundamental importance of investigating gastrointestinal motility within clinical and pharmaceutical contexts, revealing implications not just for gastrointestinal wellbeing but also for the administration of therapeutic regimens.

1.4.3. Disorders of Gastrointestinal Motility

Gastrointestinal motility disorders are a class of disorders that disrupt normal movement of the gastrointestinal tract, leading to a wide variety of symptoms that can seriously compromise quality of life. These disorders may manifest either as hypermotility, leading to diarrhea and urgency, or hypomotility, often leading to constipation and obstructive symptoms. The pathogenesis of the disorders is typically multifactorial, involving an abnormality of neuromuscular coordination of the gastrointestinal tract and abnormalities of the enteric nervous system. For example, evidence has shown that changes in electromechanical coupling at the gastroduodenal junction can compromise gastric emptying, thereby presenting a promising target for new therapeutic approaches to restore normal patterns of motility (Simmonds et al., 2024). A comprehensive understanding of the disorders requires an in-depth knowledge of gastrointestinal physiology, from the electrical signaling mediated through interstitial cells of Cajal (ICC) to the interaction of central and peripheral nervous system effects on gastrointestinal function. The interrelationship between motility disorders and neurological disorders provides critical insights into the pathophysiology of dysfunctions of the gastrointestinal tract. Specifically, spinal cord injuries (SCI) can induce neurogenic bowel dysfunction characterized by a broad range of gastrointestinal symptoms, such as constipation and fecal incontinence. Disruption of normal neural pathways alters the motility of the bowel and colon, leading to serious complications and compromised quality of life in the affected individual (Rodriguez & Gater, 2022). Assessment and management of the condition emphasize the need to know about gastrointestinal innervation and motility dynamics. A stepwise management that involves medical management and pharmacological therapies, along with individualized bowel programs, is important for effective treatment. These strategies are not only aimed at the restoration of normal gastrointestinal function but also at the enhancement of the overall well-being and autonomy of individuals suffering from such debilitating diseases. Information gained from studies of gastrointestinal motility disorders goes beyond symptomatic relief and suggests the need for a thorough investigation of potential biomarkers for both diagnostic and therapeutic use.

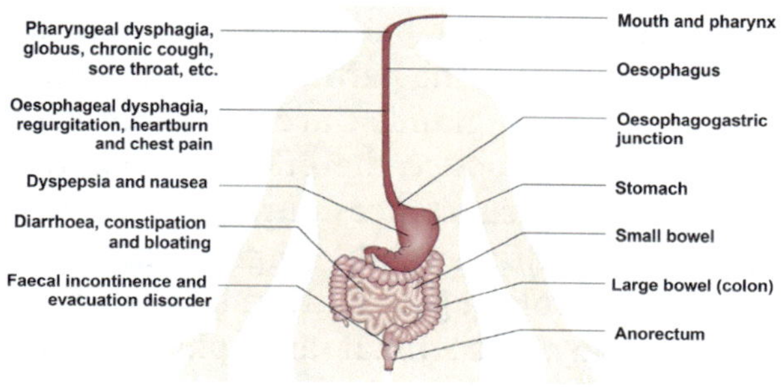

Figure 1.14. Disorders of gastrointestinal motility.

Source: https://media.springernature.com/lw1200/springer-static/image/art%3A10.1038%2Fs41575-018-0030-9/MediaObjects/41575_2018_30_Fig1_HTML.jpg.

Recent research studies have put more focus on the quest for reliable biomarkers that may offer more insight and control over gut-brain-related disorders and become the foundation of individualized therapeutic approaches (Simmonds et al., 2024). Electrophysiological techniques monitoring the bioelectrical activity of the gastrointestinal tract are significant in understanding the mechanisms that lead to motility disorders. By providing an understanding of the relationship between electrical events and muscular contraction in the gastrointestinal tract, clinicians can formulate effective interventions. Studies of the pathophysiology behind motility disorders not only increase diagnostic potential but also support the development of novel therapies that target gastrointestinal health, filling vital gaps in current healthcare approaches, improving patient-centered outcomes in the treatment of gastrointestinal health (Figure 1.14).

1.5. Gastrointestinal Secretions

Gastrointestinal secretions are of fundamental significance to the process of digestion and absorption of nutrients, facilitating the complex mechanisms of human nutrition. Secretions are of varied origin in the gastrointestinal (GI) tract, such as the salivary glands, gastric mucosa, pancreas, and liver. For instance, saliva contains enzymes like amylase that start degrading carbohydrates even prior to food entering the stomach. In the stomach environment, hydrochloric acid and pepsinogen work together to denature proteins and initiate their digestion. Coordination of secretions is significant as it optimizes the digestive process and facilitates the utilization of nutrients further down the GI tract. Understanding of these secretions adds value to gastrointestinal physiology and explains the role of these secretions in maintaining overall well-being, providing a foundation for further research in gastrointestinal anatomy. The pancreas, a key organ of the digestive tract, secretes a variety of enzymes and bicarbonate that play a central role in deactivating gastric acid and digesting macronutrients. Pancreatic secretions include lipases, proteases, and amylases that break down fats, proteins, and carbohydrates, respectively, into forms that are absorbed. This enzymatic activity is most evident after the ingestion of a meal, when the presence of chyme in the duodenum stimulates the release of secretin and cholecystokinin. These hormones not only stimulate pancreatic juice production but also regulate gallbladder contraction, with the release of bile acids that further optimize digestion. Such hormonal and enzymatic interactions demonstrate the complexity of gastrointestinal physiology and highlight the significance of these secretions in optimizing digestive function. Regulation and production of gastrointestinal secretions are susceptible to a variety of physiological and pathological influences, including dietary preferences, psychological stress, and numerous disease states. Gastric acid secretion, for example, can be triggered by visual or olfactory food-related stimuli, which initiates a reflex mechanism involving the central nervous system. Alteration in secretion patterns, however, gives rise to diseases like gastroesophageal reflux disease, peptic ulcer disease, and malabsorption syndromes, highlighting the fine balance needed within this system. Recent studies have increasingly attempted to define potential therapeutic approaches directed toward enhancing secretion in patients with gastrointestinal disease. New approaches may encompass the development of oral drug delivery systems to enhance efficacy and absorption of therapeutic agents, highlighting the wider implications of gastrointestinal secretions for disease and health management (Homayun et al., 2019). Clear understanding of these processes is a prerequisite for new therapy design and has underpinned continued research into improved treatment regimens (C-Rodrigues et al., 2019) (Figure 1.15).

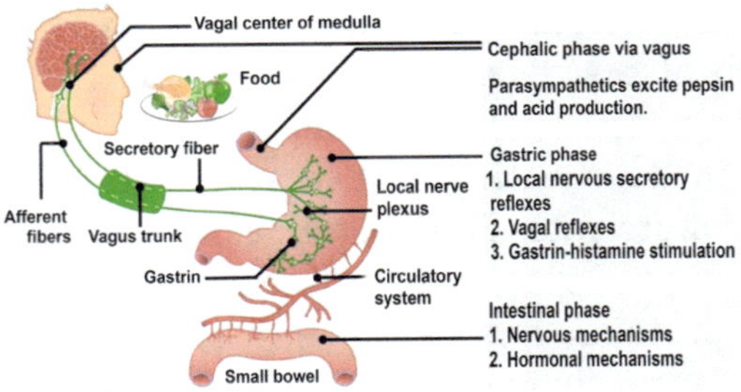

Figure 1.15. Gastrointestinal secretions.

Source: https://cdn.lecturio.com/assets/Phases-of-digestion-with-their-functional-components.jpg.

1.5.1. Salivary Secretions and Their Functions

Salivary secretions are integral to the initial digestion processes, acting as a prelude to the complex processes occurring throughout the gastrointestinal tract. Consisting mainly of water, electrolytes, and a combination of proteins, saliva facilitates the mechanical breakdown of food by moistening and lubricating boluses to facilitate swallowing. Additionally, enzymes like alpha-amylase facilitate carbohydrate digestion, breaking down carbohydrates into simpler sugars. The presence of antibacterial compounds, such as lactoferrin, further demonstrates the protective role of saliva as a defense against pathogens. The salivary glands, comprising the parotid, submandibular, and sublingual glands, are hierarchically structured to produce the effective secretion of these crucial substances during mastication and with specific stimuli, emphasizing their foundational role in gastrointestinal physiology and anatomy. Emotional and physiological stimuli significantly affect the dynamics of salivary secretion, emphasizing the synergism between the nervous system and digestive processes. Research confirms that stress can impact salivary output, such that active coping mechanisms have a tendency to enhance proteins critical to immune defense, such as MUC7 and lactoferrin. For instance, research on stressor responses suggests sympathetic activity may augment salivary secretion in response to demanding cognitive tasks, while passive coping mechanisms trigger a distinct salivary release pattern. The findings demonstrate the intricate dynamics between psychological states and physiological responses, emphasizing how salivary glands react to external and internal stimuli, thus influencing digestive efficiency and oral health (Bosch et al., 2000). This aspect of salivary secretion not only emphasizes its digestive role but also highlights its role in maintaining homeostasis. Recent research highlights the importance of salivary secretions with implications extending beyond human physiological contexts, and the research provides knowledge contributions on digestion in other animals, including insects. Research on Acheta domesticus, a domestic cricket, provides fascinating accounts of its salivary glands and their enzymatic function in the digestion process. The A. domesticus salivary glands, with parietal and zymogenic cells, secrete substances with an important role in luminal pH regulation, an element essential for optimal enzymatic activities within the gastrointestinal tract. The presence of carbonic anhydrase in the glands attests to the function of salivary secretions in creating an alkaline environment that enhances digestion. Such interdisciplinarity not only deepens our insight into digestive processes but also encourages a holistic approach towards the evolutionary origin and function of salivary secretions in different organisms (Holm et al., 2020). Such an insight deepens our knowledge of the intricacies involved in gastrointestinal physiology (Figure 1.16).

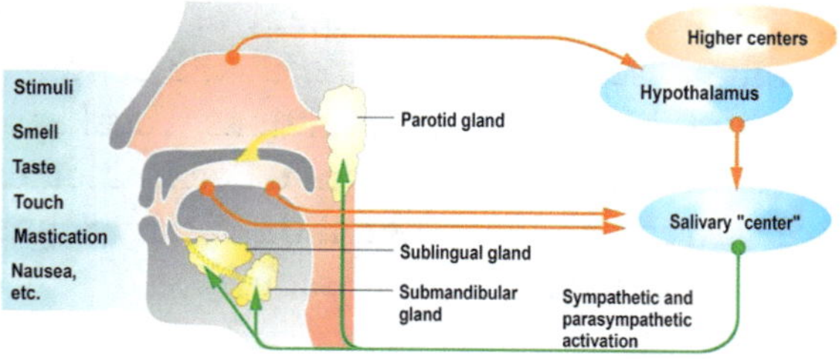

Figure 1.16. Salivary secretions and their functions.

Source: https://books.lib.uoguelph.ca/app/uploads/sites/13/2020/02/image200.jpg.

1.5.2. Gastric Secretions and Their Role in Digestion

The digestive process is closely linked with gastric secretions that are essential for the denaturation of proteins, emulsification of fats, and uptake of nutrients. The important constituents of gastric secretions are hydrochloric acid, pepsinogen, intrinsic factor, and mucus substances. Hydrochloric acid creates an acidic environment that is indispensable for pepsinogen activation to pepsin, an enzyme essential to protein digestion. Moreover, the acidic state is also essential in sterilizing ingested food, thus reducing the burden of pathogens and increasing the solubility of some minerals and vitamins. By sustaining the acidic state, gastric secretions also control the transit of chyme to the small intestine, enabling efficient use of digestive enzymes in a more neutral environment, thus allowing maximum uptake of nutrients. The composition of gastric secretions can be controlled by numerous factors, such as dietary content and physiological state. For instance, dietary supplementation with non-starch polysaccharides (NSP) has been reported to alter gastrointestinal dynamics, affecting both digestibility and absorption of nutrients. High NSP concentration can lead to increased retention of organic matter and reduced digestibility in the small intestine, as supported by swine nutrition studies. As dietary fiber alters digestive kinetics, it also emphasizes the function of gastric secretions in controlling varied dietary sources. Such interactions not only affect the digestive process but also have implications for the gut as a whole, as they can affect microbial populations and the intestinal microenvironment, emphasizing the sensitive relationship between secretion composition and digestion. Moreover, dysfunction in gastric secretions can lead to severe gastrointestinal disorders, including dysmotility and inflammation. Studies have shown that spinal cord injury can exacerbate such complications by compromising the circulating of blood to intestinal tissue, thereby causing visceral hypoperfusion and inflammation. For example, in thoracic spinal cord injury, there is an abrupt decline in vital blood flow to the superior mesenteric artery (SMA), which negatively affects nutrient absorption and gut integrity. The resultant ischemia and inflammation can initiate disturbances in gastric secretions, thereby worsening conditions such as nausea, vomiting, or appetite loss. The understanding of such pathological effects highlights the absolute importance of balanced gastric secretions, not just in digestion but also in maintaining gastrointestinal health in different physiological states, thereby indicating their critical importance in the domain of gastrointestinal physiology and anatomy.

1.5.3. Pancreatic and Biliary Secretions

Synthesis and secretion of pancreatic and biliary fluid are fundamental processes of gastrointestinal physiology responsible for the digestion and absorption of nutrients. The pancreas plays a critical role in that it secretes a variety of enzymes , such as amylase, lipase, and proteases, for carbohydrate, fat, and protein hydrolysis, respectively. The enzymes are secreted in an inactive form in order to prevent autodigestion of the pancreatic gland. Furthermore, bicarbonate ions are secreted from the pancreas to neutralize gastric acid and create an ideal pH for enzymatic function in the small intestine. All the above secretions are regulated by hormonal stimuli , such as secretin and cholecystokinin, which are stimulated by the arrival of acidic chyme in the duodenum so that digestive enzymes are secreted at the right time for optimal digestion. Meanwhile, the biliary apparatus, or the gallbladder and liver, plays a critical role in lipid metabolism through the secretion and storage of bile. Bile consists of bile acids, cholesterol, bilirubin, and phospholipids, which together permit emulsification and absorption of dietary lipids. Bile is secreted when stimulated by cholecystokinin, which, in turn, squeezes the gallbladder and forces it to expel bile into the duodenum. Furthermore, enterohepatic circulation allows for the recycling of bile acids, enhancing their utilization towards digestion. The complex process involving pancreatic and bile secretions serves to emphasize the importance of these systems towards digestive health and nutrient absorption. Understanding the dynamics of such secretions is an appreciated advancement in gastrointestinal anatomy and physiology as a whole. The clinical importance of pancreatic and biliary secretions is tremendous, particularly with regard to their role in metabolic disease. Interference with these secretions can lead to conditions like pancreatitis, cholestasis, and obesity. For instance, interference with pancreatic enzyme production can lead to malabsorption syndromes, whereas distension of biliary ducts results in jaundice and liver failure. Recent research on endoluminal therapy aims to present a solution to these issues by exploring new treatments targeting gastrointestinal secretions and their physiologic routes. The future of such developments in obesity management and related metabolic diseases appears promising, with emerging technologies like gastric mucosal devitalization showing potential in inducing weight-independent optimization of metabolic parameters (Kumbhari, 2019). As advancements in gastrointestinal physiology unfold, understanding and management of pancreatic and biliary secretions remain at the center of successful therapeutic interventions (Focal Spot, Fall/Winter 2010/2011. Bernard Becker Medical Library Archives. Washington University School of Medicine, Saint Louis, Missouri).

1.6. Common Gastrointestinal Disorders

The human GI system has a critical role in the digestion of food, nutrient absorption, and waste elimination. However, some of the frequent gastrointestinal disorders can interfere with these essential processes to cause significant discomfort and health problems. Diseases like gastroesophageal reflux disease (GERD), irritable bowel syndrome (IBS), and inflammatory bowel disease (IBD) are prevalent and can present a range of symptoms. For instance, GERD, characterized by chronic regurgitation and heartburn, occurs when stomach acid regularly backs up into the esophagus, which may cause damage to the esophagus. Similarly, IBS, a functional gastrointestinal disorder syndrome, may produce a variety of symptoms like abdominal pain, bloating, and changes in bowel habits, proposing a complex interplay of physiological and psychological processes in its pathogenesis. Understanding these disorders in the context of gastrointestinal physiology is crucial to effective management and treatment. Beyond symptomatic control, nutrition's role in relation to gastrointestinal integrity underlies the management of common disorders. Dietary choices directly impact symptomatology and overall gastrointestinal function. Scientific research indicates that some dietary therapies can cause cellular homeostasis and quell symptoms associated with disorders like IBS and GERD. For instance, a diet rich in fiber can promote bowel regularity and alleviate constipation dominance in IBS patients. Moreover, low-acidity foods can be advantageous for GERD patients because they minimize irritation of the mucosa of the esophagus. The potential of functional food and prebiotics in the control of gut microbiota presents a new avenue for patients suffering from gastrointestinal disorders, as new evidence has shown their ability to restore balance and improve gut health (Sarmidi, 2012). Such findings are significant in favor of incorporating nutritional counseling into conventional treatment practices. In addition, rehabilitative interventions are now also serving as useful adjuvants in the treatment of specific gastrointestinal conditions, particularly swallowing disorders. Dysphagia, or swallowing difficulty, may have a profound impact on patients with certain gastrointestinal diseases, complicating the provision of nutrition. Current research has investigated rehabilitation exercises for the strengthening of pharyngeal muscles, which are integral in the act of swallowing. Using resistance training in swallowing, researchers have shown the promise for enhancing pharyngeal contractile function, leading eventually to the augmentation of the mechanism of swallowing (Shaker et al., 2016). This innovation reiterates the importance of understanding the dynamic anatomy and physiology of the gastrointestinal tract so as to more effectively utilize site-specific treatments that address underlying dysfunctions, thus providing a more holistic treatment for common gastrointestinal diseases (Figure 1.17).

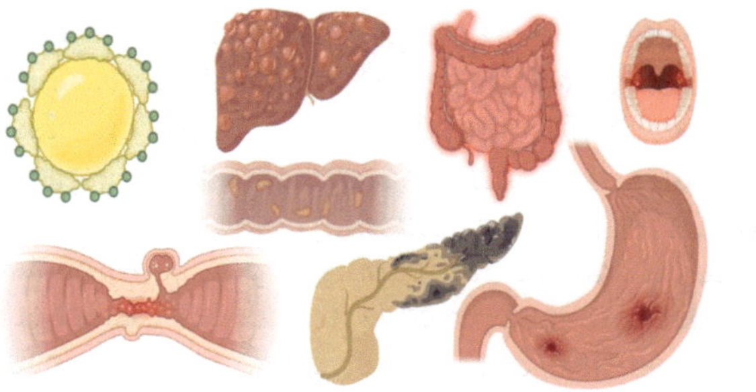

Figure 1.17. Common gastrointestinal disorders.

Source: https://microbenotes.com/wp-content/uploads/2019/03/Disorders-and-Diseases-of-the-Human-Digestive-System.jpeg.

1.6.1. Overview of Functional Disorders

Functional gastrointestinal disorders are a complex interaction of dysregulation of physiology and subjective symptomology that makes them challenging to comprehend and manage. IBS and IBD are quintessential in that they are characterized by chronic pain in the abdomen, bloating, diarrhea, and constipation. The episodic quality of such symptoms can be taken as indicative of underlying oscillations in bodily state or hormonal cueing, which would suggest that variability in gastrointestinal function could have a major impact on patient experience. The pathophysiology of these functional disorders requires not only an understanding of gut anatomy and physiology but also an understanding of how such factors interact with psychological and hormonal influences, as the latter can modify or potentiate symptoms and therefore calls for a holistic approach in diagnosis and treatment (Linson, 2013). The pathophysiology of functional gastrointestinal disorders has significant relevance to their management and choice of therapy. For instance, constipation is defined by specific criteria , such as straining and reduced frequency of defecation, with sensations of incomplete evacuation. The understanding of such functional mechanisms accentuates the importance of colonic transit and the defecation process towards ensuring regular bowel. Regimens for treatment are likely to be complemented by patient-specific lifestyle modification and pharmacotherapy, especially when there are co-existing comorbid conditions. The literature increasingly puts emphasis on evidence-based practice in informing therapeutic intervention and prescribing, with a focus on symptom relief as well as on understanding the underlying processes engaged (Gardiner & Hilton, 2016). Moreover, the therapeutic environment in functional disorders is evolving, and increasing recognition is being afforded to the impact that hormonal influences may have on disorders like IBS. Current data indicate that hormones, particularly progesterone, may influence gastrointestinal motility and symptom expression, and therefore open up new therapeutic options. Targeting the manipulation of hormonal fluctuations can represent a promise of the shift in treatment plans from symptom mitigation to addressing the underlying pathogeneses of functional disorders. As a result, a multidisciplinary plan, combining gastroenterological, endocrinological, and psychosocial considerations, is essential for advancing knowledge and therapeutic intervention in functional gastrointestinal disorders. By integrating these various aspects, we can move towards more holistic and effective health strategies for patients impacted by the complexity of functional gastrointestinal disorders (Linson, 2013).

1.6.2. Structural Disorders and Their Implications

Understanding structural disorders of the gastrointestinal tract is crucial to fully realizing their vast health implications. These disorders, which could be caused by congenital abnormalities, trauma, or degenerative disease, can disrupt regular physiological functioning. Esophageal structural abnormalities, for instance, like strictures and diverticula, can result in dysphagia and significantly affect nutritional absorption. In light of the gastrointestinal tract's pivotal position in digestion and nutrient acquisition, disruptions brought about by structural malformations can result in more complex metabolic problems, affecting homeostasis. This interplay between structural integrity and functional competence stresses the importance of a holistic solution that considers both anatomical and physiological paradigms in the management of gastrointestinal conditions, as provided in studies that underscore food and nutrition's role in human well-being and metabolism (Sarmidi, 2012). The implications of structural disorders extend beyond isolated issues. Patients suffering from these disorders typically manifest with multifaceted problems, including dysphagia, which significantly disables swallowing as well as adds to additional nutritional deficits. The prevalence of dysphagia is especially common in neurologic patients, where swallowing disorders can add to enhanced morbidity, e.g., dehydration and malnutrition, thus reducing the quality of life. It is particularly noteworthy to employ methods like videofluorographic swallowing studies in order to evaluate dysphagia accurately, so that clinicians are able to make feeding regimes tailored to each individual patient. Early treatment and diagnosis are not merely likely to enhance the prognosis of a patient but are also likely to enhance quality of life in general, highlighting the intense bond between structural disorders and cascading impact on health outcomes (Focal Spot, Fall/

Winter 2010/2011. Bernard Becker Medical Library Archives. Washington University School of Medicine, Saint Louis, Missouri). Thus, the management of structural disorders of the gastrointestinal tract involves multidisciplinary care integrating inputs from various specialties , such as medicine, nutrition, and rehabilitation. Through keen observation and management of these conditions, clinicians are better equipped to handle complexities arising due to such disorders. A thorough knowledge of the anatomy and physiology of the gastrointestinal tract is also crucial for planning effective intervention strategies capable of combating threats from structural aberrations. Because nutrition stands at the core of health promotion, along with the management of metabolic disease, biochemistry integration with anatomical data can restore homeostasis. Lastly, this intricate insight is testament to the wide-ranging impact structural disease has on gut health and merits a preventive and informed approach to fortifying patient outcomes (Sarmidi, 2012).

1.6.3. Impact of Lifestyle on Gastrointestinal Health

The complex interaction between lifestyle and gastrointestinal health is a subject of increasing significance in the field of medicine and health science. Physical activity, diet, and behavioral variables all impact gastrointestinal function and well-being. A fiber-rich diet consisting of fruits, vegetables, and whole grains is linked to enhanced bowel regularity and reduced symptoms of gastrointestinal disorders like constipation and diverticulitis. On the other hand, excessive intake of processed foods and sugars may disrupt gut microbiota, leading to dysbiosis, which has been associated with inflammatory bowel disease (IBD) and other chronic gastrointestinal illnesses. A recognition of these interactions serves to demonstrate the importance of health education programs that promote healthful lifestyle habits as a means of preventing gastrointestinal disease and inducing digestive health, and, by so doing, demonstrates the role of diet and lifestyle in gaining homeostasis in the GI tract. Engaging in regular physical activity is also an important component in promoting gastrointestinal health.

Physical activity has been proven to enhance gut motility, thus lowering the incidence of constipation and other related disorders. Exercise also fosters emotional well-being, which in turn can influence gastrointestinal health via the gut-brain axis. Stress and anxiety have negative impacts on gastrointestinal function, often leading to symptoms , such as irritable bowel syndrome (IBS). Hence, physical activity is not only beneficial for physical health but can also relieve stress-related gastrointestinal ailments. Recognizing the multi-dimensional impact of lifestyle choices allows for a potential avenue of promoting health, as interventions encouraging exercise show better outcomes for patients with gastrointestinal illness, leading eventually to an integrated wellness approach. Education programs that offer an understanding of the connection between lifestyle and gastrointestinal well-being have a significant impact on patient outcomes, too. Literature suggests that individuals who are more aware of their situation have better management skills and adherence to treatment regimens. Knowledge about the etiologic contribution of lifestyle factors to diseases like IBD is vital in the promotion of healthy coping strategies and active management of health. Programs , such as Katalyst, designed for fifth graders to experience body systems through experiential learning, highlight the efficacy of education in imparting required health knowledge early on. Interventions , such as these can generate competent individuals who are more capable of making well-informed nutrition and lifestyle choices, thereby suppressing the prevalence of gastrointestinal diseases and optimizing general health trajectories within communities. Closing knowledge gaps not only benefits the health of individuals but can also have broader ramifications for public health through the alleviation of the health burden of gastrointestinal disease to healthcare systems (Figure 1.18).

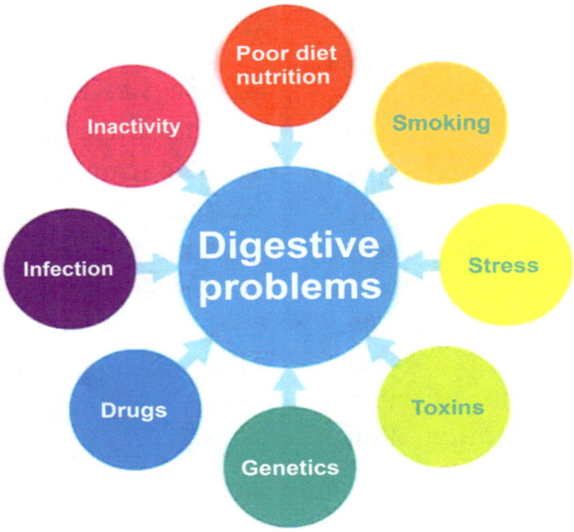

Figure 1.18. Impact of lifestyle on gastrointestinal health.

Source: https://cdhf.ca/wp-content/uploads/2022/06/digestionproblems.png.

SUMMARY

In short, a study of basic gastrointestinal anatomy and physiology gives one a full overview of the intricate systems that are involved in the digestion and absorption of nutrients. Through the intricate combination of the gastrointestinal tract's numerous elements, it is possible to comprehend the astonishing efficiency of the process by which the body digests food. The comprehension of such physiological mechanisms not just accounts for the normal physiology of the GI tract but also emphasizes the pathophysiological implications relevant to GI disorders. The issue of constipation is a classic example, which shows the importance of colonic transit and defecation mechanism, which further signifies the importance of a harmonious management approach taking into account symptomatic relief as well as etiology (Gardiner & Hilton, 2016). This information is the foundation for therapeutic methods and the improvement of patient treatment in the context of gastrointestinal health. Furthermore, anatomical structures of the gastrointestinal tract are the foundation of knowledge for how individual organs work in coordination to provide digestion. From the esophagus to the rectum, each part of the division plays a distinct role in the process of food digestion, and any disruption has critical clinical applications. Structural and functional differences between species also give insight into evolutionary adaptations that enhance digestive efficiency. Furthermore, the anatomic method enhances the understanding of diagnostic techniques and interventions utilized during clinical practice. For example, determining the effectiveness of different pharmacological agents for the treatment of constipation is crucial in optimal patient management (Broad et al., 2018). This union of physiology and anatomy highlights the value of a holistic educational and practice strategy in the field of gastrointestinal health. Ultimately, an understanding of the fundamentals of gastrointestinal physiology and anatomy is key to both students and practitioners who want to improve healthcare outcomes. The more research is incorporated into revised practices, the more its importance to healthcare. This ongoing research holds the promise of opening new doors on digestive health and new therapeutic paths to gastrointestinal disease. Emphasizing the importance of anatomical form as well as physiological function lends added appreciation to the body's complexity. Subsequent research that unites these fields will serve both to further clinical practice and to inform a more substantive knowledge base upon which the next generation of healthcare practitioners will rely. Therefore, the end of this journey is not merely a summary but a call to further exploration and advancement in the study of gastrointestinal anatomy and physiology.

The gastrointestinal tract is a complex dance of anatomical structures and physiological functions required for breakdown and nutrient absorption. It begins in the oral cavity, where mechanical digestion through mastication and enzymatic digestion by saliva initiate the digestive process. Food travels through the esophagus by the muscular contractions of peristalsis to the stomach. In the stomach, hydrochloric acid and digestive enzymes enable food to be digested to chyme, a semi-fluid that can be further processed in the intestines. This process puts into perspective the importance of each anatomical structure since the effectiveness of digestion lies in the proper functioning and coordination of its structures. Understanding these basic processes is critical to appreciating the complexities of gastrointestinal physiology and thus, is a significant area to study both in health and disease. The chyme proceeds from the stomach to the small intestine, and the role of the small intestine is to absorb nutrients. The small intestine has three segments: the duodenum, jejunum, and ileum. Pancreatic enzymatic secretions and bile from the liver also contribute to digestion so that macronutrients are broken down into units ready to be absorbed. The microvilli and villi greatly increase the surface area of the small intestine, with optimal absorption by diffusion and active transport mechanisms. This intricate system highlights coordination among organs and the value of anatomical specialization in optimizing digestive efficiency. As research continues to uncover the complexity of nutrient uptake, implications for gastrointestinal disease, nutrition, and well-being are even more apparent, substantiating the relevance of these principles to clinical care. In the past few years, curricula emphasizing instruction in gastrointestinal anatomy and physiology have gained popularity. Projects , such as those described in Anatomical Academy showcase the double dividend of enhanced pedagogical skills among mentors and science literacy for young students. Active learning approaches enable mentors to not only deepen their expertise in key areas of anatomy and physiology but also engage students in effective communication on matters regarding health and diet. Findings of the same indicate high levels of mentor confidence and knowledge retention by students, a sign of a mutually positive association between learning and instruction. Since such learning environments have put a focus on knowledge transfer of gastrointestinal health is paramount, particularly in developing a future generation of people who embrace the fundamental principles of physiology and nutrition well-being, as evidenced in the objectives and outcomes of the programs (Diaz et al., 2019).

CLOSER LOOK

GASTROINTESTINAL PHYSIOLOGY AND ANATOMY

The gastrointestinal (GI) system is a long, continuous passageway, approximately 30 feet (9 meters) in length in a living person, extending from the mouth to the anus, responsible for ingestion, digestion, absorption, and elimination. It consists of the hollow GI tract organs—the mouth, pharynx, esophagus, stomach, small intestine, and large intestine—as well as accessory organs like the salivary glands, liver, gallbladder, and pancreas which secrete essential enzymes and bile.

Food begins its journey in the mouth, where mechanical digestion (chewing) and the chemical breakdown of carbohydrates (via salivary amylase) begin. The chewed food, or bolus, is then propelled through the pharynx and esophagus into the stomach by a wave-like muscular contraction called peristalsis. In the stomach, strong muscular churning (mechanical digestion) mixes the food with highly acidic gastric juices (hydrochloric acid and pepsin) to form a semi-liquid mixture called chyme, initiating protein digestion and destroying most pathogens.

The chyme is released gradually into the small intestine, the primary site for chemical digestion and nutrient absorption. Here, it mixes with bile from the liver and gallbladder (for fat emulsification) and numerous enzymes from the pancreas (for further breakdown of proteins, fats, and carbohydrates). The small intestine's inner lining is covered in millions of microscopic, finger-like projections called villi and microvilli, which vastly increase the surface area for efficient absorption of nutrients into the bloodstream and lymphatic system.

Undigested waste then moves into the large intestine, where the main functions are the absorption of remaining water, electrolytes, and some vitamins produced by symbiotic bacteria. The waste material is converted into feces, stored in the rectum, and eventually eliminated from the body through the anal canal and anus during defecation. The entire process is regulated by a complex system of neural controls, including the enteric nervous system (the "brain of the gut"), and various hormones.

REFERENCES

1. Broad, J., Kung, V. W. S., Palmer, A., Elahi, S., Karami, A., Darreh-Shori, T., Ahmed, S., Thaha, M. A., Carroll, R., Chin-Aleong, J., Martin, J. E., Saffrey, M. J., Knowles, C. H., & Sanger, G. J. (2019). Changes in neuromuscular structure and functions of human colon during ageing are region-dependent. *Gut, 68*(7), 1210–1223. https://doi.org/10.1136/gutjnl-2018-316279(accessed on 15th July 2025).
2. Bailey, B., Cox, D., Darwich, A., Dorey, G., Duwal, S., Ette, E., et al. (2018). *Population variability in animal health: Influence on dose-exposure-response relationships: Part II: Modelling and simulation.* https://core.ac.uk/download/159992803.pdf (accessed on 15th July 2025).
3. Shaker, R., Sanvanson, P., Balasubramanian, G., Kern, M., Wuerl, A., & Hyngstrom, A. (2016). Effects of laryngeal restriction on pharyngeal peristalsis and biomechanics: Clinical implications. *American journal of physiology. Gastrointestinal and liver physiology, 310*(11), G1036–G1043. https://doi.org/10.1152/ajpgi.00010.2016 (accessed on 15th July 2025).
4. Balick, M., Bischoff, M., Blumenthal, M., Bortoft, A., Bott, S., Cookson, C., Doe, J., et al. (1997). *Anthroposophic Perspectives in Primary Care.* https://core.ac.uk/download/46965261.pdf (accessed on 15th July 2025).
5. Balters, S., Steinert, M. (2017). *Capturing emotion reactivity through physiology measurement as a foundation for affective engineering in engineering design science and engineering practices.* https://core.ac.uk/download/636669831.pdf (accessed on 15th July 2025).
6. Besecker, E. S., Cooper, T. K., Deiter, G. M., Holmes, J., et al. (2016). *Mesenteric vascular dysregulation and intestinal inflammation accompanies experimental spinal cord injury.* https://cupola.gettysburg.edu/cgi/viewcontent.cgi?article=1073&context=healthfac (accessed on 15th July 2025).
7. Bosch, J. A., de Geus, E. J. C., Hoogstraten, J., Nieuw Amerongen, A. V., et al. (2000). *Innate secretory immunity in response to laboratory stressors that evoke distinct patterns of cardiac autonomic activity.* https://core.ac.uk/download/pdf/15457442.pdf (accessed on 15th July 2025).
8. Breit, S., Kupferberg, A., Rogler, G., Hasler, G. (2018). Vagus nerve as modulator of the brain–gut axis in psychiatric and inflammatory disorders. *Frontiers in Psychiatry, 9.* https://doi.org/10.3389/fpsyt.2018.00044 (accessed on 15th July 2025).
9. Christensen, W. (2006). *The Evolutionary Origins of Volition.* https://core.ac.uk/download/pdf/87234.pdf (accessed on 15th July 2025).
10. Coaten, J. (2024). *How to assess and examine a patient with abdominal symptoms.* https://core.ac.uk/download/617025296.pdf (accessed on 15th July 2025).
11. Cornell University. (1995). *College of Veterinary Medicine.* https://ecommons.cornell.edu/bitstream/handle/1813/38405/COS_v87_1995_96_16.pdf?sequence=1&isAllowed=y (accessed on 15th July 2025).
12. Cornell University. (2000). *College of Veterinary Medicine.* https://ecommons.cornell.edu/bitstream/handle/1813/38477/COS_v91_1999_2000_16.pdf?sequence=1&isAllowed=y (accessed on 15th July 2025).
13. Danaei, M., Dehghankhold, M., Ataei, S., Hasanzadeh Davarani, F., Javanmard, R., Dokhani, A., Khorasani, S., et al. (2018). Impact of particle size and polydispersity index on the clinical

applications of lipidic nanocarrier systems. *Pharmaceutics, 10*, 57. https://doi.org/10.3390/pharmaceutics10020057 (accessed on 15th July 2025).

14. Diaz, M. M., Lassetter, J., Mageno, A., McCleve, B., et al. (2019). *Who is the teacher and who is the student? The dual service- and engaged-learning pedagogical model of Anatomy Academy.* https://core.ac.uk/download/288117085.pdf (accessed on 15th July 2025).

15. Dong, J., Zhang, H., Ai, X., Dong, Q., Shi, X., Zhao, X., Zhong, C., et al. (2024). Improving chilling tolerance of peanut seedlings by enhancing antioxidant-modulated ROS scavenging ability, alleviating photosynthetic inhibition, and mobilizing nutrient absorption. *Plant Biology.* https://www.semanticscholar.org/paper/6d0ff0cbfadfaa2be12c02618ba9ff0ebe982af5 (accessed on 15th July 2025).

16. Dunton, F. (1963). *Science concepts: Nursing care of patients with bleeding esophageal varices.* https://open.bu.edu/bitstream/2144/4581/1/Dunton_1963_web.pdf (accessed on 15th July 2025).

17. Eklund, G. (2003). *Cadmium in Newborns.* https://core.ac.uk/download/11694662.pdf (accessed on 15th July 2025).

18. Flint, A., Peeters, A., Butland, B., Challis, B., Abbott, C., Byrne, C., Byrne, C., et al. (2019). *A study protocol for a randomized crossover study evaluating the effect of diets differing in carbohydrate quality on ileal content and appetite regulation in healthy humans.* https://core.ac.uk/download/286269689.pdf (accessed on 15th July 2025).

19. Flood, P., Hanrahan, N., Nally, K., Melgar, S. (2023). Human intestinal organoids: Modeling gastrointestinal physiology and immunopathology — Current applications and limitations. *European Journal of Immunology, 54.* https://www.semanticscholar.org/paper/0c8a1861163cdf78f546d38df45f8eaa512cf7c9 (accessed on 15th July 2025).

20. Gardiner, A., Hilton, A. (2016). *Managing Constipation in adults with Co-Morbidities.* https://www.magonlinelibrary.com/doi/abs/10.12968/indn.2016.10.21#:~:text=Treatment%20is%20normally%20started%20for,the%20person%20still%20has%20difficulty.. https://core.ac.uk/download/151161237.pdf (accessed on 15th July 2025).

21. Hagedorn, R. L., Baker, K., DeJarnett, S. E., Hendricks, T., McGowan, M., Joseph, L., Olfert, M. (2018). Katalyst Pilot Study: Using interactive activities in anatomy and physiology to teach children the scientific foundation of healthy lifestyles. *Children, 5.* https://www.semanticscholar.org/paper/3221974e3ec32c2f56c6d6701d2aec03542630dc (accessed on 15th July 2025).

22. Holm, L., Jansson, A., Thorsson, E., Vaga, M., et al. (2020). *Histochemical localization of carbonic anhydrase in the digestive tract and salivary glands of the house cricket, Acheta domesticus.* https://core.ac.uk/download/335350171.pdf (accessed on 15th July 2025).

23. Homayun, B., Lin, X., & Choi, H. J. (2019). Challenges and recent progress in oral drug delivery systems for biopharmaceuticals. *Pharmaceutics, 11*, 129. https://doi.org/10.3390/pharmaceutics11030129 (accessed on 15th July 2025).

24. Kanmani, S., & Koo, B. S. (2020). Gut–brain axis: Role of gut microbiota on neurological disorders and how probiotics/prebiotics beneficially modulate microbial and immune pathways to improve brain functions. *International Journal of Molecular Sciences, 21*, 7551. https://doi.org/10.3390/ijms21207551 (accessed on 15th July 2025).

25. Keet, A. D. (1974). *An anatomico physiological principle governing the direction of the gastrointestinal mucosal folds during life.* https://core.ac.uk/download/37329238.pdf (accessed on 15th July 2025).

26. Kumbhari, V. (2019). *Endoluminal weight loss and metabolic therapies: Current and future techniques.* https://core.ac.uk/download/286559630.pdf (accessed on 15th July 2025).

27. Linson, E. A. (2013). *The interplay between hormones and irritable bowel disease.* B.S., Emory University, 2010 Submitted in partial fulfillment of the requirements for the degree of Master of Arts 2013 https://open.bu.edu/bitstream/2144/12149/6/Linson_Elyse_2013_nosig_nocv.pdf (accessed on 15th July 2025).

28. Liu, S. L. (2022). *Reduced ileum peristaltic contractility in cystic fibrosis swine.* https://core.ac.uk/download/523375968.pdf (accessed on 15th July 2025).

29. Liu, X. (2023). *Verification and validation of numerical modelling approaches pertinent to stomach modelling.* https://core.ac.uk/download/559247572.pdf (accessed on 15th July 2025).

30. Focal Spot, Fall/Winter 2010/2011. Bernard Becker Medical Library Archives. Washington University School of Medicine, Saint Louis, Missouri(accessed on 15th July 2025).

31. Regev, A., Teichmann, S. A., Lander, E. S., Amit, I., Benoist, C., Birney, E., Bodenmiller, B., et al. (2017). The human cell Atlas. *eLife, 6.* https://doi.org/10.7554/elife.27041 (accessed on 15th July 2025).

32. Rodriguez, G., Gater, D. (2022). Neurogenic bowel and management after spinal cord injury: A narrative review. *Journal of Personalized Medicine, 12.* https://www.semanticscholar.org/paper/ee2f04c2a6996eb2c0b2e45a349a42b99cadabc7 (accessed on 15th July 2025).

33. Roma-Rodrigues, C., Mendes, R., Baptista, P. V., & Fernandes, A. R. (2019). Targeting tumor microenvironment for cancer therapy. *International Journal of Molecular Sciences, 20,* 840. https://doi.org/10.3390/ijms20040840 (accessed on 15th July 2025).

34. Sarmidi, M. R. (2012). *Food Is Our Medicine.* https://core.ac.uk/download/11801185.pdf (accessed on 15th July 2025).

35. Schmidt, C. K., Medina-Sánchez, M., Edmondson, R. J., & Schmidt, O. G. (2020). Engineering microrobots for targeted cancer therapies from a medical perspective. *Nature Communications, 11.* https://doi.org/10.1038/s41467-020-19322-7 (accessed on 15th July 2025).

36. Sequeira, C., Santos, I., Coelho, M., Teixeira, C., Mangualde, J., Cremers, I., Oliveira, A. (2022). P210 Assessment of disease specific knowledge and quality of life among patients with inflammatory bowel disease. *Journal of Crohn's and Colitis.* https://www.semanticscholar.org/paper/840791334648211f215f0d86d2a1120791c528a7 (accessed on 15th July 2025).

37. Simmonds, S., Matthee, A., Dowrick, J. M., Taberner, A., Du, P., & Angeli-Gordon, T. R. (2024). Electromechanical coupling and anatomy of the in-vivo gastroduodenal junction. *American Journal of Physiology. Gastrointestinal and Liver Physiology.* https://www.semanticscholar.org/paper/b3de8887834e5f11fbfc1dba5a71e6f57a6e2c99 (accessed on 15th July 2025).

38. University of Nebraska College of Medicine. (1966). *Bulletin of the University of Nebraska: Annual catalog of the College of Medicine, 1966–1967.* https://core.ac.uk/download/268251847.pdf (accessed on 15th July 2025).

39. Vijay, M. N. (2020). *A multi-compartmental mathematical model of the postprandial human stomach: A thesis presented in partial fulfilment of the requirements for the degree of Doctor*

of Philosophy in Anatomy and Physiology at Massey University, Palmerston North, New Zealand. https://core.ac.uk/download/519744837.pdf (accessed on 15th July 2025).

40. Vinarov, Z., Abdallah, M., Agúndez, J. A. G., Allegaert, K., Basit, A. W., Braeckmans, M., Ceulemans, J., et al. (2021). Impact of gastrointestinal tract variability on oral drug absorption and pharmacokinetics: An UNGAP review. *European Journal of Pharmaceutical Sciences, 162,* 105812. https://doi.org/10.1016/j.ejps.2021.105812 (accessed on 15th July 2025).

41. White, R. J. (2025). *Acid-Base Homeostasis in the Human System.* https://core.ac.uk/download/pdf/42869639.pdf (accessed on 15th July 2025).

42. Yacoubi, N. (2016). *Water-soluble short-chain arabinoxylans produced by enzymatic treatment of wheat grain improve growth performance and intestinal health of broilers.* https://core.ac.uk/download/74662445.pdf (accessed on 15th July 2025).

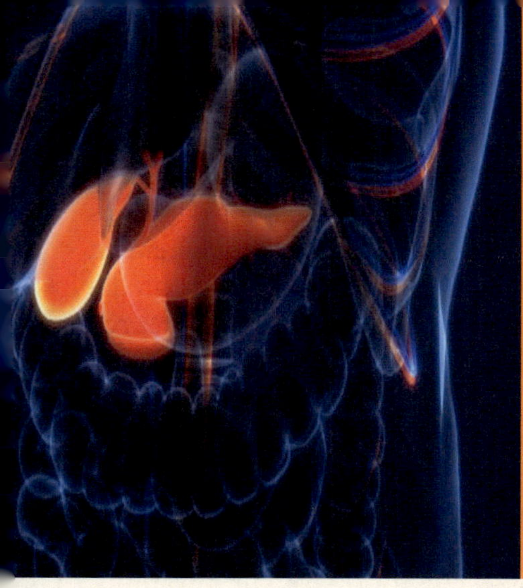

Chapter 2

DIAGNOSTIC TECHNIQUES IN GASTROENTEROLOGY

Contents

Introduction

In gastroenterology, proper diagnosis is paramount because of the nature of gastrointestinal disease. Familiarity with the wide range of diagnostic techniques is important for doctors who want to optimize patient results. The technology and methods have evolved significantly, leading to improved diagnostic efficiency, and physicians are now able to diagnose and treat everything from typical gastrointestinal complaints to rare, multifaceted disorders. For instance, imaging technology innovation , such as endoscopy and MRI, has revolutionized diagnostic potential. However, despite all these innovations, there are challenges in differentiating among diseases with similar symptoms since such diagnostic overlap may cause misdiagnosis, delayed treatment, and morbidity among patients. In addition, the inclusion of biomarkers in gastroenterological diagnostics can enhance clinical decision-making. There have been recent discoveries in research that emphasize the need to find biological markers associated with specific gastrointestinal diseases, thereby contributing to the diagnostic process.

The exploration of genetic, biochemical, and neuroimaging biomarkers offers a possible avenue towards improving the accuracy of diagnosis, for example, in research that emphasizes the demands for additional research in these areas (Parlatini et al., 2024). Yet, achieving real advancement in this area requires the resolution of vast hurdles, including the biological heterogeneity of the majority of gastrointestinal diseases and methodological dissimilarity that can stagnate research momentum. As diagnostic technology progresses, adherence to accepted clinical guidelines remains central to the provision of effective patient care. For instance, the European Society for Paediatric Gastroenterology, Hepatology and Nutrition (ESPGHAN) has proposed no-biopsy strategies for conditions like coeliac disease, evidencing significant shifts in diagnostic techniques (Rižnik et al., 2024). Diagnostic approaches, particularly across various populations, show that diagnostic standards need to be adaptable to use. This adaptation not only enhances the quality of care for patients but also decreases the risk of diagnostic delay and improves overall treatment durations. As the specialty evolves further, greater collaboration between practitioners and scientists will be needed in order to refine the diagnostic technique and its application in clinical practice further (Figure 2.1).

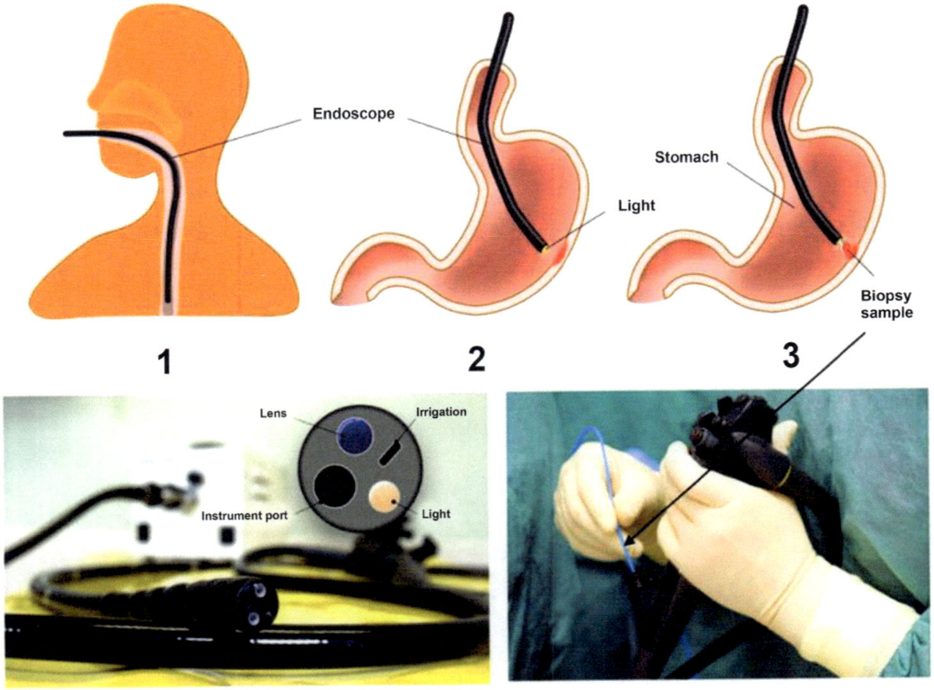

Figure 2.1. Diagnostic techniques in gastroenterology.

Source: https://www.bayousurgery.com/wp-content/uploads/2020/07/Gastroenterology-upper-GI-endoscopy-768x696.jpg.

Definition of Gastroenterology

Gastroenterology is a branch of medicine that treats and diagnoses diseases in the GI tract and associated organs , such as the liver and pancreas. Gastroenterology encompasses a broad range of conditions, including but not limited to inflammatory bowel disease , such as Crohn's disease and ulcerative colitis, functional gastrointestinal disease, liver disease, and GI cancer. As gastroenterology becomes central in the management of these typically intricate conditions, the inclusion of proper diagnostic procedures is of the highest consequence. Proper diagnosis is necessary in terms of determining the appropriate treatment and assisting in minimizing the impact of gastrointestinal conditions on the life of the patient, thereby suggesting the significance of quality improvement in diagnostic procedures under this medical specialty. The gastroenterology diagnostic setting has rapidly evolved, with technology and research leading the way. Traditional methods , such as endoscopy or colonoscopy, remain essential in tissue sampling and viewing of abnormalities within the GI tract. But innovations , such as non-invasive imaging technologies and biomarkers have deepened the pool of diagnostic tools. Such advances not only enhance the quality and validity of diagnoses but also aid in more individualized therapeutic methods. The establishment of professional guidelines grounded on systematic review of the literature and consensus among experts is notable in streamlining the process of diagnosis. As noted in respective gastroenterological societies' clinical guidelines, these guidelines allow clinicians to make evidence-based care a reality in patients with many GI disorders with an optimization of health outcomes (Chalasani et al., 2017; Rosen et al., 2018). Moreover, a greater understanding of gastrointestinal illness further reiterates the need for comprehensive diagnostic approaches. For instance, the increasing incidence of nonalcoholic fatty liver disease (NAFLD) has the urgency of a thorough assessment that includes clinical evaluation, biomarkers, and imaging tests. While the gastrointestinal tract continues to encounter escalating rates of diseases like NAFLD, timely diagnosis assumes increasing importance. In this regard, continual updates to clinical guidelines and diagnostic criteria, derived from recent clinical studies and expert panel consensus, continue to further delineate our ability to identify at-risk populations and maximize patient management. In doing so, the definition of gastroenterology not only encompasses treatment of GI disease but, importantly, emphasizes the vital function of diagnostic innovation in the delivery of effective health care outcomes in this significant area of medicine.

Importance of Diagnostic Techniques

In gastroenterology, the role of diagnostic techniques cannot be overemphasized since they form the pillar of effective disease control and treatment interventions. Early and accurate diagnosis has a significant impact on patient outcomes, particularly in chronic illnesses , such as liver disease and inflammatory bowel disease. The ambiguity of these diseases tends to mask their presence, making precise diagnostic techniques imperative. For instance, in pediatric patients, the lack of obvious symptoms can lead to delayed diagnosis, with the significance of heightened awareness and sensitive diagnostic methods. By utilizing techniques , such as imaging, serology, and endoscopy, physicians can more effectively diagnose these diseases early on, hence enabling early management and intervention, which is crucial in altering the course of the disease (Della Corte et al., 2016). Along with this has come the revolution in diagnostic technology, which has altered the management of gastroenterological disease to enable more subtle and less intrusive diagnostics. Techniques , such as capsule endoscopy and balloon-assisted enteroscopy have taken the central role in visualizing the small bowel, a challenging area for conventional endoscopic approaches. These techniques not only enable the diagnosis of conditions , such as Crohn's disease but also play an important role in follow-up monitoring of disease activity and response to therapy. As has been established, such imaging techniques can accurately inform patient management planning, especially in individuals who have undergone surgical resection of bowel segments, illustrating the double role of diagnostics in timely diagnosis as well as in ongoing patient care (Hausmann & Albert, 2011). Such a changing situation highlights the importance of keeping diagnostic techniques at the vanguard of gastroenterology practice. The incorporation of advanced methods of diagnosis into everyday clinical practice is directly correlated with improved outcomes for the patient. Such diseases as chronic liver diseases are so insidious, the risk of delayed diagnosis is clear. Advanced imaging and laboratory techniques allow detection of disease progression, which is not only important for clinical management but also for developing preventative strategies. These diagnostic tests generate knowledge that enhances understanding of disease pathogenesis and consequently results in the identification of new therapeutic targets and interventions. As the discipline continues to grow, therefore, a strong insistence on validating and utilizing diagnostic innovations will be paramount in overcoming difficulties resulting from complex gastrointestinal diseases and bringing enhanced health benefits for patients (Della Corte et al., 2016).

2.1. Endoscopy

Endoscopy is a milestone in gastroenterology that possesses both therapeutic and diagnostic capabilities that have significantly enhanced patient care. The minimally invasive technique uses flexible instruments fitted with cameras to view within the gastrointestinal tract to enable clinicians to identify lesions , such as tumors, ulcers, and bleeding points. Compared to traditional diagnostic methods, endoscopy provides real-time visualization and biopsy sampling, enhancing the accuracy of diagnoses. The therapeutic applications of endoscopy, such as polypectomy and hemostatic control of bleeding lesions, demonstrate the two-fold advantage of endoscopy in therapy and diagnosis. With advancing technology, newer endoscopic devices and procedures are emerging, which need critical evaluation of their safety and efficacy before their widespread use in clinical practice (Bhandari et al., 2019). Such strict screening is important to ensure that innovations are commensurate with approved clinical guidelines and optimize patient outcomes. The use of capsule endoscopy (CE) has revolutionized the evaluation of occult gastrointestinal bleeding (OGIB) and small bowel disease. Standard diagnostic methods were usually unsatisfactory, especially for the small intestine, due to the challenges of intubation with conventional endoscopes. However, recent technological advancements have enabled CE to provide non-invasive and comprehensive imaging of the small bowel. The diagnostic yield of CE for patients suspected of small bowel bleeding ranges from 38% to 83%, making it a crucial tool in modern gastroenterological practice. Besides, the complementary function of CE and other endoscopic techniques , such as single-balloon enteroscopy (SBE) enhances diagnosis through allowing clinicians a platform to enhance the precision of their techniques based on the findings obtained from the use of CE (Lee, 2016). Therefore, CE is a vital tool for uncovering diagnoses that otherwise cannot be identified, testifying to the excellence of technological development in gastroenterology. Despite the evident benefits of endoscopic technology, there is a need for rigorous evaluation of new devices and techniques before use in clinical practice. Variations in diagnostic yield and complications of endoscopic technologies necessitate a proper framework of clinical evaluation. This is especially important in the situation of newer technologies, where uptake may be in advance of safety and efficacy knowledge. Comparative effectiveness research provides an attractive paradigm for evaluating innovative endoscopic procedures so that strengths and limitations versus best available care can be determined (Bhandari et al., 2019).

By fostering a culture of rigorous evaluation and standardization, societies , such as the British Society of Gastroenterology can facilitate new technique application in a safe way. This formal strategy not only benefits clinicians in embracing innovations but also guarantees that patient safety is an overarching concern in the changing gastroenterology world (Figure 2.2).

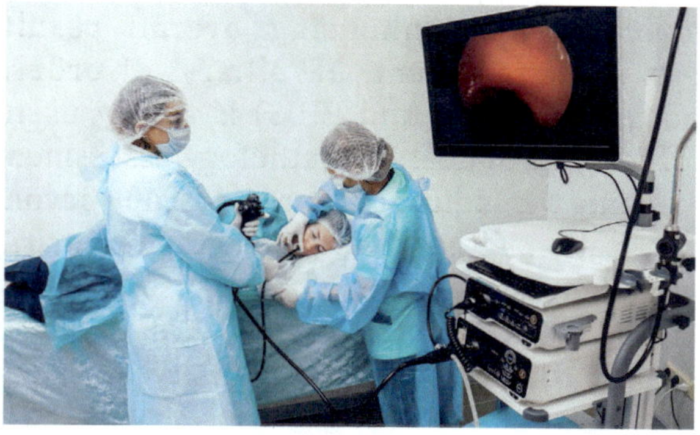

Figure 2.2. Endoscopy.

Source: https://www.cvskl.com/wp-content/uploads/2023/02/Upper-Gastrointestinal-Endoscopy1.jpg.

2.1.1. Types of Endoscopic Procedures

Endoscopy is an important intervention in gastroenterology, with numerous procedures modified to diagnose and treat diseases prevalent in the gastrointestinal tract. Among these are esophagogastroduodenoscopy (EGD), a widely performed procedure that allows direct visualization of the esophagus, stomach, and duodenum. Through a flexible endoscope with a camera, clinicians can identify abnormalities , such as ulcers, polyps, or malignancies. The technique also enables biopsies to be recovered for histopathological study, enabling a better diagnosis of diseases like gastric cancer, which receives a poor prognosis upon detection at an advanced stage (Ajani et al., 2022). EGD may even be used therapeutically to manage esophageal varices or strictures through the facilitation of treatment maneuvers like dilation or band ligation. This dual role of diagnosis and treatment reaffirms the fundamental significance of EGD in the overall care of gastrointestinal disease. Another important endoscopic procedure is colonoscopy, a necessary tool for diagnosing colorectal disease and for screening for colorectal cancer. Colonoscopy enables health care providers to reach the entire colonic mucosa, allowing complete examination of polyps or lesions that could signal cancer. The American Society of Colon and Rectal Surgeons (ASCRS) highlights the preventive aspect of colonoscopy, particularly since most colorectal cancer occurs in asymptomatic patients above the age of 50 years (Vogel et al., 2021).

Not only does it enable diagnosis, but it also enables therapeutic interventions , such as polypectomy, where suspicious polyps can be excised during the same visit. Thus, the addition of colonoscopy to regular screening protocols has profoundly changed early detection and patient outcomes in the battle against colorectal cancer. In addition to EGD and colonoscopy, endoscopic retrograde cholangiopancreatography (ERCP) is a valuable modality for the diagnosis and treatment of bile and pancreatic duct disorders. This involves the use of fluoroscopy and endoscopy combined to visualize these ducts and identify strictures or blockages caused by disease states , such as gallstones or tumors. ERCP is particularly useful because it can serve both therapeutic and diagnostic purposes, e.g., stone extraction and placement of stents to relieve these obstructions. The value of ERCP is apparent in the situation of dealing with complications secondary to disorders , such as pancreatitis, where prompt intervention can avoid substantial morbidity. The utility of ERCP in both the diagnosis and treatment of biliary and pancreatic disease emphasizes its central position in the armamentarium of endoscopic techniques utilized in gastroenterology (Figure 2.3).

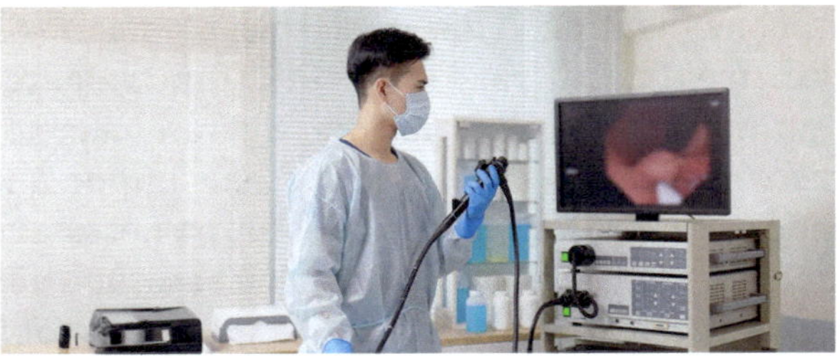

Figure 2.3. Types of endoscopic procedures.

Source: https://medicalblogs.co.uk/wp-content/uploads/2024/04/Different-Types-of-Endoscopy-Procedures_11zon.webp.

2.1.2. Indications for Endoscopy

In gastroenterology, endoscopy is a cornerstone investigative tool underlined by a wide range of clinical indications. One of the most relevant indications for endoscopy is dyspepsia with symptoms of upper abdominal pain, bloating, and nausea. The multicausal nature of dyspepsia with a long list of potential underlying pathologies necessitates adequate evaluation to rule out sinister conditions , such as peptic ulcer disease and malignancies. Initial assessments prioritize symptomatic treatment, but recurrent or complicated dyspepsia will typically trigger more investigation and treatments, including upper gastrointestinal endoscopy. This uncomplicated gastroscopy not only permits direct mucosal visualization but also facilitates targeted biopsies where indicated, significantly enhancing diagnostic sensitivity in distinguishing between benign and premalignant lesions and directing follow-up management plans (Talkhan et al., 2024). Endoscopic retrograde cholangiopancreatography (ERCP) is another extremely critical indication for endoscopic treatment, particularly in the context of biliary obstruction. ERCP has undergone much development since its inception and is now the treatment of choice as a first-line modality in the management of extrahepatic biliary obstruction. ERCP can provide both therapeutic and diagnostic opportunities with the ability to visualize the bile duct, along with procedures , such as stone extraction and stenting. Despite its high success rates of up to 95%, complications are still possible, necessitating the performance of alternative techniques in some proportion of patients when ERCP fails to achieve successful cannulation (Rai et al., 2023). Therefore, awareness of the indications of ERCP and optimizing patient selection is important in reducing associated morbidity and enhancing overall results in the management of biliary disorders. Endoscopic ultrasound (EUS) is a very useful tool for gastrointestinal pathology assessment, extending the indications for endoscopy beyond visualization. Although originally used primarily for diagnostic purposes, EUS is currently a valuable component in the treatment of complex conditions , such as pancreatitis and pancreaticobiliary malignancies. Particularly, EUS-directed interventions like fine-needle aspiration and biliary drainage have emerged more prominently due to their potential to surpass the shortfalls of the standard practices , such as ERCP and percutaneous drainage.

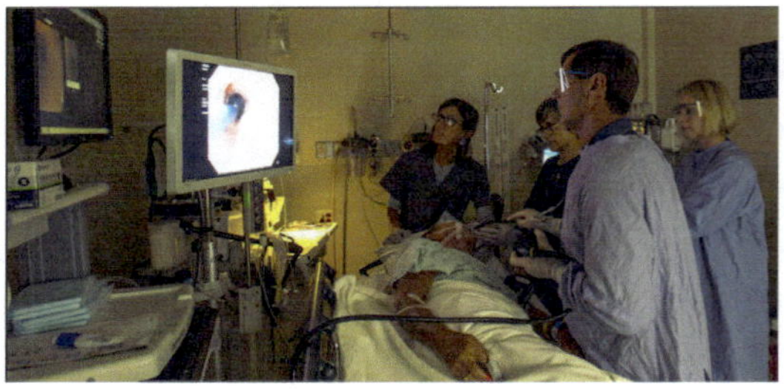

Figure 2.4. Indications for endoscopy.

Source: https://www.cooleydickinson.org/wp-content/uploads/2016/07/Endo-Gastro-OVERVIEW-BrandCanvas-scaled.jpg.

Moreover, the EUS's potential to assess layers of tissue non-invasively provides valuable information regarding staging and treatment planning for the majority of gastrointestinal tumors (Rai et al., 2023; Talkhan et al., 2024). As techniques in gastroenterology become progressively sophisticated, the part played by endoscopy increases and requires a sophisticated comprehension of its indications in providing the best patient care (Figure 2.4).

2.1.3. Risks and Benefits of Endoscopy

Endoscopy is a critical diagnostic tool in gastroenterology, offering an opening into the gastrointestinal tract that can contribute significantly to the diagnosis of many conditions. The benefit of endoscopy is significantly high, particularly in the identification of cancerous tissue, preneoplastic polyps, and inflammatory disease. Such recognition is necessary for proper treatment regimens and can ultimately improve patient outcomes by permitting early interventions. Besides, the method provides direct visualization and biopsy of lesions, which are essential in providing histopathological information. However, there has been a concern that many endoscopic interventions, particularly lower gastrointestinal endoscopy, have been performed among patients with low risk, which may lead to minimal clinical outcomes, citing the need for appropriate patient selection for maximizing their benefits (Beaton et al., 2024). Despite its many benefits, endoscopy carries risks that warrant careful consideration when used in clinical practice. Potential complications include reactions to sedation, bleeding, and perforation of the gastrointestinal tract, though rare. These risks justify the necessity for a proper pre-procedure assessment to ensure that the potential benefits outweigh the risks for the patient. Furthermore, with the majority of endoscopic tests being performed to diagnose dyspepsia and other similar conditions, practitioners must reconcile the need to obtain full diagnostic data with the responsibility to avoid exposing patients unnecessarily to harm. It is important that providers understand the reconciliation of risks and benefits to improve patient care and make gastrointestinal diagnostics more efficient overall. An important component of the diagnostic utility of endoscopy lies in its application for evaluation of dyspepsia, a common gastrointestinal ailment whose symptoms include pain or discomfort in the upper abdomen. Initial assessments preferentially seek to identify immediate causes, such as peptic ulcers or drug reactions, and also screen for serious underlying diseases , such as cancers (Talkhan et al., 2024). Gastroscopy remains a principal modality for these assessments, with the ability to target visualization and intervention. Furthermore, imaging modalities , such as endoscopic ultrasonography (EUS) have provided the entry to additional diagnostic capabilities, such as improved visualization and accurate staging of various gastrointestinal lesions. Such advancement solidifies endoscopy as a diagnostic and therapeutic device, reiterating the importance of gauging risk versus benefit within gastroenterology facilities (Figure 2.5).

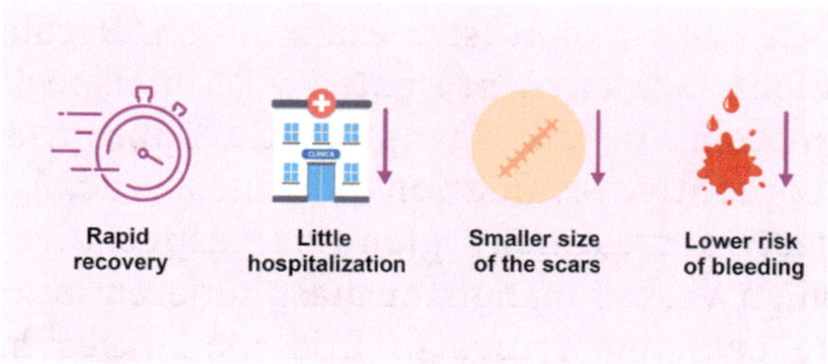

Figure 2.5. Risks and benefits of endoscopy.

Source: https://www.invitra.com/en/wp-content/uploads/2015/02/benefits-surgery-through-endoscopy-2048x870.png.

2.2. Imaging Techniques

Imaging modalities play an important role in gastroenterology, playing a major role in diagnosing gastrointestinal diseases. Among the various modalities available, intestinal ultrasound (IUS) has also emerged as a front runner, becoming more popular due to the fact that it is noninvasive and allows for real-time imaging. Recent advancements have provided

IUS as a useful imaging modality for diagnosing Crohn's disease (CD) with very good sensitivity and specificity in the demonstration of key markers , such as bowel wall thickening and blood flow. As characterized by recent studies, IUS can provide important information about disease activity and complications and hence be an invaluable tool for clinicians when dealing with and following CD. This minimally invasive technique not only increases the comfort of the patient but also lowers the need for even more invasive techniques, and it is creating a paradigm change in the management and assessment of gastrointestinal diseases in clinical practice (Wild et al., 2025). Except IUS, endoscopic ultrasonography (EUS) is also very popular due to its diagnostic value, particularly in assessing pelvic masses affecting intestinal structures. EUS is unique because it can provide high-resolution imaging of subepithelial lesions and surrounding tissue with noninvasive examination. Because patients are often presented with nonspecific symptoms or are asymptomatic, appropriate preoperative evaluation becomes crucial in effective treatment planning, especially in benign versus malignant mass differentiation. The evolving nature of EUS modalities has significantly enhanced diagnostic accuracy, enabling the clinician to estimate disease depth and histology accurately. Besides, EUS is an excellent guide to therapeutic interventions, a testament to its flexibility in the overall context of gastroenterological diagnostic tools (She et al., 2023). Use of various imaging modalities in gastroenterology not only enables accurate diagnosis but also enables enhancement in disease progression and therapeutic response understanding. With the advancement of the specialty, the combination of imaging experts with gastroenterologists becomes increasingly important in maximizing the outcomes of the patients. Standardization of imaging protocols, as well as enhanced training among practitioners, will need to be studied in the future so that technology revolutions like IUS and EUS can be fully exploited in clinical practice. This ongoing quest for excellence in imaging will not merely increase diagnostic precision but will also contribute toward the development of individualized therapeutic strategies for the management of patients with complex gastrointestinal diseases. By embracing new-generation imaging technologies, gastroenterology can ride its path toward a more efficient, patient-centered model of care that addresses both short-term and long-term needs of the patient (Figure 2.6).

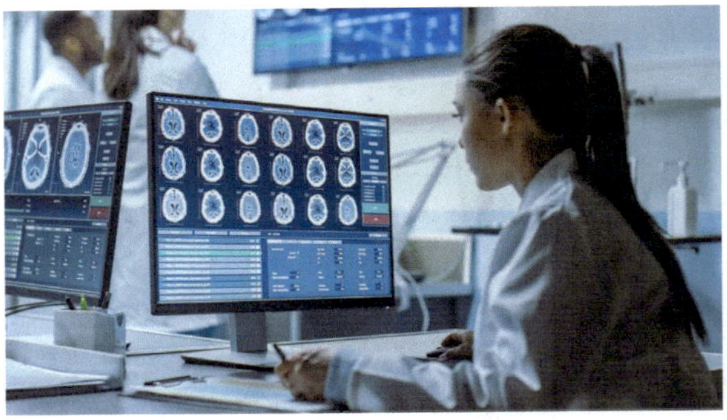

Figure 2.6. Imaging techniques.

Source: https://duckduckgo.com/?q=Imaging+Techniques&t=h_&iar=images&iai=https%3A%2F%2Fwww.healthcarebusinesstoday.com%2Fwp-content%2Fuploads%2F2020%2F07%2Fimage1.jpg.

2.2.1. X-Rays and Fluoroscopy

The application of X-rays and fluoroscopy has had a tremendous influence on the procedures involved in gastroenterology diagnosis, achieving real-time imaging that is immensely helpful for internal anatomy visualization. X-rays, an electromagnetic wave, offer for the inspection of gastrointestinal anatomy and the identification of pathological changes. Used in conjunction with fluoroscopy, which obtains dynamic images by continuous acquisition of X-rays, these procedures enable the clinician to see the gastrointestinal tract in motion. This is especially useful in procedures like barium swallow studies or gastrointestinal tract angiography, where movement of contrast material through the system may demonstrate evidence of functional abnormality. The capacity of real-time monitoring not only supports diagnosis but also assists in guiding therapeutic intervention and hence plays an essential part in gastroenterology patient management. Fluoroscopy, with its capacity to generate high-resolution images during procedure execution, has become pivotal in the application of endoscopic evaluation and intervention. Fluoroscopic guidance is commonly employed in gastroenterology for precise localization and intervention in pathologies like gastrointestinal obstructions, tumors, or strictures. Refined methods like digital subtraction angiography continue to advance the visualization of blood vessels of the gut, allowing detection and management of vascular disorders that might threaten gut blood supply. Increasing reliance on these imaging procedures does present concerns about radiation exposure in patients as well as healthcare workers. Recommended practice emphasizes the need for adherence to the ALARA (As Low As Reasonably Achievable) principle in minimizing radiation doses while maintaining diagnostic quality. Therefore, an awareness and implementation of best practices in radiation safety are essential in maximizing the benefits of these imaging modalities in gastroenterology. While the contributions of X-rays and fluoroscopy in gastroenterology are immense, the dangers of ionizing radiation should not be discounted. Long-term exposure can result in deterministic effects, for instance, skin damage and more profound stochastic effects, including increased lifetime cancer risk. As underlined by studies, knowledge and information on radiation protection strategies are critical both for patients and practitioners. The ever-evolving nature of technology calls for a constant re-evaluation and adjustment of current guidelines to reduce such risks. Coordination among health care professionals, e.g., gastroenterologists and medical physicists, ensures that radiation exposure is minimized while ensuring effectiveness in diagnostic imaging. As it continues to develop, future improvements of these techniques will strive to enhance imaging capacity at the behest of the safety and well-being of all concerned, in accordance with clinical performance and risk management principles (Figure 2.7).

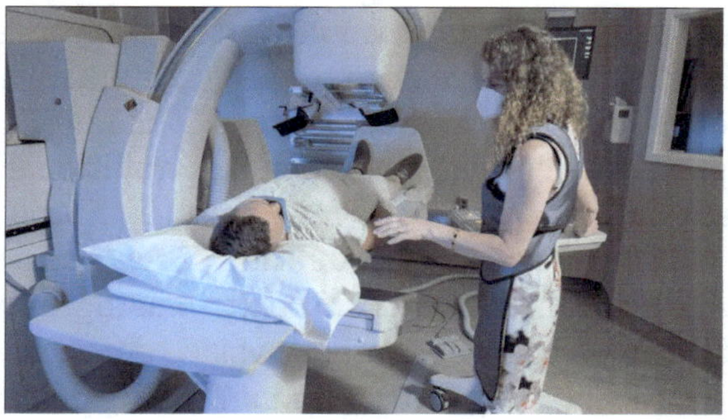

Figure 2.7. X-rays and fluoroscopy.

Source: https://www.gritman.org/wp-content/uploads/Advanced-Technology-Flouroscopy-Dominant.jpg.

2.2.2. Ultrasound in Gastroenterology

In the specialty of gastroenterology, ultrasound has emerged as an essential diagnostic tool in that it offers a non-invasive means of evaluating numerous gastrointestinal conditions. It employs high-frequency sound waves to produce real-time images of internal structures, allowing physicians to examine organs , such as the liver, gallbladder, pancreas, and kidneys. Compared to conventional imaging techniques, ultrasound is non-ionizing, which means it does not harm patients with ionizing radiation, and therefore, it is used for repeated monitoring, particularly in patient populations that need prolonged follow-up. The specificities and sensitivities of abdominal ultrasound have rendered it a valuable tool for the diagnosis of conditions like cholelithiasis, hepatic steatosis, and even hepatocellular carcinoma (HCC). Ultrasound's ability to give instant feedback can assist therapeutic intervention, highlighting the modality's potential as a cornerstone diagnostic tool in gastroenterology. The application of ultrasound extends to routine diagnostic imaging and more advanced techniques , such as elastography, which provides measurements of liver stiffness. This type of technique is significant in that it can quantify fibrosis, a common result of chronic liver disease. Measuring stiffness, elastography can be used to diagnose cirrhosis of the liver early, and physicians can identify patients who would be ideal candidates for surveillance or treatment. While liver biopsy has traditionally been the gold standard for assessing fibrosis, it is an invasive technique that poses risks of complications. In this context, elastography offers itself as a useful non-invasive alternative since the industry focuses on minimizing patient risk and discomfort while maintaining diagnostic quality. The ability to risk-stratify patients based on their fibrosis stage carries implications of profound importance to treatment planning and resource utilization. Additionally, the application of ultrasound to guide interventions further proves its significance in gastroenterology practice. Techniques , such as ultrasound-guided drainage and biopsy are just some examples of how ultrasound adds to procedural success with reduced risks involved. For instance, lesion localization for biopsy is greatly improved because the real-time imaging allows proper orientation, lessening the risk of complications , such as bleeding and infection. Furthermore, technical improvements in ultrasound, such as contrast-enhanced ultrasound, offer novel possibilities for liver mass characterization and discrimination between benign and malignant disease. These innovations not only increase diagnostic confidence but also facilitate the delivery of individualized treatment planning in the management of patients with complex gastrointestinal disease. Therefore, the addition of ultrasound to routine practice not only enriches the diagnostic arsenal but also emphasizes a patient-focused policy in the management of gastrointestinal disorders, reinforcing its pivotal role in modern gastroenterology (Figure 2.8).

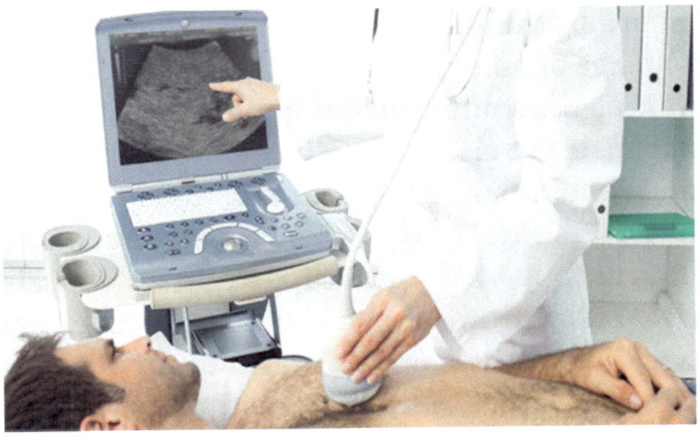

Figure 2.8. Ultrasound in gastroenterology.

Source: https://6ada39ab3e4e4dfd9962-0915b3b9e650afef6a84b370287eeb00.ssl.cf5.rackcdn.com/endoscopic-ultrasound-2-georgia.jpg.

2.2.3. MRI and CT Scans

The addition of MRI and CT scans to the diagnostic regimen for gastroenterology has revolutionized the evaluation of many gastrointestinal diseases. CT scan, with its rapidity in image acquisition and sensitivity to differences in tissue density, provides accurate cross-sectional images that are extremely valuable in the detection of tumor, abscess, or obstruction in the gut. Use of contrast also enhances delineation of vascular structures and potential lesions, useful for cancer staging or assessment of inflammatory conditions. Availability and relative speed of CT imaging also establish it as an instant diagnostic modality in acute settings where rapid decision-making is critical to patient outcomes. Therefore, it is critical for gastroenterologists to be aware of the advantages and disadvantages of CT imaging so that diagnostic accuracy and treatment planning in patients with complex gastrointestinal disorders can be maximized, particularly during colorectal cancer screening and staging (Vogel et al., 2021). Used less commonly than CT to diagnose the gastrointestinal tract, MRI possesses its own unique advantages that work well with the strengths of CT scans. One benefit of MRI is that it has the ability to provide better soft tissue contrast, which is particularly valuable for the elucidation of liver lesions, pancreatic neoplasms, and biliary system abnormalities. MRI does not use ionizing radiation like CT, and thus it is a beneficial choice for certain patient populations , such as those in whom repeat imaging studies are required over time. Apart from that, advanced-technology MRI techniques, including diffusion-weighted imaging and MR cholangiopancreatography (MRCP), have also enhanced the imaging and characterization of bile duct disease and focal liver lesions. With the growing relevance of MRI in gastrointestinal diagnostics, clinicians need to stay informed on the newest imaging technology and how it could be effectively used in combination with CT imaging (Benson et al., 2021).

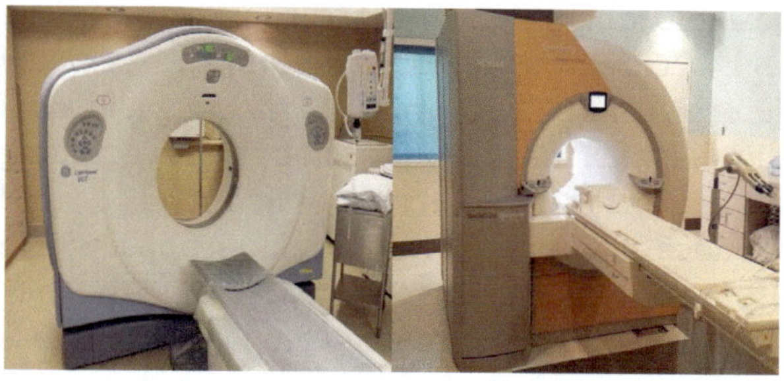

Figure 2.9. MRI and CT scans.

Source: https://i.pinimg.com/originals/8b/7e/2b/8b7e2b93840bdb1d0e4b631e360ec4fe.jpg.

In practice, the choice between MRI and CT scans would typically be based on the clinical question involved, the patient characteristics, and the need for emergent intervention. For instance, while CT scans become standard as part of the initial evaluation of acute abdominal pain or in suspected malignancies during staging, MRI might be preferred when patients have chronic liver disease or complex biliary disease assessment. Collaboration within an interdisciplinary team can enhance diagnostic precision by vast percentages; e.g., discussing imaging findings with radiologists optimizes interpretation and is integrated with patient history and lab results. With the gastroenterology profession embracing emerging advances in imaging technologies, continued assessment of MRI and CT scan appropriateness and effectiveness will play a critical role in offering excellent patient care as well as improving outcomes of gastrointestinal disease (Benson et al., 2021; Vogel et al., 2021) (Figure 2.9).

2.3. Biopsy Procedures

Biopsy tests form a core component of the diagnostic technology in gastroenterology, offering critical information regarding numerous gastrointestinal disorders. The principal role of a biopsy is to include a tissue sample for histological examination, which can either rule in or rule out conditions , such as cancer, inflammatory disease, and infection. There are various biopsy methods, including endoscopic biopsies, percutaneous biopsies, and surgical biopsies, each tailored for specific clinical conditions. Among them, endoscopic biopsy procedures are exceptional due to their minimality of invasiveness and precision of target acquisition, allowing clinicians to obtain tissue samples from the target locations immediately during procedures like endoscopies. This targeted approach is essential for accurate diagnosis, enabling interventions to be made in good time to significantly improve gastroenterological disease patient care. New technologies in imaging have revolutionized the procedural environment for biopsy, in terms of efficiency as well as accuracy of tissue sampling. Volumetric laser endomicroscopy (VLE) is such a development, enabling microscopic, real-time visualization of the gastrointestinal tract. In a multi-center registry trial, VLE had an unprecedented improvement in diagnostic yield for neoplasia by identifying areas of suspicion not visible on routine white light endoscopy in 59% of patients. Furthermore, VLE-guided tissue acquisition led to a staggering 700% improvement in neoplasia detection compared with random biopsy sampling. By integrating

VLE into biopsy protocols, healthcare providers can offer higher-quality samples and more well-informed decision-making processes, significant in the management of conditions like Barrett's esophagus and evaluating neoplastic potential (Smith et al., 2019).

In pediatric gastroenterology, biopsy procedures assume additional significance because of the complexities encountered in diagnosing liver disease in children. Chronic liver disease is usually underdiagnosed in children and must be identified with accurate diagnostic methods to avoid the development of advanced complications like cirrhosis and hepatocellular carcinoma. Biopsy is still a cornerstone in the diagnosis of liver diseases in children, allowing for histological investigations that guide treatment. Further, advances in diagnostic methods have opened ways to better comprehend liver pathogenesis, which can improve the management of the condition. As the awareness grows regarding the incidence of liver diseases among children, the role of biopsy procedures cannot be overstated; they play a crucial role in identifying early-stage diseases and preventing long-term health consequences (Della Corte et al., 2016) (Figure 2.10).

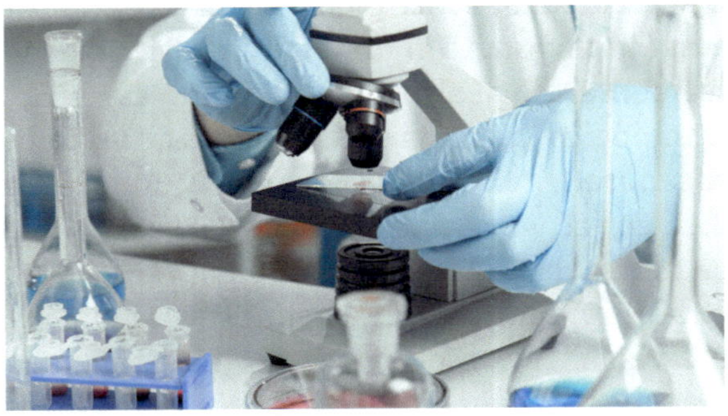

Figure 2.10. Biopsy procedures.

Source: https://www.sbmf.org/wp-content/uploads/2021/09/SBM_BiopsyProcedures-1080x600.png.

2.3.1. Types of Biopsies in Gastroenterology

In gastroenterology, there are also different types of biopsies utilized for obtaining tissue specimens for diagnostic purposes, each applicable to the respective clinical setting and target site within the GI tract. Endoscopic biopsies are one of the most common procedures, employing flexible scopes to directly examine and take tissue samples from most sites, such as the esophagus, stomach, and intestines. This technique is invaluable for the diagnosis of numerous conditions, such as inflammatory conditions and cancers, as it makes targeted biopsy of visually abnormal-appearing lesions possible during endoscopic examination. The high accuracy of endoscopic biopsies is a key determinant of their great diagnostic yield, as it allows clinicians to make assumptions regarding conditions like Barrett's esophagus and adenocarcinoma, thereby making appropriate therapeutic measures possible. Another fascinating gastroenterology biopsy technique is fine needle aspiration (FNA) which is frequently utilized to biopsy masses or suspicious liver, pancreatic, and lymph node lesions. FNA employs extremely fine needles to obtain cell material for cytological analysis, which provides the clinician with real-time information regarding the nature of a lesion. Its minimal invasive nature is a valuable advantage as it is usually feasible to perform it under ultrasound or CT control, with accuracy in sampling without requiring more extensive surgery. The procedure is of great utility in the assessment of pancreatic lesions, where early distinction between benign and malignant illness can significantly impact patient management. Thus, FNA is a valuable tool in the gastroenterologist's diagnostic toolbox, allowing for rapid and effective patient management. More advanced modalities, such as liquid biopsies, are gaining popularity in gastroenterology, primarily for surveillance in colorectal cancer. Liquid biopsies comprise an array of tests analyzing circulating tumor products, such as circulating tumor DNA (ctDNA), which have the potential to provide important biomarkers for cancer treatment. This surgery-free technique avoids some of the disadvantages with standard tissue biopsy sampling, making it available to patients who may already have had major surgeries in the past. The examination of these circulating biomarkers may inform clinicians about tumor dynamics, track responses to treatment, and detect recurrences more easily. The integration of liquid biopsies into standard practice is the evolving landscape of gastroenterology diagnosis, which shows the need for new strategies to maximize patient outcomes, especially in the management of colorectal cancer (Calborean et al., 2018). Furthermore, techniques like volumetric laser endomicroscopy (VLE) are revolutionizing biopsy acquisition in Barrett's esophagus, reflecting improvements to enable diagnostic yield and management planning (Smith et al., 2019).

2.3.2. Indications for Performing a Biopsy

The reason behind the biopsy in gastroenterology is the need for a definitive tissue diagnosis that will guide subsequent management. A biopsy is warranted where non-invasive imaging techniques suggest malignancy, significant pathology, or in the presence of persistent clinical signs despite conservative management. For example, patients with unexplained abdominal pain, weight loss, or gastrointestinal bleeding may qualify for endoscopic biopsies to identify underlying conditions , such as infection, inflammatory bowel disease, or malignancies. Biopsy results may be crucial in understanding histological features of the lesions and differentiating between malignant and benign processes and in planning treatment. Hence, biopsies are an essential component of the diagnostic process and play a major role in affecting outcomes clinically through early diagnosis and specific therapy. Some gastrointestinal conditions also need biopsies in their diagnostic evaluation. Conditions , such as esophagitis, gastritis, and peptic ulcer disease can be assessed with tissue biopsy to rule out malignancy or to test for underlying etiology. For instance, in premalignant conditions like Barrett's esophagus, associated with chronic gastroesophageal reflux disease, serial biopsies must be performed during routine follow-up for the appearance of dysplasia or carcinoma. The clinical practice guidelines are interested in the biopsy role in this context because not only does the histological acquisition help in diagnosis, but also in prognostication and risk stratification. Furthermore, inflammatory bowel disease (IBD) patients typically require biopsies to determine disease status and guide therapy, so that algorithms of treatment can be tailored to the patient (Tringali et al., 2017). Finally, biopsy use is recommended in specific cases with foreign body studies or unexplained gastrointestinal symptoms in children. In kids, for example, biopsies may be indicated to investigate the potential of eosinophilic esophagitis or manage corrosive ingestion complications, contributing to the significance of proper tissue examination. Endoscopic techniques enable doctors to obtain tissue samples from various sites in the gastrointestinal tract, including the esophagus, stomach, and colon, increasing the extent of diagnostic potential. Besides, as emphasized in recent literature, integration of biopsy findings into the broader clinical context enhances the clinician's ability to treat difficult gastrointestinal disorders, ultimately towards optimal patient care (Al-Haddad et al., 2014). All these points reflect the multifaceted role of biopsy in gastroenterology in keeping diagnostic practice robust and effective.

2.3.3. Interpretation of Biopsy Results

Biopsy results interpretation constitutes a pillar in the workup for diagnosis in gastroenterology, particularly in delineating conditions , such as coeliac disease and liver pathology. Diagnosis relies on histological examination, where tissue architecture and cellular defects are assessed. An example includes where there is a suspicion of coeliac disease, a duodenal biopsy has been termed the gold standard for the diagnosis of the condition. Diagnosis is often guided by the Marsh classification system, permitting pathologists to grade the extent of mucosal damage and guide subsequent clinical management. A recent study proved that patients with high tTG IgA levels could validate their diagnosis without resorting to invasive therapy, further fueling controversy about the necessity for standard biopsy protocols, lengthening the time before patients start dietetic modifications that are the basis of recovery (Ranjan et al., 2019). In addition to coeliac disease, liver biopsy findings create special challenges and opportunities in gastroenterology. Liver biopsy plays a crucial role in the evaluation of hepatitis to cirrhosis; however, the complexity of hepatic histology necessitates rigorous analysis. Research into mechanisms underlying liver stiffness by both transient elastography and magnetic resonance elastography has confirmed that tissue elasticity is linearly related to the progression of fibrosis. These advanced imaging devices have been shown to correlate with biopsy findings, enhancing diagnostic accuracy and prediction. By quantification of liver stiffness, such methods essentially replace the invasive biopsy procedure in the majority of patients, particularly chronic liver disease patients. As the application of biopsy continues to advance, there is still a need for proper interpretation, which remains valid for the successful management of patients (Talwalkar, 2008). Moreover, the interpretation of biopsy results highlights the requirement for interprofessional collaboration between radiologists, gastroenterologists, and pathologists. The course of gastrointestinal disorders requires an interdepartmental strategy, wherein every specialty contributes its expertise towards the diagnosis and treatment of the patients to achieve a precise diagnosis and optimal patient care. Pathologists must communicate effectively with clinicians, who must incorporate these results into a general appreciation of the state of the patient, often refining provisional diagnoses with consensus wisdom. With improved diagnostic gastroenterology technology, more emphasis will be placed on accurate biopsy interpretation, augmented by new imaging modalities, to further enhance clinical outcomes. This multidisciplinary collaboration reinforces the role of pathology as it continues patient care and assures its role as a fundamental building block in diagnosing and treating gastrointestinal disease (Talwalkar, 2008).

2.4. Laboratory Tests

The role of laboratory testing in gastroenterology lies at the heart of accurate diagnosis and management of gastrointestinal disease. The application of biomarkers in inflammatory bowel diseases (IBD), such as ulcerative colitis (UC), has been a significant focus area. Traditional assessments are extremely reliant on clinical features, which may poorly reflect disease activity. In an effort to circumvent such a limitation, contemporary research is untangling novel biomarkers, and circulating microRNAs are in competition as the top candidates. Various profiles of these microRNAs have been discovered in research, not only separating UC patients from controls, but also with significant correlation with disease activity, thus providing clinicians with important information not provided by traditional markers (e.g., C-reactive protein) (Touroutoglou et al., 2015). Such innovation in the science of biomarker discovery would advance patient screening and disease management, further entrenching the position of laboratory testing in clinical gastroenterology. Aside from new biomarkers, genetic testing is now a precious tool in gastrointestinal diagnostics. With the vast increase in knowledge of genetically important variants, high-throughput diagnostic approaches have been able to offer extended genetic profiles to patients. The diagnostics make it possible to monitor for many mutations as for thousands at once and thereby allow personalized therapy. Pharmacogenomics, or the application of drug therapy tailored to the individual's genetic makeup, has emerged as a valuable means for gastroenterological use of genetic testing (Wiita & Schrijver, 2011).

The capabilities not only enhance diagnostic performance but also allow for more individualized treatment protocols, leading to enhanced patient outcomes. However, complexity in translating genetic variants to clinical interpretation proves difficult for the incorporation of these tests into daily clinical practice, and thus, it is necessary for healthcare professionals to remain well-informed about developments in diagnostic technology. Incorporation of laboratory testing into gastroenterological practices remains a vital element in enhancing patient care and outcomes. With advancements in processes, healthcare professionals increasingly employ laboratory diagnostics in guiding clinical decision-making. For instance, employing high-throughput genetic testing and screening of novel biomarkers will transform the diagnosis and therapy of gastrointestinal disease. However, the efficacy of such tests hinges upon strict clinical validation and clinical interpretation of test results, particularly for complex diseases like IBD. The ongoing collaboration between clinicians and researchers is necessary not only to refine such laboratory studies but also to establish good guidelines for their application in patient management. With new technology being developed, it is critical that the gastroenterology community be adaptable to ensure that laboratory studies continue to fine-tune diagnostic accuracy and improve patient care (Figure 2.11).

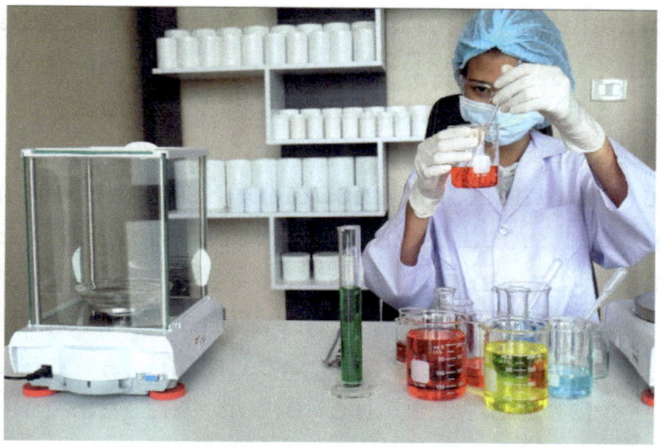

Figure 2.11. Laboratory tests.

Source: https://www.healthc.in/image/catalog/Home-Lab-Test1.jpg.

2.4.1. Blood Tests for Gastrointestinal Disorders

Blood testing is also key to the diagnosis and management of gastrointestinal disorders, offering a minimally invasive method of obtaining valuable information about a patient's health. Blood testing may measure the amount of various biomarkers, for instance, liver enzymes, complete blood counts, and inflammatory markers, which, respectively, may indicate the presence of underlying conditions like liver disease, infection, or inflammatory bowel disease. By monitoring levels of liver-specific enzymes, physicians can ascertain the liver's function and detect potential disorders , such as hepatitis or cirrhosis. Also, elevated inflammatory markers can be used among the initial testing of Crohn's disease or ulcerative colitis, allowing prompt intervention to take place. Collectively, these blood markers are important markers that guide further imaging studies and therapeutic measures specific to the patient's unique gastrointestinal pathology. Among the myriad of gastrointestinal diseases, some blood tests have shown exceptional promise for managing more virulent diseases , such as gastric cancer and hepatocellular carcinoma (HCC). For gastric cancer, biomarker testing is now routine, particularly in the assessment of HER2 status, microsatellite instability, and PD-L1 expression, which can assist in selecting candidates for agents , such as trastuzumab and nivolumab. Incorporation into the oncologic model of gastrointestinal illness of blood tests is in progress, with these biomarkers not merely serving a diagnostic purpose but also as predictors of clinical results and response to treatment. As gastric adenocarcinomas are often diagnosed at advanced stages of disease, explanation of such molecular characteristics by blood testing is critical in order to optimize patient management options and potentially modify survival (Ajani et al., 2022). Hepatocellular carcinoma is also representative of the significance of blood tests in gastrointestinal disease. The cancer is especially prevalent in the Asia-Pacific region, and this represents a serious public health emergency.

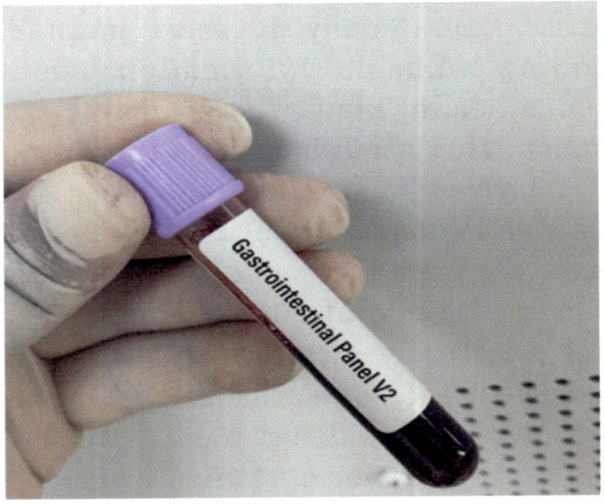

Figure 2.12. Blood tests for gastrointestinal disorders.

Source: https://media.istockphoto.com/id/1421511175/photo/blood-sample-for-gastrointestinal-panel-v2-pcr-test-to-diagnosis-of-gastrointestinal-disorder.jpg?s=170667a&w=0&k=20&c=gBH7ApPwnZefxI_UkiViXac4R2tKxqrdV8ShpnIZDVo=.

The application of blood biomarkers , such as alpha-fetoprotein (AFP), assists in the early diagnosis and monitoring of the disease because raised levels are evidence of the presence of a tumor. Furthermore, the priority set by organizations like the Asia-Pacific Association for the Study of the Liver in new guidelines supports the use of evidence-based treatment universally, with particular emphasis placed on blood testing within comprehensive management regimens. A multi-dimensional approach involving both laboratory markers and clinical assessment is aimed at the multi-dimensional nature of HCC to ensure improved results through timely intervention (Omata et al., 2017) (Figure 2.12).

2.4.2. Stool Tests and Their Significance

Stool testing has emerged as a key gastroenterology diagnostic tool, particularly in diagnosing and monitoring of inflammatory bowel disease (IBD). Stool testing provides valuable information regarding intestinal inflammation by measuring fecal biomarkers. For instance, fecal calprotectin (FC) is a perfect non-invasive mucosal healing and disease activity marker. There have been studies that have proven increased FC levels to be linked to enhanced endoscopic activity of disease in patients with conditions , such as Crohn's disease and ulcerative colitis, hence being an integral component of monitoring strategies clinically. As more gastroenterologists embrace evidence-based practice, integration of stool tests into diagnostic pathways allows for timely therapeutic optimization and improves patient outcomes (Wilkens et al., 2022). The function of stool tests is not merely to detect inflammation; they have a significant role in the management of IBD through ongoing monitoring of disease activity. They are crucial for effective strategies for remission achievement and maintenance and the avoidance of disease exacerbation. In the clinical setting, regular measurement of FC levels allows practitioners to predict future relapses and change treatment regimens. Moreover, new telemedicine models have made stool testing more convenient. Home-testing kits can be used by patients to measure FC, enabling them to become proactively engaged in the management of their disease. This model not only empowers the patients but also reduces the healthcare burden on resources as the monitoring process is made easier (Gaebler et al., 2021). Tests on the stool other than fecal calprotectin may give microbiome composition information, an emerging area in gastroenterology. Gut microbiota plays a critical role in immunity and inflammation, and influences the IBD course. Fecal sampling will be used to diagnose dysbiosis and guide decisions regarding the use of probiotics or dietary manipulation. As research continues to enlighten us regarding the gut microbiota-GI health relationship, stool tests can be at the center of developing individualized treatment options. Lastly, the integration of these tests in diagnostic systems enhances the efficiency of IBD management through enhanced personalized care to patients and further understanding of gastrointestinal diseases (Wilkens et al., 2022) (Figure 2.13).

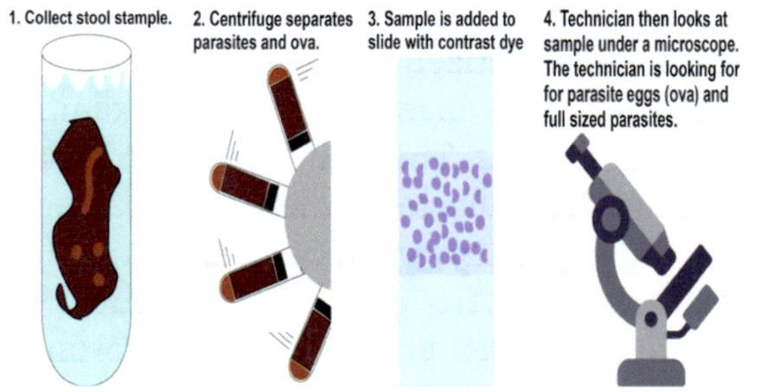

Figure 2.13. Stool tests and their significance.

Source: https://www.parasites.org/images/ova-parasite-stool-test-large-1024x537.png.

2.4.3. Breath Tests for Specific Conditions

Breath testing has emerged as a prominent diagnostic tool in the field of gastroenterology, particularly for diagnosing conditions , such as small intestinal bacterial overgrowth (SIBO) and carbohydrate malabsorption. As they are non-invasive, the tests are advantageous to both patients and physicians as a less invasive procedure than endoscopy or jejunal fluid aspiration. Breath tests typically involve quantification of specific gases in expired breath, such as hydrogen or methane, that are produced as a side reaction of microbial fermentation in the gut. As increasing research is conducted, the significance of the correlation between breath test results and functional gastrointestinal disorders becomes increasingly relevant, particularly in patients presenting with symptoms , such as bloating, diarrhea, or abdominal pain. Importantly, their standardization and elaboration have rendered these tests clinically more useful in the assessment of conditions that are often characterized by cumulative symptoms and by amenability to diagnosis. The application of breath tests in gastroenterology is radically influenced by the recognition of microbial dysbiosis as an extremely significant aspect of many gastrointestinal conditions. For instance, disturbances in the intestinal microbiota have been identified to be associated with diseases like irritable bowel syndrome (IBS) and functional dyspepsia (FD), highlighting accurate diagnosis of these diseases through proper testing. Emerging evidence verifies that SIBO, which is defined by inappropriate bacterial loads within the small intestine, may cause or be caused by symptoms in patients presenting with functional gastrointestinal disorders. Hence, breath tests, with the potential to provide information on the presence of SIBO, play a crucial role in guiding treatment and patient management. Though their value is recognized, the tests are not without limitations regarding sensitivity and specificity, making continued refinement and validation in clinical application warranted, as emphasized by recent clinical guidelines (Tornkvist et al., 2022). Furthermore, the evolving approach to breath testing reflects the ongoing necessity to familiarize and utilize a series of diagnostic techniques within the overall background of gastroenterological practice. As much as traditional means of SIBO diagnosis, such as jejunal fluid culture, have been determined to be non-feasible for routine use due to their invasive and complicating nature, breath tests are an obvious substitute. Despite this, however, controversy continues to surround their diagnostic accuracy and effectiveness and therefore their use is problematic (Shah et al., 2022). Next-generation sequencing and molecular methods have brought with them promising solutions for further refining SIBO diagnostics and analyzing gut microbiome dysbiosis in more depth. Last but not least, as research continues to explore the link between breath analysis and digestive health, these methods can provide critical data to enhance diagnostics and maximize treatment potential within gastroenterology (Figure 2.14).

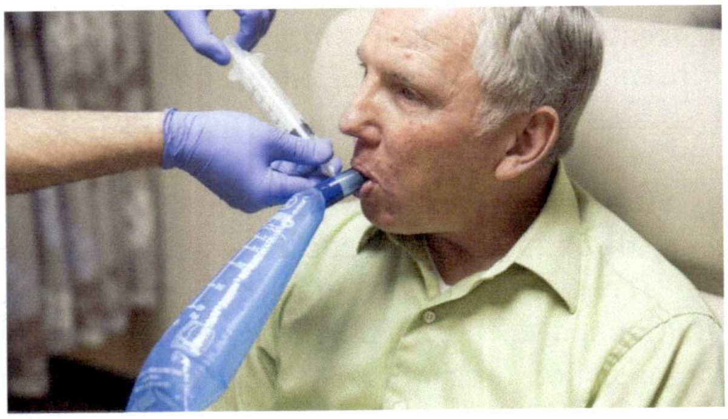

Figure 2.14. Breath tests for specific conditions.

Source: https://www.uofmhealth.org/sites/default/files/styles/full_size_image/public/HydrogenBreathTestImage-crop.jpg?itok=-F7OC-vb.

2.5. Functional Testing

Functional testing is a central function in gastroenterology that offers information not usually found by traditional means of diagnosis. Functional testing assesses the physiological and biochemical activity of the gastrointestinal (GI) tract, enabling medical professionals to identify underlying problems that may be causing symptoms or disease. In diseases , such as cholangiocarcinoma, in which it occurs in a heterogeneous and asymptomatic manner, the functional tests, in addition to detecting abnormalities, also offer a more elaborate understanding of the pathological processes underway. As the incidence of biliary cancers grows, the enhancement of functional testing becomes increasingly vital in ensuring the validity of diagnosis and patient prognosis, particularly in response to the failure of non-invasive approaches to effectively diagnose such aggressive types of the disease (Bañales et al., 2020). Furthermore, enhanced incorporation of deep learning algorithms in functional testing platforms is forthcoming as a vital part of modern gastroenterology diagnostics. By the use of convolutional neural networks (CNNs), researchers have been exploring how such new technologies can detect hidden patterns from diagnostic imaging that might result in earlier and more precise diagnosis of gastrointestinal illnesses. Functional tests have always relied on interpretation by the clinician, but with AI now entering the scene, not only does access become democratized to expert-level analysis, but the inherent biases in human examiners are also mitigated. This shift reflects a broader trend in gastroenterology where the intersection of technology and functional testing achieves optimal diagnostic performance such that clinicians are presented with the best information to manage their patients (Nagendran et al., 2020). The future of functional testing also emphasizes the need for ongoing research into its effectiveness and application in clinical use. With growing consciousness of the truth that artificial intelligence has revolutionary promise, but realizing these benefits are subject to rigorous scrutiny through potential research and rigorous compliance with reporting standards, the implications of these novel diagnostic techniques are in their acceptance among physicians and therefore necessitate broad investigations to establish their clinical utility in real-world clinical practice. The gastroenterology landscape continues to evolve, and with it, the necessity to refine functional testing protocols that enhance diagnostic accuracy and eventually contribute to improved patient outcomes is an intrinsic part of ongoing research and clinical practice (Bañales et al., 2020; Nagendran et al., 2020) (Figure 2.15).

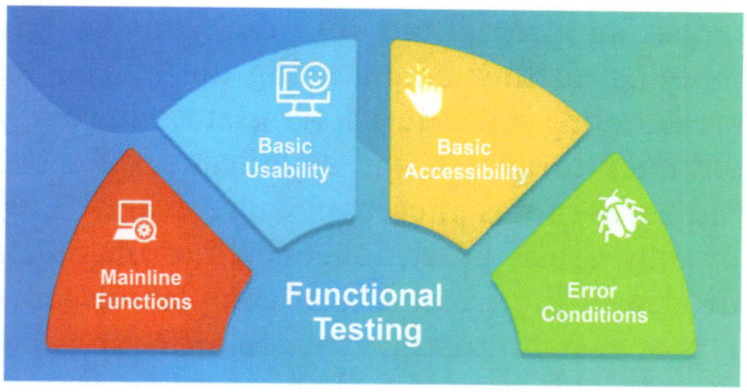

Figure 2.15. Functional testing.

Source: https://www.qatouch.com/wp-content/uploads/2019/12/Functional-Testing.jpg.

2.5.1. Esophageal Motility Studies

Esophageal motility testing and, in particular, esophageal manometry have emerged as central gastroenterologic diagnostic technologies utilized mainly to assess disorders , such as achalasia and pseudoachalasia. The tests apply various mechanisms to measure the pressures and profiles of muscle contractions within the esophagus and thereby acquire information regarding the intricate esophageal motility mechanisms. High-resolution manometry (HRM) has come a great distance in propagating the science, making it possible to undergo minute scrutiny of esophageal pressure topography (EPT). This technique not only enhances sensitivity for the diagnosis of motility disorders but also permits subtyping of achalasia. Correct identification of these conditions is significant since they present differently clinically and are managed differently. Finally, utilization of esophageal motility studies is pivotal in making a correct diagnosis and optimal management planning in patients with esophageal dysmotility and dysphagia and thus signifies their key role in modern gastroenterological practice. Recent literature has highlighted the potential for complications of laparoscopic adjustable gastric banding (LAGB), including esophageal motility disorders. Khan et al. present a case of the development of pseudoachalasia in patients who have undergone LAGB, as indicated by symptoms , such as dysphagia and regurgitation. Esophageal manometry revealed absent peristalsis in the patients, leading to a diagnosis similar to achalasia with major implications for patient treatment. The proper assessment with esophageal motility tests in such a case is critical in differentiating primary and secondary achalasia, particularly when the obstruction location is not the lower esophageal sphincter. The differentiation can play an important role in treatment, and can lead to band deflation or removal, and thus the need for gastroenterologists to remain vigilant regarding esophageal motility during bariatric surgery, as the findings of this study indicated (Roman & Kahrilas, 2011). Within the overall framework of functional gastrointestinal disorders (FGIDs), esophageal motility tests have become significant since they can aid in delineating underlying pathophysiological mechanisms. Dilation of conceptual models now positions FGIDs within a biopsychosocial model so that a broadened view of symptoms like dysphagia can be comprehended. Such a paradigm shift fosters an awareness of disturbances of motility as true disorders, making symptoms usually overlooked in standard gastroenterological practice more valid. Furthermore, advances in investigational modalities, including high-tech motility evaluation and imaging, have stimulated interest in FGIDs. Therefore, Rome Committees established diagnostic criteria that call for adequate motility studies. The integration of esophageal motility tests' results into the practice of medicine eventually makes a more comprehensive strategy for managing

FGIDs possible, verifying the importance of such diagnostic procedures in current gastroenterology (Sheth, 2007).

2.5.2. Gastric Emptying Studies

Gastric emptying tests are of utmost relevance in the diagnosis of a variety of gastrointestinal syndromes. Tests are particularly valuable in the assessment of patients presenting with symptoms of early satiation, nausea, and bloating after meals, suggesting gastroparesis or delayed gastric emptying. The gastric scintigraphy, being the most commonly utilized test in this respect, is a long-standing and reliable technique that allows the clinician to quantitatively determine the rate of gastric emptying. During this procedure, a patient ingests a radiolabeled meal, and subsequent imaging captures the progress of the gastric contents along the gastrointestinal tract. Although gastric scintigraphy is highly informative, its utility could be affected by several factors, including patient compliance and the homogeneity of the composition of the meal, which may not precisely reflect physiological states under usual modes of eating. Although gastric scintigraphy is still a leading technique used to assess gastric emptying, other modalities have also been developed to improve the accuracy of diagnosis. The advent of breath testing has provided a non-invasive approach that has the potential to simplify the diagnostic process. They examine breath samples after meal ingestion for certain metabolites that serve as indicators of digestion efficiency. However, breath testing is still criticized for its specificity and sensitivity relative to scintigraphy, especially in the accurate detection of gastroesophageal reflux symptoms. Gastric emptying tests should also often be supplemented with other diagnostic modalities for a broader evaluation. For instance, incorporation of gastric emptying assessment with esophageal pH monitoring provides a broader overview of gastrointestinal motility and reflux pathophysiology, which ultimately guides individualized treatment planning for diseases like GERD. The relevance of gastric emptying tests is more than just their value in terms of diagnosis; they also provide significant therapeutic decision-making information. For example, in gastroesophageal reflux disease (GERD), the rate of gastric emptying will influence treatment strategies like dietary modification or surgery. Procedures like transoral incisionless fundoplication (TIF) can be provided to those patients whose symptoms result from mechanical issues supplemented by delayed gastric emptying, further emphasizing the efficacy of correct study procedures. As gastroenterology continues to evolve, the significance of these studies becomes increasingly relevant. They not only assist practitioners in the diagnosis but also in the treatment of complex diseases of the gastrointestinal tract, affirming the indispensable role of gastric emptying studies in the overall field of diagnostic procedures in gastroenterology (Dranove, 2008; Fanous et al., 2018) (Figure 2.16).

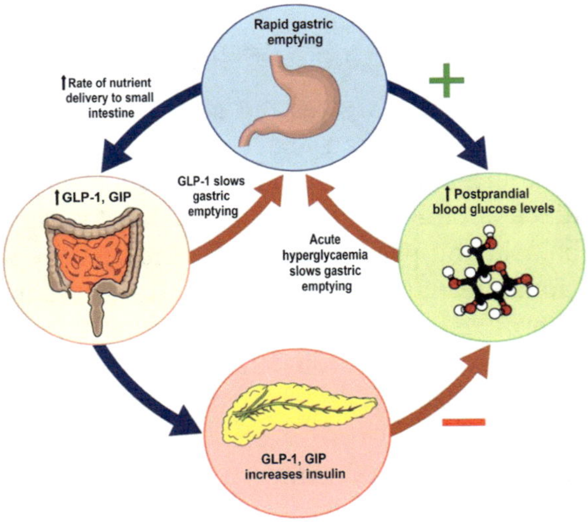

Figure 2.16. Gastric emptying studies.

Source: https://www.researchgate.net/publication/364152758/figure/fig3/AS:11431281094258746@1667443747888/Schema-of-the-interdependent-relationships-of-gastric-emptying-incretin-hormones-and.png.

2.5.3. pH Monitoring for Acid Reflux

Of the several methods applied in the diagnosis of GERD, pH monitoring is significant among them. The method records intra-esophageal pH over time, usually a 24-hour period, to identify acid reflux events. This test, at times supplemented with impedance monitoring, provides a good means of learning about the nature of the reflux, the frequency, and the duration of acid exposure in the esophagus. The continuous character of the monitoring allows clinicians to superimpose symptoms upon reflux events and yield useful information about the success of therapeutic interventions. Literature is in support of an appreciable decrease in the frequency of reflux episodes when utilizing structured feeding methods in certain patient groups, such as preterm infants, and illustrates the applicability of the methods in clinical decision-making (Martini et al., 2024). In addition, the integration of pH monitoring with high-resolution manometry and other modalities enhances diagnostic accuracy in patients with suspected GERD. While pH monitoring measures acid exposure directly, the use of other methods allows a broader assessment of esophageal motility and structural disease. A landmark study contrasting the Functional Luminal Imaging Probe (FLIP) with existing techniques supports the need for using multiple assessments while determining a diagnosis of an esophageal disorder with precision. Although FLIP yields beneficial information about esophageal function, FLIP correlation with pH monitoring is poor and is therefore still a foundation for the diagnosis of reflux-associated conditions (Miller et al., 2024). The use of pH monitoring transcends uncomplicated diagnosis; it is a basic instrument in therapeutic modalities. With its status as an objective measure of the presence and intensity of acid reflux, the technique allows for focused therapeutic intervention, e.g., diet modification or pharmacotherapy. In children, for instance, research has indicated that the use of continuous feeding methods is able to reduce instances of acid reflux, indicating an applied role of pH monitoring data to guide feeding protocols (Martini et al., 2024). As such, the utility of pH monitoring is not just to diagnose GERD, but to influence treatment modalities suited to the specific needs of the patient. This multi-modal approach reflects the face of gastroenterological diagnosis changing, highlighting the role of integrated assessment to improve patient care.

2.6. Emerging Diagnostic Technologies

The development of gastroenterological diagnostic technologies has also played a central role in enhancing patient treatment and management. The traditional diagnostic methods rely on clinical symptoms and standard biomarkers that do not accurately represent the actual disease state. Therefore, it is needed to find valid and new biomarkers to enhance the screening and therapy of diseases , such as IBD. Recent research indicates the potential of circulating microRNAs as novel diagnostic markers, capable of differentiating between active patients with ulcerative colitis and controls or patients in remission. The promise of a given signature of twelve circulating microRNAs, numerous which have high correlation with disease activity, is an indication of the prospective role these biomarkers can play in the clinical setting, being more sensitive and specific than other traditional diagnostic methods , such as C-reactive protein levels (Touroutoglou et al., 2015). The implementation of new technologies in the gastroenterological diagnostic sector is also expressed in the evolving techniques of endoscopy. New methods, including chromoendoscopy and magnifying endoscopy, have greatly improved the visualization of small neoplastic lesions, which is crucial for successful colorectal cancer screening programs. These new methods improve the examination of the gastrointestinal tract, enhancing the accuracy of diagnoses and reducing the risk of missed lesions. Further, simulator-based training programs have been introduced to enhance the skills of doctors in colonoscopy so that they can deal with complicated cases effectively. The transformation of endoscopic practice, typified by state-of-the-art methodology and enhanced training, is a testament to the necessity for an ongoing transformation in the direction of better patient outcomes (Arebi et al., 2005). Besides endoscopic and laboratory advances, the use of new technologies in the diagnosis of the gastrointestinal tract is also being introduced to non-invasive techniques, providing patients with safer alternatives.

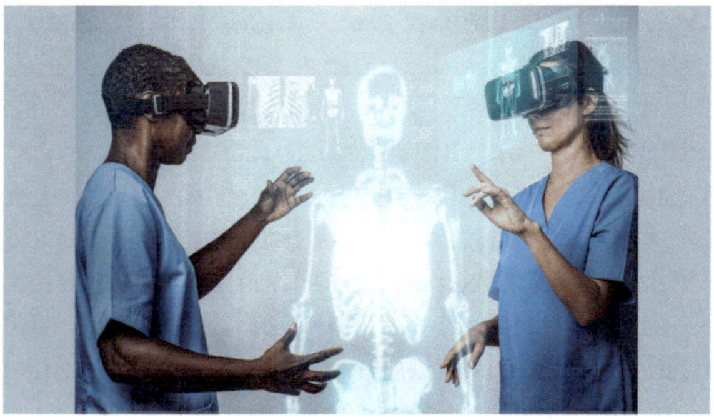

Figure 2.17. Emerging diagnostic technologies.

Source: https://innohealthmagazine.com/wp-content/uploads/2023/08/Ai-driven-medical-diagnostics-%E2%80%93-The-new-reality-1.png.

Capsule endoscopy, for instance, has revolutionized the diagnosis of small bowel disease with complete visualization without the interference of invasive procedures. Not only does the technology enhance the comfort of the patient, but it also improves compliance with screening regimens. In addition, the creation of advanced therapeutic devices, like those combined with double balloon enteroscopy, has increased the therapeutic flexibility for patients suffering from complicated gastrointestinal disorders. While these novel diagnostic technologies are being increasingly applied, they may potentially revolutionize gastroenterological practices in the long run, culminating in better management of patients as well as improved patient outcomes across different gastrointestinal conditions (Figure 2.17).

2.6.1. Capsule Endoscopy

In gastroenterology, capsule endoscopy is a revolutionary diagnostic modality that has forever altered the face of gastrointestinal evaluation. It is a minimally invasive procedure where a very small, swallowable capsule that contains cameras takes high-quality pictures of the entire gastrointestinal tract, including areas that cannot be reached via standard endoscopic access. The capability of the technology to provide a comprehensive view of the small intestine, where conventional endoscopy may be time-consuming, has drastically improved the diagnostic capability of doctors. Physicians are ever more reliant on capsule endoscopy to evaluate conditions like small bowel bleeding, inflammatory bowel disease, and cancers, thereby helping make timely and accurate diagnoses that have the potential to make a critical difference in patient outcomes. Whereas having several advantages, capsule endoscopy also has its disadvantages. One of its most dominant shortcomings is the difficulty of precisely locating the capsule inside the delicately three-dimensional (3D) gastrointestinal tract. Real-time tracking properly is critical in building a clear 3D map of internal organs, which can lead clinicians to more intuitive diagnoses. State-of-the-art advancements, such as the development of robotic active capsule endoscopes, are aimed at addressing these challenges with innovative technologies like visual simultaneous localization and mapping (SLAM). The new technology applies RGB-Depth SLAM methods to develop globally consistent dense maps in real-time, thereby facilitating more complex navigation and visualization of the GI anatomy. These advances have a high promise of enhancing the clinical usefulness of capsule endoscopy for both patient comfort and safety as well as for diagnostic precision (Almalioglu et al., 2017). Progress in capsule endoscopy predicts a fascinating future for gastroenterology's diagnostic tool of choice. With ongoing technological advancement, the use of capsule endoscopy in combination with artificial intelligence (AI) and machine learning can also change the imaging examination, with automatic detection of abnormalities and ease of diagnosis. In addition, advancements in capsules themselves, including possibly live video and advanced imaging modalities, can broaden even further the diseases that could be diagnosed effectively. Lastly, these breakthroughs highlight the necessity for continuous research and development in this promising area. The use of these advanced diagnostic modalities holds the potential to make a profound impact on patient care and is a step in support of the assertion that gastroenterology's future is more reliant on sophisticated, non-invasive technologies like capsule endoscopy (Ho et al., 2011).

2.6.2. Artificial Intelligence in Diagnostics

The use of artificial intelligence (AI) in gastroenterology diagnostic procedures is a significant advancement in medical processes. Machine learning algorithms and deep learning models are employed by AI to enhance the accuracy and timeliness of various diagnostic procedures, such as endoscopy and imaging tests. For example, AI systems have been used to aid in colonoscopy procedures to increase adenoma detection rates, which play critical roles in detecting early colorectal cancer. With advancing technology, its applications in both malignant and benign lesion identification have led to increased reliable diagnostic results. Additionally, AI's capability to process enormous amounts of data allows for an increased understanding of patient conditions, which ultimately translates into better patient management practices in gastroenterology, as seen in the case of biliopancreatic disorders (Robles-Medranda et al., 2025). The value of AI use in diagnosis extends beyond simple identification; it also plays a significant role in enhancing prognostic assessment and treatment planning in gastrointestinal diseases. AI has been particularly helpful in pancreatic lesion characterization, a factor that contributes to the early diagnosis and treatment of pancreatic cancer. Advanced imaging tools, including computed tomography and magnetic resonance imaging, utilize AI to sift through scans with high precision, identifying features too faint for human vision. By assisting doctors with deciding whether a tumor can be resected and guiding treatment plans tailored to the patient, AI has the potential to transform outcomes in gastroenterology. Besides, the AI method synthesizes natural language processing and deep learning to process clinical data and deliver a combined model of patient diagnosis and care (Sridhar et al., 2024). The inclusion of AI in routine diagnostic practice has many benefits, yet some challenges must be surmounted to apply it optimally in gastroenterology. Consistency in the performance of AI programs in multiple clinical settings mandates rigorous validation to yield uniform results. Second, ethical issues arise, particularly concerning data privacy and algorithmic bias. These must be tackled very carefully as clinicians and researchers try to strike a balance between leading-edge technological innovation and regulation. As the field aims to further standardize AI's capability with clinical evidence, highlighting training healthcare providers in the design of these tools will become of utmost importance. Encouraging multidisciplinary practice will aid in maximizing AI's potential for diagnostics as a strong collaborator in gastroenterological disorders management (Robles-Medranda et al., 2025) (Figure 2.18).

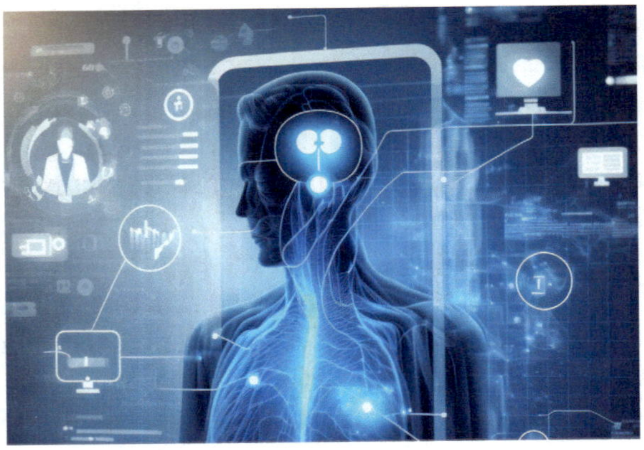

Figure 2.18. Artificial intelligence in diagnostics.

Source: https://static.scientificamerican.com/sciam/cache/file/01C9741F-6F6D-4882-8217D92370325AA7_*source.jpg*.

2.6.3. Genetic Testing in Gastroenterology

Gastroenterology has discovered genetic testing to be a significant diagnostic means for the field, particularly for inherited gastrointestinal disease. Genetic testing makes possible the identification of mutations for diseases , such as colorectal cancer syndromes, familial adenomatous polyposis, and Lynch syndrome. The genetic tests provide significant information that informs surveillance guidelines as well as treatment. For instance, individuals with a proven genetic predisposition to colorectal cancer can be assisted by more vigorous and earlier investigation, which could lower their chance of progression to advanced disease by quite a margin. The active approach expresses the paradigm-breaking potential of genetic testing for the management of inherited conditions, in that it rearranges the paradigm from cure to prevention, with early detection being the focus in order to optimize patient benefit. Moreover, genetic testing yields insights into pharmacogenomics that can refine treatment modalities for patients with gastrointestinal disease. By examining a specific genetic marker, doctors can better predict an individual's response to drugs and tailor treatments to a patient's unique genetic makeup. This is particularly applicable in diseases , such as inflammatory bowel disease (IBD), where a number of biological therapies are available. Genotyping may help clinicians select the best therapy, thereby increasing efficacy and minimizing side effects. As pharmacogenomic testing becomes more integrated into clinical practice, the tailored approach mirrors the evolving interface of genetic testing in gastroenterology, foreshadowing safer and more effective therapy protocols that are tailored to individual patient needs. Despite its numerous benefits, the application of genetic testing to gastroenterology faces with challenges that need to be addressed. Ethical considerations involving genetic privacy, discrimination, and the psychological impact of testing outcomes become critical concerns that will not be ignored. Some other concerns are ongoing disparities in access to genetic testing and counseling services, particularly among marginalized populations. Such barriers highlight the necessity for widespread education and policy reform to ensure equal access to genetic testing in gastroenterology. As information regarding genetic risk factors in gastrointestinal disease further develops, impending research and education will be imperative for addressing these challenges. The expanding science of genetic testing thus promises and incurs responsibility in gastroenterology and will necessitate judicious wayfinding to ensure that its maximum benefits accrue to all.

SUMMARY

In short, the technological evolution in gastroenterological diagnosis heralds a revolutionary time for the specialty, enhancing clinicians' capacity to diagnose and treat many gastrointestinal diseases. As argued in the course of this essay, techniques , such as endoscopic imaging, breath tests, and artificial intelligence platforms, including ChatGPT-4 -4 yield robust solutions to traditional diagnostic challenges. Specifically, the use of artificial intelligence in image interpretation can revolutionize diagnosis, but so far is only demonstrating variable success rates for different investigations, needing to be honed before being of utility in clinical practice (Saraiva et al., 2025). It highlights the fact that further research needs to be undertaken to optimize these new technologies so that they are able to augment existing methods effectively. Moreover, the diagnostic difficulty inherent in conditions like small intestinal bacterial overgrowth (SIBO) necessitates well-determined guidelines and standardized gastroenterology procedures. The overlap of signs and symptoms between SIBO, irritable bowel syndrome (IBS), and inflammatory bowel disease (IBD) complicates accurate diagnosis, thus the necessity for uniform non-invasive tests like lactulose and glucose breath tests. While these tests are the essence of SIBO diagnosis, their shortcomings certify the imperative to create more effective methodologies for the minimization of false positives and negatives (da Silva et al., 2025). It is imperative to standardize diagnostic procedures in order to enhance patient care, particularly in heterogeneous healthcare systems that could be subject to unusual diagnostic delays. In the end, the conclusion drawn about diagnostic practices in gastroenterology underscores an actual need for innovation combined with tried-and-true procedures. As ongoing studies into new treatment practices continue to look for other options, medical professionals must be watchful in their approach to integrating new technology with long-standing procedures. The road to optimal diagnostic utility in gastroenterology goes on, with emerging innovations that will more closely direct and sharpen clinical practice. This not only enhances outcomes for patients but also helps eliminate unequal access to care and quality, where all patients receive accurate and timely diagnoses that meet contemporary medical standards.

In gastroenterology, various diagnostic techniques are applied for the evaluation and treatment of gastrointestinal illness effectively. Colonoscopy is one of the most important procedures for the identification and removal of colorectal lesions. By using this technique, the colonic mucosa is visualized directly, whereby polyps and malignant lesions can be detected. The effectiveness of colonoscopy is substantiated by research findings that demonstrate considerable reductions in incidence and mortality from colorectal cancer when adenomatous polyps are eradicated as part of screening examinations. Specifically, the National Polyp Study proved that polypectomy is associated with up to a 50% decrease in mortality from colorectal cancer compared to population controls, and has solidified colonoscopy as the gold standard of prevention of colorectal cancer (Kaltenbach et al., 2020). In addition, advances in imaging technology have expanded the armamentarium of diagnostic modalities within gastroenterology. Techniques , such as endoscopic mucosal resection (EMR) and narrow-band imaging (NBI) improve polyp characterization and removal accuracy. EMR is particularly valuable for larger, non-pedunculated lesions because it allows removal of such lesions with the potential for complete histological examination. NBI, meanwhile, employs narrow-band light to maximize the visual identification of vascular patterns and mucosal surface characteristics, allowing endoscopists to identify neoplastic versus non-neoplastic lesions. The incorporation of such advanced techniques not only enhances the accuracy of diagnosis but also optimizes therapeutic performance, a significant leap forward in the treatment of gastroenterology (Rosen et al., 2018). The second important aspect in gastroenterology diagnostic techniques includes the diagnosis of gastroesophageal reflux disease (GERD) in pediatric populations. The recent guideline update recommends a multifactorial assessment, both endoscopic and clinical, to provide an integrated view of GERD in infants and children. Systematic review of literature indicates that clinical presentation can be inadequate to render a diagnosis definitive, and diagnostic procedures , such as pH monitoring and esophageal manometry must be included. Moreover, evidence-based guideline suggestions enable uniform therapy, thus ensuring that GERD management and assessment are set with the most up-to-date evidence and expertise. This integrated system is a promise of improved patient outcomes and manifests the importance of individualized diagnostic approaches in managing complex gastrointestinal disorders (Rosen et al., 2018; Kaltenbach et al., 2020).

CLOSER LOOK

LIVER BIOPSY FINDINGS:

Liver biopsy provides one of the most definitive methods for evaluating hepatic pathology, offering direct visualization of cellular architecture, patterns of injury, and the extent of fibrosis. A closer look at liver biopsy findings reveals how subtle morphological changes can guide diagnosis, assess disease severity, and shape treatment decisions. Although imaging and laboratory tests have advanced significantly, biopsy remains crucial when the etiology of liver dysfunction is uncertain or when staging disease is essential for management. Microscopically, liver biopsy findings are typically assessed across several domains: inflammation, steatosis, hepatocellular injury, cholestasis, and fibrosis. The presence, distribution, and severity of these features help differentiate among various liver conditions. For example, inflammatory infiltrates—often composed of lymphocytes, plasma cells, or neutrophils—can indicate viral hepatitis, autoimmune hepatitis, or acute injury. The pattern of inflammation, whether portal, periportal, or lobular, provides additional diagnostic clues.

Hepatocellular injury, observed as ballooning degeneration, necrosis, or apoptosis, is another key feature. Ballooning, characterized by swollen hepatocytes with rarefied cytoplasm, is a hallmark of nonalcoholic steatohepatitis (NASH). In contrast, widespread necrosis might point toward severe drug-induced liver injury or fulminant viral hepatitis. Steatosis, or fat accumulation within hepatocytes, is graded by its extent and distribution. Macrovesicular steatosis—large fat droplets displacing the nucleus—is commonly seen in nonalcoholic fatty liver disease and alcohol-related liver disease, whereas microvesicular steatosis may suggest more acute metabolic disturbances such as Reye syndrome or certain drug toxicities.

Cholestasis appears as bile plugs within canaliculi or bile pigment in hepatocytes, indicating impaired bile flow. Its presence can distinguish cholestatic liver diseases from primarily hepatocellular injuries.

One of the most critical components of biopsy interpretation is the assessment of fibrosis, which reflects chronic injury. Fibrosis is staged according to its location and progression, from portal fibrosis to bridging fibrosis and ultimately cirrhosis. Identifying early fibrosis is essential, as interventions can still prevent progression to irreversible liver scarring.

Collectively, liver biopsy findings provide a comprehensive picture of hepatic health. They not only confirm diagnoses but also help predict prognosis and guide therapeutic decisions. Despite being an invasive procedure, biopsy remains a cornerstone in hepatology due to the depth and precision of information it offers.

REFERENCES

1. Tringali, A., Thomson, M., Dumonceau, J. M., Tavares, M., Tabbers, M. M., Furlano, R., Spaander, M., Hassan, C., Tzvinikos, C., Ijsselstijn, H., Viala, J., Dall'Oglio, L., Benninga, M., Orel, R., Vandenplas, Y., Keil, R., Romano, C., Brownstone, E., Hlava, Š., Gerner, P., ... Zambelli, A. (2017). Pediatric gastrointestinal endoscopy: European Society of Gastrointestinal Endoscopy (ESGE) and European Society for Paediatric Gastroenterology Hepatology and Nutrition (ESPGHAN) Guideline Executive summary. *Endoscopy*, *49*(1), 83–91. https://doi.org/10.1055/s-0042-111002 (accessed on 15th July 2025).

2. Ajani, J. A., D'Amico, T. A., Bentrem, D. J., Chao, J., Cooke, D. T., Corvera, C. U., Das, P., et al. (2022). Gastric cancer, version 2.2022, NCCN clinical practice guidelines in oncology. *Journal of the National Comprehensive Cancer Network, 20*, 167–192. https://doi.org/10.6004/jnccn.2022.0008 (accessed on 15th July 2025).

3. Hausmann J, Albert JG (2011) Detecting and Managing Small Bowel Crohn's Disease – Capsule Endoscopy Becoming a First Line Diagnostic Method? J Gastroint Dig Syst S1:002. doi:10.4172/2161-069X.S1-002(accessed on 15th July 2025).

4. Al-Haddad, A., Anand, R., Baron, T., Berg, B., Bhutani, M., Bottrell, R., Boyle, et al. (2014). *Clinical evaluation, imaging studies, indications for cytologic study, and preprocedural requirements for duct brushing studies and pancreatic FNA: The Papanicolaou Society of Cytopathology recommendations for pancreatic and biliary cytology.* https://deepblue.lib.umich.edu/bitstream/2027.42/106723/1/dc23095.pdf (accessed on 15th July 2025).

5. Della Corte, C., Mosca, A., Vania, A., Alterio, A., Alisi, A., & Nobili, V. (2016). Pediatric liver diseases: current challenges and future perspectives. *Expert review of gastroenterology & hepatology*, *10*(2), 255–265. https://doi.org/10.1586/17474124.2016.1129274 (accessed on 15th July 2025).

6. Almalioglu, Y., Araujo, H., Konukoglu, E., Sitti, et al. (2017). *A non-rigid map fusion-based RGB-depth SLAM method for endoscopic capsule robots.* http://arxiv.org/abs/1705.05444 (accessed on 15th July 2025).

7. Arebi, N., Saunders, B. P., & Surgical Procedures, Endoscopic. (2005). *Endoscopy: An Evolving Specialty.* https://core.ac.uk/download/46602009.pdf (accessed on 15th July 2025).

8. Bañales, J. M., Marín, J. J. G., Lamarca, Á., Rodrigues, P. M., Khan, S. A., Roberts, L. R., Cardinale, V., et al. (2020). Cholangiocarcinoma 2020: The next horizon in mechanisms and management. Nature Reviews Gastroenterology & Hepatology, 17, 557–588. https://doi.org/10.1038/s41575-020-0310-z (accessed on 15th July 2025).

9. Beaton, D., Sharp, L., Lu, L., Trudgill, N., Thoufeeq, M., Nicholson, B., Rogers, P., et al. (2024). Diagnostic yield from symptomatic lower gastrointestinal endoscopy in the UK: A British Society of Gastroenterology analysis using data from the National Endoscopy Database. *Alimentary Pharmacology & Therapeutics, 59*, 1589–1603. https://www.semanticscholar.org/paper/fe102f12d223f5ef56b79df3e5eac13d5cc82e1f (accessed on 15th July 2025).

10. Benson, A. B., D'Angelica, M. I., Abbott, D. E., Anaya, D. A., Anders, R. A., Are, C., Bachini, M., et al. (2021). Hepatobiliary cancers, version 2.2021, NCCN clinical practice guidelines in oncology. *Journal of the National Comprehensive Cancer Network, 19*, 541–565. https://doi.org/10.6004/jnccn.2021.0022 (accessed on 15th July 2025).

11. Smith, M. S., Cash, B., Konda, V., Trindade, A. J., Gordon, S., DeMeester, S., Joshi, V., Diehl, D., Ganguly, E., Mashimo, H., Singh, S., Jobe, B., McKinley, M., Wallace, M., Komatsu, Y., Thakkar, S., Schnoll-Sussman, F., Sharaiha, R., Kahaleh, M., Tarnasky, P., ... Chang, K. (2019). Volumetric laser endomicroscopy and its application to Barrett's esophagus: results from a 1,000 patient registry. *Diseases of the esophagus : official journal of the International Society for Diseases of the Esophagus, 32*(9), doz029. https://doi.org/10.1093/dote/doz029(accessed on 15th July 2025).

12. Bhandari, P., Subramaniam, S., & East, J. (2019). British Society of Gastroenterology Endoscopy Quality Improvement Program (BSG EQIP): Implementing new endoscopic techniques and technologies into clinical practice. Frontline Gastroenterology, 10, 155–159. https://www.semanticscholar.org/paper/3618a0e3e3773de61a045a7f4a5e5dfcc5e5296b (accessed on 15th July 2025).

13. Busuttil, R. W., Faltermeier, C., & Zarrinpar, A. (2015). *A surgical perspective on targeted therapy of hepatocellular carcinoma.* https://core.ac.uk/download/323077917.pdf (accessed on 15th July 2025).

14. Calborean, V., Miscoci, A., Pirvu, C. D., Pădureanu, et al. (2018). *The importance of circulating tumor products as "liquid biopsies" in colorectal cancer.* https://core.ac.uk/download/216808108.pdf (accessed on 15th July 2025).

15. Crossan, C., Tsochatzis, E. A., Longworth, L., Gurusamy, K., Davidson, B., Rodríguez-Perálvarez, M., Mantzoukis, K., O'Brien, J., Thalassinos, E., Papastergiou, V., & Burroughs, A. (2015). Cost-effectiveness of non-invasive methods for assessment and monitoring of liver fibrosis and cirrhosis in patients with chronic liver disease: systematic review and economic evaluation. *Health technology assessment (Winchester, England), 19*(9), 1–vi. https://doi.org/10.3310/hta19090 (accessed on 15th July 2025).

16. Chalasani, N., Younossi, Z. M., Lavine, J. E., Charlton, M., Cusi, K., Rinella, M. E., Harrison, S. A., et al. (2017). The diagnosis and management of nonalcoholic fatty liver disease: Practice guidance from the American Association for the Study of Liver Diseases. Hepatology, 67, 328–357. https://doi.org/10.1002/hep.29367 (accessed on 15th July 2025).

17. Chiorean, E. G., Nandakumar, G., Fadelu, T., Temin, S., Alarcon-Rozas, A. E., Bejarano, S., Croitoru, A. E., et al. (2020). Treatment of patients with late-stage colorectal cancer: ASCO resource-stratified guideline. *JCO Global Oncology.* https://doi.org/10.1200/jgo.19.00367 (accessed on 15th July 2025).

18. da Silva, B. C., Ramos, G. P., Barros, L. L., Ramos, A., Domingues, G., Chinzon, D., Passos, M. (2025). Diagnosis and treatment of small intestinal bacterial overgrowth: An official position paper from the Brazilian Federation of Gastroenterology. *Arquivos de Gastroenterologia, 62.* https://www.semanticscholar.org/paper/ed9dcbde0b87d9ace2e6982504f9166ca4e104f5 (accessed on 15th July 2025).

19. Dranove, J. (2008). Focus on diagnosis: New technologies for the diagnosis of gastroesophageal reflux disease. *Pediatrics in Review, 29*(9), 317–320. https://www.semanticscholar.org/paper/54fcb70ec05b8d7a52a5c5d48c0a4f59a054bda4 (accessed on 15th July 2025).

20. Fanous, M., Jaehne, A., Lorenson, D., & Williams, S. (2018). Impact of endoscopic training for surgeons on endolumenal and laparoscopic treatment for gastroesophageal reflux disease: Data from a rural, high-volume anti-reflux program. The American Surgeon, 84, 245–247.

https://www.semanticscholar.org/paper/dc8dcf3149172519f37aa21445195be2c7e42201 (accessed on 15th July 2025).

21. Gaebler, C., Wang, Z., Lorenzi, J. C. C., Muecksch, F., Finkin, S., Tokuyama, M., Cho, A., et al. (2021). Evolution of antibody immunity to SARS-CoV-2. *Nature, 591*, 639–644. https://doi.org/10.1038/s41586-021-03207-w (accessed on 15th July 2025).

22. Ho, K. Y., Kencana, A. P., Lin, L., & Phee, et al. (2011). *Therapeutic capsule endoscopy: Opportunities and challenges*. https://core.ac.uk/download/48818860.pdf (accessed on 15th July 2025).

23. Jacob, A., & Zacharia, G. S. (2025). DRESS' from a gastroenterology & hepatology perspective. *Japanese Journal of Gastroenterology and Hepatology*. https://www.semanticscholar.org/paper/5fa117aefe4d07ccb2628bdd38dad0064202c8f0 (accessed on 15th July 2025).

24. Kaltenbach, T., Anderson, J. C., Burke, C. A., Dominitz, J. A., Gupta, S., Lieberman, D. A., Robertson, D. J., et al. (2020). Endoscopic removal of colorectal lesions: Recommendations by the US Multi-Society Task Force on Colorectal Cancer. The American Journal of Gastroenterology, 115, 435–464. https://doi.org/10.14309/ajg.0000000000000555 (accessed on 15th July 2025).

25. Lee, B. I. (2016). Obscure gastrointestinal bleeding: Capsule or balloon? *Clinical Endoscopy, 49*, 4, 5. https://www.semanticscholar.org/paper/e442d2bfdbd363acbba5a036f2c70e138531539e (accessed on 15th July 2025).

26. Martini, S., Meneghin, F., Aceti, A., Cerchierini, N., Beghetti, I., Lista, G., & Corvaglia, L. (2024). Effect of different tube feeding methods on gastroesophageal reflux features in preterm infants: A pH-impedance monitoring study. European Journal of Pediatrics, 183, 4755–4762. https://www.semanticscholar.org/paper/2ac1721f5d4b195752fa5c4bfd2730c2e9f35fa6 (accessed on 15th July 2025).

27. Miller, J. D., Kemple, B., Evans, J. K., & Clayton, S. B. (2024). A comparison of functional luminal imaging probe with high-resolution manometry, timed barium esophagram, and pH impedance testing to evaluate functional luminal imaging probe's diagnostic capabilities. *Journal of Clinical Gastroenterology, 58*, 981–988. https://www.semanticscholar.org/paper/48dc5ccdc650d096efe1b6c7f68b915fbac3edb6 (accessed on 15th July 2025).

28. Modarai, B., Haulon, S., Ainsbury, E., Böckler, D., Vañó-Carruana, E., Dawson, J., Farber, M. A., et al. (2022). Editor's Choice – European Society for Vascular Surgery (ESVS) 2023 clinical practice guidelines on radiation safety. *European Journal of Vascular and Endovascular Surgery, 65*, 171–222. https://doi.org/10.1016/j.ejvs.2022.09.005 (accessed on 15th July 2025).

29. Nagendran, M., Chen, Y., Lovejoy, C. A., Gordon, A., Komorowski, M., Harvey, H., Topol, E. J., et al. (2020). Artificial intelligence versus clinicians: Systematic review of design, reporting standards, and claims of deep learning studies. BMJ. https://doi.org/10.1136/bmj.m689 (accessed on 15th July 2025).

30. Omata, M., Cheng, A. L., Kokudo, N., Kudo, M., Lee, J. M., Jia, J., Tateishi, R., et al. (2017). Asia–Pacific clinical practice guidelines on the management of hepatocellular carcinoma: A 2017 update. Hepatology International, 11, 317–370. https://doi.org/10.1007/s12072-017-9799-9 (accessed on 15th July 2025).

31. Parlatini, V., Bellato, A., Gabellone, A., Margari, L., Marzulli, L., Matera, E., Petruzzelli, M., et al. (2024). A state-of-the-art overview of candidate diagnostic biomarkers for attention-deficit/hyperactivity disorder (ADHD). Expert Review of Molecular Diagnostics, 24, 259–271. https://

www.semanticscholar.org/paper/417284bc4daf18e4bbb12f3d446ffa7d33605784 (accessed on 15th July 2025).

32. Rai, P., Udawat, P., Chowdhary, S., Gunjan, D., Samanta, J., Bhatia, V., Singla, V., et al. (2023). Society of Gastrointestinal Endoscopy of India Consensus Guidelines on Endoscopic Ultrasound-Guided Biliary Drainage: Part I (Indications, Outcomes, Comparative Evaluations, Training). Journal of Digestive Endoscopy, 14, 30–40. https://www.semanticscholar.org/paper/ec295c315f7b032a8ec294970fb80fa50886a633 (accessed on 15th July 2025).

33. Ranjan, R., Dallal, H., Dragos, C., & Gaston-Ross, J. (2019). PWE-032 Can you diagnose adult coeliac disease without the need for a duodenal biopsy? Gut, 68, A166–A167. https://www.semanticscholar.org/paper/09a3374be26eb9e4c5adc348d4e05758293759d8 (accessed on 15th July 2025).

34. Rižnik, P., Trop, T. K., Klemenak, M., Krenčnik, T., Milanič-Koron, T., Mojškerc, E. M., Pavlin, T., et al. (2024). Insights into coeliac disease diagnosis: A 2021–2023 overview of diagnostic approach and delays in children in Slovenia. Wiener Medizinische Wochenschrift (1946), 174, 257–261. https://www.semanticscholar.org/paper/9f9bc57c87396058ed846b4a2cfb667e689267b0 (accessed on 15th July 2025).

35. Robles-Medranda, C., Verpalen, I., Schulz, D., & Spadaccini, M. (2025). Artificial intelligence in biliopancreatic disorders: Applications in cross-imaging and endoscopy. *Gastroenterology.* https://www.semanticscholar.org/paper/7cb1ac77dd384794e6b1763af4012e6c028dd7f5 (accessed on 15th July 2025).

36. Roman, S., & Kahrilas, P. (2011). Pseudoachalasia and laparoscopic gastric banding. Journal of Clinical Gastroenterology, 45(9), 745–747. https://www.semanticscholar.org/paper/8952b222fdf11a5c80694968aa20dc7201f9602f (accessed on 15th July 2025).

37. Rosen, R., Vandenplas, Y., Singendonk, M., Cabana, M. D., DiLorenzo, C., Gottrand, F., Gupta, S. K., et al. (2018). Pediatric gastroesophageal reflux clinical practice guidelines. Journal of Pediatric Gastroenterology and Nutrition, 66, 516–554. https://doi.org/10.1097/mpg.0000000000001889 (accessed on 15th July 2025).

38. Saraiva, M., Ribeiro, T., Agudo, B., Afonso, J., Mendes, F., Martins, M., Cardoso, P., et al. (2025). Evaluating ChatGPT-4 for the interpretation of images from several diagnostic techniques in gastroenterology. Journal of Clinical Medicine, 14. https://www.semanticscholar.org/paper/24d5a1c708229603da8202c1167a52ed6c9bbcc4 (accessed on 15th July 2025).

39. Wiita, A. P., & Schrijver, I. (2011). Clinical application of high throughput molecular screening techniques for pharmacogenomics. *Pharmacogenomics and personalized medicine, 4,* 109–121. https://doi.org/10.2147/PGPM.S15302 (accessed on 15th July 2025).

40. Shah, A., Talley, N., & Holtmann, G. (2022). Current and future approaches for diagnosing small intestinal dysbiosis in patients with symptoms of functional dyspepsia. *Frontiers in Neuroscience, 16.* https://www.semanticscholar.org/paper/44850e389b8dde8cc7d678e0ec298fd22b8f00f3 (accessed on 15th July 2025).

41. She, Y., & Ge, N. (2023). Diagnostic value of endoscopic ultrasonography in pelvic masses with bowel involvement. Therapeutic Advances in Gastroenterology, 16. https://www.semanticscholar.org/paper/804382d0a38eefc97ef4aad303c0b9ebbb65321e (accessed on 15th July 2025).

42. Sheth, A. (2007). ROME III: The functional gastrointestinal disorders. *Journal of Clinical Gastroenterology, 41*, 867. https://www.semanticscholar.org/paper/203840105233296c2f769f68790990f981831d0b (accessed on 15th July 2025).

43. Sridhar, G., Prasad, A. V. S., & Lakshmi, G. (2024). Scope and caveats: Artificial intelligence in gastroenterology. *Artificial Intelligence in Gastroenterology.* https://www.semanticscholar.org/paper/8f53b866c1e14f4e8cc6b889e8d513bb74d51354 (accessed on 15th July 2025).

44. Talkhan, M. G., & Elsayed, M. O. K. (2024). Assessment of dyspepsia in the era of endoscopic ultrasonography. Gastroenterology and Functional Medicine. https://www.semanticscholar.org/paper/d1b55d39d5c91fa8ba746a876b075d2a35c17295 (accessed on 15th July 2025).

45. Talwalkar, J. (2008). Elastography for detecting hepatic fibrosis: Options and considerations. *Gastroenterology, 135*(1), 299–302. https://www.semanticscholar.org/paper/923068dd7ab1d480799f63aec062d687cd738183 (accessed on 15th July 2025).

46. Tornkvist, N., & Törnblom, H. (2022). European guidelines on functional bowel disorders with diarrhea: United European Gastroenterology (UEG) and European Society for Neurogastroenterology and Motility (ESNM) statements and recommendations. United European Gastroenterology Journal, 10, 615–616. https://www.semanticscholar.org/paper/6c3a2ef15a7746794aa5309966eba2faaae99067 (accessed on 15th July 2025).

47. Touroutoglou, A., Oikonomopoulos, A., Baltimore, Baumgart, Cho, Polytarchou, C., CramaBohbouth, et al. (2015). *Assessment of circulating microRNAs for the diagnosis and disease activity evaluation in patients with ulcerative colitis by using the Nanostring technology.* https://core.ac.uk/download/30650084.pdf (accessed on 15th July 2025).

48. Umitzhanov, M., Abdiramanova, B., Abutalip, A., Bakirov, N., & Sarimbekova, S. (2023). Comparative assessment of regulated methods and PCR in the diagnosis of trichophytosis in veterinary mycology. Open Veterinary Journal, 13, 1614–1622. https://www.semanticscholar.org/paper/3578f6b60ffc24d5b88a582b45ddb1d5d627d1a1 (accessed on 15th July 2025).

49. Vogel, J. D., Felder, S., Bhama, A. R., Hawkins, A. T., Langenfeld, S. J., Shaffer, V., Thorsen, A. J., et al. (2021). The American Society of Colon and Rectal Surgeons Clinical Practice Guidelines for the Management of Colon Cancer. Diseases of the Colon & Rectum, 65, 148–177. https://doi.org/10.1097/dcr.0000000000002323 (accessed on 15th July 2025).

50. Wild, J., Nandi, N., Chew, T. S., Rea, B., & Sidhu, R. (2025). Small bowel ultrasound: Friend or foe? *Current Opinion in Gastroenterology, 41*, 154–163. https://www.semanticscholar.org/paper/582cd1767b4e65a94c08214bf221514d522a2fb4 (accessed on 15th July 2025).

51. Wilkens, R., Dolinger, M. T., Burisch, J., & Maaser, C. (2022). Point-of-care testing and home testing: Pragmatic considerations for widespread incorporation of stool tests, serum tests, and intestinal ultrasound. Gastroenterology, 162, 1476–1492. https://doi.org/10.1053/j.gastro.2021.10.052 (accessed on 15th July 2025).

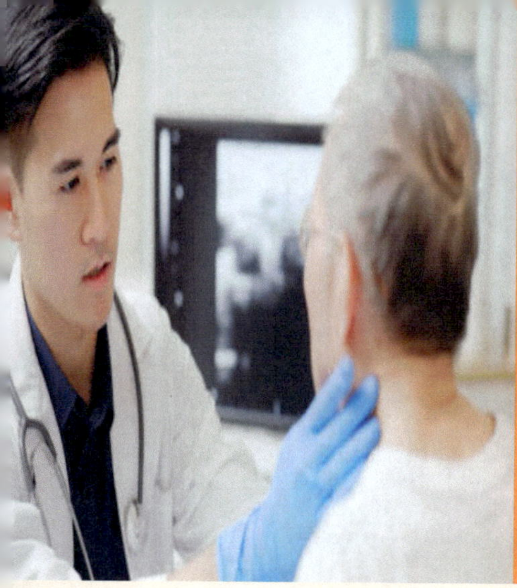

Chapter 3

DISORDERS OF THE ESOPHAGUS

Contents

Introduction

The esophageal diseases are a daunting problem in gastroenterology practice, affecting a huge number of individuals and with extreme diversity in severity and symptomology. From gastroesophageal reflux disease (GERD) to achalasia, all these can have a very dramatic effect on the quality of life of an individual, inducing discomfort and complications that can interfere with daily functioning. GERD, or the backflow of stomach contents into the esophagus, is extremely prevalent and will produce symptoms , such as heartburn and regurgitation. Disorders , such as achalasia are due to a failure of the esophagus to properly deliver food to the stomach due to defects in neural control. Therefore, etiologic knowledge of the disorders, their symptoms and treatment are important for both patients and clinicians, since timely intervention can circumvent to a great extent the bad effects on health and well-being. Pathophysiology of esophageal disorders is intricate and complex, involving frequently complicated interactions between anatomical structures, neurological function, and biochemical events. For instance, motility disorders

, such as achalasia are believed to result from degeneration of myenteric plexus ganglion cells, leading to abnormal peristalsis and esophageal blockage. Further, GERD can be aggravated by a plethora of factors , such as lifestyle, obesity, and hiatal hernia. This heterogeneity of etiological factors serves to highlight the importance of personalized diagnosis and treatment modalities.

The patient may present with a wide array of symptoms from nonspecific discomfort to complications , such as esophagitis or Barrett's esophagus with high chances of esophageal cancer. Hence, adequate knowledge of both the mechanism and the symptoms of the patient is important for effective management modalities. In bringing together management modalities for esophageal disorders, a multidisciplinary approach must be employed involving lifestyle modification, medical therapy, and, in some cases, surgery. Pharmacotherapy, like proton pump inhibitors (PPIs), has been instrumental in managing GERD symptoms and promoting mucosal healing, with dilation treatment or myotomy surgery being reserved for those achalasia patients with refractoriness to less invasive therapy.

In addition, increased use of endoscopic approaches highlights the movement toward updating treatment strategies to serve the patient better. Educational efforts that promote awareness of esophageal diseases and their symptoms are essential to early diagnosis and care. As additional research progresses toward an enhanced understanding of the pathophysiology and efficacy of treatment, attention must also be paid to novel therapies that hold the potential to redefine management paradigms. Through these developments, combined with ongoing patient education and research, patients' quality of life can be optimized (Figure 3.1).

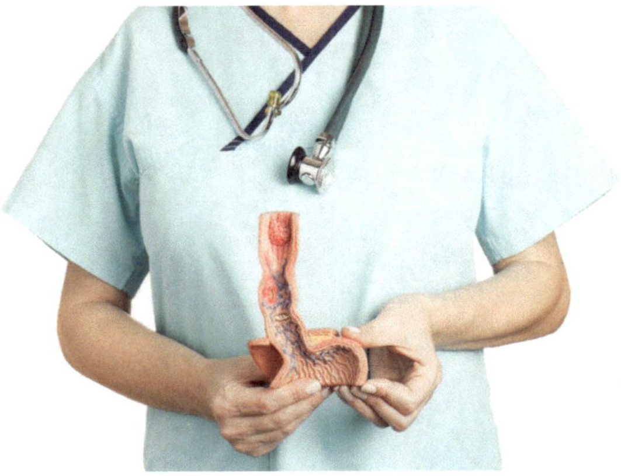

Figure 3.1. Disorders of the esophagus.

Source: https://www.verywellhealth.com/thmb/EKqi41yIhvhu06Igt9TeeGcyWxI=/1100x0/filters:no_upscale():max_bytes(150000):strip_icc()/esophagus-illnesses-155358910-80080ca477514ff3851688885feefdbf.jpg.

Definition of Esophageal Disorders

Esophageal diseases represent a vast array of conditions that affect the esophagus' structure and function, a muscular tube that conveys food from the throat to the stomach. The esophageal diseases may develop due to congenital disease, infections, inflammatory processes, or mechanical obstruction and, depending on the cause, have different symptoms , such as dysphagia, pain in the chest, or regurgitation. A global approach needs to be employed when classifying such disorders, as it involves encompassing both the physical symptoms as well as the etiologies that influence these symptoms and impact esophageal health. It is vital to comprehend the extensive variability of dysfunction within the esophagus, as the disorders can have very extensive consequences on nutritional metabolism and quality of life for the patient. One of the significant challenges of diagnosing and classifying esophageal disorders is the overlapping presentation and complexities. These conditions, such as eosinophilic esophagitis, gastroesophageal reflux disease (GERD), and achalasia, may share overlapping clinical presentations but are rooted in distinct pathological processes. For instance, eosinophilic esophagitis is an immune process, while GERD is primarily a reflection of an incompetent lower esophageal sphincter that fails to prevent acid reflux. According to the design of established classification systems, such as the World Health Organization International Classification of Functioning, Disability, and Health, a more open diagnostic perspective. It integrates functional impairment and psychosocial factors and allows for a thorough understanding of patient needs and informs the creation of useful interventions (Browne et al., 2019). In addition, an essential component of esophageal disorders is the requirement for accurate imaging and evaluation methods to discriminate between conditions. Swallowing fluoroscopic studies are critical in examining esophageal function, especially in complicated cases when conventional tests are not sufficient. From these studies, the following pattern of esophageal dysfunctions may be observed: pharyngoesophageal webs or abnormal impressions that may be indicative of disease (Gordon et al., 2010). These advanced diagnostic techniques not only assist in accurate classification but also enhance the formulation of customized management plans. With increased understanding of the disorders of the esophagus, acceptance of multidimensional definitions that include medical, anatomical, and psychosocial aspects is the key to enhancing clinical success for individuals presenting with these problems.

Importance of Understanding Esophageal Health

It is crucial to comprehend the health of the esophagus not only to prevent disorders but also to understand the intricate relationship between the structure and function of the esophagus. The esophagus is a vital component of the digestive system that facilitates the passage of food from the mouth to the stomach. Any malfunction of the organ can lead to serious complications, such as gastroesophageal reflux disease (GERD) and esophageal cancers. By examining the elementary architecture of the esophagus, as a series of the lower esophageal sphincter (LES) and accompanying musculature, researchers can discover the function that these structures have in achieving the best esophageal performance. The helical arrangement of circular muscle fascicles throughout the LES, for instance, indicates the importance of muscular coordination in preventing reflux (Cheng et al., 2017). Therefore, the knowledge of esophageal anatomy and physiology is directly applied to clinical practice and interventions that will minimize the incidence of esophageal disorders. Furthermore, the scientific community has found profound links between esophageal disorders and cancer, which is strong evidence of the necessity of extensive esophageal health education. Esophageal squamous cell carcinoma (SCC) is one of the predominant types of malignancy with high health implications. It has been studied that mutations in signaling pathways, i.e., the Notch pathway, play a key role in the tumorigenesis of SCC (Biswas et al., 2016). It is important to discover these genetic causes for early diagnosis and designing targeted therapy in affected individuals. In addition, educational interventions concerning esophageal health can promote awareness of prevention strategies, such as dietary modifications and lifestyle modifications that can reduce the risk of esophageal diseases and cancers. Establishing such knowledge can empower individuals to make decisions regarding their health and promote preventive healthcare. Lastly, given the vast prevalence of esophageal disorders across the globe, it is essential to ensure that the general public and healthcare professionals help maintain esophageal health. Early intervention and individualized treatment regimens improve patient outcomes substantially and can prevent the deterioration of diseases that originate from untreated disorders. This project involves expanding the knowledge of disease-related risk factors , such as Barrett's esophagus, which turns cancerous if not diagnosed and treated on time.

Furthermore, research on the anatomical and physiological characteristics of the esophagus can guide interventions, advancing medical and therapeutic interventions. As knowledge of esophageal health expands, so grows the necessity for interdisciplinary coordination among researchers, clinicians, and patients, a factor that underscores the necessity to approach the resolution of esophageal health and disease intricacies through an integrative framework (Figure 3.2).

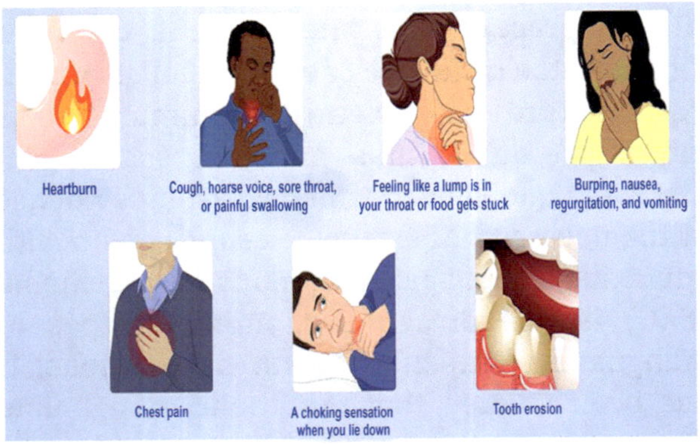

Figure 3.2. Importance of understanding esophageal health.

Source: https://external-content.duckduckgo.com/iu/?u=https%3A%2F%2Fwww.youandesophagealcancer.com%2Fen-ec%2Fslides%2Funderstanding-esophageal-cancer-gerd-and-barretts-esophagus%2Fec01-slides-m1_slide_12%24jpg&f=1&nofb=1&ipt=293d94ec3ee13b74cbe77c33161b9d68086f017a76b62db3901e101813592264.

Overview of Common Disorders

The esophagus is susceptible to a range of disorders, one of the most prevalent of these being gastroesophageal reflux disease (GERD). A disease in which stomach contents reflux into the esophagus, GERD occurs in the majority of the population and has a range of complications if untreated. The signs usually are heartburn, regurgitation, and dysphagia. Recurrent reflux may cause inflammation and progress to Barrett's esophagus, a condition in which the squamous lining of the esophagus is replaced with columnar cells by metaplasia. While Barrett's esophagus itself is not usually symptomatic, it increases the risk of developing esophageal adenocarcinoma, one of the most incurable types of cancer, so early diagnosis and treatment of GERD are essential to prevent more severe complications (Palmese, 2016). Another very common disorder affecting the esophagus is esophagitis, which is an inflammation of the lining of the esophagus. There are various etiologies of this condition, including infection, irritants like chemicals or drugs, and immune responses. Swallowing pain, chest pain, and dysphagia are noted in this condition's patient, significantly impairing the patient's quality of life. Fungal infections, particularly in immunocompromised hosts, and viral infections are also key in producing esophagitis. The management of esophagitis is most often the identification and management of the underlying causes, for example, dietary modification or the use of drugs to reduce inflammation. As esophagitis is a potential precursor to complications, understanding its etiology and management helps prevent complications like esophageal scarring and stricture. Achalasia and diffuse esophageal spasm, though less common, are also important esophageal motility disorders. Achalasia is a disease characterized by the inability of the lower esophageal sphincter to relax normally, leading to dysphagia and food regurgitation. Chest pain and significant weight loss due to dysphagia may occur and contribute to morbidity in patients. Similarly, diffuse esophageal spasm is manifested by repetitive muscle contractions in the esophagus that produce chest pain and dysphagia that may mimic heart disease symptoms. These motility disorders can be diagnosed with the aid of advanced tests , such as esophageal manometry, in most instances. Treatment involves drug therapy, endoscopic management, or surgery if necessary. Unraveling the complexities of such disorders is critical to further improving the prognosis and quality of life of the afflicted (Adashek et al., 2020).

3.1. Anatomy and Physiology of the Esophagus

The esophagus, a muscular tube approximately 25 centimeters in length, is the conduit from the throat to the stomach. The esophagus's structural content includes an exterior adventitia layer, a middle layer consisting of circular and longitudinal fibers, and an innermost mucosal coat for food passage. The esophagus has three anatomically distinct parts: cervical, thoracic, and abdominal. This special anatomy of the building permits the esophagus to perform its important role of transporting food efficiently while providing a flexible, durable pathway through the chest space. Dysfunctions or pathologies in any part of this complex anatomy may lead to such conditions, underscoring the importance of understanding the esophagus physiology as a foundation for diagnosing and treating these conditions. One of the most important aspects of esophageal physiology is that sphincters exist, the upper and lower esophageal sphincters. The upper esophageal sphincter (UES) plays a crucial role in controlling entry to the esophagus and ensuring cessation of air regurgitation during breathing. Recent studies have revealed the UES's new anatomical arrangement, aligning with age-old assumptions about shape and mechanism. Researchers have indicated that the UES is not a round-shaped entity, hence the need to reexamine methods used in addressing diseases of this area (Belafsky, 2024). With increased understanding of the physiology of the area around the UES, it is understood that diseases related to this sphincter have a significant effect on the functioning of the esophagus, calling for enhanced diagnostic and treatment techniques. Furthermore, the lower esophageal sphincter (LES) helps maintain the esophagus separated from the stomach and guards against gastroesophageal reflux. Physiology of the UES and LES is subject to many factors, including the anatomic relationship and the intrinsic motility patterns governing the motion of the esophagus. EGJ disorders may arise from multiple pathophysiologic mechanisms, but their mechanisms are not well understood (Vahedi et al., 2023). This underlines the necessity for ongoing research that will provide an understanding of the distinctive characteristics of patients with EGJ outflow disorders and their normal motility counterparts. Accurate comprehension of the complex interplay among the esophagus' physiological and anatomical forms is critical in the effective management of disorders of the esophagus.

3.1.1. Structure of the Esophagus

The esophagus is an important muscular tube employed as a conduit for food and liquids between the throat and stomach. It measures approximately 25 centimeters in length in adults and contains four distinct layers: the mucosa, submucosa, muscularis, and adventitia. The mucosa, which is lined with stratified squamous epithelium, envelops and shields from abrasion by food particles. Under this lies the submucosa, containing connective tissue, blood vessels, and nerve fibers that supply the esophagus. The muscularis is the crucial layer, containing striated muscles in the upper esophagus to provide voluntary control and smooth muscles in the lower esophagus to contract automatically. This enables peristalsis, the coordinated contraction that propels food into the stomach. The structure of the esophagus is paramount to its fundamental operation, but any defect can cause severe disorders as outlined in the following sections. Physiologically, the esophagus has sophisticated mechanisms that facilitate its operation. The lower esophageal sphincter (LES), a delicate muscular ring located at the nexus of the esophagus and the stomach, functions to keep gastroesophageal reflux at bay. Under normal functioning, the LES remains contracted to avoid reflux of the contents of the stomach into the esophagus. The operation of the LES is subject to change through various factors, including obesity, pregnancy, and some medications, which to induce conditions like gastroesophageal reflux disease (GERD). The peristalsis of the esophagus is also subject to control from a wide range of factors, from the biomechanical properties of the muscular coat to nervous command over the motor activity. Interference with this organized process can result in motility disorders, which demonstrate the way in which the structure of the esophagus is intimately associated with its function and susceptibility to disorder.

The complexity of the structure of the esophagus is more than just layered, with sophisticated relationships to adjacent anatomical structures. Its close proximity to critical structures like the trachea and the aorta emphasizes its importance and vulnerability. In addition, the esophagus exhibits major structural differences along different parts; i.e., cervical and thoracic parts have typical muscular arrangements that determine motility. In pathological conditions, e.g., in strictures or malignancy of the esophagus, structural differences lead to severely impaired function. The clinical relevance of familiarizing oneself with esophageal anatomy is exacerbated by the growing incidence of esophageal diseases, which implies that medical professionals should consider anatomical variations and their implications on diagnostics and treatment. A complete understanding of the esophagus anatomy thus offers a basis for the comprehension of the numerous disorders that impact this critical organ, such as those viewed in the broad context of gastrointestinal health (Hunt et al., 2017; Yamamoto et al., 2018) (Figure 3.3).

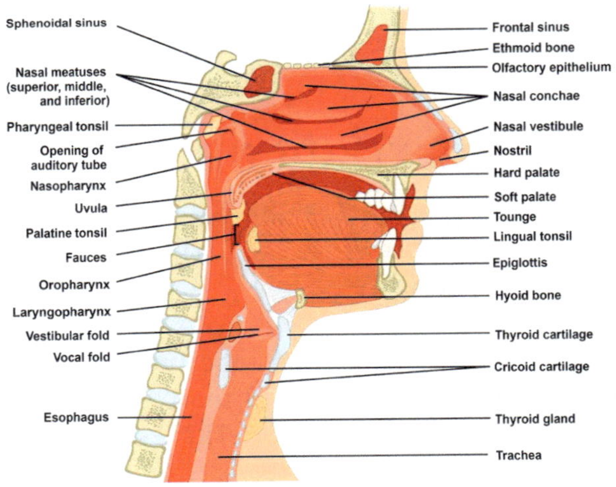

Figure 3.3. Structure of the esophagus.

Source: https://medicinebtg.com/wp-content/uploads/2017/06/de-Esophagus-Function-And-Structure-mar-webmds-esophagus-anatomy-page-provides-a-detailed-picture-and-the-which-may.jpg.

3.1.2. Function of the Esophagus in Digestion

The esophagus has a crucial function in the digestive system, with its role being essentially that of a transport tube from the mouth into the stomach. After consuming food, it travels down the esophagus through a series of coordinated muscular contractions, which is the essence of peristalsis. Through such rhythmic contractions, the food bolus gets transported to the lower gastrointestinal tract with ease. The lower esophageal sphincter (LES) is an important valve located at the esophagogastric junction, which prevents gastric contents from entering the esophagus. Its anatomical arrangement, characterized by particular myo-architectural organization, contributes to fulfilling this function. As the literature explains, the muscle fascicles that surround the LES form a noose-like structure around the esophagus, which facilitates effective pressure and closure and plays the key role in preventing the reflux events that could result in diseases , such as GERD (Cheng et al., 2017). In addition to its mechanical role, the esophagus also secretes mucus, which serves an essential protective function during digestion. Mucus is secreted by the epithelial lining of the esophagus and creates a lubricating covering that cushions the passage of food while also shielding the subjacent tissues from acidic gastric contents.

This mucus layer plays a crucial role in maintaining the integrity of the lining of the esophagus by preventing mucosal damage and subsequent inflammation. Recent studies highlight the importance of the mucins, or the glycoproteins of the mucus, and their role in forming a gel-like protective barrier. The type of these mucins, in particular their pore size and charge, dictates what is able to pass through to the epithelial surface and thereby maintain esophageal function and health (Macierzanka et al., 2012). Dysfunction of this defense system can lead to severe disorders like Barrett's esophagus or esophagitis. The interrelatedness of the structure and function of the esophagus and its involvement in the digestion process expose it to various disorders. Achalasia, where the esophagus is unable to relax normally, greatly compromises the esophageal ability for effective food transportation. Similarly, stricture and malignancy of the esophagus may lead to obstruction with resultant swallowing difficulty (dysphagia) or chronic gastroesophageal reflux. With decreasing overall health and function of the esophagus, there is an increased risk of the occurrence of secondary complications , such as malnutrition or aspiration. This underlines the importance of a coordinated perspective of the esophageal function in digestion to determine and treat potential disorders. With research continuing to evolve, the results will continue to illuminate the complex processes that define esophageal health within the larger context of gastrointestinal function (Figure 3.4).

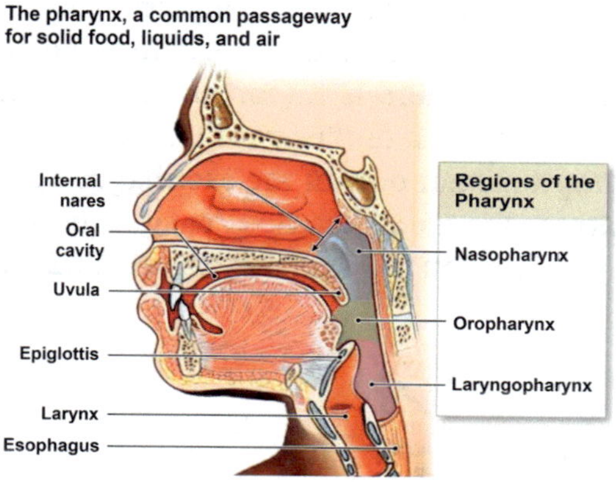

Figure 3.4. Function of the esophagus in digestion.

Source: https://medicinebtg.com/wp-content/uploads/2017/06/torso-esophagus-the-Esophagus-Function-In-The-Digestive-System-esophagus-seems-to-have-only-one-important-function-in-body.jpg.

3.1.3. Role of the Esophageal Sphincters

The esophagus is a critical passageway between the stomach and the mouth, and the esophageal sphincters play an important role in maintaining physiological integrity. The upper (UES) and lower (LES) esophageal sphincters control the passage of substances in the esophagus without refluxing gastric contents and protecting the airway. The UES, comprised of a collection of muscles, allows for the regulated passage of food and liquid while also preventing air from entering the digestive system. Conversely, the LES is a sphincter that is open to allow food into the stomach but maintains a tonic contraction to prevent reflux of the stomach into the esophagus, which is at the center of most esophageal disorders , such as gastroesophageal reflux disease (GERD) (Chen et al., 2023). Sphincter disorders, dependent on the functioning of the sphincters, can lead to significant clinical presentations. UES dysfunction may result in dysphagia and aspiration, whereas compromised function of the LES may result in acid reflux and subsequent chronic symptoms of GERD. The pathophysiological interaction between the two sphincters is important because their dysfunction has a tendency to trigger a cascade of symptoms not only of the esophagus but also of extraesophageal diseases , such as laryngitis and chronic cough (Yadlapati et al., 2020).

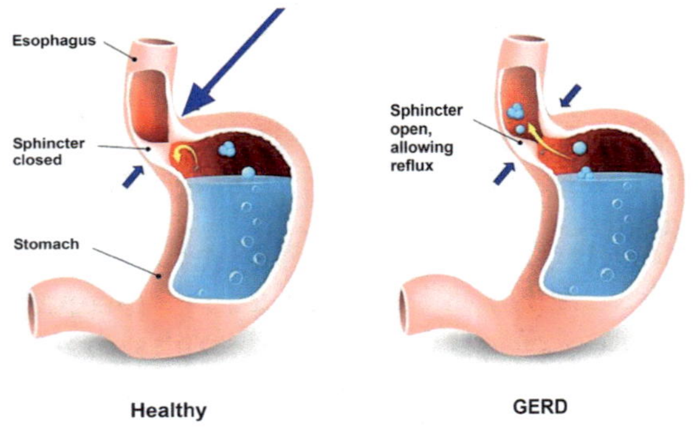

Figure 3.5. Role of the esophageal sphincters.

Source: https://healthjade.net/wp-content/uploads/2020/07/Lower-Esophageal-Sphincter.jpg.

Understanding the mechanism behind these sphincters allows targeted diagnostic approaches and treatment interventions, and therefore, it is essential for health professionals to know their function in overall esophageal health. At a wider level, technological advances in diagnostic tools , such as high-resolution manometry, allow monitoring of sphincter and esophageal motility function, enabling improved identification of proper diagnosis. The Classification of Chicago system now more accurately describes esophageal motility disorders so that clinicians may discriminate between diseases , such as achalasia, outflow obstruction of the esophagogastric junction, and ineffective motility of the esophagus. These diseases may involve alterations in sphincter tone or peristalsis abnormalities, thereby causing symptoms of esophageal disease (Chen et al., 2023). By further specifying the diagnostic criteria, medical professionals can implement more focused treatment protocols that directly address both the symptoms and the sphincter dysfunction of the esophagus, a significant milestone in the treatment of esophageal disorders (Figure 3.5).

3.2. Gastroesophageal Reflux Disease (GERD)

Gastroesophageal Reflux Disease (GERD) is a serious pathological process characterized by retrograde esophageal flow of gastric contents, which evolves into multiple clinical presentations, with the majority being heartburn. This retrosternal burning can readily be confused with cardiac manifestations, thus highlighting the necessity for early and accurate diagnosis. Epidemiologically, GERD affects a significant proportion of the population and, left untreated, can lead to chronic complications. Although most patients have mild symptoms, some develop severe esophagitis and complications requiring long-term therapeutic management. It is important to consider GERD as a chronic condition rather than an inconvenient temporary affliction in order to approach management and patient education effectively. This understanding supports the creation of extensive treatment plans based on the unique needs of each patient, with the possibility of improving lifestyle changes along with drug therapy. The therapeutic approach for GERD has evolved significantly, adopting many therapies in the direction of reducing gastric acidity and preventing mucosal damage. Proton pump inhibitors , such as omeprazole are the mainstay of pharmacologic therapy due to their ability to effectively prevent symptoms as well as esophagitis healing. But long-term PPI therapy is associated with gripes from malabsorption of nutrients, up through an increased risk of gastrointestinal infections, calling for careful monitoring of patients and potential alternative treatment. It seems from recent studies that even improving associated conditions, such as chronic constipation, can enhance GERD symptoms, illustrating the call for an integrated treatment strategy. Understanding the interaction between these gastrointestinal conditions is important to optimize therapeutic outcomes and reduce medication side effects (Hosseini et al., 2015).

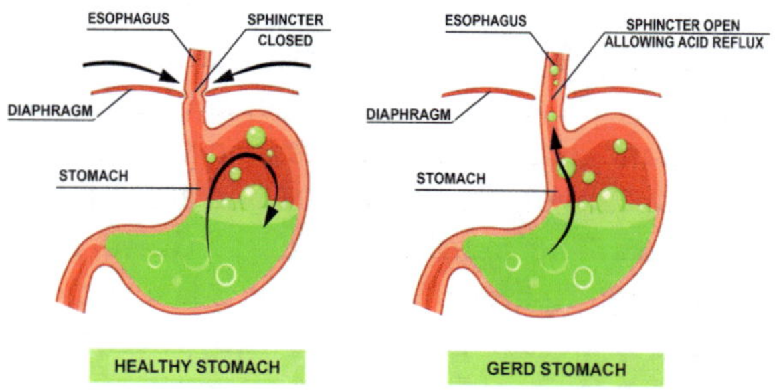

Figure 3.6. Gastroesophageal reflux disease (GERD).

Source: https://img.freepik.com/premium-vector/gastroesophageal-reflux-disease-acid-reflux-heartburn-gerd-infographic-with-medical-vector-illustration-healthy-sick-stomach-medicine-anatomy-healthy-organ-illness-gerd-infographic_499433-86.jpg?w=1480.

In addition to pharmacological treatment, lifestyle modification is an important part of GERD treatment. Patients can be asked to implement measures , such as weight loss, dietary alteration, and alteration in body position that can potentially reduce reflux remarkably. Employment of less harmful operative techniques, i.e., advances in procedures like Nissen fundoplication, has improved prognosis in patients as well, including those who are refractory to medical therapy. Chronicity of GERD necessitates utilization of a multidimensional plan of management in consideration of both the physiological pathophysiology of the disease as well as psychological aspects influencing patients. Since medical providers continue to explore newer therapies and training programs, they should always consider the pathophysiology of GERD and its implications on long-term patient care (Wall & Jacoby, 2002). A good understanding of these processes is essential in addressing this prevalent esophageal disease (Figure 3.6).

3.2.1. Definition and Causes of GERD

Gastroesophageal reflux disease (GERD) is a chronic condition in which there is abnormal reflux of stomach contents into the esophagus, causing distressful symptoms and potential complications. The condition occurs when the lower esophageal sphincter (LES), the muscle that separates the stomach from the esophagus, is weak or dysfunctional and cannot prevent gastric acid and contents from flowing upwards. Backflow could result in symptoms , such as heartburn, regurgitation, and dysphagia. If left untreated, GERD is also a cause of advanced diseases like esophagitis, Barrett's esophagus, and adenocarcinoma of the esophagus, a disease related to prolonged gastric reflux that leads to modification of the cellular composition of the esophagus (Palmese, 2016). The pathogenesis of GERD is multifactorial and is accounted for by a combination of lifestyle factors, anatomical disorders, and physiologic changes. Obesity is also a significant risk factor because increased weight can increase the pressure within the abdomen, which again tends to induce reflux. Further, certain lifestyle factors , such as smoking, alcohol, and some of the triggering foods can exacerbate the symptoms of GERD by either relaxing the LES or increasing acid secretion. Structural issues , such as hiatal hernias, can also impair the function of the LES, causing the reflux episodes to become more frequent. In children, liquids, recumbency, and infantile esophageal function are responsible for the prevalence and severity of gastroesophageal reflux (Borrelli et al., 2017). It is important to know these causes to treat GERD effectively. Therapy could involve changes to lifestyle and diet that minimize symptoms, along with medication that decreases gastric acidity or increases the motility of the gastrointestinal tract. In severe cases, surgical interventions may be done to correct anatomical defects that cause the disorder. An assessment of the potential long-term effects of neglecting GERD, such as the development of more serious disorders like Barrett's esophagus, that may lead to adenocarcinoma of the esophagus (Palmese, 2016), should also be considered. By addressing both the causes and symptoms of GERD, healthcare professionals can significantly improve the quality of life in patients and reduce the risk of severe complications associated with this esophageal disorder (Figure 3.7).

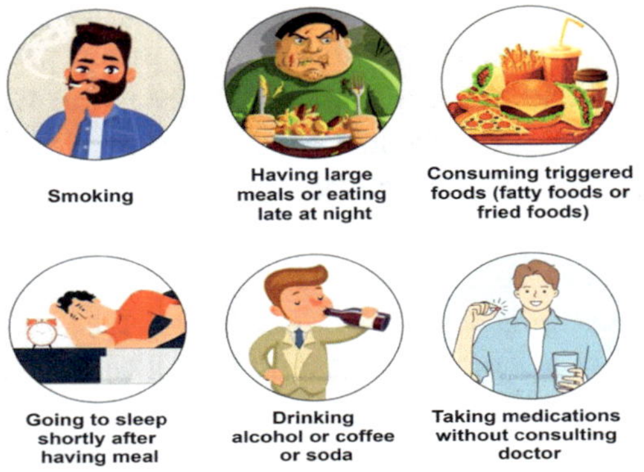

Figure 3.7. Definition and causes of GERD

Source: https://lirp.cdn-website.com/69c0b277/dms3rep/multi/opt/Risk+factors+for+GERD+(Gastroesophageal+reflux+disease)+or+chronic+acid+reflux-1920w.jpg.

3.2.2. Symptoms and Complications of GERD

Gastroesophageal reflux disease (GERD) also has a broad range of symptoms that can significantly compromise the quality of life of a patient. The typical symptoms are chronic heartburn, acid regurgitation, and dysphagia, which may result in distress and discomfort. However, the complexity of GERD is beyond the classical presentation. The majority of the patients have abnormal presentations , such as chronic cough, laryngitis, and asthma, making diagnosis more challenging, as these symptoms can be mistaken for other illnesses. Moreover, patients are not always ready with the typical symptoms of heartburn or regurgitation, so physicians should remain vigilant and aggressive in evaluating the potential connection of these symptoms with gastroesophageal reflux (Chen et al., 2023). The clouded presentation renders crucial the imperative of an inclusive approach in the management of patients who present with any symptom of esophageal or extraesophageal symptoms. The manifestations of GERD range from benign to life-threatening disease. Chronic gastroesophageal reflux has the potential to result in esophagitis, Barrett's esophagus, and adenocarcinoma of the esophagus. Esophagitis, which includes inflammation and damage to the lining of the esophagus, may lead to painful symptoms along with increased susceptibility to infection. Barrett's esophagus, which is pre-cancerous for esophageal cancer, happens when the esophagus's usual squamous cells are transformed into columnar cells after prolonged exposure to stomach acid, significantly increasing the risk of malignancy significantly (Lin et al., 2019). Moreover, the multifactorial pathogenesis of GERD-related complications necessitates an interdisciplinary treatment, given that management of the condition typically involves the services of gastroenterologists, pulmonologists, and otolaryngologists to effectively counteract its system-wide ramifications. In the management of GERD-related symptoms and consequential complications, nonetheless, a synthesis of lifestyle modifications, pharmacology, and, in some cases, surgery is required. Proton pump inhibitors (PPIs) are generally prescribed to reduce acid secretion and relieve symptoms, but variability of patient response can complicate treatment. Despite aggressive treatment, most with GERD continue to experience persistent symptoms or develop additional extraesophageal complications , such as chronic cough or laryngitis, implying the need for other alternative therapies (Chen et al., 2023). Therefore, present-day clinical practice and research focus on building total treatment regimens that combine both lifestyle and medical treatments appropriate to the particular needs of each patient, demonstrating the dynamic nature of GERD as a complex esophageal illness (Figure 3.8).

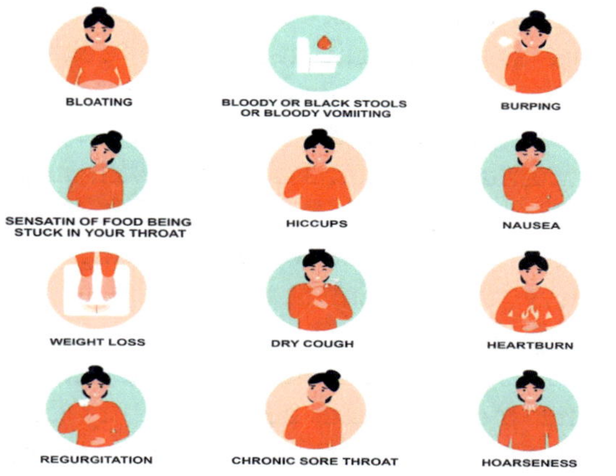

Figure 3.8. Symptoms and complications of GERD.

Source: https://gastro-md.com/wp-content/uploads/2013/08/GERD3-scaled.jpg.

3.2.3. Treatment Options for GERD

The treatment of gastroesophageal reflux disease (GERD) involves a multimodal approach that incorporates lifestyle modification, pharmacologic management, and surgery. Lifestyle change is usually the first line and encompasses dietary adjustment, weight loss, and elevation of the head, which can benefit mild symptoms in the majority of patients. Abstaining from some provocations like caffeine, alcohol, and spicy foods may significantly limit the occurrence of reflux. If lifestyle modification is not sufficient, pharmacologic therapy, with proton pump inhibitors (PPIs) as central treatment, is generally advised to effectively block gastric acid secretion. Although PPIs can be effective in reducing heartburn and other esophageal-specific symptoms, they are less effective against conditions , such as volume regurgitation, which is often a manifestation of mechanical issues at the esophagogastric junction and increased transient lower esophageal sphincter relaxations (TLESRs) (Patel et al., 2024). Therefore, treatment selection needs to be based on an accurate individualization of each patient's symptoms and pathophysiology. When medical treatments are not adequately relieving symptoms, more invasive therapies need to be used. Fundoplication and other surgical procedures assist in tightening the lower esophageal sphincter (LES) and thereby reduce the frequency of reflux. These treatments are typically reserved in patients with severe GERD or its complications, such as esophagitis or Barrett's esophagus. Furthermore, new endoscopic technologies have been developed that provide alternatives to surgery to offer less invasive ways of attaining similar outcomes. These endoluminal approaches typically function to enhance the function of the LES or reduce gastric reflux by various mechanisms, such as tissue manipulation or prosthetic devices. As surgical and endoscopic therapies may have different risk profiles and benefits, the choice of therapy should be patient-centered, keeping in mind the patient's background and severity of the disease (Aleman et al., 2020). The rising epidemic of obesity has complicated the management of GERD, particularly in bariatric surgery patients, which has been associated with the pathogenesis of de novo GERD. The altered anatomy resulting from such interventions is an etiology of a unique pattern of complications, which demands close observation and customized interventions for affected patients. Management strategies in such situations are often based on a combination of non-operative, endoluminal, and operative interventions with the goal of symptom and complication reduction. Therefore, post-operative management of GERD must consider both short- and long-term effects of various interventions. With the emergence of the specialty based on novel surgical techniques and modalities of treatment, the clinicians will need to hone their procedures further to optimize the quality of care, emphasizing the imperative for treatment plans with each patient's specificity and responsive to the idiosyncrasies of that patient's condition (Aleman et al., 2020) (Figure 3.9).

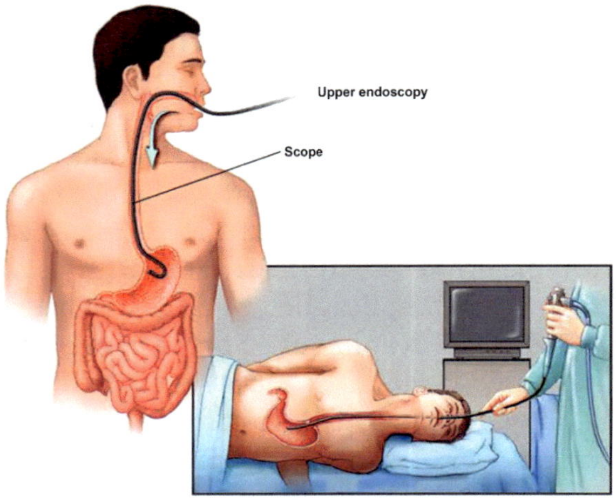

Figure 3.9. Treatment options for GERD.

Source: https://www.mayoclinic.org/-/media/kcms/gbs/patient-consumer/images/2016/05/02/14/44/mcdc7_endoscopy-8col.jpg.

3.3. Esophageal Motility Disorders

Esophageal motility disorders are a range of dysfunctions caused by defects in the coordinated muscle contractions that enable the passage of food along the esophagus. Achalasia, distal esophageal spasm, and jackhammer esophagus all share abnormal or disrupted motor patterns leading to marked esophageal dysphagia, which is difficult to diagnose and treat. These disorders are often diagnosed with high-resolution manometry (HRM), which has changed our understanding of esophageal motor function and types, allowing more precise descriptions of such complex conditions. Because they are rare and present subtly, successful treatment and diagnosis rely on a detailed understanding of the mechanisms involved and the treatment modalities available for presentation to clinicians treating such cohorts (Feng et al., 2019). The evolution of treatment for esophageal motility disorders comes as a growing body of work seeks to utilize minimally invasive techniques. Among these, peroral endoscopic myotomy (POEM) is now an important avenue for treatment, particularly for achalasia. The procedure is intended to minimize the invasiveness that has traditionally been associated with surgical myotomy and provides a means of eliminating obstructive symptoms while enhancing patient recovery time. POEM has been productive in treating not only achalasia but also other spastic esophageal conditions and achieving normal motility and better quality of life for involved patients. However, care must always be exercised against post-procedure complications, particularly an augmented risk of gastroesophageal reflux disease (GERD) that may impact long-term patient outcomes. More research will be needed to illuminate the total efficacy of POEM in the overall treatment of esophageal motility disorder (Feng et al., 2019). Comprehending the correlation between gastroesophageal reflux disease (GERD) and esophageal motility disorders will also be crucial when creating treatment plans. Symptoms for most esophageal motility disorders are comparable or can overlap with symptoms of GERD, complicating the diagnosis process for physicians. This point of intersection needs an informed evaluation of patients, particularly in the case of the use of pharmacological therapy , such as proton pump inhibitors, which are commonly employed in treating GERD. While treatments , such as calcium channel blockers and nitrates are common for spastic motility disorders, the efficacy of these medications may vary with patient profiles and the disorder. Thus, management involving gastroenterologists and primary care physicians is necessary to enable appropriate diagnosis, the best choice of treatment, and optimal care of esophageal motility disorders (Lang et al., 2019) (Figure 3.10).

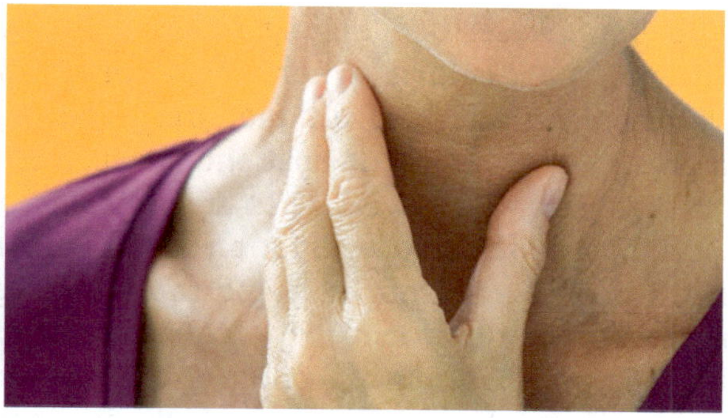

Figure 3.10. Esophageal motility disorders.

Source: https://s3-us-west-2.amazonaws.com/utsw-patientcare-web-production/original_images/esophageal-motility-disorders-600x338.jpg.

3.3.1. Types of Motility Disorders (e.g., Achalasia, Diffuse Esophageal Spasm)

Esophageal motility disorders are a class of dysfunctions secondary to peristalsis dysregulation, leading to systemic disease in involved patients. Among these, achalasia is one such primary disorder with failure of the lower esophageal sphincter to relax adequately, leading to obstruction and profound dysphagia. Achalasia has been postulated to be related to ganglion cell degeneration of the myenteric plexus, which inhibits normal coordination between muscular contractions. Consequently, the patients can experience chest pain and regurgitation, significantly impairing their quality of life. Diagnosis is usually made on the basis of esophageal manometry, showing an elevated resting pressure of the lower esophageal sphincter. Imaging studies, such as barium swallow examinations, can also show characteristic dilatation of the esophagus, making the diagnosis of achalasia and serving as a basis for potential treatment modalities. The other significant motility disorder is diffuse esophageal spasm, which is typified by uncoordinated, frequently forceful, intermittent contractions. Diffuse esophageal spasm lacks an obstruction, as opposed to achalasia, but rather takes the form of incapacitating chest pain and retrosternal pain on swallowing. The spasms can be uncomfortable enough to result in ineffective passage of food down the esophagus and thus cause dysphagia and even regurgitation. The underlying pathophysiologic mechanisms of them are still being explored, though other studies indicate a possible connection with esophageal hyperreactivity or nerve damage. Diagnosis more often involves esophageal manometry, which identifies these spasmodic contractions, and symptom-provoking tests might be necessary for certain diagnoses. Effective treatment can involve dietary alterations and pharmacologic therapy aimed at relaxing the musculature of the esophagus, which has the potential to alleviate symptoms for patients suffering from this debilitating condition. Epiphrenic diverticula also present as a major problem when motility disorders are being considered, particularly in achalasia or diffuse esophageal spasm. Epiphrenic diverticula are a form of dysmotility that may cause chronic symptoms , such as regurgitation, aspiration, and cough, which tend to be exacerbated by the underlying esophageal disorder. While they are false diverticula, formed by the weakness of the wall of the esophagus, symptomatic presentation usually necessitates treatment directed both at diverticula and at the associated motility disorder. Surgical intervention, such as myotomy, and more recent endoscopic interventions like peroral endoscopic myotomy (POEM) have been successful, thus essentially equating management of diverticula with management of the underlying disorder of motility. Notably, Nitsa et al. (2025) reports that the effective management of epiphrenic diverticula is highly effective in improving symptomatology in affected patients. Further,

Kim et al. (2020) reports that POEM is proving to be a useful intervention for various esophageal motility disorders, citing its efficacy in achieving symptom relief with an acceptable safety profile.

3.3.2. Symptoms and Diagnosis of Motility Disorders

The symptoms of esophageal motility disorders are variable or overt, typically making clinical diagnosis difficult. Dysphagia, the feeling of food being stuck in the chest or throat, is caused by abnormal peristalsis, where usual muscle contractions are interrupted. Painful swallowing, regurgitation, and reflux are some of the additional symptoms. Of significance is the fact that dysmotility at times can be nonsymptomatic, particularly in the case of severe obesity, whereby high-resolution manometry tests have shown the association of considerable motility disorders without apparent clinical manifestations (Difante et al., 2024). Therefore, a complete dependence on symptomatology can lead to underdiagnosis or misdiagnosis of underlying motility disorders and therefore, emphasizes the necessity of proper evaluation. The clinical diagnosis of esophageal motility disorders has also been revolutionized, with the advent of high-resolution manometry (HREM) as the gold standard. HREM yields detailed esophageal pressure patterns that allow accurate diagnosis of numerous motility disorders, including achalasia and nonachalasia disorders (Jain, 2023). To confirm a diagnosis, clinicians are likely to combine HREM information with clinical presentation and other imaging techniques, e.g., timed barium esophagogram and functional lumen imaging probe, which offer additional information concerning esophageal function. Moreover, adjunctive studies in the form of multiple rapid swallows and rapid drink challenges are increasingly recognized for their potential in enhancing the diagnostic accuracy, particularly when primary symptoms are not discovered in straightforward forms typical of well-defined motility disorder patterns. Despite the advancement in diagnostic modalities, the clinical application of findings in motility disorders is often wide and can vary considerably between patients. For instance, prevalent cases of esophageal motility disorders have been described among severely obese patients, particularly where most of them are asymptomatic before undergoing surgical interventions, complicating patient management and care (Difante et al., 2024). In these instances, precise preoperative evaluation with HREM has a pivotal role, not only for the planning of the surgery but also for the prediction of the postoperative course, including the risk for dysphagia or other postoperative complications related to motility following bariatric surgery. As the science of motility disorders advances, there is more and more emphasis upon integrating both clinical and diagnostic paradigms to further optimize patient outcomes in the management of esophageal disorder symptoms (Figure 3.11).

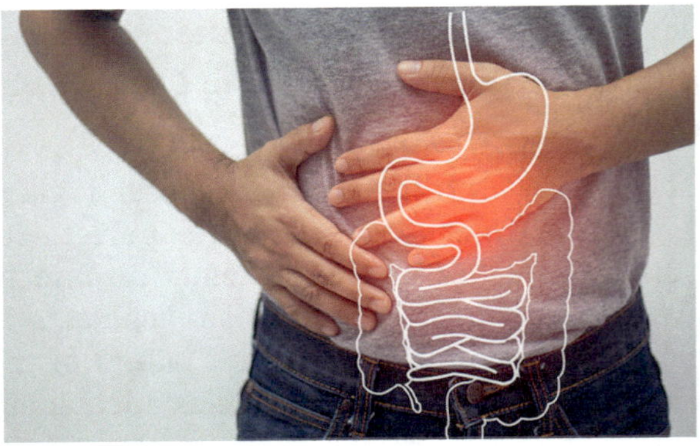

Figure 3.11. Symptoms and diagnosis of motility disorders.

Source: https://backoffice.lepetitjournal.com/sites/default/files/2023-08/Motilite-Bumrungrad.jpg.

3.3.3. Management and Treatment Strategies

Effective management and treatment of esophageal disorders are holistic and require a systemic approach in every patient. The initial step is a complete assessment consisting of medical history, physical examination, and laboratory investigation to detect specific dysfunctions associated with esophageal disorders. For instance, in the case of pediatric feeding disorders, therapists might adopt the model of the World Health Organization International Classification of Functioning, Disability, and Health to inform practice so that medical, nutritional, and psychosocial aspects are merged in an understanding of the patient's requirements. By focusing on these diverse domains, medical practitioners can provide interventions that not only influence the esophageal symptoms but also the overall quality of life (Browne et al., 2019). Pharmacologic treatments have a significant role to play in managing esophageal disorders, particularly those with motility issues or acid reflux. Medications , such as proton pump inhibitors (PPIs) are most commonly prescribed to reduce the production of gastric acid, thus alleviating symptoms of gastroesophageal reflux disease (GERD). In addition to drug therapy, changes in lifestyle, including dietary modification and weight loss, are also necessary to optimize response to treatment. These methods are essential in correcting the underlying causes of the disorders and minimizing complications of medication overuse, particularly in vulnerable populations , such as the elderly or those with a complex health history (Meltzer et al., 2025). Surgery can become essential where conservative treatment fails to relieve symptoms or where there is pronounced structural deformity. Procedures , such as fundoplication for GERD or dilatation for esophageal strictures are just a couple of examples of how surgical means can actually restore function and reduce symptoms. Also, frequent monitoring of patient outcomes of these surgical techniques is required in order to optimize long-term success. This integrated strategy of uniting surgical techniques with stringent follow-up highlights the necessity for a proactive healthcare policy that adapts to the complexity of managing esophageal illnesses in order to promote efficiency as well as qualitative care in the management techniques employed in clinical practice (Browne et al., 2019).

3.4. Esophagitis

Esophagitis, a condition characterized by inflammation of the esophagus, occurs in a number of different ways, with gastroesophageal reflux disease (GERD) and eosinophilic esophagitis (EoE) being the most significant. EoE, an immune-mediated disorder, results in eosinophilic infiltration of the mucosa of the esophagus, which creates marked dysphagia and food impaction. Its prevalence has increased since its original description in the 1990s, and it is now a focus area in gastrointestinal health. The criteria for the diagnosis of EoE are visualization of more than 15 eosinophils per high-power field in esophageal biopsies and clinical evidence of esophageal dysfunction. GERD, on the contrary, is a more common cause of esophagitis where stomach contents reflux into the esophagus, causing inflammation and mucosal damage. The diagnosis of both conditions is important to the proper treatment and diagnosis of esophageal disorders in the clinical environment (Pastuszka et al., 2025). The differentiation between GERD and EoE is still a complex issue in the clinical environment because both conditions can share common symptoms, but should be treated separately. EoE is often comorbid with other allergic conditions and necessitates careful evaluation involving dietary modification, proton pump inhibitors (PPIs), and topical corticosteroids. Nevertheless, GERD itself is usually treatable with lifestyle changes and medications of standard practice, and an accurate diagnosis is thus paramount. Current evidence indicates that a percentage of patients with refractory GERD may be hosting occult EoE, justifying a strict adherence to endoscopic and histologic criteria in endoscopic evaluations. In a research study with Egyptian patients, EoE prevalence was reported in 4%

of those who were non-responders to GERD treatment. The observation highlights the necessity for differential diagnoses in patients with persistent esophageal symptoms (Gadallah et al., 2025).

Treatment of esophagitis requires a multi-dimensional approach that is specific to the etiology and chronicity of the condition. Long-term management is particularly crucial in EoE, recognized as a chronic illness where ongoing therapeutic interventions are required to modulate symptoms and esophageal remodeling. Elimination diets with pharmacologic therapies yield promising outcomes; however, these halt disease progression altogether. Novel biologic therapies targeting some inflammatory pathways hold thrilling potential, though much more research is necessary to maximize these. For GERD, focus is directed towards symptomatic control and prevention of chronic reflux-related complications. Both diseases necessitate aggressive management of patients to improve quality of life and prevent potential esophageal complications, further establishing the need for sophisticated understanding and ongoing research in the field of esophageal disease (Pastuszka et al., 2025) (Figure 3.12).

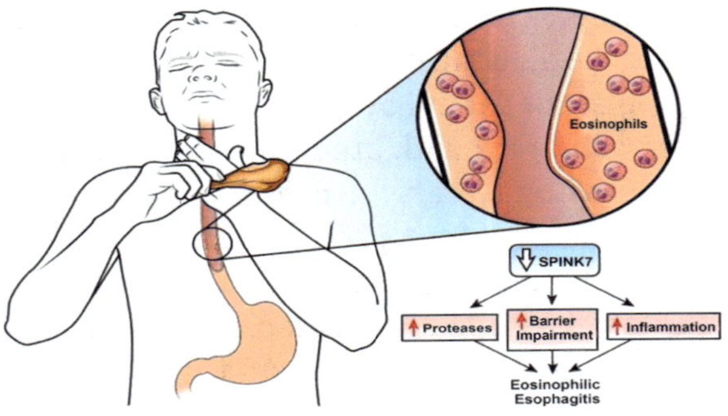

Figure 3.12. Esophagitis.

Source: https://www.homenaturalcures.com/wp-content/uploads/Eosinophilic-esophagitis-1068x641.jpg.

3.4.1. Definition and Types of Esophagitis (e.g., Reflux, Infectious)

Esophagitis is a condition of inflammation of the esophagus that can be caused by various etiologic factors and has a variety of clinical manifestations. Gastroesophageal reflux disease (GERD), the most frequent manifestation of esophagitis, is defined as retrograde backflow of stomach contents into the esophagus. Backflow can provoke an inflammatory response, manifesting as mucosal damage, erosions, and sometimes ulcerations. Clinically, patients usually come in with symptoms , such as heartburn, regurgitation, and dysphagia. Chronic inflammation may result in esophageal lining damage and, if untreated, subsequent complications , such as esophageal strictures or Barrett's esophagus, a precancerous condition secondary to long-term acid gastric content exposure (Cairns & Kang, 2022). Understanding the pathophysiology of reflux esophagitis is important in instituting effective prevention and management policies. Other than reflux esophagitis, infectious esophagitis is also a major category of the condition, particularly in immunocompromised patients. The offending pathogens most likely to be responsible include Candida spp., herpes simplex virus (HSV), and cytomegalovirus (CMV). With the offending pathogen, presentation varies depending on the pathogen, with the patient experiencing dysphagia, odynophagia, and retrosternal chest pain. Diagnostic evaluation is typically performed by endoscopy to establish visual examination of esophageal mucosa and yield biopsies for histology, which is particularly useful in distinguishing between the infectious pathogens (Pouw et al., 2021). When viral esophagitis is suspected, it is best to take a few target biopsies in order to identify the pathogen causing it accurately, thereby permitting appropriate therapeutic interventions. Infectious esophagitis should be managed with prompt diagnosis and targeted antimicrobial treatment depending upon the etiology. Eosinophilic esophagitis (EoE) is another newly recognized entity of esophagitis in patients with atopy or food allergy. It is defined by the presence of greater eosinophilic infiltrate in the esophageal epithelium and can lead to severe dysfunction of the esophagus, e.g., dysphagia and food impaction. Clinical suspicion would prompt endoscopic evaluation, where biopsies are obtained from the distal and proximal esophagus to establish the eosinophil content—vital to a firm diagnosis (Pouw et al., 2021). As awareness of EoE increases, it is more important to be mindful and study its pathophysiology, its predisposing factors, and optimal management. Together, these categories of esophagitis highlight the heterogeneity and complexity of the disease of the esophagus and demand a keen awareness of prudent clinical stewardship.

3.4.2. Causes and Risk Factors for Esophagitis

Esophagitis, or esophagitis inflammation, can be caused by several factors that largely affect the prevalence of the condition. One significant factor is gastroesophageal reflux disease (GERD), where stomach acids frequently flow back into the esophagus, causing damage and inflammation of the mucosa. Lifestyle factors , such as diet, obesity, and smoking, however, make the condition worse by being a possible cause of increased abdominal pressure and acid production. In addition, certain medications, particularly the non-steroidal anti-inflammatory drugs (NSAIDs) and antibiotics, tend to cause chemical irritation and damage the esophageal lining. The interaction of these factors creates a complex interface of esophagitis that demands deep insights into environmental and physiological components that can exacerbate or mitigate this disease. Infectious esophagitis is another significant category of esophagitis that typically occurs following infection with opportunistic pathogens in immunocompromised hosts but increasingly also in immunocompetent hosts. Candida, herpes simplex virus, and cytomegalovirus are the most common pathogens infecting the esophagus, each with particular diagnostic and therapeutic challenges. The rise in prevalence of such infections can be attributed to various risk factors, including the usage of antibiotics, which disrupt the natural flora, and underlying conditions like diabetes and HIV. Patients presenting with odynophagia or dysphagia should be evaluated for these infections, as this emphasizes the importance of early diagnosis and treatment to prevent complications of uncomplicated esophageal infections (Hoversten et al., 2018).

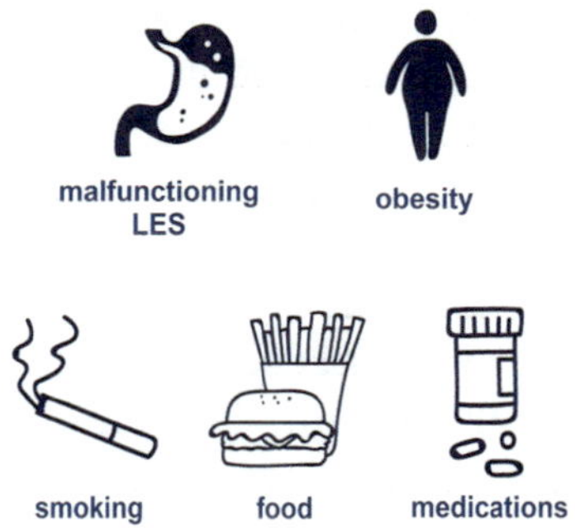

Figure 3.13. Causes and risk factors for esophagitis.

Source: https://www.drsamratjankar.com/wp-content/uploads/2022/03/risk-factors-of-esophagitis-1.jpg.

Also, structural esophageal defects can predispose a patient to major esophagitis. Achalasia, or difficulty in swallowing due to malfunction of the esophageal muscles, is one such disorder that provides an environment where the esophagus is prone to irritation and resulting inflammation. Esophageal food stasis results in bacterial overgrowth and mucosal damage, creating frank esophagitis. It has been shown through research that achalasia patients present more pronounced histological alterations and a higher proliferation index, indicating a higher risk of neoplastic development in the long term (Lee et al., 2020). These structural risk factors are important to identify for clinicians as they determine clinical management strategies that are directed towards symptom relief and avoidance of further development of more serious esophageal disease (Figure 3.13).

3.4.3. Treatment and Prevention of Esophagitis

Its treatment and prevention also rest on getting the proper diagnosis of the root cause, which may be conditions like exposure to an irritant, infection, or gastroesophageal reflux disease (GERD). In esophagitis whose major cause is GERD, treatment often starts with modification of lifestyle , such as dietary regulations and weight control, to control symptoms. In addition, medications like proton pump inhibitors (PPIs) are often used to suppress the formation of stomach acid and allow healing to take place in the esophageal mucosa. The effectiveness of these interventions is demonstrated in a systematic review of literature assessing therapeutic interventions in children and adults with esophagitis secondary to GERD, emphasizing the importance of individually tailored management strategies according to patient-specific features (Nicholas et al., 2018). If the etiology of esophagitis is infectious, e.g., from candidiasis or herpes simplex virus, antifungal and antiviral agents take prominent roles in treatment. Moreover, identification of potentially injurious substances, such as specific medications or corrosives, plays a crucial role in prevention and management strategies. Patients are educated about the avoidance of known offending drugs as well as compliance with proper medication schedules. The development of chronic primary pain as a result of untreated esophagitis can be approached with the biopsychosocial method, whereby care is not just thorough in eliminating symptoms but also includes emotional and functional impact (Nicholas et al., 2018). This kind of holistic care is vital in achieving optimal recovery and prevention of recurrence. Prevention of esophagitis mainly relies on risk factor control of its various causes. For individuals predisposed to GERD, anticipatory measures like smaller meals, avoidance of offending foods, and remaining upright after meals will significantly lower the chances of inflammation of the esophagus. Regular medical follow-up, coupled with appropriate screenings in the higher-risk patient for infectious esophagitis, are preventive supports to identify impending issues early on. Educating patients in the areas of maintaining a healthy diet and lifestyle can ensure long-term esophageal health. Additionally, ongoing research on esophageal disorders management validates the refinement of prevention strategies and the development of guidelines to reduce the incidence of esophagitis among different groups (Rosen et al., 2018). Through collaborative treatment and prevention programs, esophagitis burden can be effectively overcome (Figure 3.14).

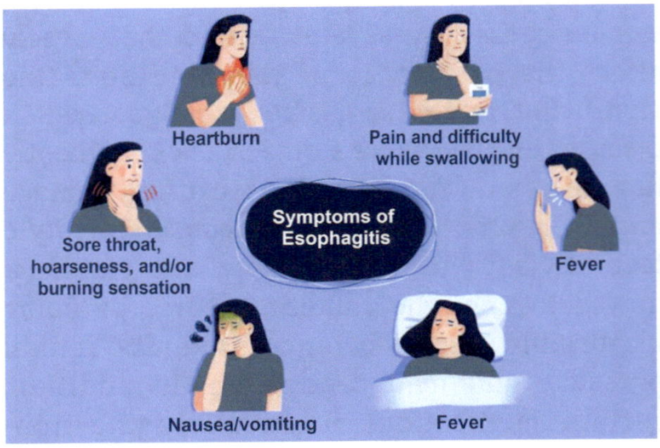

Figure 3.14. Treatment and prevention of esophagitis

Source: https://www.dravinashtank.in/wp-content/uploads/2023/06/Esophagitis-e1693901048235.png.

3.5. Esophageal Cancer

Esophageal cancer represents a severe disease, being one of the more aggressive forms of malignancies occurring in the gastrointestinal tract. The disease most often occurs in two types of histology: adenocarcinoma and squamous cell carcinoma. Squamous cell carcinoma is most often related to risk factors of heavy alcohol consumption and tobacco use, while adenocarcinoma has increasingly been associated with gastroesophageal reflux disease and obesity. The development from Barrett's esophagus, a precancerous state occurring as a result of chronic GERD, is the quintessential example of how chronic irritation may predispose to dysplastic alterations in the lining of the esophagus, thus elevating cancer risk. Early diagnosis is essential, but for symptoms , such as dysphagia, which usually occur only in late stages, makes surgical management difficult. The challenge here highlights the urgency for better screening methods and education to the public regarding the risks of esophageal cancer and its precursors. Progressive esophageal cancer is a clinical challenge in that the patients usually come with an acute impairment of swallowing, known as dysphagia. Such complications severely restrict the quality of life because the patient has trouble feeding and nutrition. The treatment is based on the stage of the cancer, but stenting with self-expanding metallic stents (SEMS) has been the most widely used palliative treatment to reduce malignant dysphagia. Where gastric cancer extends to the distal esophagus, for instance, SEMS stenting will immediately alleviate symptoms, as evidenced by recent patient case series. Effective stenting not only corrects dysphagia but also permits patients to continue receiving essential nutritional interventions while undergoing the remaining course of their treatment. This approach reflects the necessity of palliative care as a critical component of managing esophageal cancer, helping patients live a sense of normalcy and what it is despite their unfavorable prognosis (Amarendra et al., 2013). The intersection of esophageal cancer and gastroesophageal reflux disease (GERD) highlights the necessity for early detection and intervention practices. The increasing trend of GERD has been a subject of concern, especially given its association with esophageal cancers. The condition is especially insidious since it may lead to silent reflux and thus dental erosion and other complications that may go unnoticed by clinicians. Clinical suspicion of these associations is vital since unexplained dental erosion may be the precursor of an acid-related disorder. Given that studies more and more prove GERD's relationship with esophageal cancer, practitioners are urged to adopt holistic management approaches aimed at dental as well as enteric health in patients with reflux symptoms. The interconnectedness betrays the need for a holistic approach to knowing and combating esophageal disorders (Ranjitkar et al., 2011) (Figure 3.15).

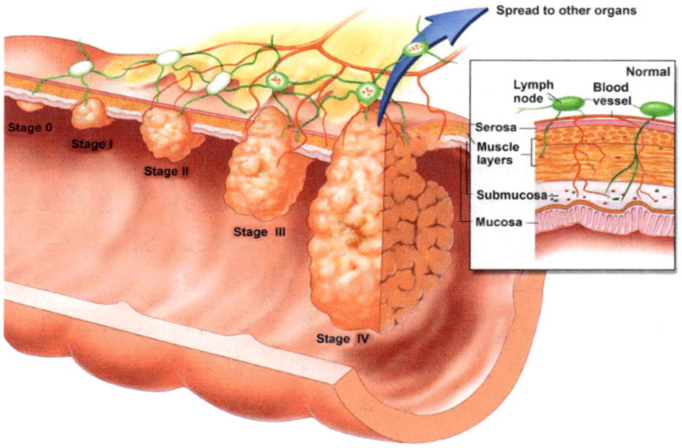

Figure 3.15. Esophageal cancer.

Source: https://healthjade.com/wp-content/uploads/2018/01/esophageal-cancer.jpg.

3.5.1. Types of Esophageal Cancer (e.g., Squamous Cell Carcinoma, Adenocarcinoma)

Categorization of esophageal cancer predominantly consists of two principal forms: squamous cell carcinoma (SCC) and adenocarcinoma. Squamous cell carcinoma is the type that originates from the squamous cells lining the esophagus and is prevalent in regions with high incidence rates of tobacco and alcohol consumption. Adenocarcinoma, however, arises from the glandular cells at the lower end of the esophagus, which is typically associated with chronic gastroesophageal reflux disease (GERD) and Barrett's esophagus. The surge in obesity rates has also grown the incidence of adenocarcinoma, as it is associated with the rising rate of acid reflux diseases that erode the esophagus lining. Being aware of these distinctions is crucial because they influence clinical management and therapeutic strategies employed for victims of these cancers. Having a clear knowledge of the risk factors of these cancers can lead to more effective prevention and early detection. Trends in populations of esophageal cancer reflect wide variations in incidence as well as survival between the two forms. SCC affects mainly older persons and is more commonly found in men, particularly in Asian and African populations. Epidemiological studies show a negative correlation between allergic inflammation and cancer risk, and the existence of certain allergic diseases would lead to reduced incidence of esophageal SCC (Kabir et al., 2021). Adenocarcinoma, however, has shown rising incidence in Western countries, especially in young men, which may be due to alterations in lifestyle that have led to higher rates of obesity and GERD. This epidemiologic transition calls for a twofold strategy of preventive interventions targeted towards high-risk groups and targeted screening programs to detect esophageal adenocarcinoma in its early stages. Enhanced information and education about such forms, considering demographic variables, are essential for effective public health measures. The prognosis for diagnosed esophageal cancer varies dramatically between SCC and adenocarcinoma based on the stage of diagnosis, as well as the underlying biology of the tumors. Both are characterized by aggressiveness and poor survival, but evidence indicates that adenocarcinoma has a poorer prognosis following diagnosis. Effective treatments include surgical excision, chemotherapy, and radiotherapy, tailored based on the histological type and stage of the cancer. Research still investigates the relationship between metabolic avidity and the nature of tumors, as is evident from research in associated sciences, e.g., lung carcinoma (Divisi et al., 2021). These findings highlight the relevance of novel therapies targeted at specific pathways of cancer. As further studies try to unravel the biological mechanisms of esophageal cancer, the medical community must remain aware of differences between cancers. This could maximize treatment options and move patient success considerably in this challenging area.

3.5.2. Risk Factors and Symptoms of Esophageal Cancer

Esophageal cancer is a severe health issue, particularly due to its complex interdependence of risk factors. Most prominent among these is lifestyle, with smoking and excessive alcohol consumption the primary contributors. The carcinogenicity of tobacco and the capacity of alcohol to damage cells further increase the risk of esophageal cell mutation. In addition, obesity has also emerged as an important risk factor, and it is linked to gastroesophageal reflux disease (GERD), which subsequently may lead to Barrett's esophagus—a premalignant lesion. Environmental exposure, such as exposure to certain chemicals, is also involved, particularly in occupational settings. Moreover, human papillomavirus (HPV) was also reported to be linked with certain subtypes of esophageal cancer, proving the multifactorial etiology of the disease. Individually and collectively, these conditions are responsible for the rising incidence of esophageal cancer, emphasizing the importance of preventive targeting and early detection among these risk groups. The symptomatology of esophageal cancer most frequently is such that it profoundly impacts patients' quality of life. It can involve dysphagia, or swallowing disturbance, the feeling of food stuck in the throat or chest. This symptom is particularly distressing and can cause weight loss and malnutrition, further complicating the patient's underlying health problems. Pain in the chest, heartburn, and unintentional weight loss are some other common symptoms. Patients also have a complaint of cough or hoarseness, which, if accompanied by these other symptoms, can indicate more severe disease. In one study evaluating patients with esophageal cancer, it was discovered that a large percentage had accompanying gastrointestinal symptoms that reflect the interrelated character of esophageal health and general physical well-being (Luo et al., 2023).

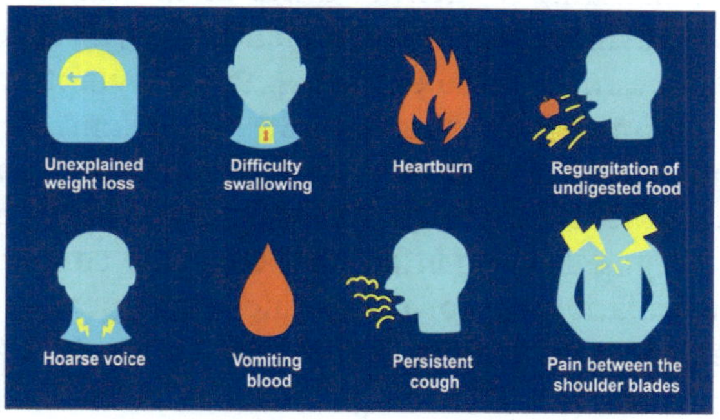

Figure 3.16. Risk factors and symptoms of esophageal cancer.

Source: https://www.verywellhealth.com/thmb/XDtf1Fg0U7XCcO5AFrFQpXN-iAE=/1500x0/filters:no_upscale():max_bytes(150000):strip_icc()/esophageal-cancer-overview-1741801_final-01-1e72286507304912b6cca0f73b1e85dd.jpg.

These symptoms tend to trigger mental health problems as well, compounding the psychological burden on suffering individuals. The psychological implications of esophageal cancer must not be underestimated, especially at the peri-radiotherapy stage. Research sets the fact that there is a high percentage of patients who experience negative feelings of depression and anxiety, which play a critical role in influencing their nutritional status and treatment outcomes. Specifically, results indicate that approximately 18.3% of patients experienced negative feelings during treatment, resulting in malnutrition rates of 41.9% (Luo et al., 2023). Factors , such as economic status, aggressiveness of cancer (TNM stage), and comorbid disease have been identified as independent predictors of these negative emotional states. This suggests that physical and psychological health are strongly interconnected in the care of esophageal cancer. Thus, providing whole patient care to address psychological and nutritional needs is the utmost priority to improve prognoses in patients and quality of life in a stressful treatment regimen (Figure 3.16).

3.5.3. Diagnosis and Treatment Options for Esophageal Cancer

Diagnosis of esophageal cancer is a multifaceted endeavor and most commonly begins with a thorough clinical evaluation of the patient's history and symptoms that are presented, commonly including dysphagia, weight loss, and chest discomfort. Diagnostic imaging plays a central role in the detection and staging of esophageal cancer; imaging tests like computed tomography (CT) scans and endoscopic ultrasound (EUS) are commonly utilized. Endoscopy is particularly valuable, with the option of direct visualization of the esophagus lining and biopsy sampling for histological analysis. High-resolution manometry can be employed to check for esophageal motility, differentiating cancer from other diseases, such as achalasia, that present similarly (Han et al., 2023). A comprehensive diagnosis is imperative in an attempt to create an appropriate treatment plan and rule out other conditions that could present similarly to esophageal cancer and ultimately influence the patient's management and prognosis. The treatment of esophageal cancer relies on the location and stage of the tumors, and a multidisciplinary approach is often required for optimal outcomes in patients. Surgical resection is the primary curative therapy for localized carcinoma of the esophagus, most commonly with esophagectomy. A few are not surgical candidates due to comorbidities or extensive disease. In such cases, neoadjuvant therapy, including chemoradiation, may be employed to reduce the tumor before surgery or palliate symptoms in advanced cases. The incorporation of targeted drugs and immunotherapy, including therapies directed against the HER2 and PD-L1 targets, has provided access to novel therapeutic methods for metastatic disease (Ajani et al., 2022).

Multimodal therapies aim to maximize survival and improve the quality of life, underlining the importance of tailoring therapies to the individual clinical presentation of the patient. Endoscopic interventions have emerged as the standard of care for esophageal cancer in the role of definitive treatment as palliation, particularly in patients no longer considered surgical candidates for curative resection. Endoscopic mucosal resection (EMR) and endoscopic submucosal dissection (ESD) are techniques through which early cancers may be excised with minimal invasiveness but preserve esophageal function. Palliative endoscopic stenting also serves to alleviate dysphagia secondary to occluding tumors, thereby improving the quality of life for patients with advanced disease. Although the role of regular endoscopic follow-up in high-risk populations, such as achalasia patients, is not clearly established, there is hope for early detection and intervention with advances in endoscopic instrumentation, which would avoid further evolution to malignancy (Han et al., 2023). Continuous research and clinical trials will be required to establish the best practices and guidelines for the management of esophageal cancer, given the dynamic and evolving nature of treatments available.

3.6. Other Esophageal Disorders

Various esophageal illnesses fall outside the better-known conditions like gastroesophageal reflux disease (GERD) and esophagitis, for which an impeccable, comprehensive understanding is required to manage them. Of such illnesses, extraesophageal presentations of GERD or extraesophageal reflux (EER) present a number of diagnostic and therapeutic challenges. The usual symptoms may include persistent cough, laryngitis, and even dental erosions, which make it challenging to identify GERD as the cause. As noted in more recent recommendations, a proper evaluation of these extraesophageal symptoms is paramount for treating GERD clinicians. This multi-factorial approach demands coordination with other specialties, including pulmonology and otolaryngology, to effectively treat the complex interrelationship of reflux and other potential pathological conditions (Chen et al., 2023). Furthermore, EER diagnosis is typically also complicated by the lack of a solitary definitive test, again pointing up the usefulness of a full clinical assessment that incorporates symptom evaluation along with diagnostic evaluation. Along with EER, another significant esophageal disease includes Barrett's esophagus, a disorder that is premalignant as a consequence of chronic acid exposure. This condition presents as a metaplastic transformation of the esophagus lining and is generally asymptomatic, so that early treatment is difficult. Due to its association with adenocarcinoma of the esophagus, patients with Barrett's esophagus must be evaluated frequently by endoscopy to check for dysplasia. The guidelines point out the necessity of informing the patient about his disease, risk, and the necessity of surveillance. Significantly, recent studies have begun to concentrate on the function of chemerin and its receptors in gastrointestinal illness, including Barrett's esophagus. Chemerin has been implicated in immune-modulating reactions with esophageal pathologies, which suggests increasing interest in the potential for it to be used as a drug target or biomarker (Jacenik et al., 2020). Lastly, motility disorders of the esophagus, such as achalasia and esophageal spasm, finish the list of diseases of the esophagus. Achalasia, secondary to an inability of the lower esophageal sphincter to relax, often results in dysphagia, regurgitation, and weight loss. Achalasia is managed by a range of maneuvers from pneumatic dilation to surgery like myotomy, each with its own risks and benefits. The same process, indeed, can lead to blinding chest pain and dysphagia in esophageal spasms. In understanding the pathophysiology and symptomatology responsible for such disorders, one should be capable of designing proper curative plans. Manometry and esophageal pH testing play a critical role in the diagnosis and treatment of these motility disorders, offering an evidence-based model of care. As more esophageal disorders continue to prevail, there is a need for constant investigation and clinical insight to improve patient outcomes (Figure 3.17).

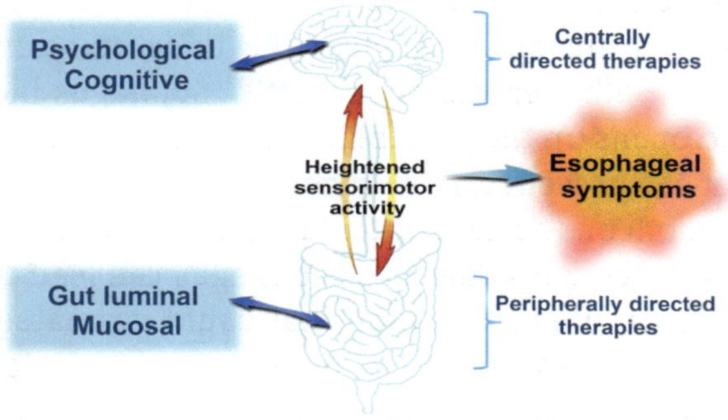

Figure 3.17. Other esophageal disorders.

Source: https://els-jbs-prod-cdn.jbs.elsevierhealth.com/cms/attachment/1039fc07-dece-453f-9662-59fc725cfced/gr1_lrg.jpg.

3.6.1. Esophageal Strictures and Their Causes

Esophageal strictures are a difficult clinical condition and are classified as a narrowing of the esophagus that impedes the flow of food and liquids. Esophageal strictures can result from a number of etiologic causes, including chronic gastroesophageal reflux disease (GERD), which leads to inflammation and scarring of the lining of the esophagus. Over time, the constant exposure to stomach acid causes a cycle of tissue injury and repair with resultant promotion of stricture formation. Esophageal strictures may also be a sign of a more complicated process of pathophysiology wherein diseases like eosinophilic esophagitis, an inflammatory condition due to food allergens, take center stage. Eosinophilic esophagitis induces invasion of immune cells and tissue remodeling that is favorable to fibrotic modifications, thus leading to severe mechanical stiffening of the esophagus, ultimately forming a stricture (Muir et al., 2018). Caustic agent ingestion is another mechanism of the formation of esophageal strictures, leading to acute and chronic esophageal mucosal damage. This injury needs to be treated due to the potential risk for extensive scarring and fibrosis, particularly when treatment has been partial or delayed. Strictures may also occur secondary to technical problems like postoperative changes or radiation for surrounding malignancies, which can complicate scarring through the mechanism of the inflammatory process (Hunt et al., 2017). In patients receiving dilatation of the esophagus, there is also a recurrence of stricture, which calls for repeated monitoring and may even call for further intervention. All these various etiologies highlight the importance of understanding the mechanisms and background in preparation to formulate effective management programs for strictures of the esophagus. Diagnosis for strictures of the esophagus is primarily obtained from a combination of patient history, symptomatology, and diagnostic imaging techniques , such as endoscopy. Endoscopy not only facilitates direct visualization of the esophageal lumen but also enables the procurement of biopsy samples, which are capable of differentiating between stricture arising from benign and malignant etiology. Treatments following diagnosis include dilation procedures for dilating the esophagus, medical treatment through topical steroids in eosinophilic esophagitis, or surgery in advanced cases (Muir et al., 2018). Lastly, management of esophageal stricture should be multidisciplinary for symptom relief and treatment of the causative underlying disease to improve quality of life and patient outcomes. With the evolving treatment modalities, so evolves the capability of improved patient care with higher diagnostic and therapeutic sophistication.

3.6.2. Barrett's Esophagus and Its Implications

Barrett's esophagus (BE) is a severe alteration of the esophageal lining and happens predominantly as a result of chronic gastroesophageal reflux disease (GERD). The disorder is characterized by the substitution of the normal squamous epithelium lining of the esophagus with a columnar epithelium, a disorder that is traditionally identified as a precursor to adenocarcinoma of the esophagus. BE patients are at increased risk of developing esophageal cancer and thus need strict control and monitoring. Early detection remains the top priority, as findings demonstrate that the incidence of Barrett's esophagus is a significant risk factor for malignancy, with the transformational process indicating an increased need for intense surveillance measures in high-risk populations. Knowledge of Barrett's esophagus risk factors and pathophysiology, therefore, becomes critical for clinicians to minimize the risk of cancerous events and to offer adequate care for patients with a similar condition. Histological intricacies of Barrett's esophagus also play a critical role in its diagnosis and subsequent management. The condition is defined by the presence of Barrett's specialized epithelium, that is, goblet cell metaplasia, which was only fully confirmed using endoscopic biopsy. The importance of careful histologic examination cannot be overemphasized, since the correct record of findings dictates prognosis and therapeutic approach. In clinical practice, successful treatment will often include repeated endoscopic follow-up to detect dysplastic change signifying increased risk of further progression to adenocarcinoma. Such prophylactic intervention is essential, particularly in young people, where the disease can silently present but has intrinsic risks that justify early treatment. Thus, the importance of Barrett's esophagus extends beyond diagnosis to a whole paradigm of long-term management and potential treatment. Growing research elucidates the molecular pathophysiology of Barrett's esophagus and suggests the involvement of claudins in disease pathology. Claudins are a family of proteins that are integral to cellular tight junctions, and their dysregulation is increasingly recognized to be involved in various gastrointestinal disorders, including Barrett's esophagus. It has been proven through research that some claudins, i.e., –1, –2, –3, –4, and –18, exhibit altered expression patterns in pre-neoplastic conditions, and these altered expression patterns may serve as biomarkers for prognosis and early detection. Identification of these molecular changes not only enhances the understanding of the pathogenesis of Barrett's esophagus but also opens up the possibility of targeted therapy that can prevent carcinogenesis. Thus, continued research on the genetic and molecular signature associated with Barrett's esophagus can lead to considerable information that could ultimately translate into improved patient outcomes for this challenging disease (Hassall, 1993; Ouban & Arabi, 2023).

3.6.3. Foreign Body Ingestion and Its Management

Foreign body ingestion is a prevailing clinical issue, especially among certain populations , such as children and elderly adults. The type of foreign bodies presented can be varied from food items, such as bones and shells, to non-food items, such as coins and small toys.

The condition can lead to severe complications like esophageal obstruction or even perforation, necessitating emergent intervention. The initial management relies on symptom severity; mild cases may be followed up, while major events typically require immediate endoscopic removal to avoid complications. Notably, the timing of management is important as it will increase the risk of morbidity and mortality in foreign body ingestion, necessitating identification and adequate training in handling the emergency in clinics (Tringali et al., 2017). Endoscopy is also the standard for both diagnosis and treatment of foreign body ingestion. In kids and teenagers, EGD is particularly useful for visualization and removal of the foreign object, as indicated in most guidelines on the subject (Tringali et al., 2017). This minimal-invasive technique allows clinicians to assess damage to esophageal mucosa safely while evacuating foreign bodies lodged in the esophagus or proximal gastrointestinal system. Furthermore, expertise in such endoscopy is essential to healthcare providers, since ongoing skills acquisition ensures timely and effective intervention, and therefore leads to improved patient outcomes. After foreign bodies have been resistant to endoscopic removal, surgery may be warranted, which highlights the dynamic and case-dependent nature of management. Along with acute management techniques, an overall method for foreign body ingestion would also involve prevention and educational aspects. For instance, educating caregivers and parents about the dangers of certain small objects can decrease the risk of ingestion, particularly among children. Moreover, implementing procedures in emergency departments and outpatient clinics can make the response to such an event effective, allowing for early detection and treatment. Radiologists play the most crucial role in diagnosing foreign body ingestion through adequate imaging, which helps to define the nature and site of the foreign bodies (Caseiro-Alves et al., 2015). Through the encouragement of collaboration between various medical professionals, the general management of foreign body ingestion can significantly improve, adhering to the best practices in esophageal disorders and improving patient safety outcomes.

SUMMARY

In summary, esophageal disorders are a heterogeneous collection of medical diseases that exert a significant impact upon patient quality of life and systemic health. By examining the clinical and physiological manifestations of such diseases, it is apparent that early diagnosis and timely management are essential in maximizing patient prognosis. Diseases like gastroesophageal reflux disease (GERD) and strictures of the esophagus can lead to more severe complications if not addressed, thus the need for healthcare professionals to have a high level of clinical suspicion. Furthermore, understanding the complex interdependence between the motility of the esophagus and the rest of the gastrointestinal tract emphasizes the need to incorporate an all-encompassing approach in treatment and diagnosis. Also. Treating the psychosocial aspects of esophageal illness is integral to comprehensive care. As noted in a study evaluating quality of life in patients with congenital facial weakness, patterns also emerge in patients with esophageal disease. These individuals report poor quality of life for their illnesses and state they feel this way about their conditions, suggesting that clinicians should take supportive care and physical therapy seriously. The findings underscore the influence of psychological well-being on adherence to treatment and overall outcomes and how the findings correlate with the conclusions drawn in studies that have dealt with psychiatric disorders influencing workplace safety (Yama et al., 2024). My conclusion is that the future direction of the management of esophageal disorders should be towards synthesizing multidisciplinary approaches that incorporate medical and psychosocial aspects. With advancements in the treatment of conditions, drug and surgical therapies will also have to be weighed against dietary control, patient education, and counseling. As an illustration, patients undergoing surgical reanimation for facial paralysis indicate results that spill over into areas outside of physical health, and thus a holistic approach to esophageal disorder management must be applied (Liberton et al., 2024). Through inter-disciplinary collaboration of gastroenterologists, dietitians, and mental health professionals, the healthcare system can make an effort towards a complete solution that will enhance the overall quality of life of esophageal disorder patients.

The pathophysiology of esophageal disorders demonstrates a complex interaction among physiological, genetic, and pathophysiologic factors. Esophageal transport, another critical function of this organ, is the coordinated effort between muscular layers to effectively move food that was consumed from the pharynx to the stomach. Dysfunction in this process may be an expression of underlying esophageal disorders. New methods for simulating esophageal dynamics, such as the immersed boundary method, have enhanced our understanding of motility and how it relates to bolus transport and muscle activation. These simulations make comprehensible the esophageal pressure dynamics, enlightening motor function of the esophagus and demonstrating how perturbations could lead to dysphagia or gastroesophageal reflux disease and thereby emphasizing the importance of examining mechanical and neural interactions in diseases of the esophagus (Bhalla et al., 2015). In addition to mechanical properties, genetic dysregulation is also the central cause of esophageal disorders. Research has highlighted the role of long non-coding RNAs, like SOX2OT, in gene regulation to maintain esophageal health. SOX2OT is a gene located on chromosome 3q26.3 and is most associated with the SOX2 gene important for stem cell pluripotency. Alterations in the pattern of SOX2OT expression have been implicated in various cancers, like esophageal squamous cell carcinoma. This finding underscores the potential that some of these genetic markers might both be used as diagnostic tools and serve as targets for therapy in the treatment of esophageal disease.

Implicating these findings further illustrates that additional research is required to uncover how genetic factors are involved in causing esophageal pathologies and how this may impact options for treatment (Jazi et al., 2015). The salient point characterization with regard to esophageal disorders is directed towards the complex nature of the diseases. A consideration of esophageal transport physiology and genetic regulation of primary biomarkers is crucial for developing effective treatment regimens. While research advances, the synergistic strategy of combining physiological modeling with genetic study has the potential to shed more light on the pathogenesis and progression of esophageal disorders. Greater insight in both areas will result in the evolution of clinical practice, from diagnosis to targeted therapies. Ultimately, an integrated approach that accounts for both biomechanical and genetic examination will be essential in addressing the needs of esophageal disease and improving patient outcomes in populations with varying backgrounds.

CLOSER LOOK

PROTON PUMP INHIBITORS (PPIS)

Proton pump inhibitors (PPIs) are among the most widely prescribed medications worldwide and play a central role in managing acid-related gastrointestinal disorders. By irreversibly inhibiting the hydrogen–potassium ATPase enzyme located in the parietal cells of the stomach, PPIs dramatically reduce gastric acid secretion. This potent acid suppression makes them highly effective for treating gastroesophageal reflux disease (GERD), peptic ulcer disease, Zollinger–Ellison syndrome, and for preventing gastrointestinal bleeding in high-risk patients using NSAIDs or anticoagulants. A closer look at PPI therapy reveals both its substantial benefits and important considerations. Clinically, PPIs relieve symptoms more effectively than H2 receptor blockers and heal erosive esophagitis in a significant proportion of patients. They also play a crucial role in combination therapy for Helicobacter pylori eradication by increasing gastric pH, thereby enhancing antibiotic stability and activity. For patients with severe erosive disease or Barrett's esophagus, long-term PPI use may be essential to maintain mucosal healing and prevent complications.

However, growing evidence highlights the need for careful prescribing. Chronic PPI use has been associated with several potential risks, although many associations remain debated. These include nutrient malabsorption such as vitamin B12, calcium, and magnesium deficiencies due to reduced gastric acidity. Long-term therapy may also alter the gut microbiome, increasing susceptibility to enteric infections like Clostridioides difficile. Other observational studies have suggested possible associations with bone fractures, chronic kidney disease, and dementia, though causality is not firmly established. Because PPIs profoundly reduce acid output, they can mask symptoms of more serious conditions if used without appropriate evaluation.

Judicious use is therefore essential. Clinical guidelines recommend prescribing PPIs at the lowest effective dose and for the shortest appropriate duration, with periodic reassessment of the need for ongoing therapy. Step-down approaches—such as transitioning to on-demand dosing or switching to H2 blockers—can be effective for patients whose symptoms have stabilized. Lifestyle modifications, including weight loss, elevation of the head during sleep, dietary adjustments, and limiting alcohol and tobacco use, can further reduce reliance on medication.

In summary, PPIs remain indispensable for managing many gastrointestinal diseases, offering strong efficacy and a favorable safety profile when used appropriately. A closer examination underscores the importance of balancing therapeutic benefits with potential risks through individualized, evidence-based prescribing.

REFERENCES

1. Tringali, A., Thomson, M., Dumonceau, J. M., Tavares, M., Tabbers, M. M., Furlano, R., Spaander, M., Hassan, C., Tzvinikos, C., Ijsselstijn, H., Viala, J., Dall'Oglio, L., Benninga, M., Orel, R., Vandenplas, Y., Keil, R., Romano, C., Brownstone, E., Hlava, Š., Gerner, P., ... Zambelli, A. (2017). Pediatric gastrointestinal endoscopy: European Society of Gastrointestinal Endoscopy (ESGE) and European Society for Paediatric Gastroenterology Hepatology and Nutrition (ESPGHAN) Guideline Executive summary. *Endoscopy*, *49*(1), 83–91. https://doi.org/10.1055/s-0042-111002(accessed on 15th July 2025).

2. Adashek, J. J., Kato, S., Lippman, S. M., & Kurzrock, R. (2020). The paradox of cancer genes in non-malignant conditions: implications for precision medicine. *Genome medicine*, *12*(1), 16. https://doi.org/10.1186/s13073-020-0714-y(accessed on 15th July 2025).

3. Ajani, J. A., D'Amico, T. A., Bentrem, D. J., Chao, J., Cooke, D. T., Corvera, C. U., Das, P., et al. (2022). Gastric cancer, version 2.2022, NCCN clinical practice guidelines in oncology. Journal of the National Comprehensive Cancer Network, 20, 167–192. https://doi.org/10.6004/jnccn.2022.0008 (accessed on 15th July 2025).

4. Aleman, R., Lo Menzo, E., Szomstein, S., & Rosenthal, R. (2020). De novo gastroesophageal reflux disease esophageal surgery in bariatrics: A literature review and analysis of the current treatment options. Annals of Translational Medicine, 9. https://www.semanticscholar.org/paper/a88f1c7f247c748e3e1c83f176dca09c9ec0af02 (accessed on 15th July 2025).

5. Amarendra, G., Pribadi, R. R., Simadibrata, M., Syam, et al. (2013). *Self-expanding metallic stent placement as a palliative therapy for an advanced gastric cancer patient.* https://media.neliti.com/media/publications/70432-EN-self-expanding-metallic-stent-placement.pdf (accessed on 15th July 2025).

6. Belafsky, P. (2024). Dilation of the upper esophageal sphincter. Foregut, 4, 487–496. https://www.semanticscholar.org/paper/0ce1f7d43511fdccea232893b92a5167f68f1db3 (accessed on 15th July 2025).

7. Bhalla, A. P. S., Griffith, B. E., Kahrilas, P. J., Kou, et al. (2015). *A fully resolved active musculo-mechanical model for esophageal transport.* http://arxiv.org/abs/1501.02010 (accessed on 15th July 2025).

8. Biswas, S., Deng, W., Gong, W., Qin, et al. (2016). *Does Notch play a tumor suppressor role across diverse squamous cell carcinomas?* https://core.ac.uk/download/323069105.pdf (accessed on 15th July 2025).

9. Borrelli, O., Pesce, M., Rybak, A., Thapar, et al. (2017). *Gastro-Esophageal Reflux in Children.* https://core.ac.uk/download/111029577.pdf (accessed on 15th July 2025).

10. Browne, J., Cohen, S. S., de Camargo, O. K., Delaney, et al. (2019). *Pediatric feeding disorder: Consensus definition and conceptual framework.* https://core.ac.uk/download/286544045.pdf (accessed on 15th July 2025).

11. Cairns, C., & Kang, K. (2022). *National Hospital Ambulatory Medical Care Survey: 2019 Emergency Department Summary Tables.* https://doi.org/10.15620/cdc:115748 (accessed on 15th July 2025).

12. Caseiro-Alves, F., De Cecco, C. N., Faggian, A., Grassi, et al. (2015). *Application of imaging*

guidelines in patients with foreign body ingestion or inhalation: Literature review. https://core.ac.uk/download/61498643.pdf (accessed on 15th July 2025).

13. Chen, J. W., Vela, M. F., Peterson, K. A., & Carlson, D. A. (2023). AGA clinical practice update on the diagnosis and management of extraesophageal gastroesophageal reflux disease: Expert review. Clinical Gastroenterology and Hepatology, 21, 1414–1421.e3. https://doi.org/10.1016/j.cgh.2023.01.040 (accessed on 15th July 2025).

14. Cheng, L. K., Kumar, D., Mittal, R. K., Zifan, et al. (2017). *Three-dimensional myoarchitecture of the lower esophageal sphincter and esophageal hiatus using optical sectioning microscopy.* https://core.ac.uk/download/323064197.pdf (accessed on 15th July 2025).

15. Divisi, D., Rinaldi, M., Necozione, S., Curcio, C., Rea, F., Zaraca, F., De Vico, A., et al. (2021). Is it possible to establish a reliable correlation between maximum standardized uptake value of 18-fluorine fluorodeoxyglucose positron emission tomography/computed tomography and histological types of non-small cell lung cancer? Analysis of the Italian VATS Group Database. Diagnostics, 11. https://www.semanticscholar.org/paper/a9fdbae4cd41fe160328b61626cf8338dbbdb6a8 (accessed on 15th July 2025).

16. Dos Santos Difante, L., Trindade, E. N., de Barros Lopes, A., Martins, E. F., Remus, I. B., & Trindade, M. (2024). Clinical relevance of esophageal motility disorders after bariatric surgery: A prospective study based on high-resolution impedance manometry. Arquivos Brasileiros de Cirurgia Digestiva: ABCD, 37. https://www.semanticscholar.org/paper/6d9776d5eaf83d9003e17e8dfb8aefd8a99b69b5 (accessed on 15th July 2025).

17. Feng, J., Ali, R. W., Hao, J., Kong, G. X., Yang, L., & Xiaojun, H. (2019). Peroral endoscopic myotomy for esophageal motility disorders. Esophagus, 17, 11–18. https://doi.org/10.1007/s10388-019-00693-w (accessed on 15th July 2025).

18. Gadallah, A., El Shayeb, E. S., Hisham, B., Abdou, A. G., & Abdalla, E. (2025). Prevalence of eosinophilic esophagitis in refractory gastroesophageal reflux disease in Egyptian patients. *The Egyptian Journal of Internal Medicine.* https://www.semanticscholar.org/paper/242217a9a70f6dee9260ac90ad756f87e52b3932 (accessed on 15th July 2025).

19. Gordon, A. R., White, C. J., Friedland, G. W., Butler, H., Allen, J. E., Clements, J. L., Nosher, J. L., et al. (2010). *Posterior cricoid region fluoroscopic findings: The posterior cricoid plication.* https://core.ac.uk/download/323068550.pdf (accessed on 15th July 2025).

20. Han, S. Y., & Youn, Y. H. (2023). Role of endoscopy in patients with achalasia. Clinical Endoscopy, 56, 537–545. https://doi.org/10.5946/ce.2023.001 (accessed on 15th July 2025).

21. Hassall, E. (1993). Barrett's esophagus: New definitions and approaches in children. Journal of Pediatric Gastroenterology and Nutrition, 16(4), 345–364. https://www.semanticscholar.org/paper/047502aaf05a98c2ac262a57596dddba01c3c289 (accessed on 15th July 2025).

22. Hosseini, M., Salari, M., & Salari, R. (2015). *Psyllium seed may be effective in the treatment of gastroesophageal reflux disease (GERD) in patients with functional constipation.* https://core.ac.uk/download/pdf/82812188.pdf (accessed on 15th July 2025).

23. Hoversten, P., Kamboj, A. K., & Katzka, D. A. (2018). Infections of the esophagus: An update on risk factors, diagnosis, and management. Diseases of the Esophagus. https://doi.org/10.1093/dote/doy094 (accessed on 15th July 2025).

24. Hunt, R. H., Armstrong, D., Katelaris, P., Afihene, M., Bane, A., Bhatia, S., Chen, M., et al. (2017).

World Gastroenterology Organization global guidelines. Journal of Clinical Gastroenterology, 51, 467–478. https://doi.org/10.1097/mcg.0000000000000854 (accessed on 15th July 2025).

25. Jacenik, D., & Fichna, J. (2020). Chemerin in immune response and gastrointestinal pathophysiology. Clinica Chimica Acta, 504, 146–153. https://doi.org/10.1016/j.cca.2020.02.008 (accessed on 15th July 2025).

26. Wall, Geoffrey & Jacoby, Henry. (2002). "Gastroesophageal reflux disease". American Journal of Pharmaceutical Education. 66. (accessed on 15th July 2025).

27. Jain, M. (2023). Diagnosis and management of esophageal motility disorders beyond achalasia. Gastroenterology, Hepatology and Endoscopy Practice, 4, 17–21. https://www.semanticscholar.org/paper/3952a58e0f2d6ebb8dbfe452f0b85e88ec9b84b2 (accessed on 15th July 2025).

28. Jazi, M. S., Mowla, S. J., Samaei, N. M., Shahryari, et al. (2015). Long non-coding RNA SOX2OT: *Expression signature, splicing patterns, and emerging roles in pluripotency and tumorigenesis.* https://core.ac.uk/download/52205708.pdf (accessed on 15th July 2025).

29. Kabir, M. F., Karami, A., Mu, A., & Whelan, K. A. (2021). Abstract 1752: Exploring the relation of eosinophilic esophagitis (EoE) with esophageal cancer. Immunology. https://www.semanticscholar.org/paper/da664a103571d61bba78acbd23632aa8e6309bcc (accessed on 15th July 2025).

30. Ranjitkar, S., Kaidonis, J. A., & Smales, R. J. (2012). Gastroesophageal reflux disease and tooth erosion. *International journal of dentistry, 2012*, 479850. https://doi.org/10.1155/2012/479850 (accessed on 15th July 2025).

31. Kim, J. Y., & Min, Y. (2020). Peroral endoscopic myotomy for esophageal motility disorders. Clinical Endoscopy, 53, 638–645. https://www.semanticscholar.org/paper/10bc1e01c47d62fed788be3319322110b8ff7640 (accessed on 15th July 2025).

32. Kombo, A. F., & Ji, X. Y. (2024). Incidence, risk factors and mortality of COVID-19 among cancer patients: A meta-analysis. *EAS Journal of Medicine and Surgery.* https://www.semanticscholar.org/paper/c38cff8edea27517fb8518664e0e4478e28f3e9a (accessed on 15th July 2025).

33. Lang, G., Gyawali, C. P., & Kahrilas, P. J. (2019). Esophageal motility disorders. In Esophageal Disorders (Chapter 3). https://doi.org/10.1002/9781119211419.ch3 (accessed on 15th July 2025).

34. Lee, B. E., Kim, G. H., Shin, N., Park, D. Y., & Song, G. A. (2020). Histopathological analysis of esophageal mucosa in patients with achalasia. *Gut and Liver, 15*, 713–722. https://doi.org/10.5009/gnl20195 (accessed on 15th July 2025).

35. Liberton, D., Almpani, K., Mishra, R., Bassim, C., Van Ryzin, C., Moebius Syndrome Research Consortium, Webb, B., et al. (2024). Oral health-related quality of life in rare disorders of congenital facial weakness. International Journal of Environmental Research and Public Health, 21. https://www.semanticscholar.org/paper/45910f00af34b863158b0cee87eb98c9ee1de4af (accessed on 15th July 2025).

36. Lin, S., Li, H., & Fang, X. (2019). Esophageal motor dysfunctions in gastroesophageal reflux disease and therapeutic perspectives. Journal of Neurogastroenterology and Motility, 25, 499–507. https://doi.org/10.5056/jnm19081 (accessed on 15th July 2025).

37. Luo, F., Lu, Y., Chen, C., Chang, D., Jiang, W., & Yin, R. (2023). Analysis of the risk factors for negative emotions in patients with esophageal cancer during the peri-radiotherapy period

and their effects on malnutrition. International Journal of General Medicine, 16, 6137–6150. https://www.semanticscholar.org/paper/e46b9e453ea18d7b99d0e9b3a93cffaba76d7110 (accessed on 15th July 2025).

38. Macierzanka, A., Corfield, A. P., Atuma, C., Taylor, C., Nordgard, C. T., Ambort, D., Thornton, D. J., et al. (2012). *The Role of the Mucus Barrier in Digestion.* https://core.ac.uk/download/9838060.pdf (accessed on 15th July 2025).

39. Meltzer, D., & Chung, J. (2025). *Effects of competition under prospective payment on hospital costs among high and low-cost admissions: Evidence from California, 1983–1993.* https://core.ac.uk/download/pdf/6822414.pdf (accessed on 15th July 2025).

40. Muir, A. B., Wang, J. X., & Nakagawa, H. (2018). Epithelial-stromal crosstalk and fibrosis in eosinophilic esophagitis. *Journal of Gastroenterology, 54,* 10–18. https://doi.org/10.1007/s00535-018-1498-3 (accessed on 15th July 2025).

41. Nicholas, M. K., Vlaeyen, J. W. S., Rief, W., Barke, A., Aziz, Q., Benoliel, R., Cohen, M., et al. (2018). The IASP classification of chronic pain for ICD-11: Chronic primary pain. Pain, 160, 28–37. https://doi.org/10.1097/j.pain.0000000000001390 (accessed on 15th July 2025).

42. Nitsa, Z., Faltsetas, S., Davakis, S., Patsouras, D., Vatrika, M., & Charalabopoulos, A. (2025). Laparoscopic Heller myotomy for symptomatic epiphrenic diverticula: A modern technique. Cureus, 17. https://www.semanticscholar.org/paper/8776810ddc1f1d43105729d5eb7fe218a998a200 (accessed on 15th July 2025).

43. Ouban, A., & Arabi, T. (2023). Expression of claudins in preneoplastic conditions of the gastrointestinal tract: A review. *Cancers, 15.* https://www.semanticscholar.org/paper/d6fac88bf0dae8ba7addda42838be9aeaf18d3d4 (accessed on 15th July 2025).

44. Palmese, S. J. (2016). An investigation of the progression from Barrett's esophagus to adenocarcinoma. https://open.bu.edu/bitstream/2144/16178/1/Palmese_bu_0017N_11143.pdf (accessed on 15th July 2025).

45. Pastuszka, A., Serwońska, K., Galanty-Ochyra, A., Węgrzyn, J., Czarnecki, A., Jabłońska, O., Zając, P., et al. (2025). Atopic condition of the esophagus – eosinophilic esophagitis – literature review. *Journal of Education, Health and Sport.* https://www.semanticscholar.org/paper/611fae1b609348e6bc60b1012130415f1721caaa (accessed on 15th July 2025).

46. Patel, P., Layne, S., & Leiman, D. (2024). Regurgitation, eructation, and supragastric belch: Retrograde esophageal motility, disorders, and treatment. Current Opinion in Gastroenterology, 40, 442–448. https://www.semanticscholar.org/paper/a5f806b1d698d5761ed86ea15e8de9c511fbf6b6 (accessed on 15th July 2025).

47. Pouw, R. E., Barret, M., Biermann, K., Bisschops, R., Czakó, L., Gecse, K., De Hertogh, G., et al. (2021). Endoscopic tissue sampling – Part 1: Upper gastrointestinal and hepatopancreatobiliary tracts. Endoscopy, 53, 1174–1188. https://doi.org/10.1055/a-1611-5091 (accessed on 15th July 2025).

48. Rosen, R., Vandenplas, Y., Singendonk, M., Cabana, M. D., DiLorenzo, C., Gottrand, F., Gupta, S. K., et al. (2018). Pediatric gastroesophageal reflux clinical practice guidelines. Journal of Pediatric Gastroenterology and Nutrition, 66, 516–554. https://doi.org/10.1097/mpg.0000000000001889 (accessed on 15th July 2025).

49. Stevens, I. (2024). The epistemological consequences of artificial intelligence, precision medicine, and implantable brain-computer interfaces. Voices in Bioethics. https://www.semanticscholar.org/paper/3fe9a784509e76c873cc40d87248bccbf7cb5eab (accessed on 15th July 2025).

50. Torres, T., Filipe, P., Brandão, F. M., Figueiredo, A., Soares, A. P., Basto, A. S., Rebelo, C., et al. (2023). Epidemiology of psoriasis in Portugal: A population-based study. Acta Medica Portuguesa. https://www.semanticscholar.org/paper/2212b929e6450009dba9de42612fb8b74f852eb1 (accessed on 15th July 2025).

51. Vahedi, F., Low, E., Kaizer, A., Fehmi, S., Hasan, A., Chang, M., Kwong, W., et al. (2023). Esophageal anatomy and physiology vary across spastic and non-spastic phenotypes of disorders of esophagogastric junction outflow. Neurogastroenterology & Motility, 36. https://www.semanticscholar.org/paper/018098e129adbbf17cca41eb830377ed087cd29b (accessed on 15th July 2025).

52. Yadlapati, R., Kahrilas, P. J., Fox, M., Bredenoord, A. J., Gyawali, C. P., Roman, S., Babaei, A., et al. (2020). Esophageal motility disorders on high-resolution manometry: Chicago classification version 4.0. Neurogastroenterology & Motility, 33. https://doi.org/10.1111/nmo.14058 (accessed on 15th July 2025).

53. Yama, A., Nagata, T., Odagami, K., Adi, N., Nagata, M., Mori, K., et al. (2024). Treatment status of psychiatric disorders and falls in the workplace among Japanese workers: A nationwide cross-sectional study. *Journal of Occupational Health, 66.* https://www.semanticscholar.org/paper/7dce4d5a4ef1216ae97dd5dc4a22d8a565352adc (accessed on 15th July 2025).

54. Yamamoto, M., Kensler, T. W., & Motohashi, H. (2018). The KEAP1-NRF2 system: A thiol-based sensor-effector apparatus for maintaining redox homeostasis. Physiological Reviews, 98, 1169–1203. https://doi.org/10.1152/physrev.00023.2017 (accessed on 15th July 2025).

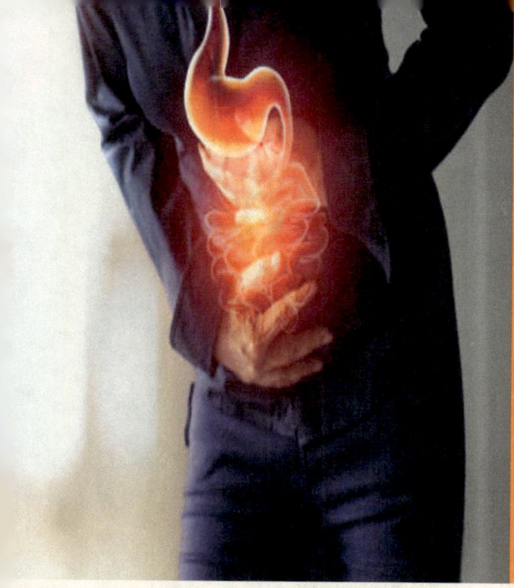

Chapter 4

GASTRIC DISORDERS

Contents

Introduction

The investigation of gastric disorders covers a wide range of conditions that affect the stomach and its functionality, leading to considerable morbidity globally. Gastric disorders may present with a wide range of symptoms, including abdominal discomfort, bloating, and alterations in appetite, considerably reducing a patient's quality of life. The cause of these disorders is sometimes multifactorial, with genetic predispositions, lifestyle factors, and environmental determinants playing important roles. Deservingly, *Helicobacter pylori* infection is now a central element in most gastric illnesses, particularly peptic ulcers and chronic gastritis. The pathophysiology of Helicobacter needs to be elucidated because not only does it lead to mucosal inflammation, but it also makes one vulnerable to even worse diseases , such as gastric cancer. Therefore, timely diagnosis of gastric diseases has a significant influence on the direction of treatment and prognosis in individuals who are affected by them. The relationship between gastric disease and hormonal regulation is another important field that also needs to be explored. There is some indication that endocrine mechanisms are involved in symptomatology and complications of most gastric illnesses. For example, recent research indicates that hormonal fluctuations , such as those in the case of progesterone, may exacerbate symptoms in individuals suffering from conditions , such as Irritable Bowel Syndrome (IBS) and Inflammatory Bowel Disease (IBD).

This involvement of hormones underlines the complexity of gastric disease, where symptoms are not only a matter of function in the gut but also influenced by broader physiological changes. Research in this field can result in new therapeutic methods aimed at treating the root causes of gastric diseases rather than alleviating their symptoms, thus providing patients with more effective treatment and improved health outcomes. Furthermore, the treatment of gastric diseases must be done through a holistic method combining medical interventions with lifestyle modifications. The treatment of conditions , such as peptic ulcers has guidelines shifting to focus on the elimination of *Helicobacter pylori* as a prevention method against subsequent complications, including gastric cancer (Obleaga et al., 2016). Similarly, treatment for conditions , such as IBS and IBD may include a multidisciplinary approach where nutritional treatment, psychological counseling, and medication are added to address both the organic and functional aspects of the condition (Linson, 2013). By embracing the holistic treatment of gastric disorders, healthcare workers are in a position to enhance patient outcomes, not only symptom relief but also overall health. This multi-disciplinary treatment not only offers the chance for personalized treatment strategies but also maintains the requirement for additional research into those interrelated factors that maintain gastric well-being (Figure 4.1).

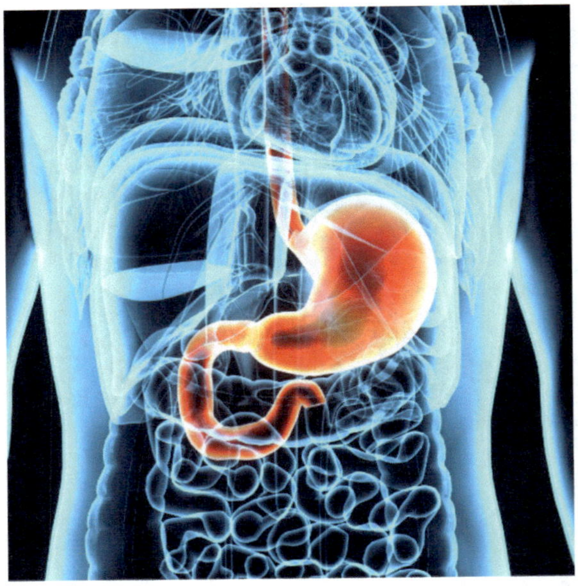

Figure 4.1. Gastric disorders.

Source: https://medlineplus.gov/images/StomachDisordersandStomachCancer_share.jpg.

Definition of Gastric Disorders

Gastric disorders are a broad category of abnormalities that affect the structure, function, and associated digestive processes of the stomach. Gastric disorders seem to occur in various ways, either as inflammation, ulceration, or gastric motility disruption, which leads to manifestations like pain, bloating, and impaired digestive function. Gastritis, gastroesophageal reflux disease (GERD), and peptic ulcers are among the common conditions under gastric disorders, each with unique pathological characteristics and complexities of treatment. It is essential to understand these disorders since they can directly influence the well-being of an individual as well as, in severe circumstances, lead to bleeding or gastric carcinoma. Gastric disease's dense etiology, that is ranging from eating and lifestyle routines to bacterial infections, demands an integrated approach to diagnosis and treatment to cure the symptoms and restore gut health. Gastric disease pathogenesis is multifactorial with intricate interplay between susceptibility, genetic, and environmental stimuli, and microbial components. Infection with *Helicobacter pylori* is a recognized risk factor for chronic gastritis and peptic ulcers, highlighting the role of microbial health in gastric disease. Factors , such as diet, stress, and nonsteroidal anti-inflammatory drugs (NSAIDs) could trigger or exacerbate gastric disease. The pathophysiologic processes of these disorders are typically changes in the production of gastric acid, mucosal integrity, and motility, which result in disabling symptoms and large healthcare expenses. A comprehension of how these factors interact is critical to devising sufficient prevention and treatment regimens in the art of medicine. Recent medical science continues to clarify the complexities of gastric disorders, particularly new strategies and technologies in therapy. For example, integration of nanomedicine is emerging as a promising field of research for the development of drug delivery systems in gastric tissue. Using nanomaterials, drugs can be designed with site-specific and drug-controlled release, which is expected to enhance the therapeutic efficacy with minimal side effects (Patra et al., 2018). In addition, more recent epidemiological research has started to measure the burden of antibiotic resistance on gastric diseases, shedding light on the role of antimicrobial resistance in complicating treatment results for individuals suffering from such conditions (Murray et al., 2022). As gastric disorders continue to be better understood, so too does the need for continuous research to better understand their multifaceted expressions, maximize therapeutic interventions, and enhance patient care.

Importance of Studying Gastric Health

Gastric well-being is significant to consider in the context of explaining the intricate relationship between digestion and well-being. The gastric system does not just carry out the mechanical and chemical breakdown of food, but also the absorption of nutrients and the immune response. Gastric well-being is studied so that clinicians and researchers can uncover the underlying mechanisms for a variety of gastric illnesses, such as gastroesophageal reflux disease (GERD), gastritis, and gastric cancer. It is essential to have a clear perception of these disorders because they are serious health risks and may lead to serious complications when left untreated. More knowledge about gastric health also assists in developing effective prevention campaigns and treatment regimens that significantly contribute to better patient care. In addition, the increasing prevalence of gastric disorders necessitates a focus on their early detection and control measures. With evidence of a substantial increase in conditions like gastritis and gastric cancer, the need to identify risk factors leading to these conditions is imperative. For instance, research has proven an alarming link between substance use disorder (SUD) with gastric cancers, with certain types showing a higher incidence of SUD, particularly in survivors of gastric and esophageal cancers (Jones et al., 2024).

These findings highlight the necessity of full care that takes into consideration both gastric health and comorbidities so that health systems may effectively allocate resources and develop specialized treatment for affected groups. Furthermore, investigating the psychological component that comes with gastric health presents a multi-chaptered intervention strategy. Emerging evidence shows that comorbid mental health significantly affects the progression of gastric conditions. For example, research indicates that individuals who have been diagnosed with conditions , such as binge-eating disorder or alcoholism are at higher risk of weight regain following bariatric surgery (Mauro et al., 2024). Understanding these connections is essential in developing holistic treatment plans that work on both body and mind. By integrating mental health care within the management of gastric issues, health care providers are able to optimize the efficacy of interventions and enhance the quality of life for patients faced with these severe challenges.

Overview of Common Gastric Disorders

Gastric illnesses encompass a wide range of conditions impacting the GI tract, with a substantial impact on individuals' quality of life. The most prevalent diseases are gastroesophageal reflux disease (GERD), gastritis, and peptic ulcers. GERD is an illness wherein stomach acid chronically backs up into the esophagus, causing irritation and resulting in further symptoms of heartburn and regurgitation. Alternatively, peptic ulcers, which are open lesions in the stomach lining or the duodenum, can cause chronic abdominal pain and complications if left untreated. Gastritis, which is inflammation of the stomach lining, has variable symptoms including vomiting and nausea, frequently as a consequence of excessive drinking, use of medications, or underlying infections. Together, these conditions emphasize the importance of understanding gastric disorders for effective management and treatment. In addition to more common gastric disorders, Barrett's esophagus and irritable bowel syndrome (IBS) are noteworthy due to their severe health implications. Barrett's esophagus is nearly entirely caused by chronic gastric reflux, which leads to metaplastic change of the esophageal lining. This transformation, while not initially symptomatic, is at heightened risk of the formation of esophageal adenocarcinoma, a challenging cancer to treat (Palmese, 2016). In contrast, IBS comprises an association between abdominal pain, bloating, and altered bowel habits that can significantly impact quality of life. The etiology of IBS is partly unknown, with hormonal changes perhaps affecting symptomology (Linson, 2013). These disorders need comprehensive clinical assessment and case-specific therapeutic modalities to prevent chronic complications and improve patient outcomes. Beyond the clinical issues involved in gastric illnesses, the psychological impact on the patient cannot be overlooked. In most instances, chronic gastric disease patients exhibit heightened anxiety, depression, and social limitations placed on them by the symptoms. For instance, the fluctuating symptoms of IBS can cause them to produce severe distress, impacting social performance and job stability. In the same way, the risk of cancer that is associated with illnesses like Barrett's esophagus can elicit excessive health- and death-related worry. Treatment regimes must therefore not only include medication but also psychological therapy, which will allow patients to manage themselves and their illness better, as well as improve their well-being. Furthermore, the current research on the pathogenetic mechanisms of these disorders, including hormonal and lifestyle factors, is still the gateway to the development of new treatment strategies that will be equal to the multidimensionality of gastric disorders.

4.1. Types of Gastric Disorders

Among the vast array of gastric diseases, gastritis is a common disorder characterized by inflammation of the stomach lining. Gastritis can be triggered by a number of factors, including heavy alcohol consumption, prolonged use of nonsteroidal anti-inflammatory drugs (NSAIDs), and *Helicobacter pylori* infection. Symptoms most commonly include abdominal pain, nausea, and bloating, which can significantly impact an individual's quality of life. Untreated chronic gastritis may lead to more severe complications , such as gastric ulcers or gastric cancer. Some types of gastritis are discovered, such as atrophic gastritis, where the stomach lining becomes thinner and can disrupt the absorption of nutrients. Understanding the causes and symptomology of gastritis is important for developing effective treatment measures to reduce its great impact on health. A second leading category of gastric disorders is gastroesophageal reflux disease (GERD), which occurs when stomach acid frequently flows into the esophagus and irritates and inflames it. Regurgitation of bitter acid up into the throat or mouth and heartburn are the primary symptoms of GERD. Long-standing GERD can cause more serious illnesses, including strictures, esophagitis, and Barrett's esophagus, a precursor to esophageal cancer. The etiology of GERD includes obesity, pregnancy, and some lifestyle factors, such as the consumption of high-fat diets and caffeine. Treatment generally involves lifestyle modifications and medication to reduce gastric acidity, such as proton pump inhibitors. Early detection is significant in identifying the multifactorial etiology of GERD in order to prevent aggravation of esophageal disease, which emphasizes the need for targeted treatment approaches. Gastric ulcers, the second common type of gastric disease, are a serious variant of peptic ulcer disease and are characterized by open sores that arise on the stomach lining. The two main causes of gastric ulcers are *Helicobacter pylori* infection and overuse of NSAIDs, leading to compromised mucosal protection and increased acid secretion. Symptoms usually consist of gnawing or burning abdominal pain and are often worsened by eating or taking certain medications. Gastric ulcers can also cause serious complications, including hemorrhage, perforation, and gastric obstruction, and prompt medical intervention is required. Although treatment approaches are generally directed at eradicating *H. pylori* infection and acid-suppressive medications, lifestyle factors should also be addressed. Appreciating the importance of gastric ulcers and how they are connected with overall gastric disease will be able to inform prevention and treatment, with the utmost emphasis on public awareness and education regarding gastrointestinal health (Figure 4.2).

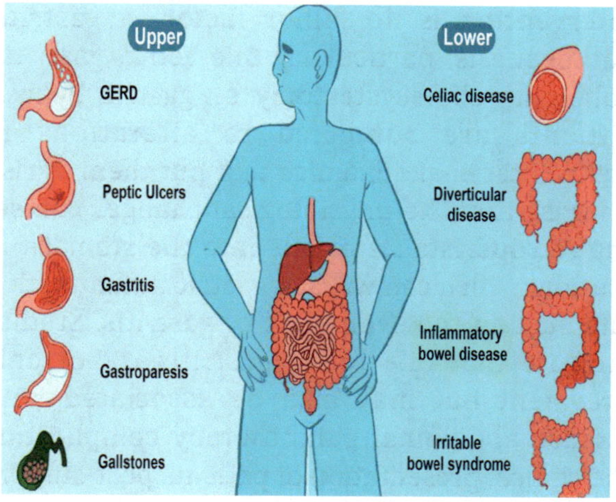

Figure 4.2. Types of gastric disorders.

Source: https://www.verywellhealth.com/thmb/JwqoTeSzGYeZqKao9Exs_fGUluw=/1500x1000/filters:no_upscale():max_bytes(150000):strip_icc()/what-is-wrong-with-my-stomach-4138111-5c454a7cc9e77c0001b21d85-5c2ddd1c5370453b8ec4ff45faefd184.png.

4.1.1. Gastritis

Gastritis, defined as inflammation of the gastric mucosa, has tremendous significance for gastrointestinal well-being. It is most often classified into acute and chronic forms, the second of which is most often linked with repetitive infections , such as *Helicobacter pylori*. In addition, other causes , such as excessive alcohol consumption, NSAIDs, and chronic stress are also reported to maintain gastric inflammation. The clinical manifestation of gastritis is varied, ranging from pain and nausea to disabling dyspepsia. A good understanding of the process behind, specifically the digestive enzyme action , such as Pachaka Pitta, is essential. As discussed, after the uncontrolled secretion of hydrochloric acid, it will lead to severe mucosal damage and subsequent complications like gastric ulcer or gastrointestinal bleeding (Patil et al., 2022). Therefore, timely management of gastritis by appropriate interventions is necessary to prevent its further progression and reduce long-term health effects. Surgical intervention is no minor factor in gastritis pathogenesis, particularly bile reflux gastritis. Following cholecystectomy or gastric bypass, patients are subjected to alterations in gastrointestinal dynamics that put them at risk for gastritis. The physiological changes can set the retroperistalsis of bile into the stomach in motion, which can worsen gastric inflammation and sustain the symptoms of gastritis. Studies indicate that bile reflux gastritis is not only prevalent but may also be associated with intense abdominal pain, thereby complicating the clinical presentation of patients post-surgery (Patil et al., 2022). Identifying the association of surgical history with gastritis highlights the need for personalized treatment protocols that consider both the history of surgery and the etiology of gastritis in order to enhance patient outcomes.

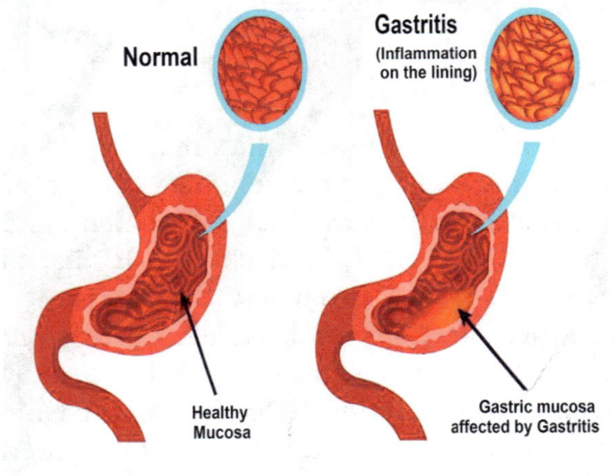

Figure 4.3. Gastritis.

Source: https://www.highcarbhealth.com/wp-content/uploads/2020/11/What-Causes-Gastritis-Highcarb-Health.jpg.

Management of gastritis is a multi-modal treatment consisting of both dietary restriction and pharmacologic management. Patients are generally advised to take a low-irritant diet, avoiding acidic, spicy, and processed foods that aggravate symptoms. Drugs , such as proton pump inhibitors and mucoprotective agents have also proven effective in managing inflammation and symptom reduction (Ho, 2022). However, the effectiveness of standard treatment options can vary based on the cause of gastritis. Hence, healthcare professionals must conduct thorough evaluations to determine the treatment course. Along with this, awareness of potential complications, such as the development of intestinal metaplasia after bile reflux gastritis, remains an essential factor in surveillance and long-term management plans, hence emphasizing the requirement for a comprehensive management plan for gastritis in the overall context of gastric diseases (Figure 4.3).

4.1.2. Peptic Ulcer Disease

Peptic Ulcer Disease (PUD) is a significant health concern, characterized by the presence of ulcers on the gastric mucosa or the proximal small intestine. The key etiologic factor for PUD is *Helicobacter pylori* infection, an organism that infects the gastric mucosa, typically acquired early in childhood. The disease caused by this pathogen leads to chronic inflammation, and the inflammation has the potential to destabilize the mucosal barrier and predispose the individual to the development of ulcers. Surprisingly, even though the majority of individuals harbor *H. pylori* asymptomatically, the interaction between the bacteria and the severity of mucosal inflammation dictates the risk for peptic ulcers. The mechanisms by which *H. pylori* causes damage is crucial for effective management of PUD and prevention of its potential complications, which could be perforation and gastrointestinal bleeding and ultimately lead the a fatal condition if not treated appropriately (Obleaga et al., 2016). Management of PUD has improved significantly, with a specific focus on the eradication of *H. pylori* through antibiotic therapy in combination with the use of proton pump inhibitors (PPIs). These latter facilitate the reduction of gastric acidity, allowing ulcerated mucosa to heal more effectively. The effectiveness of treatment is undermined, however, by increasing antibiotic resistance, which complicates management regimens and therapeutic effectiveness from time to time to be reappraised. Doctors must maintain vigilance over patients' response to therapy, along with being aware of the potential evolutionary complications from *H. pylori* infection, such as gastric lymphoma and even gastric carcinoma. Recalibration of the treatment approaches not only helps improve patient outcomes but also provides a means of knowing the mechanisms of resistance present in certain *H. pylori* strains (Obleaga et al., 2016).

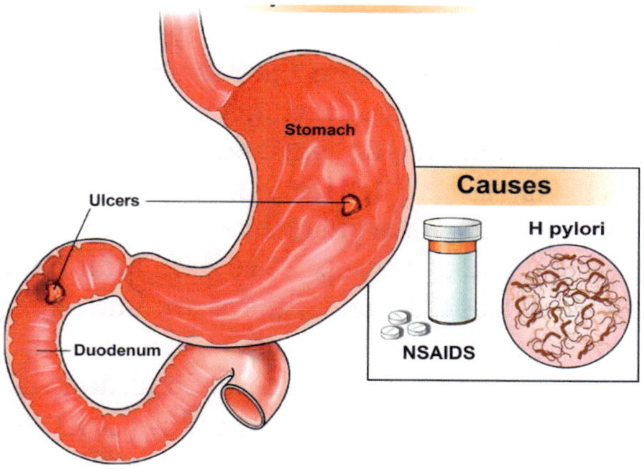

Figure 4.4. Peptic ulcer disease.

Source: https://patient.gastro.org/wp-content/uploads/2021/11/CGH_Patient-ed-ulcer_2018.jpg.

Increasing evidence continues to shed light on the intricate interactions between host components and *H. pylori* that give rise to ulcers. They also have an important function in modulating inflammatory reactions and determining the local immune environment. These factors are a contributory cause of the persistence of the bacterium and, finally, of disease consequences, demonstrating that only a minority of those infected with virulent strains eventually develop ulcers. The intricate balance of inflammation and mucosal integrity emphasizes the necessity of targeted therapeutic interventions, bearing in mind these pathogenic interactions. Given the fact that PUD remains a major global health problem, it is critical that clinicians and researchers collaborate in trying to unravel the complexity of host-pathogen interactions so that treatment improvement can be accompanied by a better understanding of its mechanisms (Robinson et al., 2015) (Figure 4.4).

4.1.3. Gastroesophageal Reflux Disease (GERD)

The prevalence of Gastroesophageal Reflux Disease (GERD) has been a key public health issue as it continues to affect a high proportion of the global population. GERD is fundamentally characterized by gastric content reflux into the esophagus, with possible causes , such as heartburn and regurgitation. Typically, as an ostensibly innocent condition, GERD actually advances to complications , such as erosive esophagitis and Barrett's esophagus, which further have the potential to progress towards esophageal malignancy. Awareness of the multifactorial pathogenesis of GERD is crucial; obesity, diet, and lifestyle contribute to its pathogenesis. Thus, effective management regimens must incorporate not only pharmacologic therapy but also lifestyle modification tailored to the patient. Advances in the pathogenesis and treatment of GERD have led to an array of therapeutic modalities on hand that alleviate symptoms and prevent complications. Proton pump inhibitors (PPIs) have become the cornerstone of medical treatment and offer impressive alleviation of acid-related symptoms by suppression of gastric acid secretion. In addition, antacids and prokinetic drugs may also be used as adjuvant therapy to enhance gastrointestinal motility and suppress gastric acids, respectively. However, prolonged use of PPIs has created problems related to supposed risks like malabsorption of nutrients and gastrointestinal infection. This has made the medical community rethink GERD treatment as seemingly a chronic illness that needs ongoing maintenance therapy to avoid symptoms and complications (Wall & Jacoby, 2002).

Surgical treatment is generally considered in refractory GERD, particularly in refractory patients in whom pharmacologic treatments fail. Fundoplication, a surgical technique specifically aimed at strengthening the lower esophageal sphincter, has been successful in alleviating symptoms in some patients. But choosing to have surgery should be cautious; predictive approaches, such as automated impedance manometry pressure-flow analysis (AIM), are being researched to find out who will benefit most from the surgery (Smits et al., 2013). Because of the complexity of GERD, as well as its symptoms, a multidisciplinary team that includes gastroenterologists, surgeons, and dietitians is needed in the optimization of treatment outcomes. Finally, awareness of the pathophysiology of GERD and knowledge of up-to-date therapeutic choices are crucial for clinicians dealing with this widespread gastric ailment (Figure 4.5).

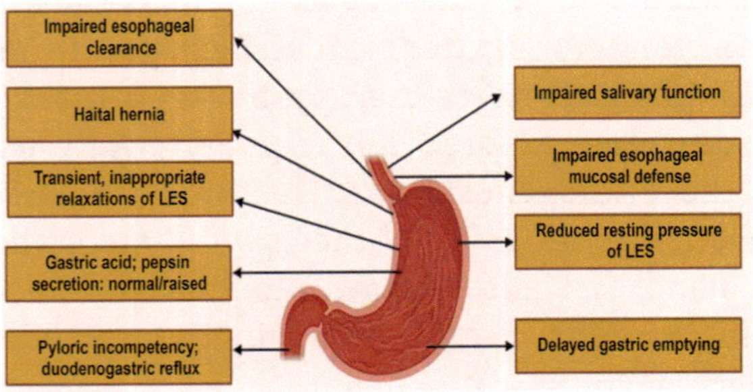

Figure 4.5. Gastroesophageal reflux disease (GERD).

Source: https://assets.cureus.com/uploads/figure/file/1130673/article_river_89c5f1b0612511efac80e19c53f42a9a-Figure-1.png.

4.2. Causes of Gastric Disorders

The multifactorial etiology of gastric disease usually resides in the synergy between genetic, environmental, and infectious factors that interact dynamically in a person. Among the most common etiologic factors reported in most studies is the bacterium *Helicobacter pylori*, or *H. pylori* stands out due to its ability to harm the gastric mucosal barrier, resulting in ailments , such as peptic ulcer disease, MALT lymphoma and gastric cancer. The correlation is especially notable given that long-term infection might pave the way for serious disorders, such as bleeding lesions and gastric lymphoma, as indicated by research on the bacterium's effect on mucosal integrity. H. clinicians ought to be vigilant when diagnosing and treating. pilor infections, as the treatment response is an important factor in avoiding more serious gastric diseases (Obleaga et al., 2016). In addition to infectious disease agents, there are underlying immunological conditions that enhance susceptibility to gastric disease. Conditions like common variable immunodeficiency (CVID) are associated with a heightened susceptibility to malignancies, including gastric cancer. Data suggest that CVID patients have higher cancer rates than the general population, particularly non-Hodgkin lymphoma and gastric cancer, as evidenced by statistical comparison with cancer registry databases. The rapid evolution from initial gastric disease to advanced cancer in this group of patients warrants aggressive surveillance regimens, highlighting the importance of timely diagnosis through the use of regular endoscopic evaluation (Pulvirenti et al., 2018). Thus, knowledge of how gastric and immune health interact is significant in treating patients who are at risk of developing such conditions. Lifestyle elements and dietary habits also have a critical role in the etiology of gastric disorders. Consumption patterns with high concentrations of irritants, such as alcohol and nonsteroidal anti-inflammatory drugs (NSAIDs), can weaken the gastric mucosa, leading to ulcers and inflammation. In addition, salt-rich, low-vegetable, and low-fruit diets have also been associated with an increased incidence of gastric cancers. These deficiencies not only compromise the body's ability to repair gastric mucosal damage but also enhance pathogen-mediated inflammation due to pathogens like *H. pylori*. In this case, knowing the different etiologic factors of gastric disease is important to apply the appropriate preventive measures and therapeutic control aimed at limiting the risk factors both of lifestyle and causative infectious agents (Obleaga et al., 2016; Pulvirenti et al., 2018) (Figure 4.6).

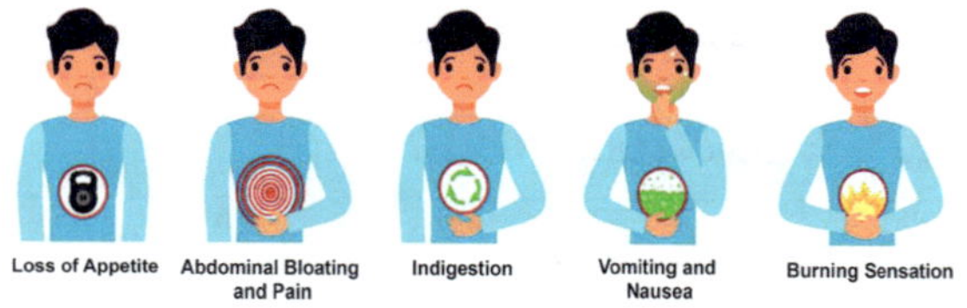

Figure 4.6. Causes of gastric disorders.

Source: https://www.manipalhospitals.com/uploads/image_gallery/symptoms-of-gastric-disorders.jpg.

4.2.1. Dietary Factors

Dietary causes and illness of the stomach have a complex and far-reaching relationship, and in certain foods are the solution to the exacerbation and alleviation of symptoms. High-fat and processed foods, for instance, have been identified as potential causatives of gastrointestinal disturbance, normally causing bloating and indigestion. Apart from that, heavy use of alcohol and caffeine may hurt gastric health and lead to acid reflux and gastritis. These dangers can be alleviated by a well-balanced fiber diet, as fiber promotes healthy digestion and easy bowel movement. A concentration on whole food sources, such as fruits, vegetables, and whole grains, can lead to normal gastric function, which confirms the necessity of proper dietary management for stomach illness. Other studies raise the significance of psychosocial factors involved in eating habits among patients suffering from gastric conditions. For example, in a study, 51.8% of morbidly obese patients exhibited anxiety and depressive disorders, which suggests that emotional well-being directly affects food consumption and diet compliance. The association points out that psychological well-being plays a highly significant role when planning meals for gastric patients. Furthermore, weight loss interventions involving holistic meal planning can lead to significant psychosocial gain, as well as improvement in quality of life.

Therefore, it is essential to grasp the psychological underpinnings of eating behavior to design effective interventions that tackle affective and physical behaviors toward gastric well-being, thereby toward more integrated healing (Kumar et al., 2010). Education and awareness in nutrition are critical to the prevention and treatment of gastric conditions. A study has reported that most horse owners interviewed had shown average levels of knowledge about the nutrition of horses, and most did not know the rules for controlling disorders related to nutrition (Stevenson et al., 2015). This is a cause for concern regarding the average public's perception of gastric requirements for the diet. Nutrition-based educational programs can potentially inform individuals to make health-conscious food decisions, thereby potentially reducing gastric disorders. With raised awareness, individuals are able to identify the role of foods in contributing to gastric health and acquire a preventive and management program approach. Thus, gaining a further understanding of the dietary factors and how these affect gastric disease is an essential method in promoting overall digestive health (Figure 4.7).

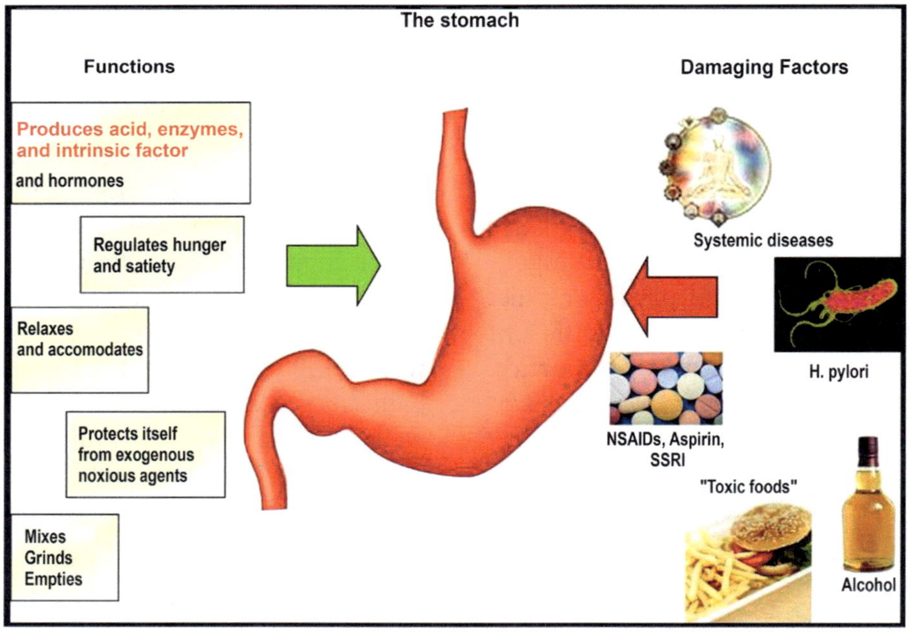

Figure 4.7. Dietary factors are complex and multifaceted, with certain foods.

Source: https://gut.bmj.com/content/gutjnl/64/10/1650/F10.large.jpg.

4.2.2. Lifestyle Choices

The link between lifestyle behaviors and gastric illness is increasingly appreciated by contemporary medical science. Central lifestyle behaviors, such as dietary patterns, exercise, and drug use, all play significant roles in disease pathogenesis of conditions , such as gastroesophageal reflux disease (GERD) and Barrett's esophagus. Chronic habits , such as fatty diets, lack of exercise, and excessive drinking or smoking may exacerbate these illnesses. These conditions of lifestyle are held accountable for the continuous production of gastric acid and lowering of the lower esophageal sphincter, leading to gastroesophageal reflux. Consequently, patients can be at a greater risk of developing Barrett's esophagus, a heightened risk for which progressing to esophageal adenocarcinoma, particularly when compounded with obesity and environmental factors (Palmese, 2016). While obesity would otherwise be considered a primary determinant influencing gastric disorders, the bigger picture of lifestyle trends encompasses much more. Individuals with an inactive lifestyle are not only at greater risk of being obese but also experience greater symptoms of reflux, as well as other gastric conditions. A helpful correlation can be drawn between changes in lifestyle and gastric recovery; i.e., weight loss consequent upon dietary alterations and increased activity have correlated with a decrease in symptoms of GERD. This suggests that the implementation of an improved lifestyle could minimize some of the adverse effects of poorly managed gastric disease. However, the intricate interaction among lifestyle choices and their biochemical implications in the gastrointestinal tract remains intricate and warrants further research to establish specific causal pathways (Dunn, 2019). Furthermore, psychological dimensions of lifestyle choices complicate the interplay between lifestyle and gastric disease. Issues , such as depression, anxiety, and stress often lead to poor eating habits, loss of interest in exercise, and even drug addiction, all of which have gastric ramifications.

Such emotional and psychological issues can provoke or exacerbate gastric symptoms, creating a vicious cycle that is hard to break. This dynamic must be understood by healthcare providers who seek to create holistic treatment plans that account for both lifestyle and mental health demands. By considering beyond the body and looking toward the psychological aspects of lifestyle decisions, practitioners can optimize patient outcomes for gastric afflictions while concurrently reducing the associated risks of developing such afflictions as esophageal adenocarcinoma (Palmese, 2016) (Figure 4.8).

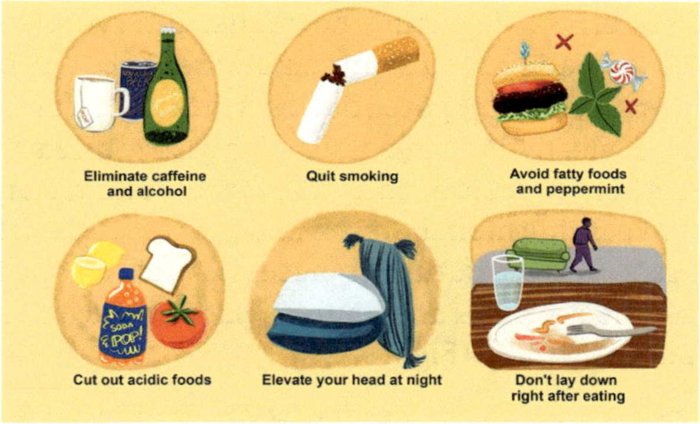

Figure 4.8. Lifestyle choices.

Source: https://www.verywellhealth.com/thmb/PeorRY1dzcVQppCBVHk2-Yp1g6w=/1500x0/filters:no_upscale():max_bytes(150000):strip_icc()/acid-reflux-headache-5191971-FINAL-db42656cedb04fd4a90ec05ec25b82a4.jpg.

4.2.3. Genetic Predispositions

Genetic predispositions are significant in the etiology and progression of gastric disease, in that they determine individuals' reactions to environmental stimuli and pathogenic microorganisms. For example, certain genetic polymorphisms may affect gastric mucosal defense, rendering individuals susceptible to *Helicobacter pylori* infection, a common cause of gastric adenocarcinoma and peptic ulcer. Research has identified individuals with specific genetic markers to be most at risk for these conditions, especially in relation to food and lifestyle factors. This highlights the complex interaction between inherited disposition and external environmental stimuli in gastric disease pathogenesis and suggests that it would require individualized approaches in prevention as well as therapy to effectively control these health ailments. Besides, variability of genetic predispositions may cause significant variation in the severity of the disease and treatment response among patients with gastric illness. For instance, patients with particular genetic backgrounds may have an increased inflammatory response to *Helicobacter pylori* infection, as reported in the context of virulence factors and host genetics of gastric disease (Lin & Koskella, 2014). This response not only accelerates the progression of gastric disease but also complicates treatment regimens due to the various responses to traditional therapies. Additionally, genetic polymorphisms control fluctuations in gastric acid secretion and mucosal barrier protection, further complicating the clinical picture. Recognition of these predispositions is crucial to developing targeted therapeutic strategies based on variation in presentation of gastric illness. Finally, the identification of genetic predispositions enables healthcare professionals to focus on at-risk groups, thereby enabling earlier intervention and better gastric disorder control. Genetic screening can also serve as a useful tool in the determination of susceptibility, thereby facilitating preventive actions targeted at individuals with high risk due to their genetics. For example, populations or breeds would have a prevalence of specific gastric diseases, such as in companion animals, in which breed-specific genetic susceptibility determines morbidity and mortality (Lewis et al., 2018). With application of knowledge of these influences on genetics, clinicians can enhance patient outcomes through personalized medicine, optimizing treatment choice and prevention measures aimed at mitigating the effects of gastric disease on the health of individuals.

4.3. Symptoms of Gastric Disorders

Symptoms of diseases of the stomach can manifest in many forms, typically leading to great discomfort and disturbance in everyday living. Common symptoms , such as abdominal pain, bloating, and abnormal bowel habits, are complained of by individuals suffering from diseases , such as Irritable Bowel Syndrome (IBS) and Inflammatory Bowel Disease (IBD). These symptoms are periodic, emphasizing the uncertain nature of gastrointestinal function. Common presentations vary from cramping and diarrhea to constipation and pain rebound, making diagnosis more complicated. Patients usually come with other signs and symptoms like nausea and even loss of weight, making their condition even more complicated. Because symptoms might mimic other conditions in the gastrointestinal tract, competent investigations should be performed for accurate diagnosis as well as best management, which is itself a reflection of increased awareness of such presentations in clinical practice. In the ageing population, the severity of gastric illnesses can be compounded further by the physiological alterations in the gastrointestinal tract with age. As age advances, the efficiency of nutrient absorption is impaired, with manifest symptoms depending on malnutrition and its overall implications. Age alters the mechanical and chemical digestive processes, resulting in diminished digestive function. For instance, motility disorders will contribute to prolonged gastric emptying times, which exacerbate sensations of fullness and distress. These alterations functionally compromise the gastric system's ability to deliver the body essential nutrients, creating a cycle that contributes to malnourishment and subsequent decline in health. This bidirectional influence between the age of gastrointestinal function and symptoms of gastric disorders accounts for the primary requirement of specialized dietary advice to consider the particular requirements of older groups (Rémond et al., 2015). Evidence has more and more signaled hormonal influence as the primary determinants of symptomatology of gastric disorders. Hormonal changes, particularly in progesterone, have been implicated in association with symptomatically related worsening of gastritis and irritable bowel symptoms. These endocrine changes may cause the onset of gastrointestinal symptoms , such as cramping and constipation, further complicating the clinical picture. Since symptoms occur cyclically, understanding the hormonal underpinning could open new doors for therapy. Exploring hormonal intervention not only attends to symptomatic relief but also causation, with potential ramifications for a more effective treatment plan for gastric disease. Further research into the interconnection between hormonal status and gastrointestinal disease in the future is necessary to advance therapeutic plans and improve patient outcomes (Linson, 2013) (Figure 4.9).

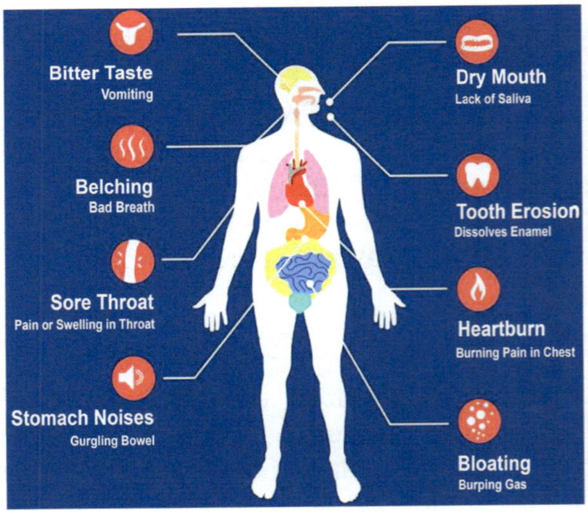

Figure 4.9. Symptoms of gastric disorders.

Source: https://www.australiawidefirstaid.com.au/media-library/symptoms-of-acid-reflux-1000w.jpg.

4.3.1. Abdominal Pain and Discomfort

Abdominal discomfort and pain a vague clinical presentations of several gastric diseases that significantly affect a patient's quality of life. The symptomatology can be due to various conditions, from functional gastrointestinal disorders like Irritable Bowel Syndrome (IBS) to structural defects like gastritis or peptic ulcer. The multidimensional nature of these conditions means that abdominal pain is not only one symptom but rather is accompanied by other gastrointestinal symptoms like bloating, nausea, and changed bowel habits. The spasmodic nature of these symptoms, particularly in IBS and Inflammatory Bowel Disease (IBD), suggests a potential correlation with hormonal fluctuations, particularly with hormones like progesterone, which exacerbate cramping and pain. Identification of , such associations is crucial in the design of effective management policies for patients with incapacitating abdominal pain (Linson, 2013). Gastroparesis, through demonstration of its delayed gastric emptying in the absence of mechanical obstruction, is another significant cause of abdominal pain and discomfort. Victims of this condition typically present with early satiety, bloating, and nausea that are both physically distressful and psychologically impairing. Due to the intricacy of gastroparesis diagnosis, with numerous possible etiologies , such as diabetes and other metabolic disorders, medical practitioners commonly face difficulties in management. As such, the treatment regimen may comprise pharmacological interventions , such as metoclopramide, which seeks to increase gastric motility and relieve symptoms. In refractory cases, specialty therapy like gastric electrical stimulation or surgery may be needed, stressing the need for a holistic, patient-centered approach to effectively address abdominal pain (Permana & Renaldi, 2018). The interaction of environmental, food, and psychological conditions is also a pivotal element in the emergence of abdominal pain and its association with gastric conditions. Food intake, such as the consumption of high-fat or high-fiber meals, can precipitate or aggravate symptoms in susceptible individuals. It has been noted in recent times that stress and psychiatric illnesses can influence gut motility and overall gut function, further contributing to conditions of abdominal pain. It is through managing these factors that full treatment programs would be created, addressing not only symptom relief but also lifestyle modifications that would lead to ultimate control and increased quality of life. Through understanding mechanisms that underlie abdominal pain and discomfort, physicians are in the position to optimize treatment regimens in a manner where not only symptoms but also the causation of gastric upset may be managed (Figure 4.10).

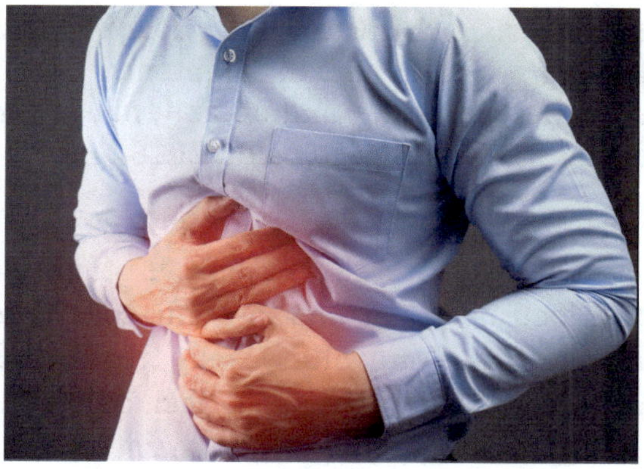

Figure 4.10. Abdominal pain and discomfort.

Source: https://images.ctfassets.net/iqo3fk8od6t9/6dL3ugQF74firSjIR9otYp/038b8c56a8d9fb59436efecb066c8a8c/man-wearing-blue-shirt-with-hand-on-upper-abdomen-pain.jpg.

4.3.2. Nausea and Vomiting

Nausea and vomiting are ubiquitous but complex symptoms that usually point to more underlying gastric illnesses. Their processes involve a sophisticated interaction between neural pathways and physiological responses. Nausea, which may usually be described as a subjective sensation of discomfort, tends to frequently prelude the act of vomiting—a complex reflex that is a mechanism for the body to expel poisonous substances. New evidence has established that not only gastrointestinal disease but also systemic disease or drug side effects lead to these types of symptoms. For example, patients undergoing chemotherapy frequently experience nausea as a side effect of treatment, highlighting the importance of understanding the multidimensional cause of these symptoms (Permana & Renaldi, 2018). This is a complication that highlights the importance of careful assessments in clinical practice because chronic nausea and vomiting can significantly impact the quality of life and the nutritional status of a patient. In diseases of the stomach, ailments , such as gastroparesis demonstrate how nausea and vomiting can present in significant, deleterious ways. Gastroparesis is characterized by delayed gastric emptying, which results in symptoms , such as early satiety, bloating, and notably, nausea and vomiting (Permana & Renaldi, 2018).

The disease is highly dangerous for malnutrition since the patient is unable to digest food normally, and in doing so, vitamin deficiency and morbidity may result. The usual techniques of diagnosis include a solid-phase gastric emptying test, which identifies the severity of the gastric motility disorder. Knowledge of gastroparesis pathophysiology is the key to successful management, as in the use of drugs like metoclopramide and, in the case of the more complicated cases, surgery. Management of nausea and vomiting in such cases not only helps in the control of symptoms but also enhances patient outcomes in general. Nausea and vomiting management should be multi-dimensional in that it tackles pharmacological as well as . Pharmacologically, there are a number of antiemetic drugs available that work on precise receptors in the emetic process. But their effectiveness is not always certain and will be based on the cause of the nausea. Non-pharmacological maneuvers , such as dietary alteration and behavioral change, can assume central positions in this process. Moreover, understanding the subjective nausea experience will optimize the effectiveness of treatment regimens; individual patient assessments are needed to develop particular therapeutic strategies (Kenward et al., 2015). As healthcare professionals become more attuned to the complexity associated with nausea and vomiting, there is an enhanced possibility for generating better therapeutic models, which translate to better control over gastric disease (Figure 4.11).

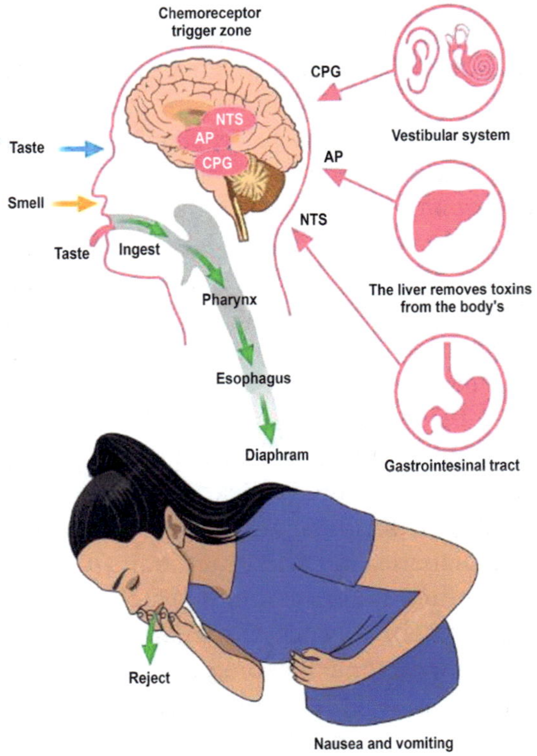

Figure 4.11. Nausea and vomiting.

Source: https://samarpanphysioclinic.com/wp-content/uploads/2023/05/Nausea-2.webp.

4.3.3. Changes in Appetite and Weight

Appetite and weight are significantly influenced by individuals with gastric disorders, typically through the presentation of a complex interaction of body and psychological reactions. Gastrointestinal alterations can lead to the disruption of hunger responses, influencing eating behaviors and consequently weight gain or loss. For example, gastroparesis can cause delayed gastric emptying that results in feeling full hours following a meal. This procedure can lead to unpredictable weight loss due to reduced caloric intake. Similarly, individuals who go for gastric bypass surgery experience remarkable changes in appetite regulation, with endocrine alterations that alter food craving. Perception of these physiological mechanisms is significant towards the development of meaningful dietetic interventions, which can aid individuals' nutritional needs and overall well-being in the treatment of their gastric disease. Besides, one must take into consideration that weight change is not only related to physiological change but also to psychological factors that usually come along with gastric diseases. Anxiety and depression, which are disorders that may exacerbate appetite change and lead to maladaptive eating, develop in the majority of patients. Emotional suffering may result in binge eating in certain individuals or loss of appetite in others. Its interaction makes treatment approaches of an all-inclusive nature consider not only the physiological causes of gastric disorders but also those of mental health. Its effective control may be through behavioral therapy, which allows patients to improve their food habits and cope with allied emotional problems of regulating appetite and weight, thus improving the quality of life. Particular attention must be paid to the elderly, in whom changes in appetite and weight can have disastrous health implications due to the compromised function of the aging gastrointestinal tract. Malnutrition has been noted to be increasing in older individuals largely due to age-related alterations in nutrient consumption, digestion, and absorption. This appears to exacerbate underlying gastric disease, making this further challenging to manage clinically. For example, in elderly patients with conditions like pancreatic exocrine insufficiency (PEI), the symptoms can be confounded with other gastric disease states and lead to undertreatment and misdiagnosis. It is important to identify the maldigestion and malabsorption clues, especially because successful intervention methods can decrease weight loss and malnutrition in this group of patients. Thus, an integrated strategy that combines dietary intervention with medical therapy is needed for healthy aging and prevention of adverse outcomes of gastric disorders in the elderly (Rémond et al., 2015; Vujasinovic et al., 2017).

4.4. Diagnosis of Gastric Disorders

Diagnosis of gastric disease typically involves a multi-component procedure that includes clinical evaluation, endoscopy, and psychiatric evaluation. Initial evaluation of the patient typically includes presenting symptoms, such as abdominal pain, dyspepsia, or change in appetite. These symptoms are often very useful in pointing to underlying disease, but they are mostly nonspecific, and therefore, investigation typically follows. Endoscopy plays an important role in the inspection of the gastric mucosa and procurement of tissue for histological examination. However, existing studies recognize that psychological factors, such as depression and anxiety, have a significant effect on gastrointestinal health and symptom reporting among patients. For instance, a study of patients undergoing upper gastrointestinal endoscopy showed high rates of psychological changes, particularly in coping styles, which in most cases have nothing to do with identifiable endoscopic findings (Angelin et al., 2015). Therefore, the relationship between psychological conditions and gastric conditions has to be considered with maximum caution during diagnosis. *Helicobacter pylori* (*H. pylori*) infection is an area of main interest in the diagnosis of gastric disease due to its association with a range of diseases, including peptic ulcer disease and gastric cancer. Sensitive detection of *H. pylori* is highly critical as it directly influences the choice of treatment and, by a continuum, patient outcomes. Traditional diagnostic strategies include urea breath tests, serology, and endoscopic biopsy with culture or histopathology. Although *H. pylori* is a well-known organism; due to its interaction with other factors, diagnosis becomes more intricate. Also, resistance to antibiotics is a newly emerging issue, as in the majority of cases, therapy does not succeed (Obleaga et al., 2016). Physicians should be vigilant about shifting patterns of resistance and modify treatment plans accordingly so that patients are provided with comprehensive care in terms of ongoing evaluation and support during treatment.

Furthermore, management of gastric disorders extends beyond diagnosis to encompass a wide view of patient health. Practitioners must appreciate that psychological factors, contributing to diagnosis, will be factors in treatment adherence and patient outcome. The frequency of psychological disturbances in gastroenterological patients underscores the need for incorporating mental health screenings into routine gastroenterological visits. Such evaluations may help identify individuals who may require extra psychological care during treatment. Good management practice should thus include discussions on possible complications of *H. pylori* infections and stress the importance of adhering to treatment regimens. Through the integration of psychological and medical understanding in gastric condition diagnosis and treatment, health professionals can facilitate an enhanced-informed approach that optimizes patient care and improves overall health outcomes (Angelin et al., 2015; Obleaga et al., 2016) (Figure 4.12).

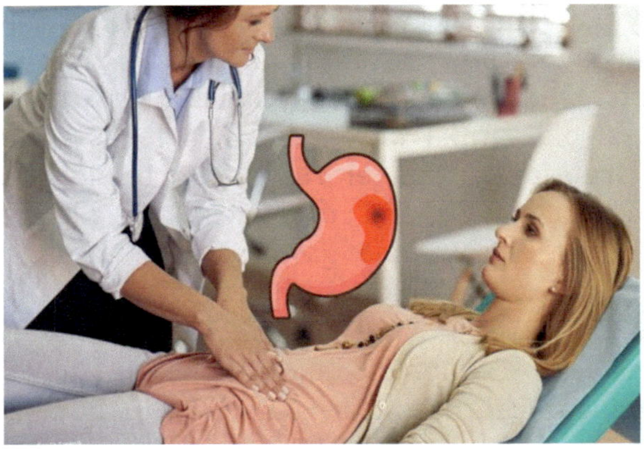

Figure 4.12. Diagnosis of gastric disorders.

Source: https://brahmhomeo.com/public/img/disease/Diagnosis-of-Gastric-Ulcers.jpg.

4.4.1. Medical History and Physical Examination

Identification of medical history is important in gastric illness diagnosis because it places symptoms into context and allows clinicians to reconstruct an accurate image of the patient's health status. Proper medical history does not only involve the patient's current symptoms, but also all previous illnesses, drug use, diet, and gastrointestinal disease family history. This is a valuable holistic method because most gastric conditions , such as gastritis or peptic ulcers, are multifactorial and involve lifestyle as well as genetic factors. It is revealed by research that patient history contributes to about 80% of a precise diagnosis, which reflects the importance of patient history in successfully diagnosing and treating gastric disorders (Fukuzawa et al., 2023). In gastrointestinal disease, an appreciation of the history of past episodes of acute GI discomfort or chronic illness may lead to more targeted and beneficial therapy regimens. The physical examination functions to add to the medical history through observation of tangible signs that pertain to gastric diseases. During the examination, clinicians check for symptoms like abdominal distension, bloating, or detected tenderness, which can indicate specific disorders like gastritis or gastric ulcers. Auscultation can also detect changes in bowel sounds, and palpation can reveal organomegaly or other abnormalities detected during history. Effective correlation of the results from the physical examination with the comprehensive medical history permits a better appreciation of the condition of the patient. Such correlation is necessary, particularly when the complexities that occur in differential diagnoses between conditions that typically have similar presentations but demand varied therapeutic interventions are being contemplated (Lahoud, 2021). Second, technological improvements, primarily the emergence of artificial intelligence (AI), can enhance diagnostic accuracy with integral medical history and physical examination. AI-based systems can review large volumes of patient information and identify patterns that even skilled clinicians may overlook. Still, technology reliance does not eradicate the necessity for fundamental clinical competencies but rather underscores the dependency on accurate patient data. Studies demonstrate that medical history diagnoses alone are good enough, but their integration into physical examination results and laboratory reports greatly improves the accuracy of diagnosis. This only serves to reinforce the continued relevance of thorough medical history and examination in spite of new diagnostic machinery coming on stream and the argument that the patient's history remains paramount even in an era coming to be increasingly reliant on machinery (Fukuzawa et al., 2023).

4.4.2. Diagnostic Tests (Endoscopy, Imaging)

The diagnosis of gastric disorders has improved significantly with the use of advanced investigative techniques, with the lead taken by endoscopy and imaging scans. Endoscopy is a valuable method of direct visualization of gastric mucosa by which clinicians not only diagnose disease abnormalities , such as erosions, ulcers, or tumors but also perform therapeutic procedures if necessary. This invasive procedure permits biopsy sampling and enables an understanding of the etiology of a range of gastric illnesses, from gastritis to malignancy. Endoscopy may also be complemented with autofluorescence imaging (AFI), which enables label-free imaging of tissues based on the intrinsic autofluorescence of endogenous molecules. This functionality potentially identifies early pathological changes, which are not detectable by routine endoscopy and thus improve diagnostic accuracy in detecting diseases that are capable of causing gastric cancer, solidifying its role further in modern gastrointestinal diagnostics (Aigner et al., 2020). Imaging modalities themselves have also experienced advancements that facilitate the evaluation of gastric disorders. Techniques , such as computed tomography (CT), magnetic resonance imaging (MRI), and wireless capsule endoscopy (WCE) are transforming gastrointestinal imaging paradigms. WCE, for example, is useful for imaging the small intestine, and its application has even been explored in pediatric settings, making it an effective non-invasive option for the assessment of gastrointestinal bleeding or suspected Crohn's disease (Bufler et al., 2009). The use of imaging offers a global view of gastric pathologies beyond endoscopy, enabling the possibility of the detection of extra-intestinal conditions affecting gastric well-being. With advances in imaging modalities, they closely trail clinical needs, offering timely and accurate diagnoses for their gastric pathology to patients. Finally, endoscopy and advanced imaging are harmonized in a comprehensive system for the diagnosis of gastric illness. The dual approaches not only enhance diagnostic precision but also provide a greater insight into gastric pathologies as a whole, thereby enhancing decisions about therapy. Nonetheless, it is important to be sensitive to the inherent limitations of each of the methods of diagnosis. While endoscopy is possible with direct vision, it is invasive and potentially perforating and infective. However, imaging techniques have the possibility of missing lesions and are operator-dependent on the skill of the radiologist. Therefore, the optimal approach to enhancing patient outcomes is a multidisciplinary one that synthesizes both endoscopic and imaging techniques such that clinicians have adequate solutions at hand to contend with the complexity of gastric ailments (Figure 4.13).

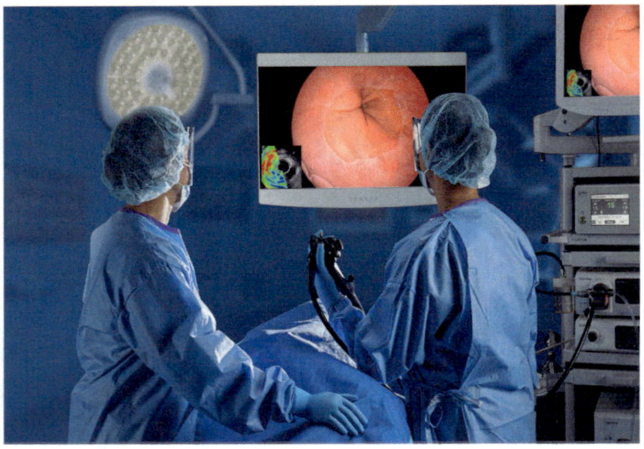

Figure 4.13. Diagnostic tests (endoscopy, imaging).

Source: https://healthcaresolutions-us.fujifilm.com/wp-content/uploads/2023/03/img_es_50-50_interventional_gastroenterology_02.jpg.

4.4.3. Laboratory Tests (Blood, Stool Analysis)

Laboratory tests, stool and blood, are of critical significance in the diagnosis of gastric disease since they assist in establishing the cause and degree of gastrointestinal malfunctioning. Blood analysis is capable of detecting a number of markers, such as the presence of specific antibodies, that are crucial to the diagnosis of autoimmune conditions , such as Coeliac disease. As described in a case study in a patient presenting with gastrointestinal symptoms, initial serologic results, including immunoglobulin A (IgA) anti-tissue transglutaminase antibodies, were instrumental in directing subsequent diagnostic steps. The clinic-laboratory correlation was a reflection of the multifaceted complexity of diagnosing conditions that could have identical presentations, hence the need for extensive blood testing before making any form of conclusion regarding gastric disorders like Coeliac disease and others, which can present with identical histological appearances (Carabottiet al., 2017). Aside from blood testing, stool testing is a significant component of gastrointestinal disease diagnosis, particularly for the identification of infectious pathogens or parasitic infections. Stool tests are capable of detecting the presence of some of these pathogens , such as Giardia, as was detected in the case hereinabove, and this led to a significant turnaround in the diagnosis of the patients. This finding emphasizes the importance of not only relying on antibody tests but also stool examinations when gastrointestinal manifestations predominate. The latter test can also identify other factors that complicate underlying diseases , such as autoimmune gastritis, like gastrointestinal infections. Both blood and stool examinations together constitute an essential laboratory picture, eventually guiding the clinician to an accurate and timely diagnosis (Carabotti et al., 2017). Also, lab tests are not just relevant to the simple identification of a pathogen; they can also reveal the existence of associated complications like anemia that frequently accompanies gastric illnesses. Autoimmune gastritis studies reveal there is a strong correlation between gastrointestinal symptoms and anemias like pernicious anemia, sometimes requiring confirmation by testing blood samples. The symptoms of such diseases can be different from case to case, and demographic factors like age and the presence of other autoimmune diseases influence the symptoms. Detection of these associations by laboratory examination enables the treating physician to plan treatment on an individual basis. Thus, the role played by blood and stool tests cannot be overstated because they form a basic ground for diagnosing gastric disorders and treating them as well as for individually designing patient therapy (Figure 4.14).

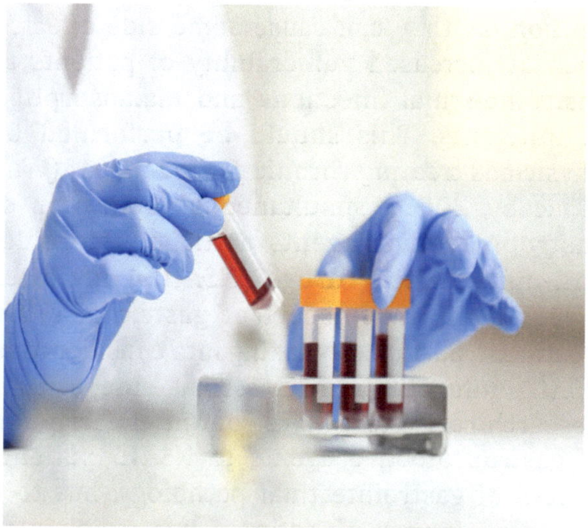

Figure 4.14. Laboratory tests (blood, stool analysis).

Source: https://precisionlabtesting.com/wp-content/uploads/2021/03/blood-test.jpg.

4.5. Treatment Options for Gastric Disorders

The treatment of gastric disorders is diverse, ranging from lifestyle modification to drug treatment. Non-drug treatment has a pillar in the form of diet modification, which helps in alleviating symptoms of various gastric disorders , such as gastroesophageal reflux disease (GERD) and peptic ulcer disease. Patients are typically advised to have small, frequent meals, reduce intake of fatty or spicy food, and avoid caffeine and alcohol to facilitate digestion. Further, weight control is also essential because gastric disease is worsened by obesity. Published literature has established that such lifestyle interventions could significantly enhance the quality of life and symptom control in patients with chronic gastric mucosal inflammation or irritation. These interventions can even fail in all patients, hence necessitating the introduction of pharmacological interventions that target the disease mechanisms more directly. Where lifestyle and diet changes fail, drug therapy is called for. Drugs , such as proton pump inhibitors (PPIs) and H2 receptor antagonists are, for instance, used to reduce gastric acid secretion and help control symptoms of acid-related disorders. The drugs have been found to be useful in the treatment of GERD and peptic ulcers, with the ultimate healing of the gastric mucosa. In addition, in the case of disorders like gastroparesis, prokinetic medications can help with the facilitation of gastric emptying as well as the improvement of the overall digestive process. However, the choice and effectiveness of such therapy largely rely on the patient, as some medications may have the best effects when used with certain gastric disorders. The sensitivity thus works to corroborate the role of customized medicine in treating gastric disorders. In pediatric populations, the management of gastric diseases can be particularly complex since there is still a lack of overall guidance. For instance, studies on gastroparesis in pediatric patients show that treatments that are effective in adults may not always achieve identical outcomes in children. The use of different pharmacologic agents has been studied, but their efficacy in managing children's symptoms is unclear, posing a critical lack of evidence-based guidelines. Recent research emphasizes the importance of conducting more research geared toward pediatric treatment protocols individually, with a call for clinical trials that establish drug efficacy and dosing levels in children. Such research is crucial to build a foundation of knowledge in order to inform subsequent therapeutic strategies so that children receive optimized care that responds to their unique needs and response to treatments (Bantu et al., 2016) (Figure 4.15).

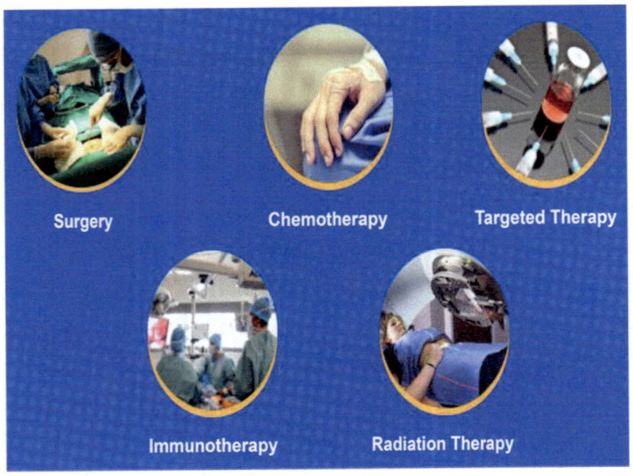

Figure 4.15. Treatment options for gastric disorders.

Source: https://actchealth.com/images/treatment/stomach-treat.png.

4.5.1. Medications (Antacids, Proton Pump Inhibitors)

Treatment of gastric disease is frequently defined by the use of antacids and proton pump inhibitors (PPIs), each serving distinct roles in the treatment of such diseases. Antacids act mainly by neutralizing stomach acid, providing symptomatic relief of diseases like gastroesophageal reflux disease (GERD) and peptic ulcers. Their mechanism involves the direct neutralization of stomach acid to raise the pH level within the gastric compartment, providing relief from pain felt through acid-induced inflammation. However, while helpful in the short run, antacids fail to address the underlying pathophysiology of gastritis or chronic acid production. In addition, antacid overuse can lead to side effects , such as skewed electrolyte balance and constipation, which points to the need for close patient education on their utilization. Proton pump inhibitors, however, provide a more comprehensive approach to managing long-term gastric illness. These drugs inhibit gastric H^+/K^+ ATPase in the stomach lining, effectively reducing gastric acid secretion. PPIs are especially beneficial in patients with recurrent episodes of GERD as they allow mucosal healing and acid reflux-induced esophagitis recurrence prophylaxis. Recent studies indicate that PPIs should be used properly, and while they perform similarly in serious conditions, therapy on a long-term basis should be administered with caution, as they can cause some side effects , such as increased vulnerability of patients to gastrointestinal infections and malabsorption of nutrients. This should be performed by physicians treating chronic gastric illness (Wall & Jacoby, 2002). Simultaneous application of gastroprotective agents with nonsteroidal anti-inflammatory drugs (NSAIDs) indicates a very significant aspect of gastric disorder treatment, particularly taking into consideration NSAID-induced gastrointestinal side effects. Research refers to a more routine prescription of gastroprotective agents to NSAID patients at risk of gastrointestinal pathology, but to a sizeable number of patients not exposed to recommended doses of these drugs (Bilušić et al., 2006). The inference from this conclusion is the presence of practice gaps at the clinical level, where potential gastric risk knowledge is not translated into optimum treatment regimens. Practitioners of medicine, therefore, need to concentrate on going back to gastroprotective approaches to ensure that vulnerable patients are adequately treated with optimal gastroprotective dosing using NSAIDs in order to prevent adverse gastrointestinal outcomes in treating patients with gastric disease.

4.5.2. Dietary Modifications

Dietary changes are central to the treatment of gastric diseases, as they can have a direct impact on symptom alleviation and general patient health. These changes usually take the form of a revision of macronutrient consumption, accompanied by selective food avoidance, designed to soothe. For example, patients who experience gastroesophageal reflux disease (GERD) are often encouraged to stay away from acidic foods, fried foods, and heavy meals, which can trigger their condition. Likewise, patients suffering from peptic ulcers may also be assisted by a low-irritant diet, for example, a low caffeinated intake and hot peppers. These dietary changes contribute towards the overall relief in gastrointestinal conditions and can even drastically decrease clinical symptoms, enabling the patient to actively engage in regular activities as well as reduce drug dependency. For more serious cases of the stomach, surgery like bariatric surgery is needed, necessitating further adjustments in diet to enable healing and prevent complications. Bariatric surgery requires patients to undergo specialized nutritional education to effectively sustain their new diet. Post-surgery, the body undergoes changes that hinder the process of nutrient absorption, thus necessitating a high-vitamin and high-mineral diet to prevent malnutrition (Azran et al., 2017). These patients must be transitioned carefully by the clinicians, emphasizing the necessity of small, nutritious meals to accommodate their altered gastrointestinal physiology. Regular monitoring of nutritional status is also required, as most patients will regain weight if dietary behavior is not adhered to after surgery, a reminder of the critical nexus between dietary behavior and successful surgery. Adults older in age most often face other difficulties in managing gastric illness due to physiological alterations brought about by aging that affect nutrient digestion and absorption. Gastric function alterations due to age can disrupt food's mechanical breakdown and compromise the intestines' capacity for nutrient absorption, posing a high risk of malnutrition (Rémond et al., 2015). Nutritional guidelines for the old must possess adapting mechanisms to conquer these impediments, such as soft and appetizing food options that facilitate easier ingestion. To conquer the result of malnutrition, it is vital to provide dietary advice that is individualized and takes into account not only the ageing GI tract but also the psychological and socio-economic determinants of food consumption. Through addressing these sophisticated needs, certain dietetic modifications can significantly promote the health of older individuals suffering from gastric diseases.

4.5.3. Surgical Interventions

Operative techniques for the management of gastric disease have gained popularity in recent years due to their efficacy in managing morbid obesity and related metabolic syndromes. Among the operative techniques, bariatric surgery has emerged as a cornerstone in the clinical management of obesity when lifestyle modification and pharmacotherapy fail. One of the popular procedures is Vertical Sleeve Gastrectomy (VSG), in which part of the stomach is removed surgically, thereby reducing its size and altering the secretion of gastrointestinal hormones. The procedure not only causes weight loss but also improves the comorbid conditions , such as type 2 diabetes and dyslipidemia. Literature currently indicates that VSG could be a possibly beneficial intervention in those with obesity due to circadian rhythm disruption, with dramatic weight reduction and metabolic improvement (Arble et al., 2015). Such findings point to the multifaceted role of surgeries as a countermeasure against hormonal and metabolic deregulations, being a component of gastric illness. The interaction between gut endocrine reactions and operations is significant to understanding the efficacy of bariatric operations. The operations induce major changes in the release of hormones like glucagon-like peptide-1 (GLP-1), which is crucial in the regulation of glycemia. As recent research focus has shown, impacting the anatomical positioning of the gastrointestinal tract, i.e., via ileal interposition, has been shown to enhance GLP-1 secretion, even in non-obese subjects (Hirata et al., 2011). What this shows is that surgery can move beyond mere weight loss, impacting physiological processes on a global level in an attempt to treat diabetes and metabolic syndromes of metabolism effectively.

Further, the research underlines the potential of such interventions to bring about long-term metabolic benefits by optimizing the secretion of hormones by gut cells, which reflects the underlying pathophysiology of gastric disease. Overall, surgical interventions are a part of the treatment protocol for gastric diseases, particularly for patients with severe obesity and associated complications.

Procedures like VSG and ileal interposition not only work for weight loss, but metabolic benefit by way of endocrine modulation is also targeted. The dual benefit identifies the critical need for clarifying the fundamental biological pathways in a bid to harness therapeutic potential. As more research is pursued, it becomes increasingly apparent that such a procedure offers new avenues of treatment for those patients previously deemed untreatable through conventional channels. The integration of surgery into the general picture of management of metabolic disease is a paradigm shift in the management of gastric diseases, promising greater care for patients and long-term benefits to health (Figure 4.16).

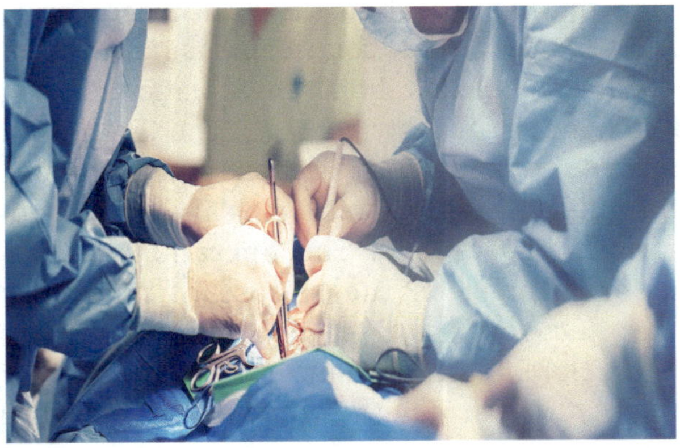

Figure 4.16. Surgical interventions.

Source: https://www.kernodle.com/wp-content/uploads/2020/02/Kernodle-OBGYN_Benefits-of-Minimally-Invasive-Surgery.jpeg.

4.6. Prevention of Gastric Disorders

Prevention of gastric illness is a multi-pronged approach that includes lifestyle modification. A well-balanced diet with high-fibre, lean-protein, and healthy-fat foods goes a long way in the prevention of the development of gastric diseases , such as gastritis and peptic ulcers. Avoid highly processed foods, high levels of caffeine, and too much consumption of fat to maintain optimal gastric health. Regular physical exercise also has a crucial part to play; it has been shown through studies that exercise not only aids in keeping weight healthy, but it can also improve digestion as a whole. By promoting these positive lifestyle changes, patients can become a very real part of gastric disorder prevention, setting them up for long-term gastrointestinal wellness. Including mental health in the prevention model for gastric disorders is also necessary. Psychological alterations, such as anxiety and depression, have been linked to the aggravation of gastrointestinal symptoms, creating a pattern that can complicate one's health further. The study emphasized coping impairment among patients with gastrointestinal disorders, supporting the reality that emotional well-being influences digestive function directly (Angelin et al., 2015). It is therefore imperative that healthcare professionals consider psychology with stress management techniques and psychotherapy. By improving coping abilities and emotional resilience, gastric symptoms can be alleviated to some extent, and gut-brain health can be ascertained. A mind-body process that integrates physical and mental well-being can substantially enhance the efficiency of gastric disorder prevention. Apart from this, education plays a crucial role in gastric disorder prevention as well. Raising awareness regarding the risk factors of such conditions makes individuals capable of making healthy decisions regarding their health. Health interventions and community projects focusing on diet education, stress-reducing activities, and periodic check-ups can lead to early diagnosis and intervention. While the prevalence of disorders like Portal Vein Thrombosis expands, it becomes critical that both physicians and patients become educated about what hidden risk factors may not always have obvious causes (Cuschieri et al., 2013). Through an active mindset towards gastrointestinal health and encouraging regular health checks, we can anticipate and thus prevent possible bouts of gastric illness from occurring and improve patient outcomes (Figure 4.17).

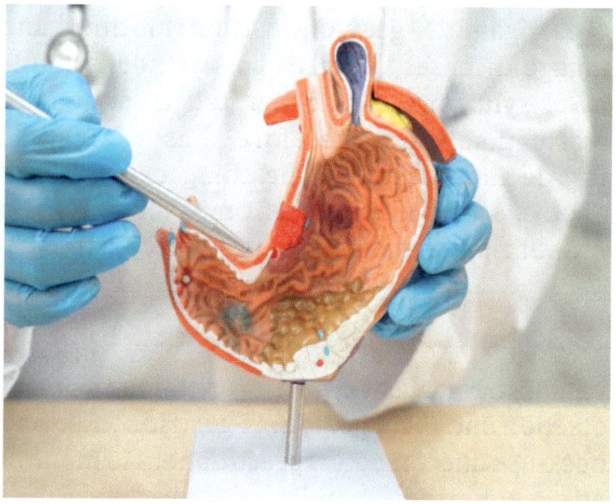

Figure 4.17. Prevention of gastric disorders.

Source: https://img.freepik.com/premium-photo/dyspepsia-gastric-disease-doctor-holding-stomach-anatomy-model-study-diagnosis-treatment-hospital_1263944-545.jpg.

4.6.1. Healthy Eating Habits

The development of good diet habits plays a crucial role in the prevention of gastric disorders, particularly in vulnerable populations , such as young people. As recent studies have reported, obesity remains a significant public health issue, oftentimes linked to an imbalance between energy intake and energy output and wrong eating habits. Increased caloric intake, without associated physical activity, promotes obesity and also diseases like Type 2 Diabetes Mellitus and Dyslipidemia. Of specific interest, adolescents can develop poor food patterns because of body image psychological stresses, which become disorders like Bulimia Nervosa or Anorexia Nervosa. Encouraging healthy dietary habits that include adequate meals and physical exercise can reduce such risk factors, highlighting the importance of integrated lifestyle interventions that foster both physical and mental well-being among youth populations (Kansra et al., 2021). Including nutrient-rich foods like eggs in the diet is an example of a measure for promoting healthy dietary habits, which can be used as protective factors against gastric disease. Eggs have been recognized to be rich in nutritional value containing all the needed macro and micronutrients, assisting in the proper body function and growth. Compared to earlier nutritional guidelines, which limited egg intake in order to prevent cardiovascular diseases, current studies establish that dietary inclusion of eggs comes with no significant contribution of egg-derived cholesterol to plasma total-cholesterol levels. Hence, eggs can be included in a healthy diet as an easily accessible and affordable food. Their nutrient density not only preserves general well-being but also shows potential in the treatment and prevention of numerous diseases, hence the importance of educating people on how to incorporate such foods into daily diets (Réhault-Godbert et al., 2019). Furthermore, healthy eating habits are more than choosing particular meals; it is about major lifestyle changes that improve general health. Effective strategies in achieving these habits include establishing an environment that fosters mindful eating, acquiring portion control, and making decisions about food intake in terms of nutritional value. Proper dietary education is key, particularly in schools, where children can be taught the impact of what they are eating on long-term health effects. In addition, engaging families in the nutrition controversy helps reinforce these habits at home and reduces the likelihood of gastric diseases. Encouraging the adoption of promotion of healthy lifestyles at a societal level, with a complementary policy for ready availability of healthy commodities, is required in combating the sly wave of obesity and associated gastric diseases (Kansra et al., 2021).

4.6.2. Stress Management Techniques

In considering how stress and gastro disorders have a relationship, it is thus important to examine effective stress management practices. Psychological factors, including anxiety and styles of coping, have been established to play a significant role in gastrointestinal function. For instance, one study revealed that a high proportion of patients undergoing upper gastrointestinal endoscopy had psychological alterations, such as poor coping, anxiety, and depression, added to the health conditions (Angelin et al., 2015). These findings underscore the importance of the application of stress management strategies appropriate for patients with gastric disorders. Stress management interventions , such as mindfulness, relaxation therapy, and cognitive-behavioral therapy can neutralize the psychological distress that inexorably exacerbates gastrointestinal symptoms, resulting in enhanced patient outcomes. Mindfulness and meditation are particularly valuable stress management interventions, as they equip patients with the capacity to effectively control their emotional reactions. By creating present-moment awareness, patients can reduce anxiety and their emotional vulnerability and this may be beneficial in the treatment of gastric symptoms. Research has indicated that mindfulness treatments can lead to greater digestion and reduced gastric pain through the relaxation and reduction of physiological processes that are associated with stress (Coleman et al., 2018). Integrating breathing exercises into everyday activities reduces heart rate and blood pressure and, as a secondary effect, stress. With regular practice, these techniques assist in developing an optimal mind-body relationship, which is so essential for the treatment of gastric disorders. An element of stress management which is equally important is the incorporation of regular exercise, which can be a prophylactic and therapeutic tool for gastric disorders. Exercise, besides guaranteeing all-around well-being, also assists in reducing stress and anxiety, which are typically precursors to gastrointestinal symptoms. For example, aerobic exercises , such as walking, jogging, or cycling stimulate the release of endorphins, mood-enhancing neurotransmitters that are also natural stress reducers. Additionally, exercise helps promote gastrointestinal motility and manage diseases , such as gastritis or irritable bowel syndrome. An integrated treatment of gastric disorders therefore, has to include lifestyle modifications, including exercise and effective stress management measures, to gain optimum patient health and quality of life.

4.6.3. Regular Medical Check-Ups

Regular medical check-ups are vital to the early detection and management of gastric conditions. Check-ups allow medical practitioners to monitor patient symptoms, conduct required tests, and examine medical histories, all of which play significant roles in diagnosis and treatment. By having a standard surveillance program, patients stand a better chance of noticing abnormal changes in their health, which might indicate underlying gastric conditions , such as ulcers or gastritis. Also, such tests can result in early interventions, thereby decreasing the chances of complications. By this early intervention, not only are patients empowered, but health outcomes in general are enhanced by preventive treatments that can stop gastric diseases from advancing. Check-ups, in this case, become particularly important to a healthcare routine for individuals fighting obesity-related gastric diseases. Obesity presents with an enhanced risk for diseases like gastroesophageal reflux disease (GERD) and peptic ulcer disease, and needs repeated follow-up. Multiple consultations provide an opportunity for education regarding weight control interventions, the option for bariatric surgery, and its gastric effects. Emerging evidence shows that bariatric surgery is efficient in clinically reducing obesity and its complications, such as diabetic gastroparesis, when appropriately utilized (Dunn, 2019). By facilitating ongoing conversations of lifestyle modifications through check-ups, medical professionals can engage patients in their care, leading to better compliance with therapeutic guidance and healthy outcomes. Routine medical check-ups are also a way to enlighten patients on the intricacies of their gastric health. These specialists can impart valuable information on food options that enhance the functioning of the stomach as well as explain the interrelationship between stomach disorders and overall health. For instance, individuals who have underlying conditions, such as cardiovascular disease, are helped by understanding how stomach health relates to their overall health (Merino et al., 2014). In addition, discussions of possible genetic predispositions and family risks involved in gastric sickness can aid in creating a more personalized healthcare regimen. By promoting a culture of open communication, regular check-ups not only lead to better treatment of existing ailments but also enhance the trust of patients in adhering to their path towards improved gastric health (Figure 4.18).

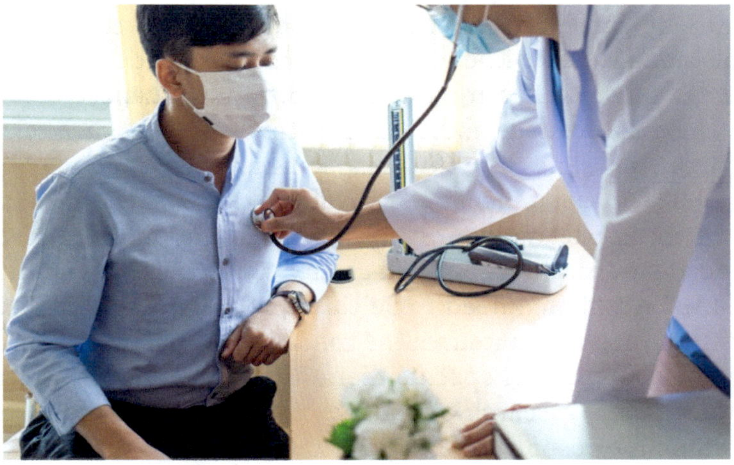

Figure 4.18. Regular medical check-ups.

Source: https://www.makatimed.net.ph/wp-content/uploads/2021/06/6-BENEFITS.jpg.

SUMMARY

With the complex etiopathogenesis of gastric disease, it is evident that treatment and diagnosis should be accomplished as an integrated scheme. Gastric disease varies in its nature, ranging from gastritis to malignancies , such as gastric MALT lymphoma. The strong correlation between chronic infections, especially by *Helicobacter pylori*, and gastric malignancy justifies an efficient mechanism of treatment. *H. pylori* also has an excellent rate of response, with studies indicating that up to 80% of patients can be cured of gastric MALT lymphoma if treated adequately. This not only presents the potential for antibacterial therapies to influence oncological outcomes but also indicates the merit in understanding the pathophysiological interactions that determine treatment regimens. The multifaceted interaction between infection and gastric health needs further study to define therapy and improve outcomes for patients. Further, the potential relationship between autoimmune disease and gastric disease offers another compelling area of study. The thyrogastric syndrome, characterized by the co-occurrence of autoimmune thyroid disease and chronic autoimmune gastritis, provides a demonstration of the complexity of autoimmune pathogenesis. Subsequent studies have shown that as many as 40% of chronic autoimmune gastritis patients may have accompanying Hashimoto's thyroiditis. Furthermore, there appears to be a common mechanism between the two conditions. , such associations must be considered by clinicians because they can affect the effectiveness of treatment and patient management. Knowledge of these associations, particularly the common immunologic and genetic substrates, can allow for more individualized treatment strategies and better patient care for these associated conditions. By acknowledging such relationships, physicians are able to ultimately make possible improved diagnosis and therapeutic effectiveness for victims of gastric disorders. Lastly, in condensing the results of the gastric disorder study, significant conclusions are drawn with implications for clinical practice and ongoing research endeavors. The documented connection of chronic infections and gastric cancers, e.g., the etiologic relation between *H. pylori* and gastric MALT lymphoma need to be carefully diagnosed and treated. In addition, the development of associations between autoimmune conditions enhances the understanding of gastric disease. Over time, the development of specific therapies addressing the gastric disease processes will be the priority. Continuous research is needed to clarify the complex associations between infectious agents, autoimmune responses, and gastric disease. With the new treatment therapies, better patient outcomes are promised, and the need for an integrative approach to treating gastric disorders becomes evident in the medical community.

The study of gastric diseases highlights numerous significant aspects that are vital in understanding their complexity and control. One such is the multi-dimensionality of obesity, presently increasingly regarded as a chronic metabolic condition that leads to a vast number of health conditions. The interconnectedness of body fat and health risk is no overstatement, as excessive body fat, particularly visceral fat, is linked to rising rates of metabolic and cardiovascular conditions. Effective management strategies should involve a thorough assessment comprising a patient's history, physical examination, and laboratory tests aimed at identifying co-morbidities. The ultimate goal of any treatment is to provide realistic weight loss and quality of life improvement for the patients. Overall approach involving dietary change, exercise, and behavioral modification plays a crucial role in achieving effective outcomes in obesity management (Busetto et al., 2015). Another important aspect in the context of gastric diseases is the role of diet in affecting gastric pH levels and gastric health. The interaction between food intake and gastric acidity is crucial to understanding the phenomena of digestion as well as the success of medical treatments. There is evidence that food intake can increase gastric pH levels quite substantially, and this can be a difficulty in sustaining the level of acidity necessary for efficient digestion. The role played by BHCl as a gastric acid supplement stems from evidence supporting its effectiveness in lowering the pH in the stomach after intake. Specifically, high intakes of BHCl have had a notable potential to reduce the time to reach baseline levels of stomach pH, bringing about the complexities medical practitioners face when treating stomach patients (Benet et al., 2019). Ultimately, multidisciplinary treatment is the key to effective management of gastric conditions , such as obesity and complications. Coordination between medical professionals—dietitians, physicians, and mental health professionals—ensures that comprehensive care is formulated based on specific needs. This may include the use of various interventions like lifestyle modifications, drug therapy, and, in severe cases, surgery. A concentration on realistic goals and ongoing support through evidence-based interventions can significantly enhance outcomes. Moreover, identifying obesity as a disease condition rather than an easy option influences more sympathetic treatment and encourages patients to engage in their care plans (Busetto et al., 2015). By briefly outlining these important points, a better understanding of gastric disorders and paths to effective management is given.

CLOSER LOOK

PROTON PUMP INHIBITORS (PPIS)

Proton pump inhibitors (PPIs) are among the most widely prescribed medications worldwide and play a central role in managing acid-related gastrointestinal disorders. By irreversibly inhibiting the hydrogen–potassium ATPase enzyme located in the parietal cells of the stomach, PPIs dramatically reduce gastric acid secretion. This potent acid suppression makes them highly effective for treating gastroesophageal reflux disease (GERD), peptic ulcer disease, Zollinger–Ellison syndrome, and for preventing gastrointestinal bleeding in high-risk patients using NSAIDs or anticoagulants. A closer look at PPI therapy reveals both its substantial benefits and important considerations. Clinically, PPIs relieve symptoms more effectively than H2 receptor blockers and heal erosive esophagitis in a significant proportion of patients. They also play a crucial role in combination therapy for Helicobacter pylori eradication by increasing gastric pH, thereby enhancing antibiotic stability and activity. For patients with severe erosive disease or Barrett's esophagus, long-term PPI use may be essential to maintain mucosal healing and prevent complications.

However, growing evidence highlights the need for careful prescribing. Chronic PPI use has been associated with several potential risks, although many associations remain debated. These include nutrient malabsorption such as vitamin B12, calcium, and magnesium deficiencies due to reduced gastric acidity. Long-term therapy may also alter the gut microbiome, increasing susceptibility to enteric infections like *Clostridioides difficile*. Other observational studies have suggested possible associations with bone fractures, chronic kidney disease, and dementia, though causality is not firmly established. Because PPIs profoundly reduce acid output, they can mask symptoms of more serious conditions if used without appropriate evaluation.

Judicious use is therefore essential. Clinical guidelines recommend prescribing PPIs at the lowest effective dose and for the shortest appropriate duration, with periodic reassessment of the need for ongoing therapy. Step-down approaches—such as transitioning to on-demand dosing or switching to H2 blockers—can be effective for patients whose symptoms have stabilized. Lifestyle modifications, including weight loss, elevation of the head during sleep, dietary adjustments, and limiting alcohol and tobacco use, can further reduce reliance on medication.

In summary, PPIs remain indispensable for managing many gastrointestinal diseases, offering strong efficacy and a favorable safety profile when used appropriately. A closer examination underscores the importance of balancing therapeutic benefits with potential risks through individualized, evidence-based prescribing.

REFERENCES

1. Kenward, H., Pelligand, L., Savary-Bataille, K., & Elliott, J. (2015). Nausea: current knowledge of mechanisms, measurement and clinical impact. *Veterinary journal (London, England : 1997)*, *203*(1), 36–43. https://doi.org/10.1016/j.tvjl.2014.10.007 (accessed on 15th July 2025).
2. Pulvirenti, F., Pecoraro, A., Cinetto, F., Milito, C., Valente, M., Santangeli, E., Crescenzi, L., Rizzo, F., Tabolli, S., Spadaro, G., Agostini, C., & Quinti, I. (2018). Gastric Cancer Is the Leading Cause of Death in Italian Adult Patients With Common Variable Immunodeficiency. *Frontiers in immunology*, *9*, 2546. https://doi.org/10.3389/fimmu.2018.02546 (accessed on 15th July 2025).
3. Aigner, F., Pratschke, J., Schumann, T., Stockmann, M., et al. (2020). *Recent advances and the potential for clinical use of autofluorescence detection of extra-ophthalmic tissues*. https://core.ac.uk/download/323257980.pdf (accessed on 15th July 2025).
4. Alarcón de la Lastra Romero, C., Castejón Martínez, M. L., Montoya García, T., Sánchez Hidalgo, M., et al. (2020). *Potential protective role exerted by secoiridoids from Olea europaea L. in cancer, cardiovascular, neurodegenerative, aging-related, and immunoinflammatory diseases*. https://core.ac.uk/download/288002452.pdf (accessed on 15th July 2025).
5. Annechini, G., D'Elia, G. M., Perrone, S., Pulsoni, A., et al. (2016). *Infectious aetiology of marginal zone lymphoma and role of anti-infective therapy*. https://core.ac.uk/download/158328504.pdf (accessed on 15th July 2025).
6. Carabotti, M., Lahner, E., Esposito, G., Sacchi, M. C., Severi, C., & Annibale, B. (2017). Upper gastrointestinal symptoms in autoimmune gastritis: A cross-sectional study. *Medicine*, *96*(1), e5784. https://doi.org/10.1097/MD.0000000000005784 (accessed on 15th July 2025).
7. Arble, D. M., Sandoval, D. A., Seeley, R. J., & Turek, F. W. (2015). *Metabolic effects of bariatric surgery in mouse models of circadian disruption*. https://core.ac.uk/download/213087641.pdf (accessed on 15th July 2025).
8. Vujasinovic, M., Valente, R., Thorell, A., Rutkowski, W., Haas, S. L., Arnelo, U., Martin, L., & Löhr, J. M. (2017). Pancreatic Exocrine Insufficiency after Bariatric Surgery. *Nutrients*, *9*(11), 1241. https://doi.org/10.3390/nu9111241(accessed on 15th July 2025).
9. Azran, C., Batterham, R. L., Busetto, L., Dicker, D., et al. (2017*). Practical recommendations of the Obesity Management Task Force of the European Association for the Study of Obesity for the post-bariatric surgery medical management*. https://core.ac.uk/download/141699962.pdf (accessed on 15th July 2025).
10. Bantu, L., Buckley, M. G., Smetana, K. S., Tillman, M., et al. (2016). *Pharmacologic treatment for pediatric gastroparesis: A review of the literature*. https://core.ac.uk/download/84831825.pdf (accessed on 15th July 2025).
11. Benet, L. Z., Frassetto, L. A., & Surofchy, D. D. (2019). *Food, acid supplementation and drug absorption – A complicated gastric mix: A randomized control trial*. https://core.ac.uk/download/286728808.pdf (accessed on 15th July 2025).
12. Smits, M. J., Loots, C. M., Benninga, M. A., Omari, T. I., & van Wijk, M. P. (2013). New insights in gastroesophageal reflux, esophageal function and gastric emptying in relation to dysphagia before and after anti-reflux surgery in children. *Current gastroenterology reports*, *15*(10), 351. https://doi.org/10.1007/s11894-013-0351-3 (accessed on 15th July 2025).

13. Bilušić, M., Erdeljić, V., Francetić, I., Huić, M., et al. (2006). *Use of gastroprotective agents in recommended doses in hospitalized patients receiving NSAIDs: A drug utilization study.* https://core.ac.uk/download/11699264.pdf (accessed on 15th July 2025).

14. Rémond, D., Shahar, D. R., Gille, D., Pinto, P., Kachal, J., Peyron, M. A., Dos Santos, C. N., Walther, B., Bordoni, A., Dupont, D., Tomás-Cobos, L., & Vergères, G. (2015). Understanding the gastrointestinal tract of the elderly to develop dietary solutions that prevent malnutrition. *Oncotarget, 6*(16), 13858–13898. https://doi.org/10.18632/oncotarget.4030(accessed on 15th July 2025).

15. Brusca, N., Capriello, S., Cellini, M., Centanni, M., et al. (2017). *Hashimoto's thyroiditis and autoimmune gastritis.* https://core.ac.uk/download/98336979.pdf (accessed on 15th July 2025).

16. Bufler, P., Fritscher-Ravens, A., Milla, P., Nuutinen, M., et al. (2009). *The feasibility of wireless capsule endoscopy in detecting small intestinal pathology in children under the age of 8 years: A multicenter European study.* https://core.ac.uk/download/12175824.pdf (accessed on 15th July 2025).

17. Busetto, L., Fried, M., Micic, D., Schindler, K., et al. (2015). *European Guidelines for Obesity Management in Adults.* https://core.ac.uk/download/53528633.pdf (accessed on 15th July 2025).

18. Cabrerizo Merino, M. del C., Cutando Soriano, A., Giménez Prats, M. J., Machuca Portillo, P., et al. (2014). *Consensus report of the XI Congress of the Spanish Society of Odontology for the Handicapped and Special Patients.* https://core.ac.uk/download/71035455.pdf (accessed on 15th July 2025).

19. Obleaga CV, Vere CC, Valcea ID, Ciorbagiu MC, Moraru E, Mirea CS. Helicobacter pylori: Types of Diseases, Diagnosis, Treatment and Causes of Therapeutic Failure. Journal of Mind and Medical Sciences. 2016; 3(2):150-161. https://doi.org/10.22543/2392-7674.1048(accessed on 15th July 2025).

20. Coleman, T. P., Gharibans, A. A., Kriegsfeld, L. J., Kunkel, D., et al. (2018). *Artifact rejection methodology enables continuous, noninvasive measurement of gastric myoelectric activity in ambulatory subjects.* https://core.ac.uk/download/323082131.pdf (accessed on 15th July 2025).

21. Cuschieri, S., Gauci, J., & Vassallo, M. (2013). *Portal vein thrombosis: A case report and literature review.* https://core.ac.uk/download/46602431.pdf (accessed on 15th July 2025).

22. Dunn, M. D. (2019). *Bariatric Surgery as a Treatment to Obesity.* https://core.ac.uk/download/212902619.pdf (accessed on 15th July 2025).

23. Lewis, T. W., Wiles, B. M., Llewellyn-Zaidi, A. M., Evans, K. M., & O'Neill, D. G. (2018). Longevity and mortality in Kennel Club registered dog breeds in the UK in 2014. *Canine genetics and epidemiology, 5,* 10. https://doi.org/10.1186/s40575-018-0066-8 (accessed on 15th July 2025).

24. Fukuzawa, F., Yanagita, Y., Yokokawa, D., Uchida, S., Yamashita, S., Li, Y., Shikino, K., et al. (2023). Importance of patient history in artificial intelligence–assisted medical diagnosis: Comparison study. JMIR Medical Education, 10. https://www.semanticscholar.org/paper/11c680ffdd149d551b35737329a0b9bca6c589c3 (accessed on 15th July 2025).

25. Hirata, A., Marigliani, B., Aguiar-Yamaguchi, G., Miguel, G., Borborema, J. F., Azevedo, J. L., et al. (2011). *Structural changes in intestinal enteroendocrine cells after ileal interposition*

in normal rats. https://core.ac.uk/download/pdf/290516.pdf (accessed on 15th July 2025).

26. Ho, K. Y. (2022). Clinical significance of post-operative bile reflux gastritis. JGH Open: An Open Access Journal of Gastroenterology and Hepatology, 6, 157–158. https://www.semanticscholar.org/paper/8087dab538b9c9fe0dbe1aed9bb9637cd179240d (accessed on 15th July 2025).
27. Wall, Geoffrey & Jacoby, Henry. (2002). "Gastroesophageal reflux disease". American Journal of Pharmaceutical Education. 66. https://core.ac.uk/download/46924346.pdf (accessed on 15th July 2025).
28. Jones, K. F., Osazuwa-Peters, O., Des Marais, A., Merlin, J. S., & Check, D. K. (2024). Substance use disorders among US adult cancer survivors. JAMA Oncology. https://www.semanticscholar.org/paper/856f240cbbf55df432ffa8cfe37c7c38aa86c153 (accessed on 15th July 2025).
29. Kansra, A. R., Lakkunarajah, S., & Jay, M. S. (2021). Childhood and adolescent obesity: A review. *Frontiers in Pediatrics, 8.* https://doi.org/10.3389/fped.2020.581461 (accessed on 15th July 2025).
30. Lin, D., & Koskella, B. (2015). Friend and foe: factors influencing the movement of the bacterium Helicobacter pylori along the parasitism-mutualism continuum. *Evolutionary applications*, *8*(1), 9–22. https://doi.org/10.1111/eva.12231 (accessed on 15th July 2025).
31. Kumar, S., Kyrou, I., Matyka, K., Osei-Assibey, G., et al. (2010). *Self-reported psychosocial health in obese patients before and after weight loss.* https://core.ac.uk/download/46368.pdf (accessed on 15th July 2025).
32. Lahoud, P. (2021). High level of suspicion based on detailed medical history and focused physical examination: Important tool to diagnose acute myocarditis. Clinical Medical Reviews and Case Reports. https://www.semanticscholar.org/paper/6161334df7df886e79689f6a90b318262f25ca74 (accessed on 15th July 2025).
33. Linson, E. A. (2013). The Interplay Between Hormones and Irritable Bowel Disease. B.S., Emory University, 2010 Submitted in partial fulfillment of the requirements for the degree of Master of Arts 2013. https://open.bu.edu/bitstream/2144/12149/6/Linson_Elyse_2013_nosig_nocv.pdf (accessed on 15th July 2025).
34. Mauro, M., Papelbaum, M., Brasil, M. A. A., Carneiro, J. R. I., Luiz, R., Hiluy, J. C., & Appolinário, J. C. (2024). Mental health and weight regain after bariatric surgery: Associations between weight regain and psychiatric and eating-related comorbidities. Archives of Endocrinology and Metabolism, 68. https://www.semanticscholar.org/paper/a004082b3e88b8d3d2bd42c4dc7ea2119c8e876e (accessed on 15th July 2025).
35. Murray, C. J. L., Ikuta, K. S., Sharara, F., Swetschinski, L. R., Robles Aguilar, G., Gray, A. P., Han, C., et al. (2022). Global burden of bacterial antimicrobial resistance in 2019: A systematic analysis. *The Lancet, 399*, 629–655. https://doi.org/10.1016/s0140-6736(21)02724-0 (accessed on 15th July 2025).
36. Palmese, S. J. (2016). An investigation of the progression from Barrett's esophagus to adenocarcinoma. https://open.bu.edu/bitstream/2144/16178/1/Palmese_bu_0017N_11143.pdf (accessed on 15th July 2025).
37. Patil, S. S., Patil, V. S., & Sontakke, A. R. (2022). A case study: An Ayurvedic management of Urdhwaga Amlapitta with special reference to hyperacidity. World Journal of Advanced Research and Reviews. https://www.semanticscholar.org/paper/0d93a8dc7cc1f56281b66a4d00dec946cd3f261d (accessed on 15th July 2025).

38. Patra, J. K., Das, G., Fraceto, L. F., Campos, E. V. R., Rodriguez-Torres, M. del P., Acosta-Torres, L. S., Díaz-Torres, L. A., et al. (2018). Nano based drug delivery systems: Recent developments and future prospects. Journal of Nanobiotechnology, 16. https://doi.org/10.1186/s12951-018-0392-8 (accessed on 15th July 2025).

39. Permana, Mustika D., and Kaka Renaldi. "Management of Gastric Motility Disorder." Indonesian Journal of Gastroenterology, Hepatology, and Digestive Endoscopy, vol. 19, no. 1, Apr. 2018, pp. 25-36, doi:10.24871/191201825-36.(accessed on 15th July 2025).

40. Réhault-Godbert, S., Guyot, N., & Nys, Y. Y. (2019). The golden egg: Nutritional value, bioactivities, and emerging benefits for human health. Nutrients, 11, 684–684. https://doi.org/10.3390/nu11030684 (accessed on 15th July 2025).

41. Robinson, K., White, J. R., & Winter, J. A. (2015). Differential inflammatory response to Helicobacter pylori infection: Etiology and clinical outcomes. https://core.ac.uk/download/30650035.pdf (accessed on 15th July 2025).

42. Stevenson, A., Becvarova, I., Bolwell, C., Buffington, T., Burk, K., Bloxham, C., Caron, J. P., et al. (2015). Equine nutrition: A survey of perceptions and practices of horse owners undertaking a massive open online course in equine nutrition. https://core.ac.uk/download/30638562.pdf (accessed on 15th July 2025).

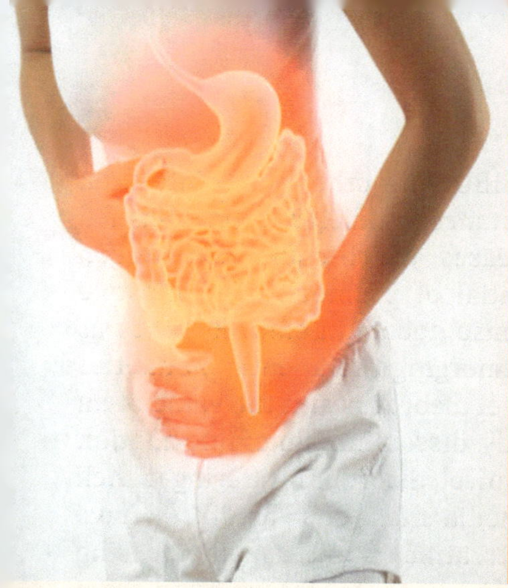

Chapter 5

SMALL BOWEL DISORDERS

Contents

Introduction

The small bowel plays a critical role in the process of digestion as the primary location of nutrient absorption following food breakdown. The delicate balance of this sophisticated process may be disrupted through disease in the small bowel, and with such disruptions, a variety of gastrointestinal disorders impacting the quality of life of an individual may ensue. Of all these disorders, small intestinal bacterial overgrowth (SIBO), irritable bowel syndrome (IBS), and intestinal methanogen overgrowth (IMO) are of particular interest due to their rising prevalence and polymorphic associations with other medical illnesses, including brain fog and chronic fatigue. Understanding the pathophysiologic mechanisms underlying these conditions and their interassociations is essential to develop effective regimens of treatment that treat not only the symptoms and signs but also the pathogenesis of small bowel diseases (Halabi et al., 2024). The creation of new diagnostic techniques and therapies has raised awareness of small bowel disease, particularly among patients who receive relief and control.

Current studies indicate that there is a significant correlation of SIBO with other gastrointestinal diseases, rendering the clinical scenario more demanding. For instance, studies have established that patients with IBS are likely to have several concomitant diseases, which could also worsen their gastrointestinal symptoms. As such, the therapeutic potential of probiotics and lifestyle changes, such as the low FODMAP diet, has been a subject of intense debate in clinical circles as potential treatment modalities (Manikandan et al., 2024). These emerging therapeutic modalities are directed towards the multi-dimensional character of small bowel disorders and the value of an integral strategy, both pharmacologic and non-pharmacologic. Lastly, dissemination of information through social media has transformed discussion about small bowel disorders, offering a rich intermixture of patient perception and clinical guidelines. Social media sites , such as TikTok have become venues for people to get their individual experiences and treatments out, usually focusing on dietary changes and non-traditional treatments. A reliance on anecdotal information from these sources presents concerns regarding the proliferation of misinformation and the absence of evidence-based advice from medical practitioners. Whereas these grassroots-level forums may provide support and awareness, it is also imperative for professionals to enter into these platforms so that accurate information can be shared, leading to further comprehension and control of small bowel disorders among the masses (Manikandan et al., 2024) (Figure 5.1).

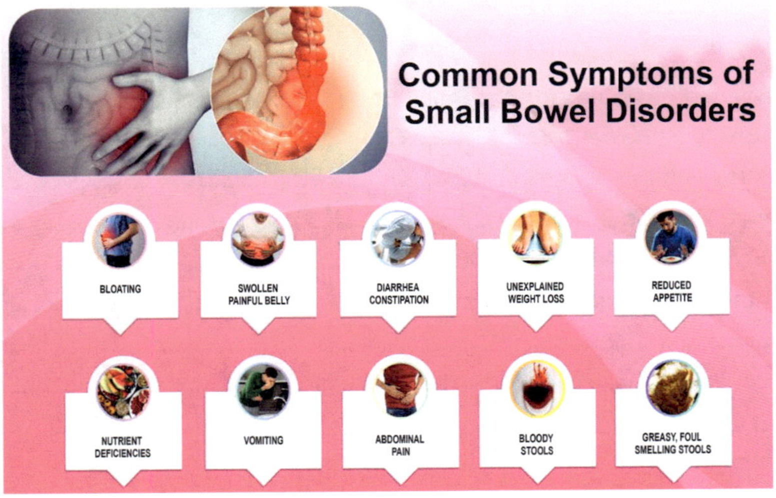

Figure 5.1. Small bowel disorders.

Source: https://thegastrosurgeon.com/wp-content/uploads/2025/04/Common-Symptoms-of-Small-Bowel-Disorders-at-Dr.-Patta-Radhakrishnan.jpg.

Definition of Small Bowel Disorders

Small bowel disease is an overarching group of disorders that affect the structure and function of the small intestine. This critical portion of the gastrointestinal (GI) tract is responsible for nutrient absorption and is fundamental to the digestive system. Small bowel disease has the potential to yield serious clinical manifestations, including malabsorption, diarrhea, and abdominal pain. These conditions are classified into various categories, such as functional disorders like irritable bowel syndrome (IBS) or organic disorders due to structural abnormalities. The complexity of the small bowels' role in digestion demands that there be an extensive understanding of these disorders in order to develop effective treatment interventions and improve patient outcomes. As researchers delve further into the interrelations between gut flora and bowel function, continuing information emerges that underlines the intricate interdependencies of the small bowel with overall health. Irritable bowel syndrome (IBS), the most commonly diagnosed disorder of the small bowel, is characterized by recurrent abdominal pain and altered bowel habits. A study shows that nearly 10% of the global population is suffering from IBS, which detects its occurrence as an issue of public health concern. Later studies have identified the potential link between small intestinal bacterial overgrowth and IBS symptoms, suggesting that alterations in gut microbiota may exacerbate gastrointestinal symptoms. In IBS patients, the identification of some of the bacterial populations, particularly *Escherichia coli*, has shown a strong correlation with symptom intensity. Furthermore, age, sex, and socio-economic status have been linked to the prevalence of IBS, which means an attempt from a multidisciplinary perspective towards determining such disorders is necessary for the best possible management and intervention (Sultan et al., 2025). Another important small bowel disorder is short bowel syndrome (SBS), which has a profound impact on nutrient absorption due to the inappropriately small size or function of the small intestine. SBS is operationally defined as a residual length of the small bowel <200 cm from the ligament of Treitz and is characterized by malabsorption, diarrhea, and nutrient deficiency. The syndrome typically develops following surgery, as in the case where most of the bowel has been lost due to disease. SBS can lead to CIF, in which patients become dependent on intravenous therapy to maintain health. Classification of SBS relies on a number of factors, including some that are anatomical length and the pathophysiological function of residual bowel. Proper classification is crucial in clinical management and treatment, acting as a standard for healthcare professionals to assess and manage the diverse presentations of SBS accordingly (Pironi, 2023).

Importance of the Small Intestine in Digestion

The small intestine is a vital component in the digestion and absorption process required for good health. The most critical site of nutrient breakdown, the small intestine, is divided into three segments: the duodenum, jejunum, and ileum, each of which makes a specialized contribution to digestion. Pancreatic enzymes and bile break down fats and continue to digest carbohydrates and proteins in the duodenum. The jejunum, which is lined with microvilli, optimizes surface area for the best nutrient absorption so that vital amino acids, fatty acids, and monosaccharides are absorbed into the circulatory system. This high rate of digestive activity reflects the small intestine's importance because any disruption, like from small bowel illnesses, will lead to malabsorption syndromes and deficiencies, which underscores the utmost significance of maintaining small intestine health. The metabolic activity in the small intestine is strongly related to intestinal gene expression unique to the diet. Nutrient composition in the diet, such as carbohydrate, fatty acids, and amino acids, has a major influence on the expression of genes and, consequently, digestibility. For instance, reduced feed consumption may be detrimental to intestinal gene expression and induce dysfunctions frequently observed after weaning in a variety of populations, like young humans and livestock. This bidirectional link between diet and gene expression provides evidence for one possible route by which dietary health might be targeted by tailored nutritional interventions. Through the modification of food ingredients, it has been suggested by scientists that one can elevate gene expression of genes encoding for digestive and absorptive proteins with the aim of maximizing functions concerning the small intestine and eradicating the impact of disorders (Bauer et al., 2011). One of the most important functions of the small intestine in the digestion process is its mucus cover that consists predominantly of mucins , such as MUC2. This layer is crucial insofar as it excludes dangerous pathogens while permitting nutrients to travel through to epithelial cells below. Structure and characteristics of this mucus are critical; charge and pore size differences determine what comes to the gut epithelium. These kinds of barriers are critical for gastrointestinal health and for enabling the correct absorption of nutrition and drugs. Any interference with such a protective layer can exacerbate small bowel disease, opening the intestine to pathogen and toxin invasion and eliciting inflammatory responses. Understanding the operation of the mucus layer and its function in nutrient distribution not only guides treatment protocols but also highlights the small intestine's vital role in digestion and overall health (Macierzanka et al., 2012).

Overview of Common Small Bowel Disorders

The small intestine is also susceptible to many disorders that can significantly influence digestive health and overall well-being. Three of the most prevalent small intestine disorders are celiac disease, Crohn's disease, and small intestine bacterial overgrowth (SIBO). Celiac disease, an immune response to gluten, results in inflammation and damage to the small intestine that results in malabsorption and many gastrointestinal symptoms , such as diarrhea and stomach pain. Similarly, Crohn's disease, an inflammatory bowel disease (IBD), has the potential to involve any part of the gastrointestinal tract but predominantly occurs in the small bowel, with patients presenting with acute abdominal pain, weight loss, and sometimes complicating symptoms , such as fistulas or strictures. Understanding these disorders different presentations is the key to successful diagnosis and patient-specific treatment methods that maximize patient outcomes. Another primary small bowel disease, small intestinal bacterial overgrowth (SIBO), has been increasingly noted with its association with conditions like irritable bowel syndrome (IBS) and non-specific inflammatory bowel diseases (IBD). SIBO is characterized by excessive bacterial overgrowth in the small intestine that produces symptoms virtually indistinguishable from those of IBS, which are bloating, flatulence, and diarrhea (Goździewska et al., 2024). The overlap in interaction between these disorders also complicates clinical management since they have overlapping symptomatology and are more likely to occur together in patients. Furthermore, the development of dietary treatments, including the low FODMAP diet, has been observed as an efficient therapy for IBS and SIBO, and this underscores the role of individualized dietary management in managing patients with these disorders.

Multidisciplinary management is useful, using pharmacotherapy, diet therapy, and possibly probiotic therapy to reestablish intestinal balance. Complications of diseases of the small bowel can be severe and deserve careful attention by medical professionals. For example, conditions , such as small vessel vasculitis can lead to severe small bowel ischemia and perforation, which typically hold a poor prognosis for the affected subjects (Gonçalves et al., 2025). Diagnosis of these diseases is difficult, and it requires high-reliability imaging modalities and endoscopic examinations to outline the extent of disease and guide appropriate interventions. Because small bowel diseases lead to severe, complicated health diseases, an interprofessional team of gastroenterologists, dietitians, and other experts must collaborate in planning optimal and effective treatment. Prevention of complications and improvement in quality of life rely on prompt detection, rightful diagnostic workup, and initiation of individualized therapeutic strategies developed according to each patient's unique presentation.

5.1. Anatomy and Physiology of the Small Bowel

The small bowel, or small intestine, is a significant component of the gastrointestinal tract and plays a role in the digestion and absorption of nutrients. It is anatomically divided into three sections: the duodenum, jejunum, and ileum. The duodenum is the shortest and is basically committed to the initial stage of digestion, in which pancreatic enzymes and bile combine with chyme. Following this, the ileum and jejunum go on to digest and absorb essential nutrients in the shapes of carbohydrates, proteins, and fats, thanks to the large surface area that comes with the villi and microvilli lining the intestinal walls. This intricate design, besides enhancing the rate of absorption, also serves to repel pathogenic microbes from the mucosa of the intestines, showing how rich and multifunctional the small intestines are in maintaining overall health and homeostasis. Physiologically, the small bowel operates via very intricate mechanical and biochemical processes. Intestinal peristalsis, or the simultaneous contraction and relaxation of intestinal muscles, propels food along the small intestine, while segmentation contractions aid in the intestinal contents mixing and absorption.

The environment of the lumens is also modified through the secretion of digestive enzymes, electrolytes, and hormones that guide digestive processes. For instance, the presence of chyme in the duodenum triggers the release of secretin and cholecystokinin, which then cause the pancreas and gallbladder to release bile and digestive juices. Nutrient uptake also occurs against a concentration gradient with the help of active transport mechanisms as well as facilitated diffusion. These processes reflect the prominent role that the small bowel plays in digestion and nutrient uptake. Although it is of critical importance, the small bowel has a propensity to a variety of disorders, which can have a significant impact on its physiological and anatomical functions. Conditions , such as Crohn's disease, celiac disease, and small bowel obstruction are only a few of the numerous small bowel disorders that can occur based on genetic, environmental, or immunological factors. These diseases are often complicated by small bowel inaccessibility, which has led to the development of advanced diagnostic modalities , such as computed tomographic enterography (CTE) and video capsule endoscopy (VCE). Diagnostic accuracy for small bowel illnesses has greatly enhanced with the advancement of these technologies and is better managed. This innovation underlines the need for more research into the anatomy and physiology of the small bowel, whose results are fundamental to implementing appropriate treatments to combat small bowel pathologies (Dhanya et al., 2024; Popa et al., 2023) (Figure 5.2).

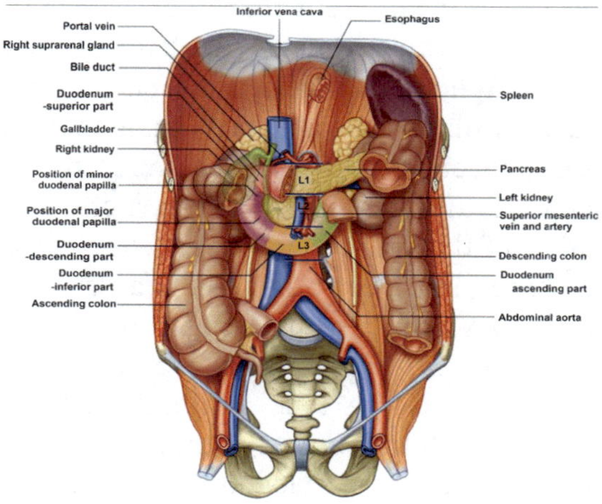

Figure 5.2. Anatomy and physiology of the small bowel

Source: https://els-jbs-prod-cdn.jbs.elsevierhealth.com/cms/attachment/2074505000/2069026008/gr2_lrg.jpg.

5.1.1. Structure of the Small Intestine

The small intestine is a vital component of the gastrointestinal tract, responsible for nutrient digestion and absorption of nutrients. It has a bifurcated structure comprising three crucial segments: duodenum, jejunum, and ileum. Each of the three segments has specialized functions and distinct structures to ensure the overall process of nutrient absorption is efficient. The first section, the duodenum, receives chyme from the stomach and is where bile and pancreatic juices are introduced to further break down carbohydrates, proteins, and fat. The jejunum has a highly vascularized lining that maximizes nutrient absorption, and the ileum further continues this action and is especially efficient at absorbing vitamin B12 and bile acids. This intricate architecture ensures that food is properly digested and the body is supplied with the best nutrients for homeostasis. In the discussion of small intestine function in the context of small bowel disorders, it is apparent that interference with its architectural structure can lead to severe health complications. Conditions , such as celiac disease, Crohn's disease, and small intestinal bacterial overgrowth (SIBO) demonstrate the impact of alterations in the structure and function of the small intestines. Celiac disease, for instance, involves immune-mediated damage leading to villous atrophy and a decrease in surface area for nutrient absorption. Crohn's disease may cause local inflammation and structuring of the bowel, further damaging nutrient absorption and leading to malnutrition. Understanding small intestine anatomy is critical in the diagnosis and management of such diseases because it enables clinicians to recognize appropriate therapeutic interventions that will restore function and abate symptoms of such conditions. New advances in imaging techniques, such as 3D cine-MRI, have provided useful information about small intestine motility and structural assessment, further contributing to our understanding of small bowel disorders. This new technology allows for observation of bowel movement and can identify abnormalities in the small intestine that will not be visible with standard imaging. The addition of machine learning to allow for automatic segmentation and centerline tracking of the intestine allows more precise measurements of motility, crucial in disorders like SIBO that can potentially affect transit time and overall gut function. As research continues to develop, the way the structure of the small intestine, its motility, and the gut-brain axis relate to one another highlights the importance of approaching the understanding and treatment of small bowel pathology in a systemic manner (Cryan et al., 2019; van Harten et al., 2022) (Figure 5.3).

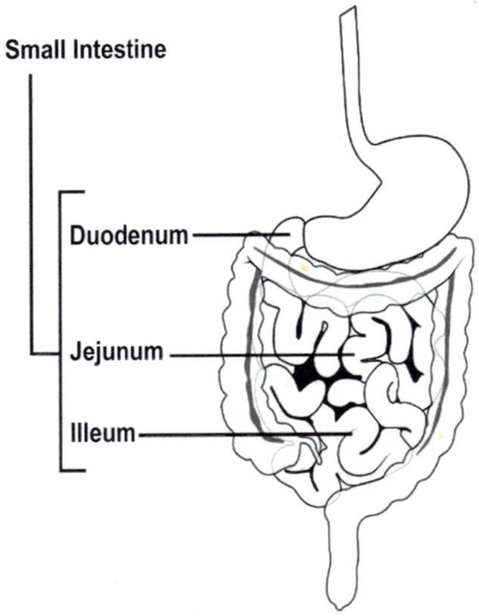

Figure 5.3. Structure of the small intestine.

Source: https://www.knowyourbody.net/wp-content/uploads/2018/04/Small-Intestine-Diagram.jpg.

5.1.2. Functions of the Small Bowel in Nutrient Absorption

The duodenum, the jejunum, and the ileum of the small intestine all play an important role in nutrient absorption from food once it has been digested. This is done by such specialized structures as microvilli and villi, which have a profound effect of increasing the surface area of the intestinal wall. This extensive surface area facilitates maximum absorption of carbohydrates, proteins, fats, vitamins, and minerals into the bloodstream. The enterocytes lining the small bowel contain an array of transporters that facilitate the selective passage of nutrients through cell membranes. Besides passive diffusion of minute molecules, it involves active transport of larger substrates. Furthermore, the rich blood supply supporting the villi ensures efficient transport of absorbed nutrients to be metabolized or stored by the body, emphasizing the significance of small bowel function towards general well-being and nutrition. Another essential characteristic of small bowel function is its interaction with gut microbiota, which plays a remarkable role in nutrient absorption. The gut's heterogeneous microbial populations are essential for fiber fermentation and the production of short-chain fatty acids, both of which are involved in energy metabolism and maintaining intestinal health. Dysbiosis of the microbial population will also directly impair nutrient absorption efficiency and may result in conditions as far-reaching as malnutrition, obesity, or type 2 diabetes. Evidence indicates that certain gut microbial metabolites have been found to improve gut barrier function and immune modulation, thereby enhancing the protective role of the small bowel against infections. As alterations in gut microbiota have been linked to several small bowel diseases, knowledge regarding the interactions is invaluable in terms of therapeutic interventions in the balance and restoration of small intestine function (de Vos et al., 2022; Ghosh et al., 2021). The small bowel absorption process is not only limited to macronutrients but also involves micronutrients, and they are important in their function to eliminate deficiencies. For instance, the ileum has a distinctive function in the absorption of vitamin B12 and bile acids, which are important for fat digestion. Malabsorption syndromes , such as celiac disease or Crohn's disease, result from the impaired lining of the intestine, thereby severely reducing the absorptive ability for nutrients and resulting in severe systemic manifestations. These patients typically present with manifestations of the resulting deficiency of nutrients, including osteoporosis and anemia. Management is by measures , such as adjustment of diet and supplementation to reverse these deficiencies by maximizing absorptive capacity for nutrients. Understanding the varied function of the small bowel in nutrient absorption signals its importance to general health and highlights how disease of the small bowel may impact an individual's well-being (Ghosh et al., 2021; de Vos et al., 2022) (Figure 5.4).

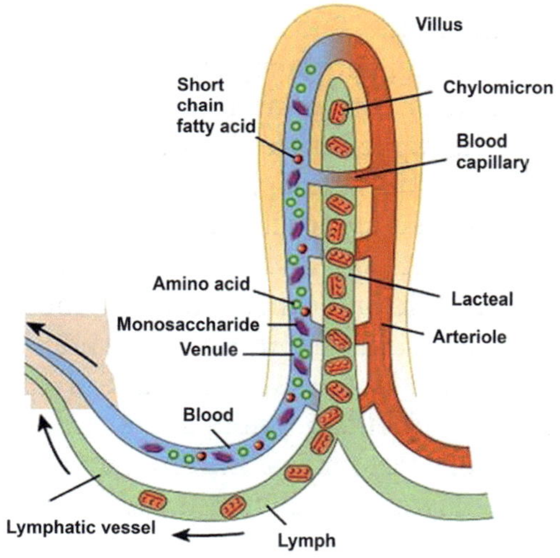

Figure 5.4. Functions of the small bowel in nutrient absorption.

Source: https://biology-igcse.weebly.com/uploads/1/5/0/7/15070316/3669884_orig.png.

5.1.3. Role of the Small Bowel in the Immune System

The small intestine occupies a pivotal place in the immune system as a key interface between gastrointestinal health and the body's immune mechanisms. This organ is responsible for maintaining homeostasis through the interaction of its epithelial cells with a broad spectrum of microbiota. The layer of intestinal epithelium serves as a physical barrier governing the passage of microorganisms and dietary antigens while allowing nutrient absorption. Interestingly, the microbiota influences the development and function of the immune system by regulating the behavior of immune cells in the mucosal layer lining the small intestine. Studies have indicated that dysbiosis, or imbalance of gut microbiota, can lead to barrier dysfunction and its resultant immune activation that can be manifest in various diseases like inflammatory bowel disease. Thus, the small bowel is not just a site for nutrient absorption but also an active participant in immunological function required to maintain health (Ghosh et al., 2021). The small bowel is also an important part in the production and regulation of immunological responses through its specialized immune cells, like lymphocytes and macrophages. These immune cells are located along the intestinal mucosa to play a strategic role and interact with dietary substances and gut microbiota to modulate immune tolerance. Microbial fermentation products also modulate immune function, tightening epithelial barriers and eliciting anti-inflammatory responses. Enteroendocrine cell hormonal signals and immune cell cytokine release serve as coordinated communication between the microbiota and the immune system. These interactions are crucial in protective immunity development as well as prevention against excessive inflammatory responses to non-pathological stimuli. Therefore, the interaction between the immune components within the small bowels and its microbiota emphasizes the role of this organ in health modulation and prevention against immune dysfunction disorders (Kayama & Takeda, 2020). In the context of small bowel pathology, understanding the immune role of this region is central in the planning of therapeutic strategies. Conditions , such as celiac disease, Crohn's disease, and other forms of enteropathy highlight the significance of disordered immune response in the small bowel. Celiac disease, for instance, is an example where the consumption of gluten triggers an inappropriate immune reaction, leading to villous atrophy and malabsorption. Alternatively, therapeutic approaches , such as fecal microbiota transplantation have been promising in redressing microbiota composition and enabling immune rebalancing. Continued studies of mechanisms of small bowel immune reactions, especially the impacts of microbiota and metabolites, may reveal new treatment methods for a spectrum of inflammatory and autoimmune conditions. Hence, the recognition of the small bowel's contribution to the immune system is vital not only in understanding pathophysiological mechanisms but also in enhancing clinical management of diseases associated with it (Ghosh et al., 2021) (Figure 5.5).

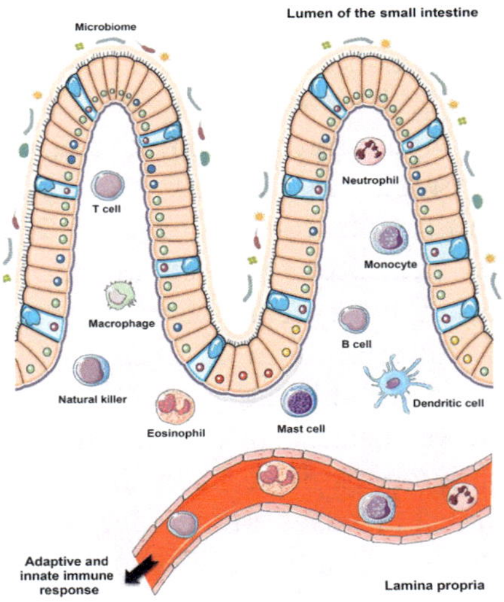

Figure 5.5. Role of the small bowel in the immune system.

Source: https://www.researchgate.net/publication/359271967/figure/fig5/AS:1154723910549521@1652319042465/The-intestinal-immune-system-physically-separated-from-the-intestinal-microbiome-The.png.

5.2. Common Small Bowel Disorders

Small bowel disease includes a variety of conditions that can seriously affect gastrointestinal health. Two of the disorders, small bowel varices and volvulus, stand out for their clinical significance and diagnostic difficulties. Small bowel varices, most commonly due to portal hypertension, are a rare but serious complication. Small bowel varices can cause gastrointestinal bleeding, such that it is important to intervene on time to avoid morbidity and mortality. The small bowel varices are at times challenging to diagnose by clinicians because symptoms are not specific and may overlap with normal gastrointestinal complaints. Furthermore, diagnostic approaches that utilize advanced endoscopic technology , such as double balloon enteroscopy (DBE) have enhanced visualization and treatment of small bowel varices with improved patient outcomes and more firm management strategies (Dolu et al., 2025). Small bowel volvulus is another severe disorder that requires emergent medical care due to its potential to cause obstructive symptoms and ischemia. Often it includes twisting of the bowel over its mesenteric axis and is also found to present acutely, mimicking a state of shock or extreme abdominal distress. The diagnostic approach is normally by radiologic studies, such as abdominal computed tomography (CT), which can ascertain the obstructive process and verify the anatomical defects present, such as an incomplete common mesentery (Manar et al., 2025). Because of the rapid onset of symptoms, prompt surgical exploration is typically needed in an attempt to decompress the obstruction and prevent sequelae like bowel necrosis. Identification of volvulus is vital for successful intervention and can significantly enhance the prognoses of patients in the event of early identification. Multidisciplinary treatment is required in the management of small bowel disorders to deal with the complex relationship of symptoms and therapeutic regimens. Small bowel varices and volvulus are classic examples of the significance of advanced diagnostic techniques and familiarity with basic pathophysiological mechanisms. The blended approach of endoscopic and surgical intervention allows for personalized treatment approaches capable of meeting individual patients' needs. Additionally, continued research into these processes is essential to increase diagnostic sensitivity and therapeutic effectiveness. As the medical device continues to advance, the ability to treat and understand these common small bowel diseases will improve further, pointing to the importance of continuing education and communication among caregivers in gastrointestinal health (Figure 5.6).

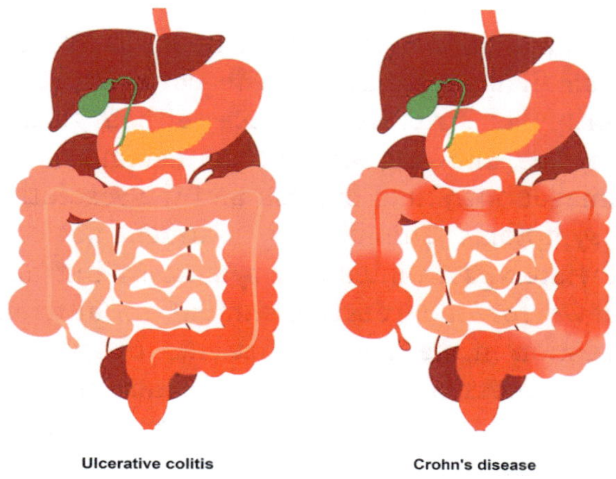

Figure 5.6. Common small bowel disorders.

Source: https://www.hopkinsmedicine.org/-/media/images/health/1_-conditions/stomach-and-gut/inflammatory-bowel-disease-graphic-large.ashx.

5.2.1. Celiac Disease

Celiac disease, an autoimmune disorder characterized by an immune reaction to gluten, has significant implications for the health of the small bowel. When an individual with celiac disease consumes gluten, which is most often found in wheat, barley, and rye, their immune system mounts an inappropriate response that includes inflammation and damage to the lining of the small intestines. This results in a set of symptoms including abdominal pain, diarrhea, and malabsorption of nutrients, compromising the health of the patients in general. Since these symptoms can also be similar to other gastrointestinal illnesses, celiac disease is sometimes hard to diagnose. In general, serologic tests to identify certain antibodies, followed by biopsy of the intestine, are performed to ascertain the severity of mucosal damage. Early diagnosis and treatment help to prevent long-term sequelae, such as nutritional malabsorption and increased risk for intestinal malignancies secondary to chronic inflammation. Furthermore, celiac disease presentation underscores the central role of dietary management in the treatment of small bowel disease. The cornerstone of therapy is strict compliance with a gluten-free diet, allowing for mucosal healing in the damaged intestinal mucosa and the resolution of symptoms. This dietary treatment not only alleviates gastrointestinal symptoms but also allows for the reestablishment of nutrient ingestion in the involved patients. Despite the effectiveness of this dietary restriction, patients have indicated prolonged symptoms despite adherence to a gluten-free diet. This is theorized to result from non-celiac gluten sensitivity or the presence of other food allergens, such as fructans or wheat germ agglutinins, that would exacerbate the symptoms. Thus, a comprehensive nutrition assessment is crucial in adults and children with celiac disease to establish other food intolerances that may require to be controlled alongside gluten exclusion (Rej et al., 2022). Compounding the challenges of the treatment of celiac disease are co-morbidities with other gastro-intestinal disorders, such as small intestinal bacterial overgrowth (SIBO). Research shows that celiac disease patients are at higher risk for SIBO development, potentially due to altered gut motility or gut microbiome change that occurs after the development of the disease. The potential significance of this association is significant due to the fact that SIBO can further exacerbate nutritional deficiencies and gastrointestinal symptoms in individuals with celiac disease. SIBO diagnosis is typically through breath tests, and then either antibiotics or changing diets, as described in a study finding increased SIBO prevalence among inflammatory bowel disease patients (Wanzl et al., 2023). This emphasizes the need for the full management strategy to consider not only celiac disease but also co-morbidities that might impact the patients' overall gut health and quality of life (Figure 5.7).

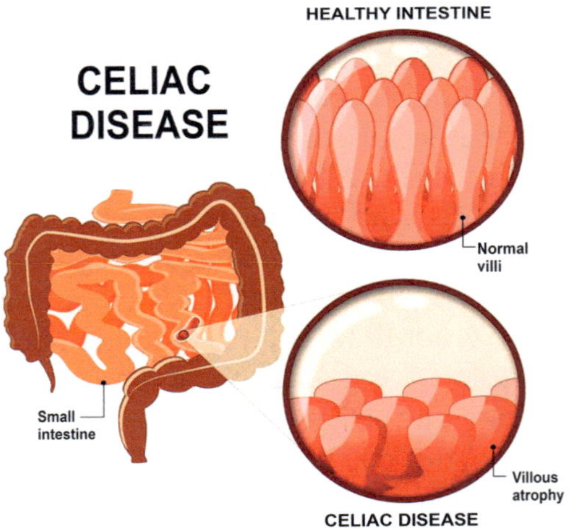

Figure 5.7. Celiac disease.

Source: https://novagastro.org/wp-content/uploads/2023/02/iStock-905599948.jpg.

5.2.2. Crohn's Disease

Crohn's disease is a complex disorder of the small bowel, characterized by chronic inflammation of the gastrointestinal tract. Crohn's disease is prevalent in the small intestines primarily, but can be found anywhere in the digestive system from the mouth all the way to the anus. Immune response dysregulation in genetically predisposed individuals suggests the multifaceted interaction of environmental, microbial, and genetic host factors resulting in widespread gastrointestinal distress and other systemic symptoms. Symptomatology of Crohn's disease is typical and includes severe abdominal pain, diarrheal stools that are often bloody, weight loss, and extraintestinal manifestations , such as skin rashes and arthralgic complaints. The relapsing and chronic course of this disease has resulted in it becoming the focus of ongoing research because it not only needs medical management but also a holistic understanding of its pathophysiology to promote patient care (Peng et al., 2024). Diagnosis of Crohn's disease needs an extensive approach, which involves clinical assessment, imaging and laboratory tests, as well as endoscopic studies. Those distinguishing characteristics that are most important in differentiating Crohn's disease from similar diseases include the recognition of ulcerations and strictures within affected portions of the intestine. Most critical is to distinguish from cryptogenic multifocal ulcerative stenosing enteritis (CMUSE), a disease with similar symptomatology but requiring distinct management paradigms. CMUSE patients will have surgeries for stenosis of the small bowel, reinforcing the utmost need for proper diagnosis. In a case report, a 62-year-old man patient presenting with abdominal pain and edema of both lower limbs, imaging and endoscopic techniques ultimately led to surgery, underscoring the need for effective diagnostic interventions in optimal care of small bowel disorders (Peng et al., 2024). Management of Crohn's disease is a multidisciplinary plan that may include conventional pharmacological treatment, biological treatment, dietary modifications, and, as a measure of last resort, surgical resection. Therapies are aimed at diminishing symptoms, causing remission, and lessening flare frequency. The pathology of Crohn's disease generally requires individualized therapy methods that account for the unique requirements of the patient and responsiveness to therapy. Although conventional treatments do exist, emerging information from integrative and holistic systems, such as Ayurveda, suggests that nonconventional treatment modalities can also prove beneficial. The above perspective considers Crohn's disease from different angles of medicine and identifies the necessity of thinking outside the box, involving a combination of conventional practices with alternative medicine, in order to improve the quality of life for patients suffering from this debilitating disease (Shah et al., 2024) (Figure 5.8).

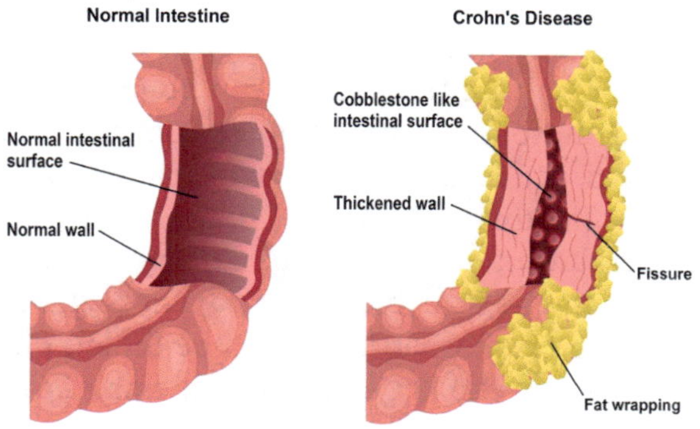

Figure 5.8. Crohn's disease.

Source: https://www.drugwatch.com/wp-content/uploads/Crohn's-Disease.jpg.

5.2.3. Small Intestinal Bacterial Overgrowth (SIBO)

Small intestinal bacterial overgrowth, or SIBO, is a disease where there is an overgrowth of bacteria in the small intestine and it can lead to significant gastrointestinal upset. The small intestine usually has very few bacteria when compared with the colon, but various factors can disrupt this homeostasis to lead to SIBO. Conditions that diminish gastric acid production, such as proton pump inhibitor therapy or gastric bypass, can allow for an adequate nidus for overgrowth of bacteria. Motility disorders also lead to the delayed movement of small intestinal contents, and the bacteria overgrow. The effects of SIBO are not restricted to mere gastrointestinal discomfort because the overgrowth also affects nutrient uptake, resulting in deficiencies that can compromise general well-being. Diagnosis of SIBO needs an immense understanding of a patient's medical history and recognition of risk factors. Doctors usually employ an accumulation of diagnostic procedures to guarantee the diagnosis of bacterial overgrowth. The most common tests are breath tests for the measurement of hydrogen or methane production after a carbohydrate substrate has been ingested and culture analysis of aspirates of the small intestine. They are utilized to establish a connection between the clinical presentation and the possibility of SIBO. It is noteworthy that the patient can be presenting with symptoms of bloating, abdominal pain, diarrhea, and malabsorption, which mimic other gastrointestinal diseases. Therefore, careful interpretation of the findings during diagnosis is paramount in a bid to avoid misdiagnosis. Thus, the diagnosis of SIBO can be difficult but significant in the larger context of small bowel disorders (Ponziani et al., 2016). The treatment of small intestine bacterial overgrowth is largely focused on managing the underlying condition, with the added removal of excessive bacteria. Therapeutic management may include the use of antibiotics targeted at those bacterial species responsible for the overgrowth. Nonetheless, pharmacologic interventions are typically supplemented by an individualized approach to the resumption of correction of the patient's nutritional deficiencies and possible underlying motility disorders. It is important that clinicians consider the patient's entire clinical profile in creating a treatment plan. SIBO patients may also be provided with dietary modifications, such as restriction of fermentable carbohydrates, that may further facilitate symptom worsening. The nature of SIBO recurrence supports the need for ongoing management measures, such as follow-up and monitoring, to prevent future recurrence and improve the quality of life in the patients (Greenson, 2015) (Figure 5.9).

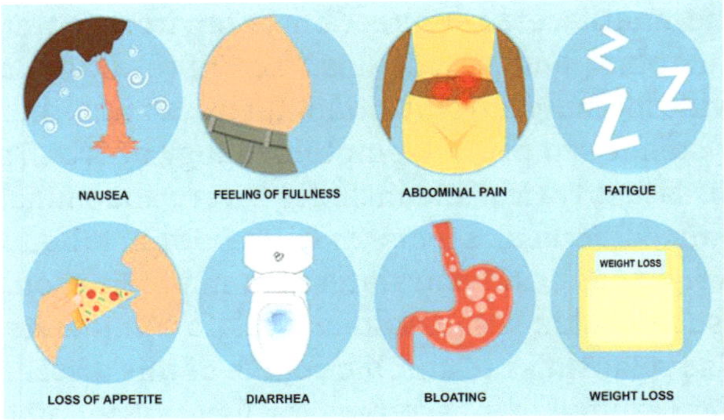

Figure 5.9. Small intestinal bacterial overgrowth (SIBO).

Source: https://jaffreykazimd.com/wp-content/uploads/2022/10/SIBO-Small-Intestinal-Bacterial-Overgrowth.jpg.

5.3. Symptoms and Diagnosis

Identification and interpretation of the symptom are critical for successful diagnosis and treatment of small bowel disease. Small bowel disease can be inferred by a wide range of symptoms, from bloating and abdominal discomfort to diarrhea and unintentional weight loss. The symptoms overlap with those of other gastrointestinal illnesses, making it harder to diagnose. For instance, small intestinal bacterial overgrowth (SIBO) displays an abnormal proliferation of bacteria within the small intestine and presents with symptoms , such as distension and malabsorption, and thus even further emphasizes the relevance of accurate diagnostic tests. To overcome these challenges, physicians use a combination of clinical evaluations and symptomatology in an attempt to get a general description of the status of the patients, thereby facilitating proper diagnostic methods and management plans (da Silva et al., 2025). Diagnosis of small bowel diseases mostly relies on non-invasive methods, importantly, breath tests, which could diagnose conditions like SIBO without the need for invasive processes. Breath tests, which include tests with glucose and lactulose, allow doctors to detect malabsorption and bacterial overgrowth by measuring hydrogen or methane in the patient's breath. These tests, however, can have their limitations, i.e., susceptibility to false positives or false negatives, and thus yield incomplete data about the underlying conditions.

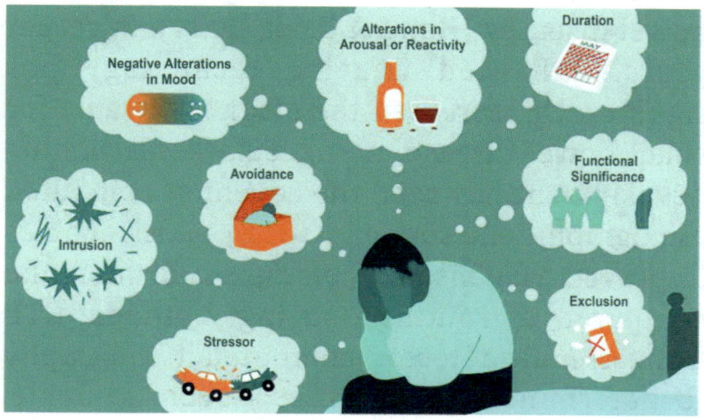

Figure 5.10. Symptoms and diagnosis.

Source: https://www.verywellmind.com/thmb/xayGVSnQ6c-C7n4XynSqErOjI58=/1500x0/filters:no_upscale():max_bytes(150000):strip_icc()/requirements-for-ptsd-diagnosis-2797637_FINAL-5c12bdac46e0fb0001e7d6b3.png.

Therefore, doctors are recommended to include symptom histories and possibly employ adjunct diagnostic techniques, e.g., imaging tests or endoscopy, particularly when preliminary tests yield inconclusive outcomes. The application of a multi-dimensional approach to diagnostic workup may significantly enhance the validity of SIBO diagnosis and other small bowel diseases (da Silva et al., 2025). Another critical component of assessing small bowel disease is distinguishing functional from structural etiologies for gastrointestinal symptoms. Disorders like chronic constipation can be caused by a multitude of physiological reasons and can have a serious effect on the quality of life of the patient. A feeling of incomplete evacuation, for example, and infrequent bowel movements are some of the symptoms. This makes it critical to ensure proper investigations. Physicians typically use the Bristol Stool Form Scale and digital rectal examination to objectively quantify symptoms and differentiate chronic constipation from other gastrointestinal conditions. Testing on physiological levels is advised to be priceless for nonresponsive individuals to first-line treatment approaches, emphasizing the importance of accurate diagnosis in dealing with small bowel disorders effectively. With adherence to set guidelines in diagnosis, physicians can improve patient outcomes and formulate interventions more specifically (Figure 5.10).

5.3.1. Common Symptoms Associated with Small Bowel Disorders

The small intestine, which forms part of the gut, is responsible for the digestion and absorption of nutrients. Once the disease occurs within this section, it will typically manifest itself in many normalizing signs that can significantly impact an individual's lifestyle. The symptom of pain in the abdomen, which can be cramping or aching, often tends to worsen upon food intake. Moreover, distention and bloating are frequent and can be painful or uncomfortable. Such complaints can be accompanied by changes in bowel habits, both constipation and diarrhea, depending on the type of small bowel disorder. The multifaceted presentation of symptoms renders it important that clinicians embrace a broad approach to diagnosis, ruling out other potential gastrointestinal conditions that can obscure the clinical picture (Ford et al., 2018). In addition to pain in the abdomen, patients with pathology of the small bowel often present with numerous gastrointestinal complaints. Diarrhea, commonly characterized by loose or watery stools, is a common consequence in conditions , such as celiac disease and small intestinal bacterial overgrowth. Conversely, some patients might complain of constipation, particularly if there is either a functional obstruction or a motility disorder of the small intestine. Nausea and vomiting are also common presentations and these precede more severe underlying conditions that demand urgent attention. These GI symptoms not only affect physical well-being but may also put a psychological strain on the patient, making them anxious or depressed as they struggle with the uncertainty of their illness (Davis et al., 2018). Nutritional deficiencies typically occur as a secondary condition in patients with small bowel disease. Due to the small bowel's principal role to absorb, diseases of its function can cause malabsorption syndromes, followed by deficiency states of major vitamins and nutrients. The consequent nutritional deficiency signs may manifest with weakness, fatigue, or involuntary weight loss, which subsequently may complicate the clinical presentation. Additionally, anemia is a frequent symptom in patients with small bowel disease, particularly when the body is not able to absorb enough iron or vitamin B12. Thus, not only do the healthcare workers need to treat acute gastrointestinal symptoms, but they also need to examine the long-term nutritional condition of the patients and apply appropriate interventions to promote overall health (Ford et al., 2018).

5.3.2. Diagnostic Tests and Procedures

Diagnosis of small bowel disease is often a multi-modal one involving multiple diagnostic tests and studies. An initial step is the performance of laboratory tests , such as serology and stool examination to search for potential inflammatory markers or infections that would be indicative of underlying diseases like inflammatory bowel disease (IBD). These tests are particularly helpful since they can be performed on an outpatient basis and results are obtained quickly, potentially guiding further diagnostic procedures. However, in the case of non-diagnostic laboratory findings, more invasive testing , such as endoscopy, becomes the need of the hour. Endoscopic procedures allow for direct visualization of intestinal mucosa and the opportunity to obtain tissue biopsies, thereby allowing further analysis of the histological activity of diseases of the small bowel. This algorithm of first laboratory tests and then invasive studies forms the foundation of the accurate diagnosis of small bowel diseases (Hong & Baek, 2024). In recent years, enhanced imaging technology has significantly increased the diagnostic value for small bowel disease. A particularly fascinating development has been the advent of computed tomographic enterography (CTE), which enables improved visualisation of the small intestine compared to routine imaging methods. CTE utilizes multidetector computed tomography to determine abnormalities , such as bowel thickening and mucosal hyperenhancement, which are critical in the diagnosis of most small intestinal diseases. In one evaluation of CTE effectiveness, there was proof that demonstrated this modality to excel in depicting intraluminal and extraintestinal pathology, rendering the modality particularly beneficial for diseases that are difficult to evaluate utilizing endoscopy alone (Dhanya et al., 2024). The accuracy and non-surgical advantages of CTE provide clinicians and patients with a reliable method with which to gauge disease progression and modify treatment plans accordingly. Endoscopic and imaging modalities are critical to the diagnosis of small bowel disease, but the integration of artificial intelligence (AI) is setting new benchmarks. Current innovation in AI technology holds the potential to make diagnosis processes more efficient with improved analysis of images and pathology results. AI algorithms are able to analyze patterns in the diagnostic images and look for minute trends that would easily escape human detection. This is particularly significant in the case of IBD, as disease activity occurring early on in the process can significantly determine the success of the treatment. Secondly, the integration of AI and established diagnostic tests would ease clinicians' decision-making with a focus on offering patients timely and appropriate interventions. In the future, the dynamics between traditional diagnostic modalities and new technologies will likely redefine the art of small bowel disorder diagnosis (Dhanya et al., 2024; Hong & Baek, 2024) (Figure 5.11).

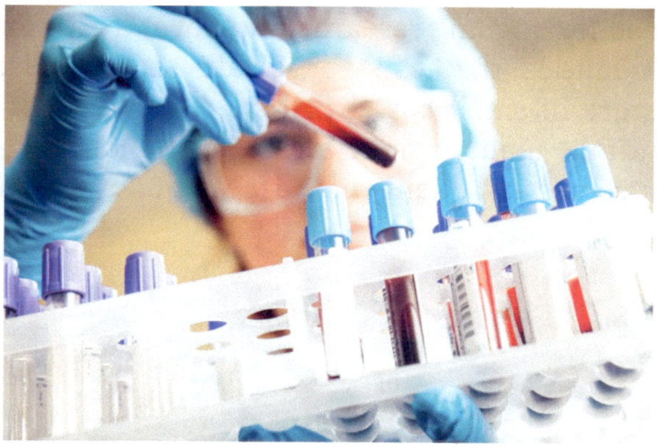

Figure 5.11. Diagnostic tests and procedures.

Source: https://familypracticecenterpc.com/wp-content/uploads/2019/09/family-practice-near-me-medical-testing-center-Atlanta-GA-x-rays-Atlanta-GA-types-of-medical-tests-blood-test.jpg.

5.3.3. Importance of Differential Diagnosis

In the setting of small bowel pathology, differential diagnosis is crucial to the appropriate diagnosis and management of a variety of gastrointestinal conditions. Small bowel pathology symptoms overlap significantly, which can complicate patient assessment. A case in point may be taken from where patients with abdominal pain, discomfort, altered bowel habits, and bloating may have heterogeneous pathologies, for instance, Irritable Bowel Syndrome (IBS) or gross structural disease like small bowel obstruction. The complexity of symptomology necessitates a broad differential diagnostic process to avoid misdiagnosis, with consequent inappropriate management regimens. Accurate assurance that health workers conduct detailed assessment and screen for a broad array of conditions is essential in order to validate diagnoses and generate effective treatment programs. The significance of differential diagnosis is further underscored by the potential co-existence of co-morbid conditions, whose presence may further blur the clinical presentation. For example, studies have shown there to be a strong association between IBS and other disorders, such as migraine, fibromyalgia, and depression, which mask or mimic the actual gastrointestinal issues. Through an analysis of health data in patients with IBS, the odds of prevalence of these comorbid diseases were found to be exponentially higher in comparison to non-IBS groups, suggesting that physicians must have a holistic view of patients' welfare. Thus, the identification of symptoms that span across several domains, psychological and gastrointestinal, for instance, is possible to achieve a correct diagnosis and a comprehensive treatment plan that targets both the small bowel syndrome and any underlying conditions and ultimately enhances patient outcomes as a whole (Cabral et al., 2006). Secondly, the application of standardized diagnostic criteria facilitates differential diagnosis and brings about clarity when interpreting symptoms. Consider, for instance, a patient with the clinical presentation of IBS, including chronic abdominal pain relieved with defecation, among other gastrointestinal manifestations like constipation and diarrhea (Zammit, 2009). Unless rigidly following differential diagnosis protocols, practitioners will overlook less common but hazardous conditions presenting with the same features, including celiac disease or inflammatory bowel disease. Through the use of a methodical process in differential diagnosis, practitioners can ensure that the overall clinical presentation is examined, leading to timely interventions that are able to counter complications and enhance quality of care provided to patients with small bowel disorders.

5.4. Treatment Options

The treatment for small bowel illnesses is diverse and generally based on the condition in question. Conservative treatment can be all that is needed in some patients who have mild to moderate presentations. The treatment often entails dietary modifications, whereby patients are advised to choose and avoid foods that trigger their symptoms. Nutritional support, such as enteral nutrition in individuals with malabsorption or marked loss of weight, also plays a crucial role in providing adequate nutrition. Pharmacologic treatment , such as anti-inflammatory medication and antibiotics, is also effective in the treatment of inflammatory bowel disease, whereas specific agents that stimulate motility can be used in dysmotility. Eventually, what is sought is to alleviate symptoms and improve the quality of life of the patients through the application of patient-based, individualized means. When conservative measures are not enough, interventional procedures and surgery can be needed. Particularly, conditions , such as small bowel obstruction or significant structural abnormalities will need surgery. Surgical treatment may range from relatively minor intervention to more extensive resections based on the nature and extent of the disorder. For instance, symptomatic Tarlov cyst patients may benefit from cyst-wrapping surgery with an aim to reduce the size of the cyst and alleviate pressure against neighboring nerve structures, thereby reducing attendant symptoms like pain and bowel and bladder control dysfunction (Mogica et al., 2023). This decision to proceed with surgery is usually based on the overall assessment of risks and benefits involved, with particular emphasis on long-term expectations and patient quality of life. New treatment modalities, particularly aimed at augmenting intestinal motility, are assuming greater significance as newer treatment options for disorders of motility , such as postoperative ileus and chronic intestinal pseudo-obstruction. The recent advancement in pacing techniques of the small intestine has been promising in modulating the contractile patterns of the intestines for improved bowel function. Research has established that the pacing parameters have the ability to alter the amplitude of segmental contractions, potentially acting as a therapeutic option for the less responsive patient group compared to conventional treatments (Nagahawatte et al., 2023). This pioneering approach emphasizes the need for ongoing research into novel treatment modalities that can appreciate the complex nature of small bowel disease to devise more optimal management strategies to optimize outcomes and quality of life for patients (Figure 5.12).

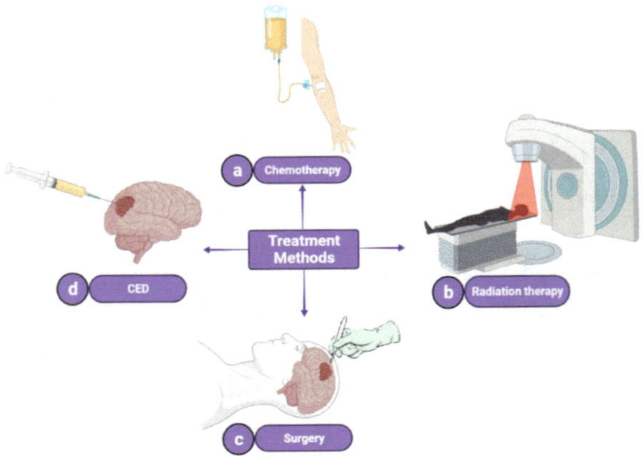

Figure 5.12. Treatment options.

Source: https://www.researchgate.net/publication/365317240/figure/fig1/AS:11431281096661553@1668226281968/Different-treatment-strategies-of-brain-tumors-In-chemotherapy-the-drug-solution-is.png.

5.4.1. Dietary Modifications and Management

Dietary modification is the core of management of small bowel diseases, particularly conditions , such as small intestinal bacterial overgrowth (SIBO) and irritable bowel syndrome (IBS). Such conditions are likely to cause debilitating symptoms , such as bloating, pain, and malabsorption, hence necessitating an integrative treatment plan. Evidence-based practice guidelines distinguish the efficacy of specific dietary treatments, including low fermentable oligosaccharides, disaccharides, monosaccharides, and polyols (FODMAPs) diets, that were effective in symptomatic reduction associated with SIBO and IBS. Through low intake of high-FODMAP foods, patients are able to avert further fermentation in the gut, thus averting painful symptoms and enhancing overall gastrointestinal functioning (da Silva et al., 2025). Such a change in diet not only helps in the control of symptoms but also allows for greater nutrient absorption, indicative of the integrated relationship between dietary lifestyles and the complexity of small bowel illnesses. Aside from low-FODMAP dietary regimens, the application of probiotics has also proven to be of potential interest in managing small bowel diseases. The gut microbiome plays a significant role in supporting gastrointestinal health and dysbiosis aggravates symptoms associated with conditions like IBS. Probiotics, in particular, certain species like Bifidobacterium and Lactobacillus, can potentially stabilize microbial balance, thereby improving the gut health and alleviating symptoms (Palaniswamy, 2025). These microorganisms support the immune system and enhance the integrity of the gut barrier, which is particularly beneficial in individuals with increased intestinal permeability. Also, dietary intervention that prefers the intake of prebiotic fiber can provoke the development of healthy microbiota, having a beneficial gut environment along with the alleviation of SIBO and IBS-associated symptoms. Long-term management of small bowel disease necessitates an interdisciplinary approach with dietary recommendations and follow-up. Follow-up is essential regularly to alter dietary interventions according to responses and concordance. A registered dietitian could play a vital role in creating individualized meal plans according to personal taste and nutritional needs to facilitate easier compliance with the diet. In addition, educating patients about the potential recurrence of symptoms, particularly in SIBO, highlights the importance of ongoing watchfulness of dietary management (da Silva et al., 2025). The interactive nature of diet management not only enables the patient but also optimizes their overall quality of life, substantiating that dietetic modification is a part of the overall small bowel disorder management (Figure 5.13).

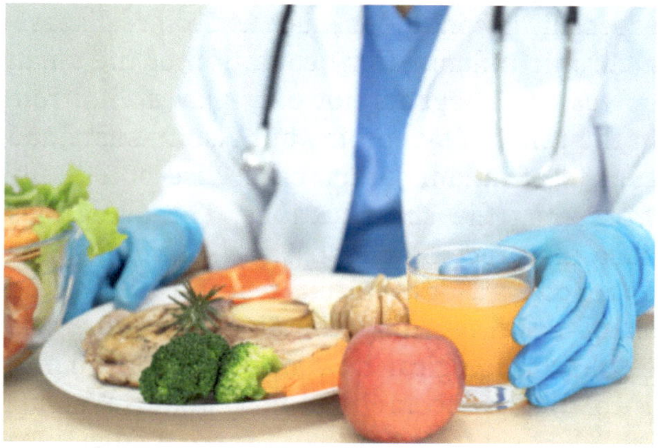

Figure 5.13. Dietary modifications and management.

Source: https://www.indexsciences.com/wp-content/uploads/2024/02/Diet-modification.webp.

5.4.2. Pharmacological Treatments

Pharmacological treatments of small bowel disease are now a pillar of the management of many gastrointestinal disorders, particularly in adhesions and intestinal well-being maintenance. Adhesive small bowel obstruction is typically secondary to prior operations and is extremely challenging due to its non-specific nature, which is comparable to other etiologies of small bowel obstruction. Although surgical options are kept in reserve for complicated situations, there is a significant role for pharmacologic modalities in conservative management. Investigations have emphasized the role of meticulous surgical techniques to minimize adhesion formation, followed by pharmacologic interventions that attempt to control healing responses and inflammation. In general, the position of pharmacological therapy in small bowel disease management demonstrates the importance of a multidisciplinary approach to balance surgical and non-surgical paradigms in managing patients (Ghimire et al., 2023). Of the variety of available pharmacological therapies, the usage of anti-inflammatory drugs and targeted medications gains popularity, especially in conditions , such as Crohn's disease, a chronic inflammatory condition of the small bowel. These agents not only play a vital role in the relief of symptoms but also in sustained control of inflammation, otherwise potentially worsening the complications. The guidelines have also recommended small-bowel capsule endoscopy as an initial test for suspected small-bowel bleeding, thereby raising the role of pharmacological treatments in consonance with diagnostic innovation (Pennazio et al., 2022). Early treatment with these medications can literally reduce the difference in patient outcome by managing symptoms and potentially preventing surgical inevitability. The evolving dynamics of drug therapy for small bowel disease promote an integrative approach, with a focus on both treatment and diagnosis. Pharmacologic treatments are also investigated for preventing complications associated with small bowel disorders. Sophisticated techniques , such as device-assisted enteroscopy, have emerged as an option to surgery for managing retained foreign bodies in small bowel obstruction patients. Pharmacologic prophylaxis becomes a key component in such conditions for maintaining intestinal motility and reducing the need for surgical intervention. Intestinal health-targeted therapies, including agents that promote motility and adhesion prevention, are found to have an increasingly important role in integrative management of patients with small bowel disorders. Continued scientific studies on the efficacy and safety of such interventions will progressively augment their adoption, ultimately leading to improved management practices with respect to patient quality of life and healthcare expenditure problems arising from small bowel issues (Pennazio et al., 2022; Ghimire et al., 2023) (Figure 5.14).

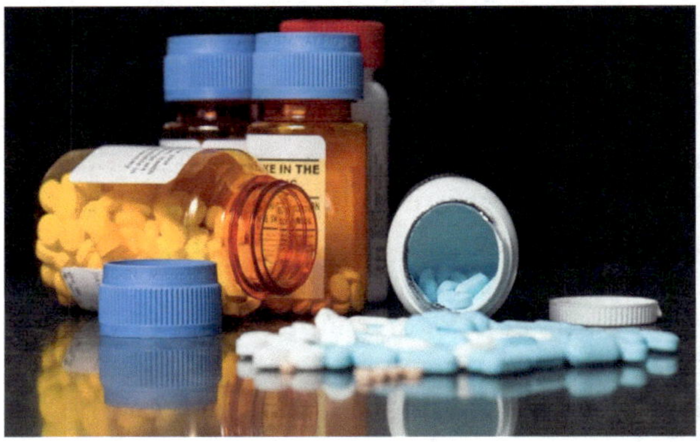

Figure 5.14. Pharmacological treatments.

Source: https://www.findatopdoc.com/var/fatd/storage/images/_aliases/fb_thumb/healthy-living/medical-advancements-new-treatments-and-perspectives-on-fibromyalgia/pharmacological-treatments/3584078-1-eng-US/Pharmacological-treatments.jpg.

5.4.3. Surgical Interventions

For the small bowel disorders, surgery is often an essential component of patient management, particularly if non-surgical interventions cannot be beneficial to the patient. Surgery plays the most important role in conditions , such as Crohn's disease, where bowel obstruction, stricture, or perforation complications can require surgery. Although the improvement in medical therapy has improved the treatment strategy, most patients with Crohn's disease ultimately require surgical intervention along the duration of the disease to address complications like severe inflammation or complication-related problems. The decision to proceed with surgery involves the correct assessment of the patient's clinical status and the potential for disease recurrence and strengthens the necessity of a proper appreciation of the unique clinical presentation and disease course of each patient in examining their treatment option (Buldukoglu et al., 2025). Adhesion disease is one of the more problematic side effects of small bowel surgery, a result of scar tissue formation after surgery. Adhesion can lead to intestinal obstruction, which will need to be managed with additional surgery to repair. Studies have proven that the likelihood of adhesions forming is significantly reduced with the use of minimally invasive laparoscopic techniques over the traditional open surgical techniques.

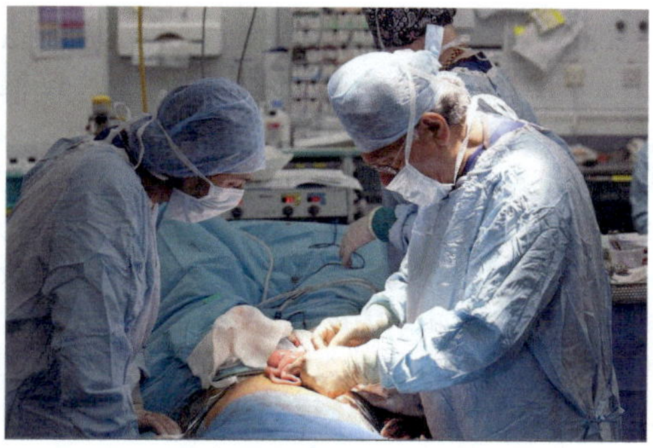

Figure 5.15. Surgical interventions.

Source: https://images.fineartamerica.com/images-medium-large-5/small-bowel-resection-surgery-mark-thomasscience-photo-library.jpg.

This emphasizes the importance of surgical technique selection in minimizing the risk of adhesions and identifies how new approaches can have a beneficial impact on patient outcomes (Savchuk & Polyovyy, 2024). Therefore, surgeons need to weigh up the benefits of such methods against the chance of necessity for reoperation due to adhesive disease occurring following surgery. Moreover, the road to establishing biomarkers, such as serum levels of GSDMD, has the capacity for disease activity measurement and surgical intervention determination in Crohn's disease. Increased serum levels of GSDMD have already been shown to indicate inflammatory activity and could be used as a non-invasive marker to decide when surgery may be needed. The use of biomarkers in treatment planning can enhance decision-making processes to enable clinicians to determine if surgery may decrease complications and the advanced nature of the disease. The application of biomarkers therefore, not only complements surgical strategies but also signifies a shift towards more personalized treatment plans in managing small bowel disease (Buldukoglu et al., 2025). It incorporates both new surgical techniques and the use of biomarkers, with the end goal of improving patient quality of life and the efficiency of therapy (Figure 5.15).

5.5. Complications of Small Bowel Disorders

Small bowel disease complications can significantly impact the outcome in the patient, particularly in those with coexisting conditions. For instance, the patients who are operated on for liver cirrhosis have an extremely high rate of postoperative complications; over 90% of such patients develop some kind of complication, as reported in studies. Serious complications like bleeding, respiratory impairment, and renal insufficiency can be exacerbated by factors like portal hypertension and impaired liver function. The challenges are particularly important in instances of emergency operations or subsequent surgical procedures, contributing to the risk associated with small bowel surgery. These findings highlight the significance of complete preoperative assessment and, if possible, preventive treatment in managing liver disorders before surgical procedures are conducted, thus maximizing patient safety and surgical outcome (Wetterkamp et al., 2020). Moreover, the link between the immune system and small bowel disease provides an additional level of sophistication in the intricacy of complications to enjoy. The gut has a primary role in housing most of the body's immune cells, which actively respond to numerous antigens and modulate immune responses.

Immune deregulation in small bowel disorders, for instance, inflammatory bowel disease, can lead to excessive inflammation, making the patient susceptible to fistula formation and bowel obstruction. Murine studies have contributed importantly to illuminating such mechanistic pathways, thus assisting health practitioners to formulate improved interventions and preventive therapies. Study of immune cell behavior in gastrointestinal inflammation allows for therapeutic targeting, which can lower symptoms and improve overall management of small bowel diseases, bringing into context the relationship between immune function and gut health (McManus et al., 2019).

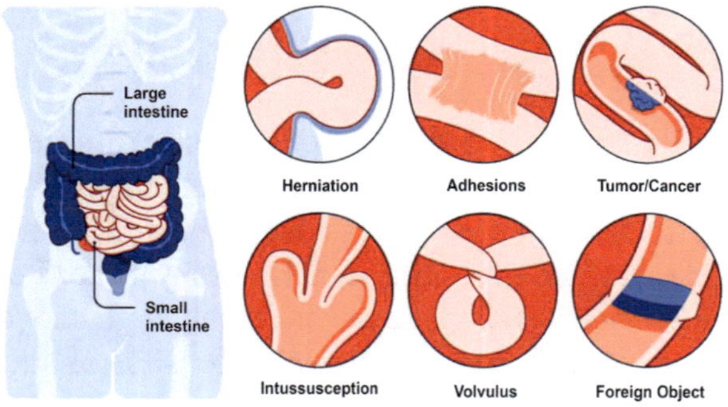

Figure 5.16. Complications of small bowel disorders.

Source: https://media.post.rvohealth.io/wp-content/uploads/sites/3/2024/01/3046713-bowel-obstruction-and-blockage_1296x889-body-1024x703.png.

Finally, the long-term impacts of complications from small bowel disease can extend way beyond the short-term risk of surgery and can impact nutritional status as well as quality of life for those affected. Malabsorption, an all-too-common result, leads to deficiencies in essential nutrients, which in turn can lead to disastrous health effects , such as osteoporosis and anemia. These complications, therefore, require treatment to be multimodal and encompass surgical correction, nutritional support, as well as ongoing monitoring for potential long-term sequelae. Identification and management of surgical and non-surgical complications of small bowel disorders are critical to improve patient outcomes. Therefore, healthcare systems need to implement appropriate follow-up practices that prioritize both surgical recovery and nutritional optimization for patients with the dilemma of small bowel disorders (Wetterkamp et al., 2020) (Figure 5.16).

5.5.1. Nutritional Deficiencies

The interplay between small bowel disease and a deficiency in diet is a delicate factor that requires comprehensive research. The absorption of nutrients is the main role of the small intestine, and any structural or functional dysfunction of the bowel can lead to severe dietary deficiencies. Celiac disease, Crohn's disease, and small intestinal bacterial overgrowth (SIBO) are classic illustrations of how damage to the small bowel can impair the absorption of macronutrients and micronutrients. Inefficient absorption of crucial elements , such as iron, vitamin B12, and folate may result in anemia, neuropathy, and other extraintestinal manifestations. Besides, small bowel disorder patients are at a higher risk for conditions associated with malnutrition, and therefore there is a need for meticulous nutritional assessments and interventions according to individual needs, especially in heterogeneous gastrointestinal pathologies. Nutritional deficiencies in patients with small bowel disorders are treated by having a clear grasp of the causative etiologies and symptoms. For instance, individuals with inflammatory bowel disease (IBD), like Crohn's disease and ulcerative colitis, may present with evidence of deficiency of nutrients due to persistent inflammation and consequent malabsorption. An elevated prevalence of SIBO has been observed by research studies in these patients with heightened bacterial overgrowth correlating with diet influences in IBD patients (Wanzl et al., 2023). As SIBO can worsen malabsorption through the use of nutrients meant for the host, treatment of this dysbiosis is crucial for the recovery of gut health. Besides this, identification of the deficiencies in nutrients among IBD patients on clinical assessment is also essential to initiate appropriate changes in diet or supplementation measures to compensate for the negative effects of such deficiencies on overall health and well-being. Blending these new diagnostic technologies, such as enteroscopy and video capsule endoscopy (VCE), has been promising to enhance the diagnosis of small bowel illnesses and resultant nutritional conditions (Popa et al., 2023). With increasing interest in using artificial intelligence to augment diagnostic yield, these modalities can aid in the early detection of pathologies that may lead to malabsorption and resultant nutritional deficiencies. For example, accurate diagnosis of lesions or functional impairment of the small intestine allows clinicians to customize nutritional therapy accordingly, thus optimizing patient outcome. Lastly, by understanding the complex interrelationship between small bowel disease and nutritional insufficiency, practitioners can adopt a more unified approach, encompassing both the gastrointestinal pathology and its systemic effects, thereby enhancing the management of those who are affected.

5.5.2. Increased Risk of Malignancy

Of note in small bowel diseases is the increased malignancy risk. Chronic conditions, such as irritable bowel syndrome (IBS) and constipation, have been of interest owing to suspected links with a variety of digestive tract cancers (DTCs). A Mendelian randomization study identified that genetically predicted constipation was strongly associated with the heightened risk of pancreatic adenocarcinoma (PAAD) (OR = 2.29, 95% CI: 1.422–3.69, P = 0.001) (Fan et al., 2024). However, IBS did not associate with a small increase in the risk of colorectal carcinoma (CRC) (OR = 1.17, 95% CI: 1–1.37, P = 0.05) (Fan et al., 2024). The findings here illustrate the necessity for monitoring of patients with long-standing gastrointestinal symptoms, as early identification and treatment of such disease may avoid possible malignant change. The relationships between small bowel disease and malignancy extend beyond gastrointestinal symptomatology, as they include systemic factors that lead to cancer. Chronic inflammatory states are a typical feature of disease , such as IBS, and this suggests that the systemic immune response will be a critical factor in tumour development. For instance, systemic autoimmune conditions , such as psoriasis, have been associated with more comorbidities , such as malignancies. In addition, therapy in such systemic conditions typically involves the administration of biologic drugs that can change inflammatory pathways. These also come with threats , such as exacerbation of existing conditions and new-onset disease, hence complicating patient management and influencing cancer risk further. The interplay between small bowel disorders and malignancy must be understood within an integrative framework that takes account of both the direct effects of these conditions and their indirect effects. Inflammatory reactions, side effects of treatment, and genetic predispositions are all potential elements within an individual's risk profile for developing cancer. Tumor necrosis factor-α inhibitors, for example, which are a common therapy for inflammatory bowel disease, have proven effective but with cautions about malignancy risks. Hence, successful patient management programs must balance the need for effective therapy against vigilant monitoring for potential malignancies. With this multifaceted comprehension, health care providers can individualize interventions so that not only can they treat the initial condition of the gastrointestinal system but also actively protect against the possible development into malignancy.

5.5.3. Intestinal Obstruction

Intestinal obstruction is a strong clinical challenge in the setting of small bowel disease, usually resulting in substantial morbidity when it goes undetected and untreated. It can result from mechanical etiology through adhesions, tumors, or strictures, and functional etiology with dysperistalsis. The presentation can be abdominal distension, vomiting, constipation, and abdominal pain, with its severity based on the site and nature of the obstruction. Such manifestations should be properly understood because ignoring the acute symptoms can lead to dreadful complications in the shape of bowel perforation or necrosis. Hence, early diagnostic imaging modalities, i.e., ultrasonography or CT scan, are of prime importance in evaluating suspected cases and formulating an effective management strategy suitable for the patient's requirements. The pathogenesis of intestinal obstruction is multifaceted, particularly in adult patients in whom it typically arises as a result of structural lesions that are identifiable. In adults, the more common etiology is intussusception, a process though not uncommon in children, can explain a significant number of cases when it does occur in the older age groups. Unlike in children, where idiopathic intussusception is prevalent, in adults, the typical lead points exist in the form of tumors or polyps and cause chronic or subacute obstruction symptomatology. This dramatic difference in presentation highlights the need for an elevated index of suspicion for potential malignancies while evaluating adult patients presenting with gastrointestinal symptoms. The early utilization of imaging techniques, in this case, CT scanning, allows for early intervention, which remains critical because non-operative adult case decreases complicate patient outcomes significantly (Aregawi & Girma, 2023). Treatment options for intestinal obstruction are heavily dependent on the underlying etiology and degree of severity. In malignancies or complicated structures, surgical treatment is typically the management of choice. General guidelines for treatment mandate exploratory surgery to be used for a direct approach to the obstruction in persistent symptoms and in imaging-diagnosed conditions. As shown in recent case histories, for instance, of patients with immunotherapy where adverse gastrointestinal reactions result in severe obstructions, an approach to treating the entire patient is important. For instance, an understanding that the majority of the complications can arise due to drug-related side effects, such as in the case of a Pembrolizumab-treated patient, serves to show the significance of interdisciplinary treatment using medical and surgical experts (Qian et al., 2024).

5.6. Current Research and Advances

Small bowel diseases are transforming in topography at a rapid rate due to tremendous innovations in medical technology and research methods. One of the most prominent areas of development is artificial intelligence (AI) in the detection and treatment of gastrointestinal illness. The recent studies have shown that machine learning algorithms , such as Artificial Neural Networks, can greatly increase the predictive capability for outcomes of lower gastrointestinal bleeding. This has a significant implication for conditions of the small bowel since early diagnosis and adequate management can prevent complications and enhance outcomes for patients. AI-based models are also being developed to assist in risk stratifying patients, thus facilitating timely interventions that are critical to effective disease management as well as preventing the risk of surgical intervention (Parikh et al., 2025). In addition to these predictive models, advances in small bowel capsule endoscopy (SBCE) have set new standards for detecting small bowel disorders. Over the past two decades, SBCE has become a pivotal tool for gastroenterologists, providing a non-invasive method for visualizing the small intestine. However, the interpretation of SBCE videos can be labor-intensive and time-consuming, posing significant challenges in clinical settings (Piccirelli et al., 2025). In order to tackle such issues, recent research has focused on integrating AI technologies to facilitate automated analysis and interpretation of capsule endoscopy videos, thereby reducing the load on health care professionals and improving diagnostic efficiency. In addition to speeding up the rate at which diagnoses are made, this integration also ensures consistency and reliability in the assessment, an important factor in dealing with complex small bowel diseases.

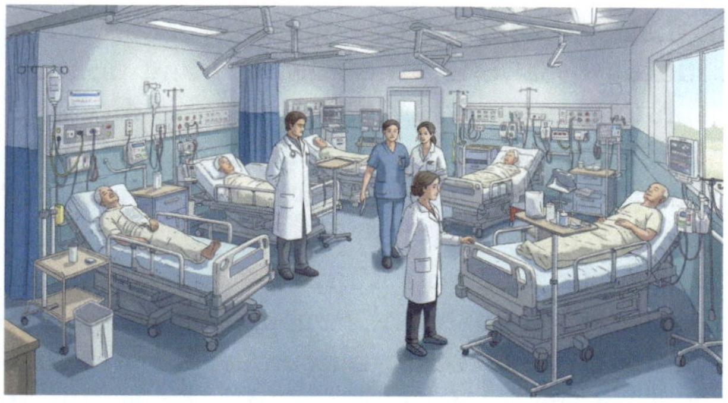

Figure 5.17. Current research and advances advancements in medical technology and research methodologies.

Source: https://149860134.v2.pressablecdn.com/wp-content/uploads/ward-1.jpg.

The research today in the area of small bowel disorders also emphasizes the need for multi-disciplinary interventions that combine technological developments with clinical wisdom. Because AI is gradually infecting all areas of gastroenterology, more studies are needed to evaluate its efficacy in real-world applications to treat small bowel disorders comprehensively. This calls for clinical trials that compare not just patient outcomes but also the competence of AI solutions in treating several gastrointestinal diseases. By doing this, the objective would be to bridge current gaps in patient care and establish a basis for future innovations that could transform treatment protocols of small bowel disease (Parikh et al., 2025; Piccirelli et al., 2025). The collaborative efforts of health professionals, researchers, and technology developers will definitely play a crucial role in shaping the next wave of developments in this field (Figure 5.17).

5.6.1. Emerging Therapies and Treatments

Treatment of small bowel disease has been revolutionized with the advent of new therapies targeting the root pathophysiological mechanisms of the disorders. Among the most important advances is biologic therapy, which harnessed the body's immune system to combat inflammation and restore gut homeostasis. As a case in point, the enhanced understanding of the pathways of signaling in inflammatory bowel disease (IBD) has led to innovative interventions. These treatments, like some of the anti-TNFs and the anti-cytokine drugs and integrin blockers, demonstrate a tailored approach that attempts to minimize the adverse effects of usual treatment, but enhance efficacy. Also, clinical research has now acknowledged the potential of novel agents with selective activity against unique pathogenetic processes, thereby opening the foundations for targeted therapy approaches specifically designed for small bowel disease (Bretto et al., 2023). One such interesting example in this context is tofacitinib, a Janus kinase (JAK) inhibitor that has been in the spotlight due to its efficacy in the management of moderate to severe ulcerative colitis (UC). Prescribed by health authorities, such as NICE, tofacitinib is an important option for those patients who have shown inadequate responses to traditional therapies. The pioneering OCTAVE trials not only emphasized its effectiveness in causing and maintaining remission but also emphasized its beneficial safety profile, making it an appropriate consideration for those with treatment challenges. Importantly, recent real-world data continue to affirm the benefits initially observed in clinical practice, demonstrating significant improvements in clinical and endoscopic response. In this regard, then, tofacitinib is a welcome addition to the treatment repertoire of IBD, particularly small bowel involvement (Liu et al., 2022). The future, however, holds that inclusion of such novel therapies implies that careful consideration must be afforded to the patient's profile and history of the disease. The future of combining therapies where JAK inhibitors , such as tofacitinib are administered alongside available biological therapies is an interesting future direction in managing small bowel disorders. Today's debate over evolving treatment paradigms places strong emphasis on the importance of personalized medicine, such that treatment modalities are customized to meet the diverse needs of a patient. Additionally, with ongoing research into next-generation JAK inhibitors and other novel agents, the prospects of small bowel disorder treatments do, in fact, appear bright. The constant evolution of these strategies not only contributes to enriching clinical results but also enhances the quality of life of patients in treating the complexity of chronic gastrointestinal diseases (Bretto et al., 2023).

5.6.2. Role of Microbiome in Small Bowel Health

The microbiome is essential for the well-being of the small bowel, impacting metabolic functions as well as immune functions. This group of diverse microorganisms is responsible for carbohydrate breakdown and nutrient uptake, refining overall digestive function. Disruptions in the microbiota can result in dysbiosis through a decrease in healthy bacteria and an increase in pathogenic organisms. These disturbances have been associated with many small bowel disorders, including small intestinal bacterial overgrowth (SIBO) and inflammatory bowel diseases (IBD). In recent studies, the gut mycobiome, which is part of the microbiome consisting of fungi, was identified as being very important, with the implication that the interaction between bacteria and fungi is essential for maintaining intestinal homeostasis and health. Understanding these interactions can lead to novel therapeutic approaches aiming to restore microbiome equilibrium and improve small bowel function. Nutritional modulation to manage microbiome composition is a growing trend for the therapy of disorders of the small bowel. A low-FODMAP diet, among others, has been used to alleviate symptoms of irritable bowel syndrome (IBS) by reducing certain fermentable oligosaccharides, disaccharides, monosaccharides, and polyols. Bloating, pain in the abdomen, and irregular bowel habits are reduced by altering the gut flora and limiting osmotic effects that are responsible for digestive discomfort. New data suggest that this dietary strategy may also treat other illnesses, including IBD and SIBO, and thus prove to be a general therapeutic agent. By prioritizing individualized changes to diet, healthcare professionals can optimize therapeutic outcomes for patients while, in the process, optimizing the health of the microbial community within the small bowel (Karoń et al., 2024). Regardless of the use of trial or regulation, the need for thorough research on the long-term effects of dietary alteration and microbial therapies reigns supreme. With treatment modalities evolving, information regarding how different diets affect microbial diversity, immune systems, and interactions with the brain will enlighten the better treatment of small bowel disorders. In addition, the interplay between dietary interventions and the mycobiome makes it imperative to consider a broad strategy in the treatment of gastrointestinal health. While exciting results are being achieved, keeping these therapy strategies sustainable and nutritionally adequate remains a continued priority. Future studies must work on the balance of microbial populations and explore possibilities for integrating dietary therapies with pharmaceutical interventions in order to create more effective, targeted therapies for patients with small bowel disease (Karoń et al., 2024).

5.6.3. Future Directions in Small Bowel Disorder Research

With increased research into small bowel disease, a crucial area of research in the future is research into the role of nuclear receptors , such as the pregnane X receptor (PXR) and constitutive androstane receptor (CAR). These transcriptional factors have come to serve as key regulators not only of drug metabolism, but also homeostatic processes within the gastrointestinal tract. The intricate interaction of these receptors with numerous endogenous and exogenous substances suggests that further research may uncover new mechanisms of signaling that would be beneficial to the understanding of inflammatory bowel diseases and other associated conditions. Studies into modulation of PXR and CAR have the potential to identify new therapeutic strategies that enhance the effectiveness of existing drugs. By examining the varied ligand-binding profiles of these receptors, scientists can formulate targeted approaches that are potentially effective for the control of small bowel disorders in the clinic (Poudel et al., 2022). Aside from receptor studies, the microbiota-gut-brain axis deserves more research as a basic element affecting small bowel diseases. The symbiotic action between gut microbiota and neurological function has been the subject of specific attention, as interest in microbial composition, not just for gastrointestinal well-being, but for broader physiological processes, has increased. Exploring the role of microbial metabolites, such as short-chain fatty acids, is one approach to understanding how gut well-being impacts brain and mental health outcomes. Since research has already confirmed correlations between the microbiota and illnesses like anxiety and autism, further work could explore microbiome-driven therapy that could alleviate symptoms in small bowel disorder (Cryan et al., 2019). The research could enable new treatments aimed at restoring microbial balance and enhancing the gut microbiota, hence the general health of individuals suffering from such disorders (Cryan et al., 2019). Finally, unraveling the dilemma of research on small bowel disorders will be crucial to progress in the future. While significant progress has been achieved during the past decade, there are still gaps in our understanding of disease etiology, especially with regard to microbiota composition-affecting variables , such as diet, medication, and environmental stressors. The convergence of advanced diagnostic techniques, such as metagenomics and bioinformatics, is able to facilitate a general improved understanding of microbial populations and their functional characteristics. In addition, longitudinal studies could provide data on how alterations in gut microbiota across phases of life could be involved in the improvement and development of small bowel disease. By isolating these influential factors, researchers are able to develop targeted interventions taking into account the complex interrelations between dietary habits, microbial diversity, and genetic predisposition, ultimately targeting optimal treatment modalities appropriate for patients' needs and status (Cryan et al., 2019; Poudel et al., 2022).

CLOSER LOOK

NON-TRADITIONAL TREATMENTS:

Non-traditional treatments, often referred to as complementary and alternative medicine (CAM), encompass a wide range of therapeutic practices that fall outside conventional Western medical approaches. A closer look at these treatments reveals both their growing popularity and the need for careful evaluation of their safety, effectiveness, and role in holistic care. Many individuals turn to non-traditional therapies seeking natural options, fewer side effects, or a more integrative approach to health—especially for chronic conditions that may not respond fully to standard treatments.

Among the most widely used non-traditional therapies are herbal and botanical supplements. Plants such as turmeric, ginger, echinacea, and ashwagandha are commonly used for inflammation, immune support, and stress reduction. While many herbs contain bioactive compounds with potential therapeutic effects, their potency can vary, interactions with medications are possible, and scientific evidence for certain claims remains limited. Therefore, guidance from trained professionals is crucial when integrating herbal remedies into care plans. Mind–body therapies form another major category. Practices such as yoga, meditation, tai chi, breathing exercises, and mindfulness-based stress reduction have demonstrated benefits for mental health, chronic pain, sleep quality, and overall well-being. These therapies work by reducing stress hormones, improving autonomic nervous system balance, and enhancing emotional regulation. Their low risk and accessibility make them appealing components of integrative care.

Manual and movement-based therapies, including acupuncture, chiropractic care, massage therapy, and osteopathic manipulation, are often used to manage musculoskeletal pain, migraines, and functional disorders. Acupuncture, rooted in traditional Chinese medicine, has gained increasing scientific support for conditions like chronic pain, nausea, and neuropathy. Chiropractic care and massage may improve mobility, reduce tension, and enhance quality of life when used appropriately and performed by licensed practitioners.

Non-traditional treatments also include energy-based therapies, such as Reiki or therapeutic touch, which focus on balancing perceived energy fields. Although scientific evidence for these modalities is limited, many individuals report subjective benefits such as relaxation and reduced stress. A growing movement toward integrative medicine emphasizes combining evidence-based non-traditional therapies with conventional care. This approach acknowledges that healing involves physical, emotional, and social dimensions. However, it also stresses the importance of scientific evaluation, professional training, and open communication between patients and healthcare providers.

Overall, non-traditional treatments can play a meaningful role in supporting health and well-being, especially when used responsibly and in conjunction with conventional medical care. A closer examination highlights the need for balanced, informed decision-making to maximize benefits while minimizing risks.

SUMMARY

In conclusion, the multigranular aspect of small bowel disorders demands a keen understanding of both their pathophysiology and management. As demonstrated, diseases , such as Crohn's disease pose exceptional challenges, particularly in the management of proximal small bowel lesions. The advent of biologic agents has new fronts in treatment to offer, but the variable success rates in achieving endoscopic healing highlight the subtleties of these diseases. Specifically, studies indicate that most patients did not achieve complete endoscopic healing after one year of biologic therapy, and thus, a need for ongoing research and treatment progress. What is clear is that personalized and optimized approaches are vital in optimizing therapeutic gains for patients with small bowel diseases (Huang et al., 2025). Furthermore, the value of appropriate prognostic assessment of small bowel tumors cannot be overstated because it has direct implications for clinical decision-making and patient management. The heterogeneity of small bowel tumors, ranging from gastrointestinal stromal tumors to adenocarcinomas, dictates careful scrutiny of multiple prognostic factors, including tumor stage and systemic inflammatory markers. The analysis of a high correlation between the stage of the tumor and survival of the patient was found to affirm the requirement for staging as a factor in prognosis. Although inflammatory markers were not statistically significant in the present research, further analysis will be important to make sure that these factors are addressed in future research and clinical practice, thereby maximizing predictive validity (Torun et al., 2025). In summary, the milieu of small bowel diseases is a heterogeneous collection of complex disorders that requires a multidimensional framework for efficacious management and treatment. As medical therapies evolve, so must our understanding of the intricate interaction between disease characteristics and outcome. Continued research into the efficacy of new treatments, along with a focused review of prognostic factors, can change the way healthcare professionals currently treat small bowel disorders. By the establishment of an integrated and interdisciplinary system, practitioners are able to better seamlessly integrate treatment with the specific needs of each patient and thereby improve the quality of care provided to this patient population. Addressing these regions not only enhances our clinical practice but also contributes to the emerging field of knowledge for disorders of the small bowel.

The small intestine, being an important component of the gastrointestinal tract, is in charge of the digestion and absorption of nutrients. Illness in this compartment can lead to serious complications to health, most commonly involving pain in the abdomen, bloating, and changes in bowel habits. An interaction of small bowel disease with systemic diseases not only presents problems for diagnosis, but also highlights the need to understand their underlying mechanisms in depth. Progress in genetic research has contributed to the understanding of associations of small bowel disease with kidney stone disease and other diseases. Specifically, studies showed that there were affirmative genetic correlations between gastrointestinal disease and kidney stone disease and that such correlations underscore the imperative to explore the correlations further for improved management and outcome of these patients (Wang et al., 2025). These results present opportunities for formulating improved treatment strategies with personalized patient profiles. Moreover, dysbiosis of the gut microbiota has been a key mechanism of pathogenesis in the majority of small bowel diseases. The gut microbiota is involved in numerous physiologic functions, including metabolic function and immune function. Dysfunctional gut microbiota can exacerbate or indeed cause conditions like Irritable Bowel Syndrome (IBS) and Small Intestinal Bacterial Overgrowth (SIBO) (Frias et al., 2025). To reverse these conditions, therapeutic approaches with the introduction of targeting the microbiota, e.g., by using rifaximin, have come into being as part of possible therapies. This antibiotic acts selectively to reduce the harmful bacteria but not by eradicating the helpful species. In doing so, rifaximin is a promising candidate for the treatment of several conditions in this part of the gastrointestinal tract that arise because of microbial imbalance, which has highlighted the strong impact of microbiota on small bowel conditions. Understanding the genetic and microbiotic determinants of small bowel disease not only informs their pathophysiology but also suggests directions for prevention and therapy. Shared common genetic architecture between gastrointestinal disease and kidney stones suggests integrative research considering the two systems simultaneously in clinical therapy (Wang et al., 2025). In parallel, ongoing investigation of the microbiota's function in maintaining health of the gut supports the therapeutic value of individualized therapies , such as rifaximin, to decrease symptoms and restore balance (Frias et al., 2025). Additional investigation in these areas will be required to advance further the pathogenesis of small bowel disease for enhanced patient outcomes and to inform public health interventions for reducing the disease burden of gastrointestinal disease.

References

1. Greenson J. K. (2015). The biopsy pathology of non-coeliac enteropathy. Histopathology, 66(1), 29–36. https://doi.org/10.1111/his.12522 (accessed on 15th July 2025).
2. Aregawi, A., & Girma, A. (2023). Case report: A closed loop obstruction secondary to idiopathic small bowel intussusception in an elderly woman. International Medical Case Reports Journal, 16, 65–72. https://www.semanticscholar.org/paper/9f068b7490d9fece51757a26d314a345cab94da4 (accessed on 15th July 2025).
3. Bauer, E., Metzler-Zebeli, B. U., Verstegen, M. W., & Mosenthin, R. (2011). Intestinal gene expression in pigs: effects of reduced feed intake during weaning and potential impact of dietary components. Nutrition research reviews, 24(2), 155–175. https://doi.org/10.1017/S0954422411000047 (accessed on 15th July 2025).
4. Bretto, E., Ribaldone, D. G., Caviglia, G. P., Saracco, G. M., Bugianesi, E., & Frara, S. (2023). Inflammatory bowel disease: Emerging therapies and future treatment strategies. *Biomedicines, 11*, 2249–2249. https://doi.org/10.3390/biomedicines11082249 (accessed on 15th July 2025).
5. Buldukoglu, O., Ocal, S., Atar, G. E., Kaya, B., Isik, M. D., Tigli, G. A., Akça, S., et al. (2025). P0349 Gasdermin D: A new inflammatory biomarker in assessing clinical disease activity in Crohn's disease. *Journal of Crohn's and Colitis.* https://www.semanticscholar.org/paper/14723107ad90a74f856df97a97f036536ae423e0 (accessed on 15th July 2025).
6. Cabral, H. J., Cole, J. A., Farraye, F. A., Rothman, K. J., et al. (2006). Migraine, fibromyalgia, and depression among people with IBS: A prevalence study. https://core.ac.uk/download/142040751.pdf (accessed on 15th July 2025).
7. Cho, Y., Lee, Y., Shin, J., Jung, H., Park, S. Y., Kang, S., Song, K. H., et al. (2023). 2022 Seoul Consensus on Clinical Practice Guidelines for Functional Constipation. *Journal of Neurogastroenterology and Motility, 29*, 271–305. https://www.semanticscholar.org/paper/41b439fd4642f850d231c22245063171c1ec62fa (accessed on 15th July 2025).
8. Cryan, J. F., O'Riordan, K. J., Cowan, C. S. M., Sandhu, K. V., Bastiaanssen, T. F. S., Boehme, M., Codagnone, M. G., et al. (2019). The microbiota-gut-brain axis. *Physiological Reviews, 99*, 1877–2013. https://doi.org/10.1152/physrev.00018.2018 (accessed on 15th July 2025).
9. da Silva, B. C., Ramos, G. P., Barros, L. L., Ramos, A., Domingues, G., Chinzon, D., & Passos, M. (2025). Diagnosis and treatment of small intestinal bacterial overgrowth: An official position paper from the Brazilian Federation of Gastroenterology. Arquivos de Gastroenterologia, 62. https://www.semanticscholar.org/paper/ed9dcbde0b87d9ace2e6982504f9166ca4e104f5 (accessed on 15th July 2025).
10. Davis, B. R., Lee-Kong, S. A., Migaly, J., Feingold, D. L., & Steele, S. R. (2018). The American Society of Colon and Rectal Surgeons clinical practice guidelines for the management of hemorrhoids. Diseases of the Colon & Rectum, 61, 284–292. https://doi.org/10.1097/dcr.0000000000001030 (accessed on 15th July 2025).
11. de Vos, W. M., Tilg, H., Van Hul, M., & Cani, P. D. (2022). Gut microbiome and health: Mechanistic insights. *Gut, 71*, 1020–1032. https://doi.org/10.1136/gutjnl-2021-326789 (accessed on 15th July 2025).
12. Dhanya, S. B., Sunil, H. C., Gowthami, G. S., Yeli, R. K., Suhas, C. N., & Kumar, M. P. (2024). Exploring the use of computed tomography enterography in the evaluation of small

bowel disease: A prospective study. Cureus, 16. https://www.semanticscholar.org/paper/d2215ed0b486e28c176baa49fddc454e812f183f (accessed on 15th July 2025).

13. Dolu, S., Arayıcı, M. E., Onem, S., Buyuktorun, I., Dongelli, H., Bengi, G., & Akarsu, M. (2025). Effectiveness of double balloon enteroscopy in the diagnosis and treatment of small bowel varices. *Diagnostics, 15.* https://www.semanticscholar.org/paper/eed94a2cccf48a5511d6a07b35b4a6c51ad5d4f9 (accessed on 15th July 2025).

14. El Halabi, M., Arwani, R., Rao, S. S. C., & Parkman, H. P. (2024). Brain fog in gastrointestinal disorders: Small intestinal bacterial overgrowth, gastroparesis, irritable bowel syndrome. *Journal of Clinical Gastroenterology.* https://www.semanticscholar.org/paper/d0c8499ce1010aa5d340272881ab3f9f87a493fd (accessed on 15th July 2025).

15. Fan, R., Zhang, J., Shen, J., Mao, C., Li, S., & Zhuang, Z. (2024). Causal relationships of chronic constipation and irritable bowel syndrome with digestive tract cancers: A Mendelian randomization study. *Recent Patents on Anti-Cancer Drug Discovery.* https://www.semanticscholar.org/paper/d13af408344c779daf1921ada6199a0f24d8db79 (accessed on 15th July 2025).

16. Ponziani, F. R., Gerardi, V., & Gasbarrini, A. (2016). Diagnosis and treatment of small intestinal bacterial overgrowth. Expert review of gastroenterology & hepatology, 10(2), 215–227. https://doi.org/10.1586/17474124.2016.1110017 (accessed on 15th July 2025).

17. Ford, A. C., Moayyedi, P., Chey, W. D., Harris, L. A., Lacy, B. E., Saito, Y. A., & Quigley, E. M. M. (2018). American College of Gastroenterology monograph on management of irritable bowel syndrome. The American Journal of Gastroenterology, 113, 1–18. https://doi.org/10.1038/s41395-018-0084-x (accessed on 15th July 2025).

18. Frias, J., Martins, M., Peixoto, A., & Macedo, G. (2025). Rifaximin as a therapeutic ally in the modulation of dysbiosis: A narrative review of its applicability in gastrointestinal disorders. *GE – Portuguese Journal of Gastroenterology.* https://www.semanticscholar.org/paper/e06281d0f75b05faf4c0176729fe413c3f7c0368 (accessed on 15th July 2025).

19. Gașpar, B. S., Roșu, O. A., Enache, R., Manciulea, M., Pavelescu, L., & Crețoiu, S. (2025). Gut mycobiome: Latest findings and current knowledge regarding its significance in human health and disease. Journal of Fungi, 11. https://www.semanticscholar.org/paper/5e830d046ad702a352217e38b7d83191b5ea07bf (accessed on 15th July 2025).

20. Ghimire, P., & Maharjan, S. (2023). Adhesive small bowel obstruction: A review. *JNMA: Journal of the Nepal Medical Association, 61*, 390–396. https://www.semanticscholar.org/paper/caccef0f26e35c3123548df75ebaeec81ce24398 (accessed on 15th July 2025).

21. Ghosh, S., Whitley, C. S., Haribabu, B., & Jala, V. R. (2021). Regulation of intestinal barrier function by microbial metabolites. *Cellular and Molecular Gastroenterology and Hepatology, 11*, 1463–1482. https://doi.org/10.1016/j.jcmgh.2021.02.007 (accessed on 15th July 2025).

22. Gonçalves, J., Rosa, B., & Cotter, J. (2025). Small bowel vasculitis? What a gastroenterologist should know – From diagnosis to management. *Current Opinion in Gastroenterology, 41*, 132–138. https://www.semanticscholar.org/paper/96ebf12137f83122eeee72fdaaca06125af360a0 (accessed on 15th July 2025).

23. Goździewska, M., Łyszczarz, A., Kaczoruk, M., & Kolarzyk, E. (2024). Relationship between SIBO and other bowel diseases and a common eating pattern for them. Part III. *Annals of Agricultural and Environmental Medicine: AAEM, 31*(3), 322–328. https://www.semanticscholar.org/paper/e6e78e207b6fc63d327c542782ae6e6a579a64ba (accessed on 15th July 2025).

24. Hong, S., & Baek, D. (2024). Diagnostic procedures for inflammatory bowel disease: Laboratory, endoscopy, pathology, imaging, and beyond. *Diagnostics, 14.* https://www.semanticscholar.org/paper/7d8abb62c26ec51ded6f041150a52fd2471d677f (accessed on 15th July 2025).

25. Huang, Z., Wang, B., Peng, B., Liu, Z., Lin, H., Yang, Q., Tang, J., et al. (2025). Effectiveness of biologics for endoscopic healing in patients with isolated proximal small bowel Crohn's disease. *World Journal of Gastroenterology, 31.* https://www.semanticscholar.org/paper/3a0cf5e667c5fee4c5d872caa5634f8a9f84d11f (accessed on 15th July 2025).

26. Jiang, Y., Chen, Y., Yu, Q., & Shi, Y. (2023). Biologic and small-molecule therapies for moderate-to-severe psoriasis: Focus on psoriasis comorbidities. *Biodrugs, 37*, 35–55. https://www.semanticscholar.org/paper/9c10cbc0304fdd7ddbdc664400dfb55ed9824d9b (accessed on 15th July 2025).

27. Karoń, Ł., Zygmunt, A., Karoń, K., Pedrycz, D., Drapała, G., Grabowski, W., & Pedrycz, E. (2024). Targeting the microbiome: The role of low-FODMAP diet in modulating gut health for IBS and inflammatory conditions. *Journal of Education, Health and Sport.* https://www.semanticscholar.org/paper/ef54f934d2e4d2ba060f5d2c7427cd24c097e93d (accessed on 15th July 2025).

28. Kayama, H., & Takeda, K. (2020). Manipulation of epithelial integrity and mucosal immunity by host and microbiota-derived metabolites. *European Journal of Immunology, 50*, 921–931. https://doi.org/10.1002/eji.201948478 (accessed on 15th July 2025).

29. Liu, E., Aslam, N., Nigam, G., & Limdi, J. K. (2022). Tofacitinib and newer JAK inhibitors in inflammatory bowel disease—Where we are and where we are going. Drugs in Context, 11, 1–17. https://doi.org/10.7573/dic.2021-11-4 (accessed on 15th July 2025).

30. Macierzanka, A., Corfield, A. P., Atuma, C., Taylor, C., Nordgard, C. T., Ambort, D., Thornton, D. J., et al. (2012). The Role of the Mucus Barrier in Digestion. https://core.ac.uk/download/9838060.pdf (accessed on 15th July 2025).

31. Manar, G., mohammed, L., Zerhouni, A., Souiki, T., Majdoub, K., Toughrai, I., & Mazaz, K. (2025). Incomplete small bowel volvulus on common mesentery – A severe and rare complication in adults: Case report. *SAS Journal of Surgery.* https://www.semanticscholar.org/paper/d8a4558523d8dc41e4340610065663ec23f8b7fa (accessed on 15th July 2025).

32. Manikandan, S., Ifrah, A., Ebeid, J., Rim, D., & Parkman, H. P. (2024). S797 Examining the relationships of small bowel and colonic bacterial burden using area under the curve to symptoms of small intestinal bacterial overgrowth (SIBO) in the lactulose breath test. *The American Journal of Gastroenterology, 119*, S549–S550. https://www.semanticscholar.org/paper/b51b8a70d5644949d4b9762e2314974ce95dfd17 (accessed on 15th July 2025).

33. McManus, D., Novaira, H., Hamers, A., & Pillai, A. B. (2019). Isolation of lamina propria mononuclear cells from murine colon using collagenase E. Journal of Visualized Experiments: JoVE, 151. https://www.semanticscholar.org/paper/8102c2f7e1f2e20ef910d8b3e3160453e780e6c4 (accessed on 15th July 2025).

34. Nagahawatte, N. D., Avci, R., Paskaranandavadivel, N., & Cheng, L. K. (2023). Evaluation of pacing parameters to induce contractions in the small intestine. *2023 45th Annual International Conference of the IEEE Engineering in Medicine & Biology Society (EMBC).* https://www.semanticscholar.org/paper/bae53753df9a37195172948ee5de5673b33fc9e4 (accessed on 15th July 2025).

35. Palaniswamy, K. R. (2025). The microbiota-gut-brain axis in irritable bowel syndrome: Expert guidance on diagnosis and management. *International Journal of Research in Medical Sciences.* https://www.semanticscholar.org/paper/ab7f8f017e1e046746e2faefe638d7f885b6b2b8 (accessed on 15th July 2025).

36. Paredes Mogica, J. A., Feigenbaum, F., Pilitsis, J., Schrot, R., Oaklander, A., & De, E. J. B. (2023). Sacral Tarlov perineurial cysts: A systematic review of treatment options. *Journal of Neurosurgery: Spine.* https://www.semanticscholar.org/paper/efbdacc4d3ce0ba4c59edad1c9a37385f08b3ecc (accessed on 15th July 2025).

37. Parikh, M., Tejaswi, S., Girotra, T., Chopra, S., Ramai, D., Tabibian, J., Jagannath, S., et al. (2025). Use of artificial intelligence in lower gastrointestinal and small bowel disorders. *Journal of Clinical Gastroenterology, 59*, 121–128. https://www.semanticscholar.org/paper/829e40d0e8a476fd822210668c6d79a619c51e26 (accessed on 15th July 2025).

38. Peng, J., Zhang, Y., Zhu, L., Zhou, H., & Yao, H. (2024). Cryptogenic multifocal ulcerating stenosing enteropathy: A rare case of small bowel stenosis. *The American Journal of Case Reports, 25*, e944218-1–e944218-8. https://www.semanticscholar.org/paper/cb5c26864bd0177f8b936668173c3bb36a9a450b (accessed on 15th July 2025).

39. Pennazio, M., Rondonotti, E., Despott, E., Dray, X., Keuchel, M., Moreels, T., Sanders, D., et al. (2022). Small-bowel capsule endoscopy and device-assisted enteroscopy for diagnosis and treatment of small-bowel disorders: European Society of Gastrointestinal Endoscopy (ESGE) Guideline – Update 2022. *Endoscopy, 55*, 58–95. https://www.semanticscholar.org/paper/63e7b56d993389a25eb3b5f74c0fdaf5d9538c4c (accessed on 15th July 2025).

40. Piccirelli, S., Salvi, D., Pugliano, C. L., Tettoni, E., Facciorusso, A., Rondonotti, E., Mussetto, A., et al. (2025). Unmet needs of artificial intelligence in small bowel capsule endoscopy. *Diagnostics, 15.* https://www.semanticscholar.org/paper/bd2cfa0483fe69a8f0962ac7b761228e5c54318b (accessed on 15th July 2025).

41. Pironi, L. (2023). Definition, classification, and causes of short bowel syndrome. *Nutrition in Clinical Practice, 38*(Suppl 1), S9–S16. https://www.semanticscholar.org/paper/707bd33274b774c9b734818e82b25e62cba15132 (accessed on 15th July 2025).

42. Popa, Ş., Stancu, B., Ismaiel, A., Turtoi, D., Brata, V. D., Duse, T., Bolchis, R., et al. (2023). Enteroscopy versus video capsule endoscopy for automatic diagnosis of small bowel disorders—A comparative analysis of artificial intelligence applications. *Biomedicines, 11.* https://www.semanticscholar.org/paper/8856e04d9cba0857df918e11c5d6f89c16e36ef4 (accessed on 15th July 2025).

43. Poudel, S., Huber, A. D., & Chen, T. (2022). Regulation of nuclear receptors PXR and CAR by small molecules and signal crosstalk: Roles in drug metabolism and beyond. *Drug Metabolism and Disposition, 51*, 228–236. https://doi.org/10.1124/dmd.122.000858 (accessed on 15th July 2025).

44. Qian, Y., Zhi, Z., Ai, J., Kang, L., Qiu, G., Huang, X., & Zhao, J. (2024). Immune-related intestinal pseudo-obstruction caused by immune checkpoint inhibitors: Case report. *Frontiers in Oncology, 14.* https://www.semanticscholar.org/paper/57855656061da5e88d30b087a8a0546b8158267e (accessed on 15th July 2025).

45. Rej, A., Potter, M., Talley, N., Shah, A., Holtmann, G., & Sanders, D. (2022). Evidence-based and emerging diet recommendations for small bowel disorders. The American Journal of Gastroenterology, 117, 958–964. https://www.semanticscholar.org/paper/99bcb68feadc43a5fdde43752070ebd978b2f32a (accessed on 15th July 2025).

46. Savchuk, A., & Polyovyy, V. (2024). Clinical characteristics of adhesion disease after surgical interventions on the peritoneal cavity organs. Kharkiv Surgical School. https://www.semanticscholar.org/paper/8712bdee766a6781889da1dfd89cfedb0c746318 (accessed on 15th July 2025).

47. Shah, S. A., Patil, A., Ghone, P. B., Rajmane, A. R., Patil, V. S., & Waware, S. S. (2024). Ayurvedic management of Ghrahani [Crohn's disease]—A single case study. Journal of Advanced Zoology. https://www.semanticscholar.org/paper/23e815a78e86707832b553fed246f184249d092d (accessed on 15th July 2025).

48. Sultan, N. M., Ali, A. A., & Mardan, H. J. (2025). Isolation and identification of the types of bacteria that cause irritable bowel syndrome. *Medical Journal of Babylon.* https://www.semanticscholar.org/paper/fd4e41b3cb2898fa0cab7124017bae5f7192f50c (accessed on 15th July 2025).

49. Torun, M., Özkan, S., Kol Özbay, D., & Özkan, E. (2025). Gastrointestinal tumors of the small bowel: Prognostic roles of tumor stage and inflammatory markers. *Anatolian Current Medical Journal.* https://www.semanticscholar.org/paper/6f1ea5d5b024c3ee0ecdd07277c0e32515c49857 (accessed on 15th July 2025).

50. van Harten, L. D., de Jonge, C. S., Beek, K., Stoker, J., & Išgum, I. (2022). Untangling and segmenting the small intestine in 3D cine-MRI using deep learning. *Medical Image Analysis, 78,* 102386–102386. https://doi.org/10.1016/j.media.2022.102386 (accessed on 15th July 2025).

51. Wang, Y., Zhao, Z., Wang, R., & Hu, X. (2025). Genetic links between gastrointestinal disorders and kidney stone disease. *Kidney360, 6,* 616–626. https://www.semanticscholar.org/paper/2f9a55cf5ba639b482fd7332b3cc477b20adc646 (accessed on 15th July 2025).

52. Wanzl, J., Gröhl, K., Kafel, A., Nagl, S., Muzalyova, A., Gölder, S., Ebigbo, A., et al. (2023). Impact of small intestinal bacterial overgrowth in patients with inflammatory bowel disease and other gastrointestinal disorders—A retrospective analysis in a tertiary single center and review of the literature. *Journal of Clinical Medicine, 12.* https://www.semanticscholar.org/paper/35065add8440c630d22f887e49be8ba7b0f01347 (accessed on 15th July 2025).

53. Wetterkamp, M., van Beekum, C. V., Willis, M., Glowka, T., Manekeller, S., Fimmers, R., Praktiknjo, M., et al. (2020). Risk factors for postoperative morbidity and mortality after small bowel surgery in patients with cirrhotic liver disease—A retrospective analysis of 76 cases in a tertiary center. *Biology, 9.* https://www.semanticscholar.org/paper/725472dc83a8572a34e534360d6c80e5d681b9e9 (accessed on 15th July 2025).

54. Zammit, E. (2009). The Irritable Bowel Syndrome. Malta Medical Journal Volume 21 Issue 02 June 2009 https://core.ac.uk/download/46602223.pdf (accessed on 15th July 2025).

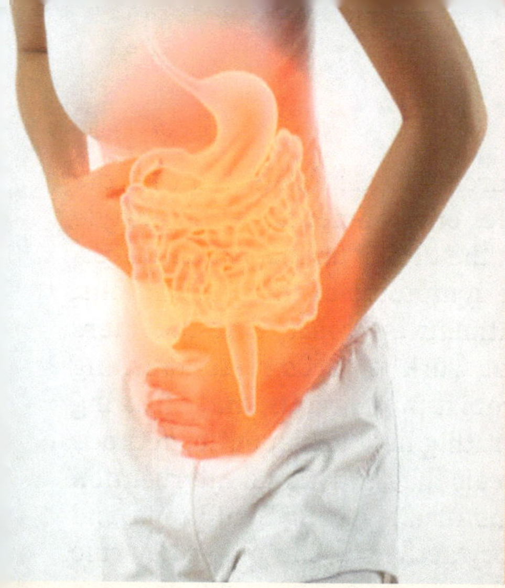

Chapter 6

DISORDERS OF THE COLON

Contents

Introduction

The colon, an integral component of the digestive system, plays a fundamental role in digestion and general health. Its functions include the absorption of water and electrolytes, the formation and storage of feces, and a habitat for an array of microorganisms known as the gut microbiota. This intricate microbial community is increasingly recognized for its critical influence on physical and psychological well-being through the microbiota-gut-brain axis, which illustrates the direct relationship between gastrointestinal health and neurological function and emotional states. The implications of this intersection are vast, considering that colon disorders have the potential to bring about far-reaching effects that extend beyond the realm of gastrointestinal discomfort to affect psychological well-being and quality of life, thus the importance of combining art and science in the management of such disorders (Cryan et al., 2019). Within the more general disease category of gastrointestinal disorders, those diseases of the colon—irritable bowel syndrome, inflammatory bowel disease, and colorectal cancer, to mention just a few—are increasing in prevalence. Research has demonstrated that the pathophysiology of these conditions is multifaceted, with genetic, environmental, and lifestyle components influencing one another in complex ways. For example, the diet of an individual, stress, and even the well-being of microbes can exacerbate or ameliorate symptoms of these conditions. With more awareness of the disorders, embracing a holistic treatment approach that considers not only symptom suppression but also lifestyle modifications that work towards re-establishing balance within the gut microbiota, ensuring a rich variety of microbial populations, and ensuring optimal colon health (Mao et al., 2019). The significance of incorporating new therapeutic methods for colon disease cannot be overemphasized. Emerging evidence reveals that nutritional intervention and functional foods, including ginger, may offer a possible means of alleviating symptoms and promoting gut health. Ginger, with antioxidant and anti-inflammatory activities, can play a key role in preserving digestive health through its bioactive compounds. By adopting a multidimensional approach incorporating both traditional medical treatments and adjunct therapies, patients and medical practitioners can work together for optimal management of colon disorders. This integrated approach not only helps address the immediate problems associated with these disorders but also promotes a proactive attitude towards overall well-being with emphasis on prevention through lifestyle and diet (Cryan et al., 2019; Mao et al., 2019) (Figure 6.1).

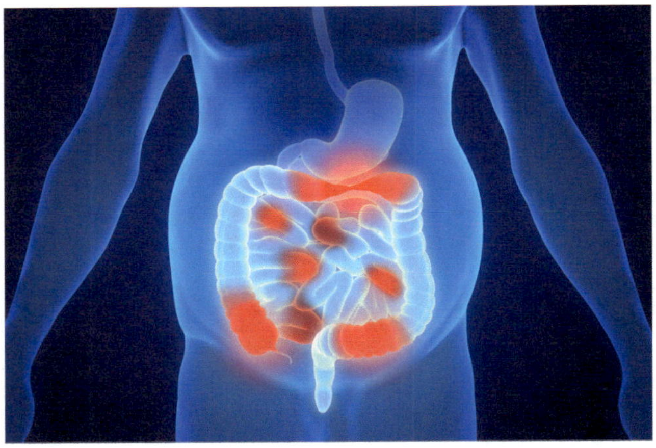

Figure 6.1. Disorders of the colon.

Source: https://kingwoodgi.com/wp-content/uploads/2017/09/Crohn's-disease.jpg.

Definition of Colon Disorders

An appreciation of colon disorders mandates an in-depth examination of their definition, etiology, and clinical significance. Colon disorders, also referred to as gastrointestinal illnesses of the colon, encompass inflammatory bowel disease (IBD), irritable bowel syndrome (IBS), diverticular disease, and colorectal cancer. These disorders will impose significant symptoms, including abdominal pain, change in bowel habit, and gastrointestinal haemorrhage, harmful to an individual's quality of life. With advances in the categorization of colon disorders, healthcare providers emphasize proper diagnosis and prevention, emphasizing how genes, environment, and lifestyle interact. Such a comprehensive system of categorization is complemented by continued research on biomarkers, opening the door to personalized therapies. The need to classify and define such disorders strongly determines therapeutic approaches and clinical outcomes in gastrointestinal health.

Colon disorder diagnosis typically involves a combination of clinical evaluation, endoscopy, and imaging tests. Physicians apply patient history and symptomatology to establish particular disorders, often following diagnostic testing in the form of a colonoscopy in order to visualize the colon and rectum directly. An example would be the diagnosis of inflammatory bowel disease by scrutinizing mucosal findings of Crohn's disease and ulcerative colitis. Molecular biology advancement is also necessary, with researchers continually striving to define diagnostic criteria and identify therapeutically actionable biomarkers, enhancing the efficacy of treatment. Such continuous enhancement enables one to apply more global applicability of colon disorder classification and management guidelines with an apparent focus on evidence-based practice (Khoury et al., 2022).

Such comprehensive knowledge of these disorders and their definitions aids both effective diagnosis and well-informed treatment strategies in clinical settings. The effects of colon disorders extend beyond acute symptoms, affecting patients' overall health and well-being. Chronic conditions , such as IBD, cause not only frequent pain and inconvenience but also potentially systemic impacts, such as nutritional deficiencies, as well as increased risks of colorectal cancer in the long term. Unveiling the burden of the disorders, it is evident that they exert pressure on healthcare systems, primarily in low-resource environments, where diagnostic facilities and good treatments may be scarce (Murray et al., 2022). The emphasis on the epidemiology and societal burden of colon disorders represents the urgent need for ongoing research, public health interventions, and health policy reforms. Through developing a deeper knowledge of these conditions, their definitions, and progression, stakeholders can develop effective solutions for maximizing patient outcomes and minimizing the public health effects of colon diseases.

Importance of Understanding Colon Health

Colon health matters since its impact on one's general well-being is enormous. The colon, also known as the large intestine, is a vital component of the digestive system, and its diseases are the cause of many diseases like colorectal cancer, inflammatory bowel disease, and irritable bowel syndrome. These not only weaken the digestion process but also negate nutrient absorption. Also, the prevalence of the above conditions highlights the need for extensive public health education and awareness on colon health. Evidence illustrates how early intervention and detection can dramatically alter outcomes, particularly in diseases like colorectal cancer, in which screening at the recommended ages reduces mortality by significant percentages. Thus, through educating an informed population on the importance of colon health, we can enhance preventive intervention alongside promoting healthier lifestyles among different populations. Additionally, colon health has a lot to do with awareness of how lifestyle determinants influence colon disorders. Factors of lifestyle, diet, and exercise directly affect the incidence and severity of colon disorder conditions. For example, high-fat, low-fiber diets and physical inactivity have been found to be related to increased risk of colon disorders. Knowing , such associations enables individuals to make choices about diet and lifestyle to lower risks. Besides, policy formulation on the basis of structural equation modeling (SEM) evidence, for example, illustrates how a set of socioeconomic factors influences colon health behaviors, and the requirement for certain public health interventions becomes clear. It is imperative that healthcare providers continue to research and learn about the impact of these lifestyle habits on the colon, eventually leading to improved patient health outcomes. Beyond individual health implications, it is also important to know about colon health at public health levels. Awareness of colon disease and prevention can lead to reduced healthcare costs associated with the management and treatment of advanced disease stages. Also, the general improvement of the population's health status by focusing on colon health can enhance worker productivity and quality of life. Similar to how mental illness can lead to numerous societal issues, a lack of proper awareness and knowledge regarding colon health can lead to persistent public health burdens. Screening and educational programs for colon health not only inform people about their risk, but they also have public policy implications to reduce the occurrence of colon diseases. It is therefore necessary to develop a culture of early intervention with colon health to maximize individual and public benefits to health consistent with overall health promotion objectives.

Overview of Common Colon Disorders

Colon disorders are of mixed etiology and presentation, frequently constituting a formidable challenge to diagnosis and management. Among the most frequent disorders are inflammatory bowel disease (IBD) in the form of Crohn's disease and ulcerative colitis, which are responsible for chronic inflammation of the gastrointestinal tract. Crohn's disease may involve any part of the gastrointestinal tract, whereas ulcerative colitis involves the colon. Symptoms are most frequently abdominal pain, rectal bleeding, and weight loss that is variable in its severity based on the patient's reaction to these chronic illnesses. Early diagnosis by endoscopy is crucial since it enables direct visual assessment of the mucosa and facilitates assessment of the disease severity and planning treatment regimens, bridging the uncertainties of subjective judgments and inter-individual variation in symptoms (González-Castro et al., 2024). Microscopic colitis is a significant colon disease, which is characterized by chronic diarrhea without the presence of relevant findings on routine endoscopic examination. Microscopic colitis is characterized by inflammatory changes in the colon revealed by histologic study of biopsies. Microscopic colitis was recently reported to be associated with celiac disease, wherein close to 6% of patients with celiac disease also have evidence of microscopic colitis (González-Castro et al., 2024). This connection emphasizes the shared autoimmune component present in both diseases and stresses screening across these patient populations. While there is similarity between the clinical presentations, it is important to recognize the distinct pathological processes and symptomatology of both diseases in an attempt at effective management and treatment strategies in the patients, particularly those that have been deemed refractory to standard therapy. Besides, the technology of diagnostic techniques, including artificial intelligence, has promise in increasing the precision in the assessment of disorders like ulcerative colitis. Emerging technologies aim to maximize the endoscopic evaluation of disease activity by providing computational aid that reduces variability and subjectivity in scoring. This incorporation of technology has a twofold benefit: it streamlines the assessment process and increases the accuracy of measuring disease severity and treatment outcomes (Zezos, 2021). As research continues, it is important that clinical professionals embrace these tools in practice to ensure proper handling of colon disorders. Emphasizing knowledge of these varied conditions and the way they interact not only aids the development of useful care plans but also facilitates increased comprehension of the complexities of gastrointestinal health.

6.1. Anatomy and Function of the Colon

The large intestine, also referred to as the colon, is a vital component of the digestive system in humans, measuring approximately five feet in length. Anatomically, it consists of four segments: the ascending colon, transverse colon, descending colon, and sigmoid colon. They are continued with each other, and separated by two flexures, the right hepatic flexure and the left splenic flexure . Each segment plays a specific role in the breakdown of waste material from the intestines. The ascending colon, too, draws water and salts out of the undigested stuff, and the transverse colon continues the process of absorption and is also a reservoir of the waste before it is passed on to the descending colon. The sigmoid colon then conditions the waste for ejection, allowing fecal matter to accumulate until defecation time. This specific anatomical organization is crucial to successful transit and absorption, and any failure in these segments will lead to serious gastrointestinal illnesses and diseases. Functionally, the colon is involved in a number of important functions aside from being used as a dumping ground for waste material. It is important for the fermentation of waste food by gut microbiota, which aids in the production of short-chain fatty acids that are beneficial to colon health. Apart from this, the colon provides for the absorption of vitamins, including vitamin K and certain B vitamins synthesized by intestinal bacteria. Its well-being also closely relates to the overall well-being of the person because abnormalities in colonic function can cause disorders , such as irritable bowel syndrome (IBS), inflammatory bowel disease (IBD), and colorectal cancer. Recognizing these interrelationships underscores the importance of nourishing a healthy colon through diet and lifestyle habits, which ultimately results in maximal digestive function and overall well-being. Furthermore, the physiology of the colon is governed by many factors, including age, nutrition, and microbiota composition. Evidence has highlighted that addressing these factors is crucial in understanding colonic disease and health. For instance, gender disparities affect the physiology of the colon, as discussed at length in the context of sex and gender differences in health outcomes. Colon diseases manifest differently based on these variables, and care approaches must therefore be approached in a more cautious manner. To this end, integration of aspects of precision medicine involving attention to individual variation can significantly contribute to enhancing care approaches. Thus, knowledge of the anatomy of the colon, its multiple functions, and the determinants of its health is critical in the management of disorders of the colon and the establishment of a healthy digestive system in populations (Jain et al., 2018; Jarvis et al., 2020) (Figure 6.2).

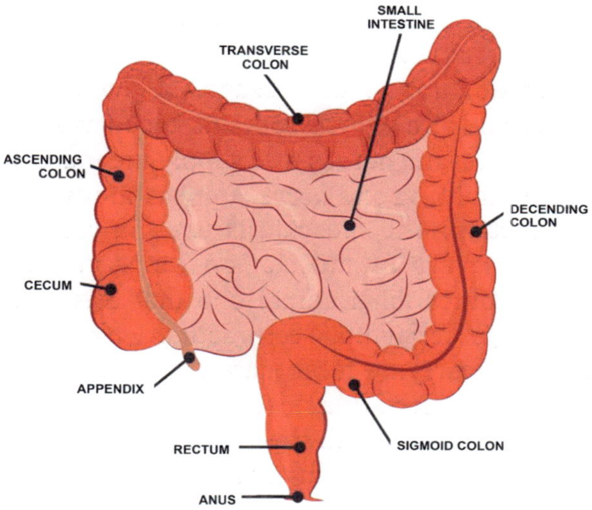

Figure 6.2. Anatomy and function of the colon.

Source: https://gastro-md.com/wp-content/uploads/2021/09/CC-Graphics2-1-scaled.jpg.

6.1.1. Structure of the Colon

The colon, a crucial component of the human intestine, extends from the cecum to the rectum and serves a significant role in water absorption, electrolyte regulation, and the creation of feces. The colon is structurally divided into four main components, i.e., the ascending colon, transverse colon, descending colon, and sigmoid colon. Each of the four components possesses certain distinct characteristics that assist in its function. The ascending colon, which begins at the intersection with the cecum, transports waste material upward along the right abdomen. The transverse colon then travels horizontally before turning into the descending colon, transporting waste downward along the left side. The sigmoid colon then stores fecal matter until it is expelled. Understanding this intricate organization is the foundation for comprehending many disorders that disrupt colon function, such as diverticulitis, colorectal cancer, and inflammatory bowel disease. Each of the four layers of the colon's wall, mucosa, submucosa, muscularis externa, and serosa, makes a special contribution to colon health and function. The mucosa, the innermost layer, is lined with epithelial cells that absorb nutrients and secrete mucus, a lubrication for stool passage. Below this is the submucosa, which contains blood vessels, lymphatics, and nerves that supply the mucosal layer with blood and nerve supply and regulate its function. The muscularis externa consists of two layers of muscle: an inner circular and an outer longitudinal one that assists in peristalsis, or rhythmic contraction, which plays a role in carrying fecal material to the colon. Lastly, the serosa encloses the colon, which provides support in the abdominal cavity. These structural components may become dysfunctional due to inflammation, infection, or tumor development, resulting in grave health conditions, ultimately forming the basis for most colon disorders. Knowledge of the structural and functional parameters of the colon is paramount to the diagnosis and management of colon disorders. New technologies in medical imaging, such as gastrointestinal ultrasound (GIUS), have enhanced the visualization of the anatomy and identification of abnormal conditions. Recent developments state that GIUS allows for the examination of normal sonoanatomical structures, providing clinicians with the information on suboptimal conditions necessitating intervention (Calabrese et al., 2016). Further, research into stem cell therapies offers a hopeful avenue for disease treatment in the case of disorders involving mucosal damage or dysfunction, pointing to the promise of regenerative medicine to treat diseases like inflammatory bowel disease and colorectal cancer (Dunn et al., 2016). This connection of anatomical knowledge to developing therapeutic procedures underscores the importance of holistically understanding the structure of the colon to effectively attack its disorders (Figure 6.3).

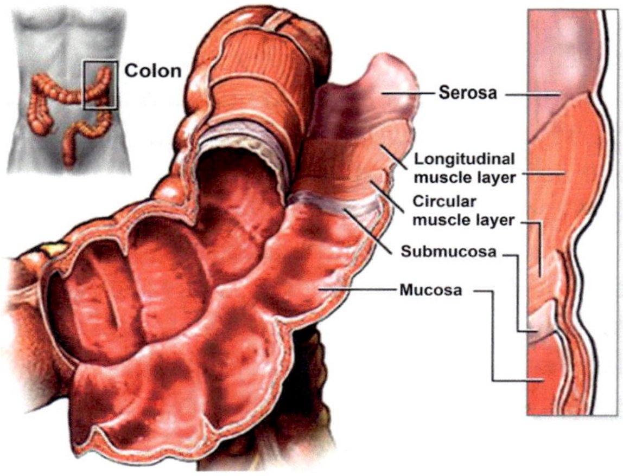

Figure 6.3. Structure of the colon.

Source: https://medlineplus.gov/ency/images/ency/fullsize/19218.jpg.

6.1.2. Role of the Colon in Digestion

The colon plays a vital role in the digestion process, particularly in the absorption of water and electrolytes needed for homeostasis in the body. As the final portion of the digestive system, the colon receives undigested food material from the food that is transmitted from the small intestine and continues to digest it. The function of this organ is not mere absorption; the colon also harbors a heterogeneous population of gut microbiota, which plays significant roles in the breakdown of complex carbohydrates and biosynthesis of essential nutrients, i.e., vitamins. These microbial interactions emphasize the host-symbiotic relationship with microorganisms, impacting both metabolic and digestive efficiency. Thus, disruption of the colon is capable of provoking many disorders, which underlines the necessity of further investigation into the impact of microbial dysbiosis and its effect on overall digestive health (de Vos et al., 2022). Beyond its function of absorption, the colon is also the location of crucial fermentation of unabsorbed substrates. The gut microbiota of the colonic gut breaks down dietary fibers, typically defined as prebiotics, and short-chain fatty acids (SCFAs) are produced as a consequence. The metabolites not only serve as energy sources for colonocytes but also play roles in regulating immune functions and the integrity of the gut barrier. The health of the colon is therefore directly related to the balance of the microbial community. Imbalances can initiate inflammatory processes or lead to conditions , such as inflammatory bowel disease (IBD), thus emphasizing the significance of microbial well-being in colonic function. Understanding the process of fermentation and their metabolic end products has the potential to inform treatment modalities for various gastrointestinal disorders (de Vos et al., 2022). Besides, the function of colons is not just to respond to immune and general body conditions, therefore making it a focal point of research in examining disorders , such as colorectal cancer and IBD. The colonic epithelium and its related immune cells have close interactions with gut microbiota, which together influence body responses against invading pathogens and inflammation. For instance, metabolites from the gut derived from microbial fermentation will induce some receptors, protecting a wide range of diseases. The existence of proteins like ACE2 in the small intestine further illustrates the mutual dependency of digestive function and immune protection, and how their disruption would have an effect on the other. Besides, the absence of certain transporters linked to amino acid transport would have systemic effects, including amino acid deficiencies and increased vulnerability to diseases like IBD. Hence, a healthy colon is part and parcel not just to effective digestion but also to the avoidance of many diseases (Figure 6.4).

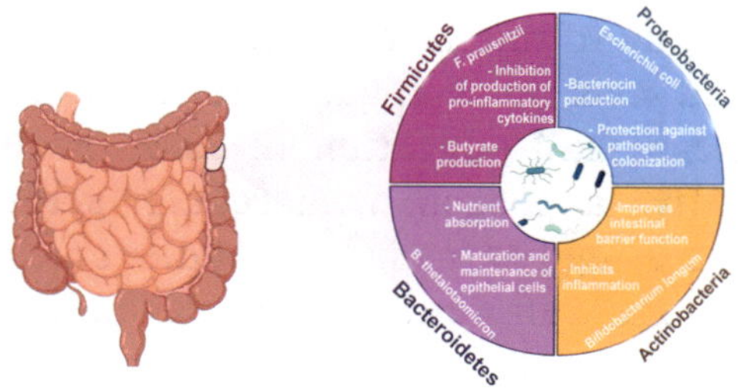

Figure 6.4. Role of the colon in digestion.

Source: Maciel-Fiuza MF, Muller GC, Campos DMS, do Socorro Silva Costa P, Peruzzo J, Bonamigo RR, Veit T and Vianna FSL (2023) Role of gut microbiota in infectious and inflammatory diseases. Front. Microbiol. 14:1098386. doi: 10.3389/fmicb.2023.1098386

6.1.3. Importance of Colon Health in Overall Well-Being

Optimal health of the colon is at the root of overall well-being since it profoundly influences not only the function of the digestive tract but also other aspects of overall systemic health. The colon is crucial in the absorption of nutrients, water balance, and elimination of waste products. A healthy colon can avoid many gastrointestinal diseases, such as irritable bowel syndrome (IBS) and inflammatory bowel disease (IBD). Moreover, if the colon is healthy, then the body is well able to perform its cleansing processes, which may be affected when toxic waste accumulates due to low digestive health. This reveals the interdependence between colonic function and general wellness, highlighting the necessity for preemptive action to maintain colonic integrity in order to prevent the onset of disorders that may impair well-being. Colon health also plays a role in the avoidance of more severe complications like colorectal cancer and other conditions. Ethnically based differences in cancer outcomes, for instance, among Maori groups, underscore how factors like access to cancer care services and patient comorbidity contribute significantly to colon health disparities. These have been underscored as pointing to the need for intervention at the targeted level through guaranteeing accessible healthcare and education in colon health. A preventive approach, with regular screening and knowledge of the impact of diet on colonic microbiota, can reduce the prevalence and death of colon disease. Evidence shows dietary practices, such as consuming high-residue foods, can lead to healthy colons and then influence cancer potential, further broadening the benefit of a healthy colon in attaining healthy results (Blakely et al., 2010). The colonic microbiota's metabolic activity, strongly diet-dependent, is crucial for sustaining the integrity of the gut and overall health. It has been shown that differences in dietary patterns cause extreme alterations in colonic content, impacting fecal output as well as gas production. As an illustration, a change from a low- to a high-residue diet will increase both the volume of fecal matter released and the frequency of bowel movements, all of which are critical in preventing the accumulation of waste within the intestines. This serves to emphasize the importance of dietary fiber for the promotion of colonic health, normal bowel function, and prevention of the risk of developing disease as a result of compromised colonic function. By understanding the connection between diet to colonic health, patients are able to have the information to make appropriate decisions that support their gastrointestinal health and overall wellness. (Garaventa et al., 2017)

6.2. Common Disorders of the Colon

Of all the diseases that affect the colon, colorectal cancer is one of the most common and dreaded conditions. The American Cancer Society estimates that in 2020, 105,000 Americans had been diagnosed with colon cancer, making it the third most common cancer in the U.S. Of specific interest is the point that, even as incidence and mortality rates in individuals aged 50 and above have been decreasing, an alarming trend indicates an increase in cases in patients under 50 years of age. This point underscores the necessity of mass screening and early diagnosis programs, specifically in light of the tendency for colorectal cancer to present asymptomatically in its initial stages. The primary method of treatment remains surgical, subsequently followed by chemotherapy at later stages. With evolutionary advancements in practice at the clinical level, including multidisciplinary consultations with a focus on individualized treatment plans, the management of colorectal cancer has also undergone significant change to allow improved patient outcomes (Vogel et al., 2021). Another extremely prevalent colonic disorder is irritable bowel syndrome (IBS), a gastrointestinal functional disorder that is linked with repeated abdominal pain and alterations in bowel habits. Although IBS is not related to identifiable structural changes in the colon, its quality of life consequences can be extremely significant, often producing extreme distress. The pathophysiologies of IBS are complex and may involve both a combination of abnormalities in gastrointestinal motility, visceral hypersensitivity, and psychosocial factors. Evidence indicates that food ingredients, such as the intake of certain forms of carbohydrates, may exacerbate symptoms, making dietary modification as a likely management option. IBS diagnosis and treatment also involve cautious diagnoses of underlying psychological diseases, including depression and anxiety. Thus, integrated treatment whereby medical as well as behavioral management is encompassed is required to optimize patient care and management (Abegaz, 2021). Diverticular disease is another frequent illness that occurs in the colon and encompasses diverticulosis and diverticulitis. Diverticulosis, which is the presence of many small pouches or diverticula in the wall of the colon, may be asymptomatic but may be preceded by diverticulitis if inflammation occurs. Low-fiber diet, obesity, and sedentary lifestyle have been postulated as etiologic factors for diverticulosis. For diverticulitis, the patients can present with fever, abdominal pain, and changed bowel habits, which might need to be treated. It can be treated in a different way, with mild cases commonly being treated with a change of diet and antibiotics, but severe cases can require surgery. Sustained research into diverticular disease pathophysiology identifies the promise of gut microbiota and inflammatory processes, highlighting the reality that comprehensive care plans should factor in dietary as well as microbial determinants of colon function (Vogel et al., 2021) (Figure 6.5).

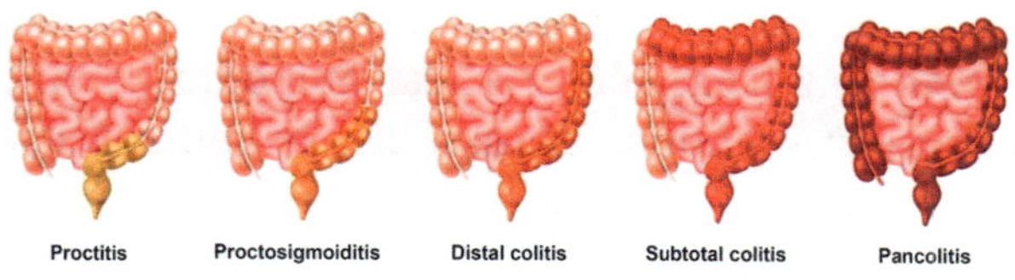

Figure 6.5. Common disorders of the colon.

Source: https://www.google.com/url?sa=i&url=https%3A%2F%2Fcaringmedical.com%2Fprolotherapy-news%2Fgerd-neck%2F&psig=AOvVaw3w84hXDT9yULEJ4Chr6tL_&ust=1750785197744000&source=images&cd=vfe&opi=89978449&ved=0CBQQjRxqFwoTCLi6jLCFiI4DFQAAAAAdAAAAABAV.

6.2.1. Irritable Bowel Syndrome (IBS)

Irritable Bowel Syndrome (IBS) is a prevalent functional gastrointestinal disorder with abdominal pain, bloating, and alteration of bowel habits, including diarrhea and constipation, as key manifestations. The Rome IV criteria, an expert-consensus diagnostic standard for gastrointestinal disorders, offer the necessary criteria for IBS diagnosis, emphasizing the necessity of recurrent abdominal pain and changes in frequency of bowel movements. IBS has a substantial impact on the quality of life of an individual, which usually culminates in absenteeism from work and heightened healthcare utilization. While IBS does not cause any anatomical alterations in the colon, its symptoms can actually influence daily functioning and psychological well-being profoundly. Treatment for IBS may include diet modification, stress management, and sometimes pharmacologic therapy, indicating that the management is multifactorial because IBS is a disease with physical and psychosocial dimensions of health (Moshiree et al., 2023). The gut microbiota is a complex collection of microbes in the gastrointestinal tract and is the core factor in IBS pathology. Dysbiosis, i.e., an imbalance in the microbial population, has been proposed as a causative factor of symptom generation in IBS patients. Dysruption of gut microbiota may lead to increased gut permeability, aberrant bile acid metabolism, and compromised intestinal motility, which may exacerbate symptoms of IBS. Emerging evidence shows that microbiota-targeted therapies, i.e., probiotics and prebiotics, are promising to restore microbially homeostatic status and alleviate symptoms. These therapies vary in their effectiveness between individuals, the difficulty of IBS treatment, and the necessity for tailoring interventions to account for the patients' own microbiome (Huang et al., 2021). It is crucial to learn about the biopsychosocial model of IBS. This model accepts the interaction among biological, psychological, and social factors in the etiology and progression of IBS. Psychiatric comorbidities, including depression and anxiety, are prevalent among IBS patients and have the potential to exacerbate gastrointestinal symptoms. Cognitive-behavioral therapy combined with medication has been an effective intervention, addressing the psychological component of the condition. Furthermore, developing a strong therapeutic relationship between healthcare providers and patients can enhance compliance and empowerment and enable global management of this multifactorial disorder. With continuous studies, the use of psychological support combined with standard medical therapy will likely improve the overall treatment of IBS patients, a significant breakthrough in ongoing research on colon disorders (Moshiree et al., 2023) (Figure 6.6).

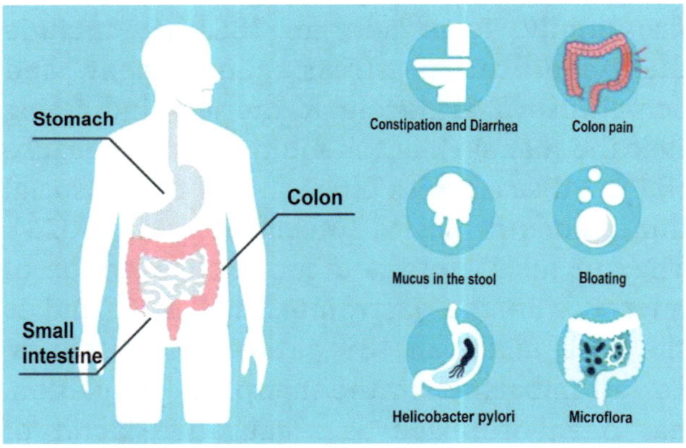

Figure 6.6. Irritable bowel syndrome (IBS).

Source: https://novagastro.org/wp-content/uploads/2023/02/iStock-965546890-1024x853.jpg.

6.2.2. Inflammatory Bowel Disease (IBD)

As a chronic gastrointestinal disease, Inflammatory Bowel Disease (IBD) encompasses two primary conditions: ulcerative colitis (UC) and Crohn's disease (CD). Both diseases are the product of a complex interaction between genetic susceptibility, environmental factors, and immune dysregulation, leading to chronic intestinal tract inflammation. Symptoms are highly varied and can significantly affect quality of life and include abdominal discomfort, chronic diarrhea, rectal bleeding, and unintended weight loss. Aside from these complications in the gastrointestinal tract, IBD is compounded by several extraintestinal complications, such as joint inflammation, skin lesions, and eye inflammation, making patient care even more challenging. The complexity of IBD requires a good comprehension of its pathogenic basis to conceptualize proper treatments addressing not only the initial gastrointestinal manifestations but also the systemic complications of the disease. IBD management remains a challenging situation founded largely on the variability of disease presentation and the limitations of conventional therapy. These conventional agents, such as aminosalicylates, immunomodulators and corticosteroids, are widely employed; however, their effectiveness diminishes in the long term, leading to relapse or the development of adverse effects. In the more recent periods, biologic agents have assumed the position of revolutionary treatment modalities for IBD, with greater specificity by acting on inflammatory processes directly. For instance, tumor necrosis factor-alpha (TNF-α)-inhibiting biologics have been shown to reduce inflammation and significantly enhance clinical outcomes. While posing tremendous therapeutic benefits, these interventions have raised concerns regarding long-term safety and availability, suggesting a basis for further investigation to establish personalized therapies that consider patient profiles and overall disease burden (Choi et al., 2024).

Increasing evidence supports the potential value of traditional medicine in IBD therapy and opens up a new prospect for future treatment strategies. A recent study explored Zanthoxyli Pericarpium (ZP), a Chinese medicinal herb, and demonstrated anti-inflammatory and antioxidant activity that may alleviate intestinal inflammation. The research found 59 bioactive molecules in ZP that targeted major IBD-associated genes, such as PTGS2 and PPARG, with powerful protective effects in colitis animal models. The results indicated ZP could decrease oxidative stress and colonic damage, which would lay a foundation for potential future applications in clinical patients. Because IBD has been challenging gastroenterology, combining the data of modern medical practice and traditional thinking is an integrative approach towards therapy of this complex disease (Choi et al., 2024) (Figure 6.7).

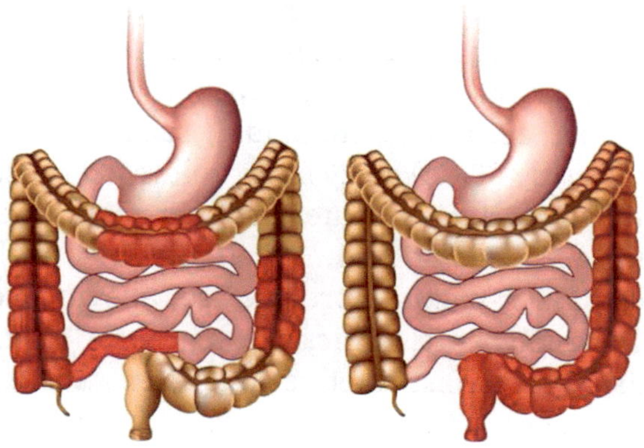

Figure 6.7. Inflammatory bowel disease (IBD).

Source: https://healthyious.com/wp-content/uploads/2020/11/Inflammatory-Bowel-Diseases-IBD-Crohn's-Disease-and-Ulcerative-Colitis-922x1024.png.

6.2.3. Colorectal Cancer

Colorectal cancer is also a significant public health concern, ranking as the third most newly diagnosed cancer and the second highest in death due to cancer in the United States. Approximately 105,000 new colon cancer and 43,000 new rectal cancer cases are projected, and with an overwhelming 53,200 deaths expected within a year. Despite a general declining trend in incidence among individuals 50 years and above due to effective screening and lifestyle modifications, there is a rising, disturbing trend in cases among individuals below the age of 50. This two-way trend highlights the necessity for high-grade screening as well as awareness campaigns, particularly among individuals below the age of 50, who may not systematically enroll for screening programs. Additionally, early diagnosis continues to be paramount, as this facilitates timely treatment that can greatly enhance prognostic results and survival rates and underscores the necessity for continued public health initiatives in augmenting awareness and preventive measures alongside increased accessibility for screening (Vogel et al., 2021). In the treatment of colorectal cancer, practice largely relies on proper staging at presentation, which is key in identifying suitable treatment modalities. The TNM of the American Joint Committee on Cancer is the standard for evaluating tumor depth, nodal status, and distant spread, making it easy for clinicians to efficiently customize management. Operative resection remains the cornerstone in the management of localized disease, often followed by adjuvant radiation or chemotherapy in advanced disease. The timing of adjuvant chemotherapy administration is critical, with evidence suggesting that commencement of therapy within eight weeks of the date of surgery will lead to better clinical outcomes. Hence, there is a necessity for multi-disciplinary intervention, including surgical, medical, and radiological services, to optimize treatment efficacy and patient survival (Yau-You et al., 2020). New clinical evidence and recommendations continue to evolve that are intended to further enhance the management of colorectal cancer. The 2021 ASCRS guidelines reflect significant treatment guideline advances, with new guidelines that emphasize the need for neoadjuvant therapy in locally advanced disease and the central role of a multidisciplinary discussion in formulating treatment. Finally, personalized medicine, including the use of molecular markers to guide therapy, represents a new, exciting frontier in colorectal cancer management. This tailor-made strategy not only enhances prognostication but also facilitates individualized care, adjusting the goals of treatment to patient-specific factors , such as genetic susceptibilities and general health status. Additional financing of such research, as well as greater public education and awareness of the risk of colorectal cancer, is key to combat this multifactorial disease and reduce its burden on the population (Vogel et al., 2021) (Figure 6.8).

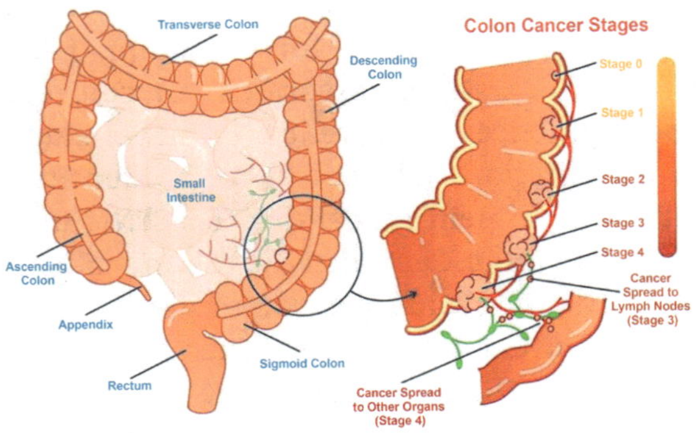

Figure 6.8. Colorectal cancer.

Source: https://a2zhealthy.com/wp-content/uploads/2019/02/shutterstock_1016095450.jpg.

6.3. Symptoms and Diagnosis

The presenting features of colon disorders can be a broad spectrum, impacting more than anything else the quality of life of an individual. Common presentations are abdominal pain, bowel habit alteration, bloating, and weight loss. They can be suggestive of irritable bowel syndrome (IBS), inflammatory bowel disease (IBD), and cancer of the colorectum. The clinician's dilemma is, however, to differentiate between these conditions, especially due to the overlap in symptoms. IBS, for instance, might often report recurrent abdominal pain and altered bowel habits, but in the absence of inflammatory markers associated with IBD. Accurate awareness of the symptomatology is therefore critical to enable accurate diagnostic investigations and appropriate treatment protocols to be instituted. Diagnosis for colon disorders is typically a stratified process involving a comprehensive patient history, clinical examination, and an array of diagnostic procedures. Early assessment is typically non-invasive and may lead to the identification of underlying conditions without exposing the patient to more invasive methods. Some of the routine diagnostic equipment includes colonoscopy, imaging studies like CT scans, and laboratory tests to identify inflammatory markers. When new technology becomes accessible, methods , such as tissue microarray (TMA) analysis for colorectal cancer gain popularity. Computer-assisted approaches, utilizing convolutional neural networks, make these assessments more precise, allowing for comprehensive classification of cancer tissue. This more sophisticated technique ensures that physicians will receive a correct diagnosis of colon illnesses, allowing them to act in time and save their patients' lives (Kızıloluk & Sert, 2022). The present research on long-term outcomes of colon disorders, particularly in the backdrop of new and emerging health issues, indicates the importance of information on both symptom and care cost. Similar to the impact observed in the management of COVID-19, patients with colon disorders will likely have increased healthcare consumption and associated costs in the long run.

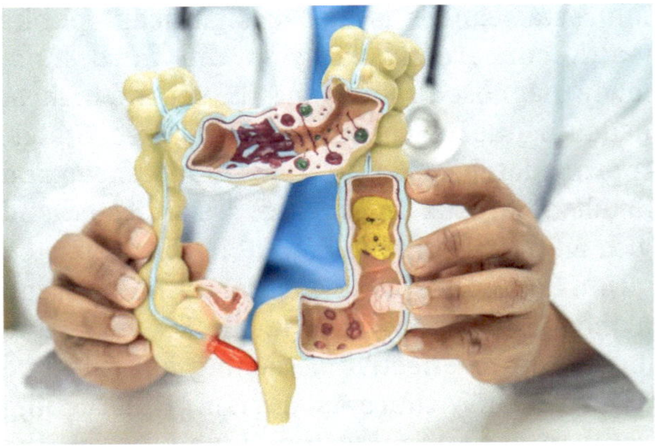

Figure 6.9. Symptoms and diagnosis.

Source: https://leicesterbowelclinic.co.uk/wp-content/uploads/2025/02/How-I-Knew-I-Had-Colon-Cancer-1024x683.jpg.

A patient-level correlation analysis determined that healthcare costs after diagnosis may extend long beyond the acute treatment period. By comparing the remaining healthcare needs of patients with colon disorders, healthcare systems are better able to utilize resources and understand the possible burden generated. Detection of such patterns not only facilitates the development of comprehensive care plans but also highlights the importance of early diagnosis and proper control in reducing long-term costs and improving patient outcomes (Koumpias et al., 2022) (Figure 6.9).

6.3.1. Common Symptoms of Colon Disorders

Symptoms of colon diseases have a tendency to present diversely depending on the condition of the gastrointestinal tract. Pain in the abdomen, from slight aching to severe cramps, is a common indicator of some conditions, such as Irritable Bowel Syndrome (IBS). The patients have a tendency to complain about alterations in bowel habits, from diarrhea to constipation or between both. In addition, stress has been recognized as a significant factor in symptom development and exacerbation and is representative of the complicated relationship between states of mind and gastrointestinal health as reflected in the interaction of stressors modulating visceral sensitivity and their role in symptom manifestation and clinical outcome (Larauche et al., 2011). Identification of such common symptoms is crucial for early diagnosis and treatment of colon disorders, ultimately leading to an improved quality of life for victims. Another important symptom often associated with colon disorders is the presence of abnormal stools, presented as altered consistency, color, or shape. Patients will observe the presence of blood in stool, which may indicate potential issues , such as inflammation or cancer in the colon. This alarming symptom always warrants immediate medical investigation. Changes in stool caliber, such as acute diarrhea or more than a few days' diarrhea or constipation, can also be signs of underlying pathology, such as infection, polyps, or cancer. Diagnostic advances, including fiberoptic endoscopy, have transformed visualization and examination of the gastrointestinal tract, facilitating better understanding and regulation of diseases affecting the colon (Camilleri, 1999). Early detection of abnormal stool presentation is thus vital to the promotion of prompt diagnosis and intervention of colon disease. Apart from the gastrointestinal manifestations, colon illnesses also present systemically, contributing to the complexity in patients. Nonspecific presentations like weight loss, weakness, and even fever can occur, typically representing a more generalized reaction to an underlying condition like inflammatory bowel disease or colorectal malignancy. The nonspecific presentations might contribute to diagnostic challenges and delay effective management. Furthermore, psychosocial implications of depression and anxiety usually accompany chronic gastrointestinal diseases, and the clinical picture becomes more complex. An understanding of the multidimensional state of colon diseases can be best elicited by a thorough evaluation of the patient, consisting of both gastrointestinal and associated systemic symptoms. Thorough evaluation is a prerequisite for the development of effective care plans, which depend on the individual case of the patient. As the study continues, there is potential for more targeted interventions that are tailored to the complexity of disorders of the colon.

6.3.2. Diagnostic Procedures (e.g., Colonoscopy)

The diagnosis of colon disease relies to a great extent on various diagnostic procedures, one of which is colonoscopy. Being minimally invasive, colonoscopy facilitates direct viewing of the colon and is important in diagnosing abnormalities , such as polyps, tumors, and inflammatory bowel disease. Colonoscopy not only aids in diagnosis but also in therapeutic procedures , such as the removal of polyps and biopsies for histopathological analysis. Of note is the rapid expansion of medical technology, which has enhanced the safety and efficacy of this intervention. As a result, physicians can obtain valuable information that guides treatment. In addition, guidelines , such as the JSCCR Guidelines 2016 highlight the necessity of regular screening using colonoscopy to assist in reducing colorectal cancer mortality, which has been rising in recent years (Watanabe et al., 2017). It is therefore crucial that it be understood in the prevention as well as management of colon disorders and hence highlight the importance of such diagnostic examinations. In addition to colonoscopy, certain diagnostic modalities complement the evaluation of colon disorders, each of which contributes in its own particular way, with advantages and disadvantages. Flexible sigmoidoscopy and double-contrast barium enema, for instance, are commonly employed when a full colonoscopy is not possible or contraindicated. These other approaches provide helpful information regarding some sections of the colon but are typically not as comprehensive as a full colonoscopy. Non-invasive imaging tests , such as CT scans, yield additional diagnostic data, particularly in circumstances where colonoscopic detection of polyps or tumors may be challenging. They are unlikely to be as revealing as visual examination and biopsy sampling, however. With the widening of diagnostic tools, clinicians can attain a comprehensive account of a patient's status and create intervention strategies to optimise outcomes for the patient, particularly with respect to evolving challenges like Clostridium difficile infection that complicates traditional diagnosis (Czepiel et al., 2019). The utility of these tests is more than mere detection; they are also employed to track disease and treatment response in colon-affected patients. As an example, periodic colonoscopies may be crucial in post-polyp resection follow-up or in colorectal cancer histories, as recommended in some clinical guidelines. By early identification of new lesions or recurrences, these interventions contribute significantly to the realization of improved survival rates. Furthermore, early diagnosis by colonoscopy and other methods facilitates proper interventions to be initiated, which may include changes in diet, modification of drugs, or even surgery. These combined strategies highlight the importance of monitoring in general, particularly during the increasing incidence of colon disorders, as testified to by medical statistics worldwide. Hence, the role of diagnostic tests in the management of colon disorders is unsurpassed in effective patient treatment and enduring health impacts (Figure 6.10).

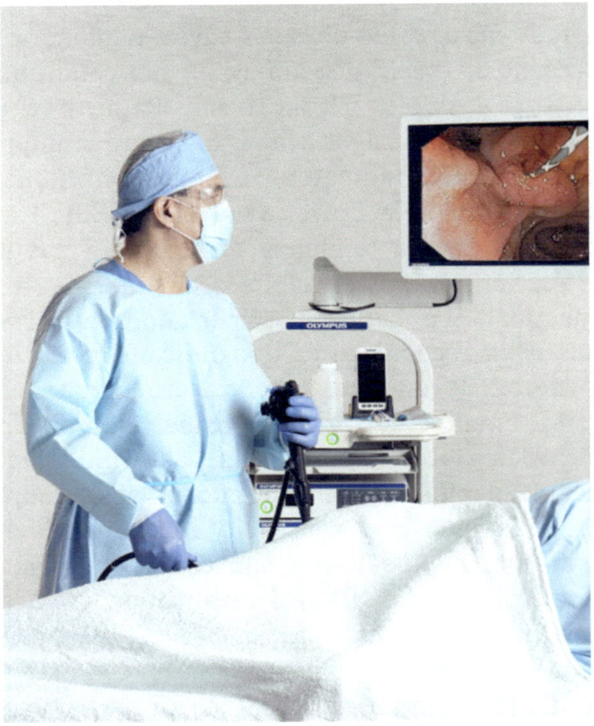

Figure 6.10. Diagnostic procedures (e.g., colonoscopy).

Source: https://www.colonoscopytoday.com/sites/default/files/inline-images/ColonCancer_Diagnosing.jpg.

6.3.3. Importance of Early Detection

The significance of early detection of colon conditions cannot be overestimated since it is crucial to improving the patient's results and the success of the treatment. Delayed diagnosis often leads to the progression of the disease and complications that could have been avoided if they were addressed early. Colorectal cancer, inflammatory bowel disease, and Hirschsprung's disease are just some of the conditions that highlight the sharp contrast in prognosis with early and late detection. For instance, survival is greatly increased for colorectal cancer when diagnosed earlier, and frequent screening as well as symptom awareness is of critical importance. Population-scale screening programs implemented in populations can maximize the chances for early diagnosis followed by treatment intervention, with ensuing health care cost savings from advanced-stage disease. As would be anticipated, the focus on education concerning these diseases is essential to developing a proactive attitude in both healthcare providers and patients. Additionally, early diagnosis has a significant impact on the treatment approaches employed for colon disorders. To give an example, when Hirschsprung's disease is diagnosed early on, patients can be provided with timely intervention that precludes the development of major complications , such as enterocolitis. The most precise example of a neonatal victim of gastrointestinal atresia, a congenital illness, demonstrates that early diagnosis and the subsequent timely and appropriate medical interventions can lead to favorable outcomes, as pointed out in recent medical research (Rathi et al., 2024). Similarly, an early diagnosis of the symptoms of inflammatory bowel disease can permit an immediate response that might minimize long-term damage to the bowel and improve the patient's quality of life. Therefore, the implementation of screening steps and public education regarding colon disease signs can guarantee that healthcare providers are well educated to recognize at-risk populations and guide them toward early diagnostic treatment. Incorporating early detection protocols into health policy forms a foundation of initiatives for better colon health results. In addition to individual advantages, early detection has far-reaching implications for public health, such as lower healthcare costs from the management of advanced diseases. As the argument in the case of Type 1 diabetes has demonstrated, early detection and treatment can provide considerable gains in health and reduce the total cost of care (Gómez-Peralta et al., 2025). By financing community education initiatives, training healthcare professionals in the importance of symptom vigilance, and stimulating regular screening, stakeholders can facilitate a culture of preventative healthcare. Therefore, the benefit of early detection extends beyond patient-level treatment and aligns ultimately with population-based health programs aimed at combating the epidemic and the social implications of colon disorders.

6.4. Risk Factors

A knowledge of inherent risk factors of colon ailments is crucial for early identification and management. These other habits of lifestyle , such as diet, physical inactivity, and obesity play a leading role in causally developing conditions , such as colorectal cancer and irritable bowel syndrome. A higher diet of red meat and processed meat and a lower intake of fruits and vegetables has been associated with increased colon cancer risk. Besides, obesity would also worsen inflammatory processes in the colon, thus enhancing disorder risks. Additionally, physical inactivity not only contributes to obesity but also has adverse effects on the motility of the gastrointestinal tract, resulting in disorders that are present in many colon diseases. The interaction between these lifestyle components underscores the need for dietary pattern policies and promoting physical activity as preventive measures against colon disorders. Psychosocial predictors also play an important role in the risk profile of colon disorders, particularly in diseases like irritable bowel syndrome (IBS). Stress and anxiety have been found to exacerbate symptoms, hence highlighting the complex interplay between body and mind. Both physical and psychological stressors were found to have the ability to affect visceral sensitivity, thus modulating the clinical presentation of IBS and other GI disorders. The mechanisms by which stress induces alterations in colon function are multifactorial, involving neural and hormonal pathways, and suggest that psychological well-being is also part of the equation in the context of gastrointestinal health. Such interconnection highlights the importance of holistic methods of therapy that consider both psychological and physical factors in treatment, thereby improving patient outcomes for colonic disorders. The multiplicity of such risk factors suggests the importance of integrated methods of prevention and care.

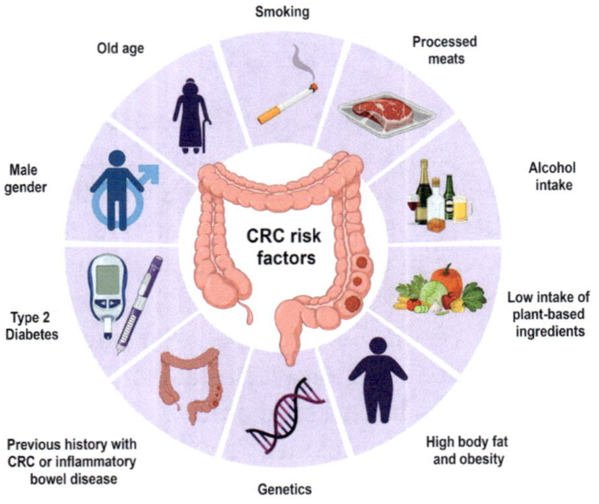

Figure 6.11. Risk factors.

Source: https://assets-global.website-files.com/621e95f9ac30687a56e4297e/64adcaec8ef58df2e228263f_V2_1685720343374_ef627b37-7b5e-491c-bfe8-c373db90ea2c_HIGH_RES.png.

Finally, demographic variation is also known to have an influence on colon disorder risk and prognosis, including colorectal cancer. It has been documented that ethnic diversity in disease incidence and survival exists, with studies demonstrating that certain groups, e.g., New Zealand's Māori, have significantly poorer outcomes from cancer compared to their non-Māori counterparts. These disparities may be the result of an interaction of biological factors, receipt of healthcare, and differing comorbidities within those affected. For instance, the presence of other disease states may complicate treatment and have negative effects on survival, most prominently in at-risk populations. The study of these population risk factors is central to understanding disparities in colon health and can inform interventions designed to address specific populations. Interventions to enhance the availability and quality of care for vulnerable populations can minimize some of those disparities, and results in colon disorder management would correspondingly improve (Blakely et al., 2010) (Figure 6.11).

6.4.1. Genetic Predisposition

The process of genetic predisposition is central to the understanding of the etiology of colon disorders, particularly when syndromes of hereditary polyp development and colorectal cancer are put in contemplation. Enormous volumes of research have aimed at the identification of numerous genetic markers of such conditions as evidence of the intricacy of inheritance patterns. Notably, families with a history of adenomatous polyposis may have an autosomal recessive inheritance pattern, pointing towards the correlation between genetic makeup and a higher risk for disease. In a classic case report, a family pedigree presented a multi-tumor predisposition syndrome, with frequent occurrence of gastrointestinal malignancies and other malignancies, highlighting the importance of genetic counseling and testing for familial risk management for colon disorders (Abdelmoula et al., 2024). Such observations can guide preventive intervention and surveillance strategies in patients at high risk. Furthermore, genetic predispositions are increasingly recognized as central to the evaluation of not only familial risk but also of implications for public health. For example, some gene variations that predispose to syndromes , such as Lynch syndrome and familial adenomatous polyposis (FAP) strongly illustrate the manner in which genetic mutations pose an increased risk for the development of colorectal adenomas or carcinomas. Research has described numerous biomarkers, e.g., mutations in the APC and MLH1 genes, that offer clinicians valuable tools for risk stratification and early intervention (Abdelmoula et al., 2024). Additionally, such information allows healthcare practitioners to individualize screening approaches with family pedigree and pattern of genetic inheritance in mind, thereby making preventive interventions against colon disorders more efficacious. Finally, the interplay between environmental factors and genetic predisposition cannot be overemphasized since the two interact to propel the expression of colon disorders. The patient with a predisposition can have increased risks in the case of certain lifestyle factors , such as diet, obesity, or smoking. Recent studies have started to investigate how genetic differences, and those associated with metabolic function, can increase these risks. For instance, obesity predispositions based on genes can increase associated conditions , such as obesity hypoventilation syndrome, which in itself may have implications for colorectal disease. As more research continues to untangle the subtleties involved, closer integration that considers both genetic factors as well as environmental factors will be critical to the development of useful treatment and prevention programs for colon disorders.

6.4.2. Lifestyle Factors (Diet, Exercise)

The relationship between lifestyle factors, i.e., diet and physical exercise, forms the crux of the understanding of colon disorders. Proper diet with high fiber, fruit, and vegetable consumption has been found to be related to a reduced risk of colorectal disease, including colorectal cancer. Epidemiological data affirm that diet and lifestyle play a significant role in gut health, with higher fiber consumption regulating gut motility and maintaining a healthy microbiota balance. Red meat and processed food diets, on the other hand, are found to be related to cancer. Regulation of diet by oneself is thus not only a preventive intervention but an integral part of treatment regimens of patients with colon disorders. Emphasis on dietary role can motivate patients to make rational choices that can minimize their risk for colon disease and enhance their well-being. Exercise forms a critical component of the prevention and management of colon disorders, a multifaceted intervention with several health benefits. Exercise has been found to reduce the risk of disease development , such as colorectal cancer, through the regulation of body weight, insulin sensitivity, and inflammation levels. Exercise is increasingly being considered as a polypill that can enhance metabolic homeostasis and reduce disease risk. Exercise is also found to have direct effects on gut health, leading to favorable changes in the composition of the microbiota that can enhance colon health. The incorporation of physical exercise in daily activity can significantly enhance the functionality and resistance of the colon to various disorders, favoring an integrated approach to well-being. The interaction of diet, exercise, and the combined impact on colon disorders is shed light on by emerging health technologies. m-Health technologies, also known as mobile health, can influence the change in lifestyle behavior by promoting dietary change and physical fitness. Research indicates that the m-health platforms can provide improved personalized interventions that teach users about healthy lifestyle choices through the application of strategies , such as gamification in an effort to enhance motivation. This new approach has the capability of making a significant impact on weight control and a healthier lifestyle, reducing the risk of colon disorders. With ongoing innovation in the area, there is a need to develop evidence-based material and strategies that will effectively educate patients on how to adopt healthy lifestyles. An interdisciplinary approach to diet and exercise interventions using technology has the capability of enhancing the health outcomes of individuals at risk for or with colon disorders (Clarke et al., 2015; Antoniou et al., 2017).

6.4.3. Environmental Influences

The complex interaction between environmental factors and colon disorders is of growing interest to research and clinical circles. Environmental toxins, toxin exposure, and socioeconomic status are some of the factors that play significant roles in the onset and development of most gastrointestinal disorders. Certain dietary patterns, most importantly those rich in processed foods and low in fiber content, have been identified as significant determinants of disorders , such as inflammatory bowel disorder (IBD) and colorectal cancer. In addition, environmental toxins , such as pesticides and industrial chemicals have been implicated in impairing gut microbiota and potentially initiating autoimmune processes. This introduces the complex interaction of factors where external factors play not only a part in the progression of symptoms but also in the intrinsic pathophysiology of colon disorders. Additionally, maternal behavior during gestation cannot be overlooked in attributing environmental factors to colon well-being. Research illustrates the role of prenatal exposure to toxins, such as tobacco, in having significant impacts on offspring growth, including gastrointestinal growth. For instance, prenatal tobacco smoke exposure in children has been reported to have impaired neurodevelopment, which, while more strongly linked with cognitive outcomes, may be applied to gastrointestinal function as well. The long-term effects of such exposures may develop in the form of a risk of colon disorders. Such evidence not only highlights the significance of public health programs aimed at smoking cessation but also suggests the potential of early interventions based on the consideration of maternal behaviors as strong predictors of children's health outcomes. Other than prenatal exposures, lifestyle factors at present, such as stress and exercise, play significant roles in colon well-being throughout life. Chronic stress has also been found to exacerbate irritable bowel syndrome (IBS) and other functional gastrointestinal disorders, as chronic stress responses have been found to alter gut motility and cause dysbiosis. Sedentary behavior will also adversely affect gut health, and so exercise is also an essential component of the prevention and management of colon disease. As more research continues to establish these correlations, interdisciplinary management of environmental etiologies of colon health is paramount. Integrating findings from current research, holistic interventions , such as diet modification, stress management, and physical activity may ultimately yield more favorable outcomes for patients with colon disease.

6.5. Treatment Options

Effective management of colonic diseases, in particular, colorectal cancer, is holistic and specific to the degree and nature of the disease. Surgical resection is the cornerstone of management, in particular for localized neoplasms, for which resection of the segment of the colon involved may be a curative procedure. In advanced colorectal cancer, multidisciplinary regimens , such as chemotherapy and radiation therapy are used. The American Society of Colon and Rectal Surgeons believes that thorough preoperative assessment, imaging, and histopathological evaluation are of immense value in establishing the optimal surgical procedure and subsequent therapeutic follow-up, since inaccuracy of disease assessment may lead to suboptimal results (Vogel et al.,

2021). Development of guidelines based on best evidence assures clinical practice to be guaranteed, ultimately maximizing patient survival and quality of life. In addition to traditional surgical and chemotherapeutic management, newer modes of treatment are increasingly being utilized in management protocols of colonic diseases. Neoadjuvant therapy, where chemotherapy or radiation is administered before surgical resection, has been found to shrink the tumor and facilitate easier and more effective resection. Furthermore, the use of immunotherapy, in particular in patients with microsatellite instability-high (MSI-H) tumors, has been a game-changer, raising expectations of therapeutic gain. The American Society of Colon and Rectal Surgeons guidelines favor the use of such advances while reiterating individualized care, pointing out that treatment decisions should be based on both clinical evidence and patient-specific factors (Yau-You et al., 2020). This shift towards personalized medicine offers opportunities afresh to patients with the challenge of colonic diseases. The advent of new technologies, such as minimally invasive surgical techniques, has revolutionized the treatment of colon disorders. The strategies, such as robot and laparoscopic surgery, are bound to lead to reduced postoperative pain, faster recovery, and less scarring compared to open surgery. There is clinical evidence to support the use of the strategies as being linked with comparable oncological results, but with enhanced patient comfort and satisfaction. Further, the application of enhanced recovery pathways following surgery has been shown to optimize outcomes through early mobilization and reduced readmission. With increasing treatment options and advancements, the integration of new technologies and strategies with standard therapies is an evolving pattern towards patient-focused and holistic management of colon disorders (Vogel et al., 2021) (Figure 6.12).

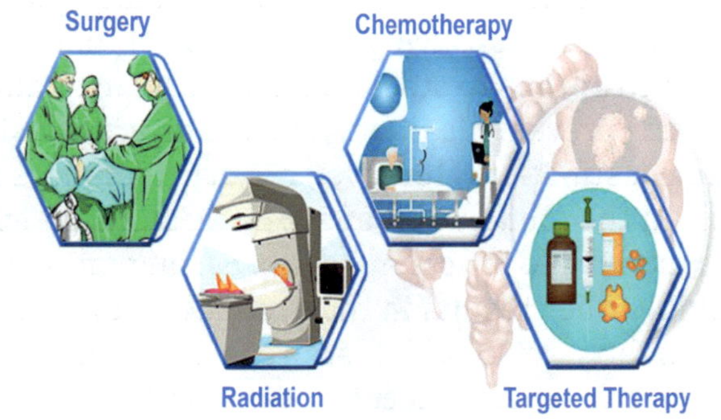

Figure 6.12. Treatment options.

Source: https://prolifecancercentre.co.in/wp-content/uploads/2019/10/Treatment-Of-Colorectal-Cancer.jpg.

6.5.1. Dietary Modifications

Dietary modifications play a crucial role in the management of various colon disorders, more so disorders , such as Irritable Bowel Syndrome (IBS). There is growing evidence to support the management of IBS by diet, and dietary modifications have been found to be very effective in the management of the disease. Among them, the low FODMAP diet has been increasingly popular in its contribution to the improvement of gastrointestinal symptoms of the disease. Outcomes have shown that patients on a low FODMAP diet reported improvement in gastrointestinal discomfort, bloating, and abdominal pain. Patients on the diet reported improvement in symptoms compared to patients who were on normal dietary advice, and outcomes showed a correlation between the diet and health status of patients with IBS (Park, 2015). Outcomes show the contribution of individualized dietary practices in the improvement of quality of life among people suffering from functional gastrointestinal disorders. Another dietary modification that is increasingly popular is the contribution of dietary intake of fiber. Clinical evidence indicates that low intake of dietary fiber is associated with various gastrointestinal disorders , such as diverticulosis and colon cancer. Fiber plays a basic role in ensuring healthy bowel function by contributing to stool bulk and regularity, and this can prevent disorders , such as diverticulosis and constipation. Moreover, dietary fiber plays a role in the modulation of gut microbiota, which is responsible for colon health. Fermentation of soluble fiber results in the production of short-chain fatty acids, which are renowned for their protective effect on colon cells and for their contribution to modulating inflammation (Lyon & Kacinik, 2012). This implies the necessity of consuming sufficient fiber in the diet because not only does it facilitate digestion, but it also bestows several health benefits that can reverse the risks of colon disorders. Successful treatment of colon disorders requires progressive dietary modifications that create short-term and long-term health benefits. Gradually shifting toward a balanced diet consisting of fruits, vegetables, whole grains, and legumes fills the system with the required nutrients while correcting prevalent gastrointestinal problems. In addition, additional dietary strategies can be incorporated into these modifications. For instance, reducing the intake of processed foods containing high sugars and unhealthy fats can improve gastrointestinal health significantly. This strategy enables a long-term transition in the direction of healthier eating, which ultimately leads to healthier colonic health. Identification of individual dietary stresses and preferences is important to success because individualized diets can enhance compliance and satisfaction. Dietary modifications, therefore, not only provide therapeutic options for the management of colon disorders but also enable the individual to have an active role in their digestive health.

6.5.2. Medications and Therapies

Management of colon disorders typically involves the use of different medications and therapies in an attempt to treat symptoms and underlying conditions. One of the major classes of treatment is pharmacological treatment, which can include anti-inflammatory drugs and antibiotics based on the condition. For instance, patients with inflammatory bowel disease (IBD) conditions, such as Crohn's disease or ulcerative colitis, respond favorably to corticosteroids for the management of inflammation. Additionally, the advancement in the discovery of biologics, which have revolutionized the treatment approach, provides targeted therapy that modulates the immune system and restricts flare-ups. As science improves, newer drugs within pharmacology continue to be discovered, and with the potential to further improve therapeutic interventions. Such continued advancement is an indicator of increasing knowledge of the biological mechanisms of these disorders as well as an indication of the need for individualized treatment plans to maximize patient outcomes, as seen in recent studies on therapeutic drug monitoring and novel biological approaches to treatment (Himmerich et al., 2024). Besides pharmacotherapy, numerous non-pharmacological interventions also play a significant role in the management of colon disorders. Dietary modification and nutritional therapy are increasingly being shown to influence gut health. For instance, some patients may benefit from the implementation of a low-FODMAP diet in an attempt to manage symptoms associated with irritable bowel syndrome (IBS). The diet is aimed at restricting fermentable oligosaccharides, disaccharides, monosaccharides, and polyols potentially causative of gastrointestinal discomfort. Similarly, probiotics and prebiotics have been shown to hold promise in rebalancing gut microbiota, particularly in those with such disorders as antibiotic-associated diarrhea. Such integrative strategies emphasize the need for an overall treatment plan that addresses not just the bodily expressions of colon disorders, but also the lifestyle and dietary considerations that might contribute to their exacerbation (Ołczyk, 2024). As gastroenterology evolves, exploration of new therapeutic modalities continues to be a developing process. New research emerging identifies the promise of microbiome therapies, aiming to leverage the gut's microbial community to establish therapeutic benefit. Utilization of new therapies like intermittent theta burst stimulation is a state-of-the-art strategy aimed at the neurobiological dimensions of colon disorders. Such developments are reflective of personalized medicine, where treatment protocols are formulated according to individual diagnostics and response to previous therapies. Furthermore, integration of various treatment modalities, drug and lifestyle therapies, can maximize overall efficacy, as evidenced by combined delivery of oral and local therapies. As we increasingly understand the complexity of colon disorders, ongoing refinement of treatment protocols will be crucial to maximizing patient care and quality of life (Himmerich et al., 2024) (Figure 6.13).

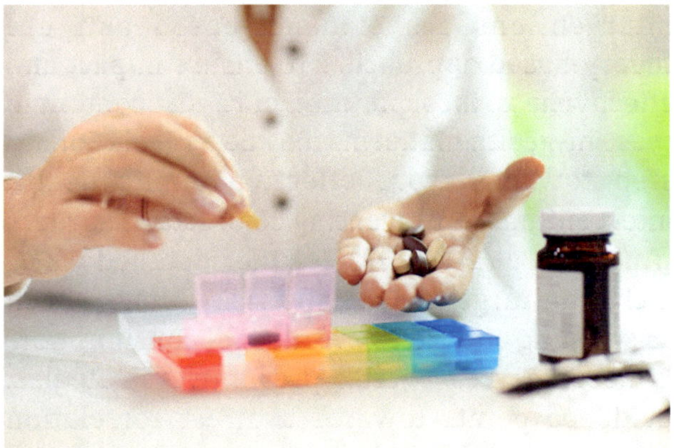

Figure 6.13. Medications and therapies.

Source: https://images.squarespace-cdn.com/content/v1/62389b1d704b5d71836403bb/94896127-7139-46b0-9967-9aa500966bf6/AdobeStock_437321912.jpeg.

6.5.3. Surgical Interventions

The surgical interventions for colon diseases play a central role in the treatment of diseases , such as colorectal cancer and diverticulitis. As colorectal cancer remains a prime public health concern, with high morbidity and mortality rates, surgical treatments are typically reserved as a last resort. Surgical resection, involving the removal of the cancerous segment of the colon and affected lymph nodes, is crucial to the possible cure of the disease. Total mesorectal excision, a technique developed to optimize oncological outcomes in rectal cancer surgery, shows that meticulous control of surgery technique is crucial to reduce local recurrence rates. The American Society of Colon and Rectal Surgeons emphasizes adopting whole guidelines for such surgical interventions, with such guidelines being aligned with the best available evidence for optimal safety in patients and best possible results (Hall et al., 2020; Yau-You et al., 2020). In addition to resection for malignant disease, surgical interventions for benign disease , such as diverticulitis, are also critical. In patients with acute complicated diverticulitis, surgical treatment may be necessary, especially in the presence of large abscess formation or perforation.

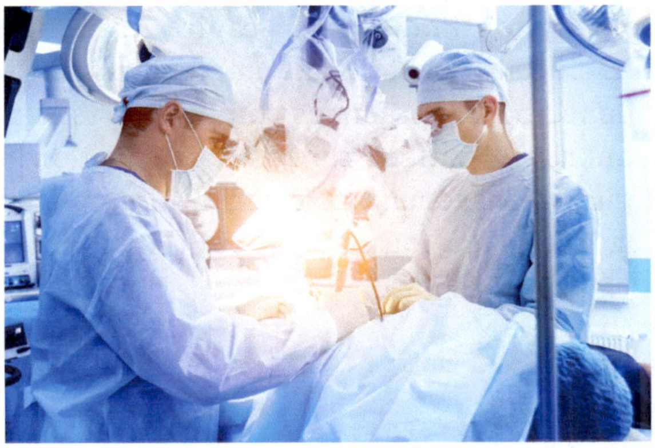

Figure 6.14. Surgical interventions.

Source: https://www.curianmedical.co.uk/wp-content/uploads/2021/10/surgery-scaled.jpg.

Laparoscopic surgery is an available option for drainage of abscesses and resection of affected bowel segments, with benefits including reduced postoperative pain and reduced recovery time. The shift in recent years towards non-operative management of uncomplicated diverticulitis reflects a strategic change in approach, but surgery remains important when complications arise or when treatments fail initially. As surgical techniques evolve, the implementation of minimally invasive techniques has revolutionized the treatment of diverticular disease, with improved postoperative outcomes and patient satisfaction overall (Hall et al., 2020; Yau-You et al., 2020).

Besides, patient selection for surgical intervention involves a comprehensive preoperative assessment to identify the ideal candidate for surgeries , such as resections and colectomies. Patient selection factors usually include age, overall health status, and comorbidities, which significantly influence surgical outcomes. Multidisciplinary care, including surgeons, gastroenterologists, and oncologists, is a significant component of revised guidelines to facilitate an integrative assessment process in managing multidimensional patient needs. The integration of healthcare providers not only optimizes per capita treatment plans but also enables the implementation of evidence-based practices, ultimately leading to improved patient care and satisfaction in surgical management of colon disorders (Hall et al., 2020; Yau-You et al., 2020) (Figure 6.14).

6.6. Prevention Strategies

Effective prevention strategies are important in lowering the incidence of colorectal disorders, including colorectal cancer and inflammatory bowel diseases. Most of the evidence indicates that lifestyle modification, most importantly diet, is able to lower the risk of development of such disorders significantly. High consumption of fresh fruits, vegetables, whole grains, and lean protein, particularly high-fiber foods, has been linked with a low risk of colorectal cancer. Exercise not only benefits health but also has been shown to lower rates of cancer development considerably. Promotion of people to consume healthier foods and exercise regularly, thus constitutes a cornerstone prevention strategy that can lower the incidence of colorectal disorders among the population and enhance patient outcomes in the long run (Antoniou et al., 2017). Another important prevention strategy is technology use, particularly mobile health (m-health) applications, which have shown potential as a tool in the provision of health behavior interventions. Use of smartphone applications with functions , such as gamification and personalized feedback can assist in engaging people and helping them adhere to healthy lifestyle modification. These apps target weight loss and enhanced behavior promotion among the population, thus some of the modifiable disease risk factors in the colon. However, it is important that the interventions are evidence-based and use theory-based approaches to ensure impact and effectiveness. Incorporation of robust content in these m-health platforms may be a revolutionary step towards more effective public health interventions in preventing colorectal disorders (Antoniou et al., 2017). Further detailed work, including targeting specific risk factors , such as smoking and excessive alcohol consumption, is necessary to overall preventive strategies. Evidence points towards a direct correlation between such lifestyle habits and a higher risk for colorectal disorders, including cancer. Public health campaigns to educate individuals about the ill effects of smoking and moderate drinking can go a long way towards disease control. Early detection campaigns, such as periodic screening of the high-risk population, also form a critical component of preventive programs. Screening campaigns are critical, as they can detect precancerous conditions, which enable intervention at the right time, culminating in a decline in mortality rates due to colorectal cancer. Hence, an interdisciplinary approach that includes lifestyle changes, public health interventions, and technological interventions will be necessary to prevent colon disorders effectively (Figure 6.15).

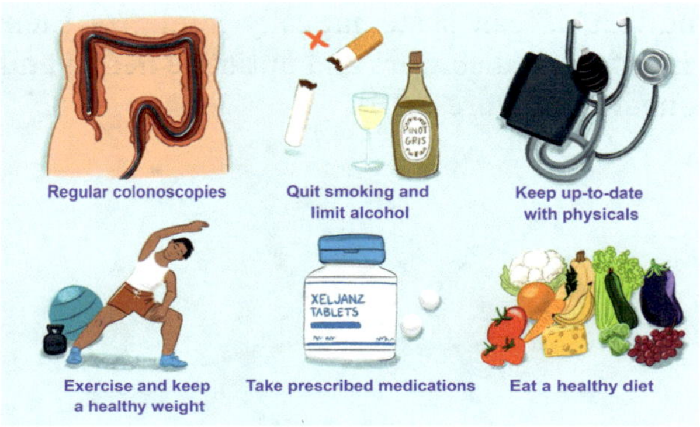

Figure 6.15. Prevention strategies.

Source: https://www.verywellhealth.com/thmb/nslSwFpobbl6tXPBG-FGrG7rwRM=/1500x0/filters:no_upscale():max_bytes(150000):strip_icc()/ulcerative-colitis-and-colon-cancer-5204560_FINAL-3ebdae59ed1f4c88a4c1ab0153f127e8.jpg.

6.6.1. Importance of Regular Screenings

Regular screenings are at the core of early diagnosis and prevention of colon disorders, and they significantly contribute to patient outcomes. Through identification of conditions , such as colorectal cancer, polyps, and other gastrointestinal tract disorders at an early stage, screenings can lead to timely intervention that is less invasive and successful. Research advocates that regular screening can reduce mortality from colorectal disease, emphasizing the need to adhere to guidelines for screening intervals. For instance, guidelines stipulate that individuals should begin regular screenings at the age of 45 or younger for individuals with risk factors, emphasizing the need for awareness and education regarding individual health history. Moreover, when unusual results are unveiled through screenings, they can be resolved early, reducing the possibility of disease progression that is usually accompanied by delayed diagnosis. Moreover, the application of technology in colorectal screening has made screenings more accessible and enhanced participation rates among various groups. Mobile health applications, as indicated in recent studies, show the significance of digital platforms in enhancing screening rates for disorders , such as colon-related complications. Patients can be reminded, provided with educational content, and supported through such technology in managing the healthcare system, ultimately leading to active participation in the control of health. The innovations reflect the potential for overcoming barriers that have previously dissuaded individuals from receiving necessary screenings, such as fear, ignorance, or misunderstanding the applicability of such tests. Through interventions for patient engagement and empowerment, the public health environment can be transformed to address preventive care and regular tests, further reducing the rates of severe outcomes for colon disorders. Despite the obvious benefits of regular screenings, public awareness and participation remain a basic concern. Many individuals may be dreading screening due to myths of pain or invasiveness, but physicians continue to insist that potential benefits are much greater than the temporary harms of such tests. Creating a culture that promotes open discussion of screening and colon health is crucial to solving such problems. Public health strategies and community outreach must focus on educating populations about the benefits of routine screening and myth-debunking to facilitate early detection. In addition, better communication from healthcare providers on risk factors and screening criteria can empower patients to take proactive action on their health. By creating a culture in which routine screenings are the standard, we can finally increase early detection and reduce the burden of colon disorders on patients and healthcare systems, resp.

6.6.2. Healthy Lifestyle Choices

A healthy lifestyle holds a central position in the prevention of colon disorders, particularly in the context of diet, physical exercise, and management of stress. A healthy diet with high levels of fruits, vegetables, whole cereals, and lean proteins has a significant role to play in the maintenance of colon health through the provision of a rich variety of gut microbiota. This variety helps to bring about superior metabolic functions, maintain gut barrier integrity, and support immune responses. A recent review informs that individuals with healthier core microbiota, determined by food intake habits and lifestyle, have less dysbiosis, which is prevalent with most intestinal diseases and disorders (Rinninella et al., 2019). Therefore, by preferring nutrient-rich foods and limiting the intake of processed foods high in sugar and fats, individuals can create a good foundation for their digestive health and well-being. In addition to food habits, regular exercise holds a significant position in ensuring colon health. Regular physical exercise has been shown to enhance gastrointestinal motility and stimulate good gut bacteria, further minimizing the risk of colon-related disorders (Rawla et al., 2019). Exercise not only helps in weight control, but also suppresses inflammation, a vital factor in most gastrointestinal disorders. Exercise has also been shown to be inversely associated with the incidence of colon cancer, indicating the role of a healthy lifestyle in prevention. Therefore, the incorporation of exercise in daily life, such as by walking, jogging, or cycling, can become a multifaceted method of enhancing digestive health. Lastly, stress management is a role normally overlooked while ensuring the health of the colon. Stress, if chronic, can disrupt the balance of gut microbiota and result in gastrointestinal disorders like irritable bowel syndrome and inflammatory bowel disease. The incorporation of mindfulness techniques like meditation and yoga can also minimize these stressors by keeping emotional health and a healthy gut environment intact. Therapy involving diet modification, exercise, and stress reduction is critical to sustaining a healthy colon. By placing a priority on these lifestyle options, individuals can systematically minimize their risk of colon disorders and optimize health and longevity (Figure 6.16).

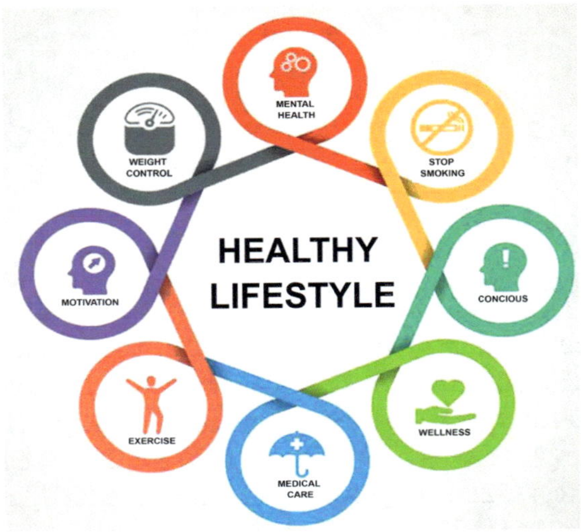

Figure 6.16. Healthy lifestyle choices.

Source: https://img.medscape.com/thumbnail_library/is_171108_lifestyle_choices_800x600.jpg.

6.6.3. Education and Awareness

Education and awareness about disorders of the colon are critical determinants for enhancing patient outcomes and public health interventions. With the increasing incidence of conditions like colorectal cancer and inflammatory bowel disease, knowledge of the signs, risk factors, and protective factors is essential. Public health interventions whose aim is to raise awareness can be a critical determinant when it comes to influencing the perception of people towards their health and the need to attend medical consultations. With increasing awareness, individuals will be more inclined towards adopting the practice of regular screening, which has been proven to decrease mortality due to such disorders. Education, thus, acts as a catalyst for active health action as well as a catalyst for preventative culture, especially among vulnerable communities. By creating an environment in which information is disseminated, healthcare systems are in a position to prepare populations to effectively fight colon disorders using the necessary knowledge. Additionally, the inclusion of education in healthcare can aid clinicians and physicians in overcoming sex and gender disparities in the diagnosis and treatment of colon disorders. Studies show that such disparities influence various aspects of disease management, such as clinical presentation and treatment response (Jarvis et al., 2020). With a focus on gender-sensitive education strategies in health curricula, future healthcare practitioners will be in a position to detect and respond to differences in practice. Additionally, with the inclusion of extensive training in applying biological and social determinants of health, the quality of care can be enhanced. Educating healthcare practitioners about the implications of sex and gender not only improves their diagnostic skills but also informs policymakers and healthcare programs working towards a response to health inequities. Therefore, the creation of a more responsive and informed healthcare workforce is key to addressing the complex requirements of colon disorder patients. Lastly, schools and community organizations are key institutions for promoting awareness and educating the public about the epidemiology of colon disorders. Research has shown that colorectal cancer, for instance, ranks as one of the top causes of cancer-related deaths, and this is an indication of the need for increased educational programs (Rawla et al., 2019). Educational workshops, seminars, and outreach programs can provide individuals with vital information on risk factors, facts, and early detection strategies. In addition, the use of social media and community leaders can also widen the scope of such programs, making information more widespread among the population. By identifying a focus on specific awareness programs aimed at specific groups, stakeholders can effectively eliminate myths and encourage preventive behavior. Therefore, an emphasis on education and awareness not only makes the public better-informed but also decreases incidence and mortality rates due to colon disorders.

CLOSER LOOK

ELECTROLYTE REGULATION:

Electrolyte regulation is fundamental to maintaining physiological stability, enabling essential processes such as nerve conduction, muscle contraction, fluid balance, and acid–base homeostasis. The body's electrolytes—primarily sodium, potassium, chloride, calcium, magnesium, phosphate, and bicarbonate—circulate in precise concentrations. Even small deviations can lead to significant clinical consequences, making tight regulation critical for overall health. A closer look reveals that the kidneys serve as the primary regulators of electrolyte balance. Through filtration, reabsorption, and secretion, the kidneys adjust electrolyte levels in response to the body's needs. Hormones such as aldosterone, antidiuretic hormone (ADH), and parathyroid hormone (PTH) finely tune this process. Aldosterone increases sodium reabsorption and potassium excretion in the distal nephron, helping maintain blood pressure and fluid balance. ADH controls water reabsorption, indirectly affecting sodium concentration by diluting or concentrating body fluids. PTH regulates calcium and phosphate levels by acting on bone, kidneys, and the intestines.

Dietary intake also plays a significant role. Electrolytes enter the body through food and fluids, and inadequate or excessive consumption can disrupt equilibrium. Conditions such as dehydration, diarrhea, vomiting, or excessive sweating can rapidly alter electrolyte concentrations. Athletes, for example, may experience sodium depletion during intense physical activity, leading to hyponatremia if losses are replaced with water alone.

Electrolyte regulation is closely linked to cellular function. Sodium and potassium gradients across cell membranes generate the electrical impulses necessary for nerve signaling and heartbeat rhythm. Calcium is essential for muscle contraction, blood clotting, and hormone release. Magnesium serves as a cofactor in numerous enzymatic reactions, while phosphate contributes to energy production through ATP. Disruptions in any of these electrolytes can impair cellular activity and lead to symptoms ranging from muscle cramps and fatigue to life-threatening arrhythmias.

The endocrine system provides additional layers of control. The renin–angiotensin–aldosterone system (RAAS) responds to changes in blood volume and pressure, while calcitonin and vitamin D regulate calcium balance. The body's acid–base status further influences electrolyte levels, as hydrogen ions exchange with potassium and calcium shifts between blood and bone depending on pH.

Overall, electrolyte regulation is a dynamic, interconnected process involving multiple organs and hormonal pathways. A closer examination underscores how essential this balance is to normal physiology and how quickly disturbances can impact health. Monitoring and maintaining electrolyte homeostasis is therefore central to medical care, especially in patients with chronic illness, acute fluid loss, or renal impairment.

SUMMARY

In compiling the complexities of colonic disorders, there is a necessity to appreciate the multifactorial etiology of the respective diseases. Various dietary habits, particularly high-fat diets, have been shown to induce widespread changes in colon motility and cause disorders , such as constipation. As an example, evidence indicates that a high-fat diet is implicated in dysregulation of gut microbiota, leading to elevated levels of inflammatory markers , such as lipopolysaccharide, which cause harmful effects on myenteric neurons of the colon. Such neurodegeneration ultimately hinders normal peristaltic movements, further complicating gastrointestinal symptoms and recognizing the role of dietary intervention as a treatment option. Identification of such correlations highlights the necessity for dietary awareness as a prophylactic treatment in the management of various colonic disorders, hence the maintenance of gastrointestinal health through nutritional intervention (Reichardt et al., 2016). Furthermore, the implication of colorectal and cancer complications, such as cachexia, offers further evidence of the inter-linkages between systemic and colonic disorders. Cachexia is not only a manifestation of the malignancy but also significantly impacts the quality of life of the patient as well as the response to treatment. Analysis of proteomic changes in muscle shows widespread alterations in metabolic and structural proteins, which highlights the complexity of nutritional deficiency in cancer patients. The concurrent analysis of the impact of chemotherapy and the presence of cancer offers critical information regarding the common biological pathways that regulate the wasting of muscle and systemic inflammation in colonic disorders. By identifying these mechanisms, therapeutic intervention may be maximized to reverse the debilitating effect of cachexia and maximize colorectal cancer treatment, underscoring the need for an integrated treatment plan for diet and disease (Barreto et al., 2016). Lastly, management of colon disorders needs an integrative approach addressing dietary habits, underlying pathologies, and the body's metabolic responses. The interaction between dietary gut microbiota alterations and systemic inflammatory mediators demonstrates the intricate interaction within the gastrointestinal tract. Moreover, the comorbidities of patients with colorectal cancer underscore the need for multimodal treatment approaches involving nutritional support, pharmacological interventions, and lifestyle changes. Lastly, a better understanding of these interactions can translate to improved patient outcomes and improved management of colon disorders. Future studies should seek to clarify the specific mechanisms and explore potential interventions on target pathways, formulating an integrative approach to gastrointestinal health (Barreto et al., 2016).

In the study of colon disorders, a critical understanding of the role of antimicrobial resistance (AMR) in the implications is necessary. Fresh research has highlighted the vast burden of AMR on public health, an estimated 4.95 million deaths in 2019 due to bacterial resistance alone. This is a chilling figure that highlights the necessity for tackling the drivers of infections to such a degree, particularly in the environment of lower resources where drug-resistant infection burden is amplified. The explicit link between the health of the colon and resistance at the microbial level highlights the necessity for strengthening preventive treatments and intervention measures for colon disease. The interventions that strengthen infection prevention through better antibiotic stewardship are pivotal to the reduction of the risk posed by AMR and, by extension, prevention of colon disorders due to resistant pathogens (Murray et al., 2022). Furthermore, the role of gut microbiota in overall regulation of health cannot be overstated, particularly in colon disorders. The gut microbiome is a focal point in modulating metabolic and immune function, with fresh research indicating a pivotal interaction between gut bacteria and neurochemical pathways through the gut-brain axis. Short-chain fatty acids (SCFAs), which are produced through the fermentation of dietary fiber by the colon, are at the core of this interaction, with implications for neuro-immunoendocrine regulation. This highlights the potential for gut microbiota disturbance as an etiology of a variety of disorders, including inflammatory bowel disease (IBD) and colorectal cancer. As research continues to chart the mechanisms of microbiota-gut-brain communication, the potential for new therapies of the gut microbiome is promising, a new frontier in the treatment of colon disorders and facilitation of holistic health (Silva et al., 2020). Lastly, giving an overall overview of key points about colon disorders entails the understanding of interrelated roles of microbial health and the effectiveness of antibiotics. The effect of AMR is not only within the immediate region of infection but also within the overall context of chronic disease in colon function. With the understanding of the complex interaction between microbial communities, diet, drug resistance, and gut health, health practitioners can promote a more preventive way of handling colon disorders. Effective communication between researchers, clinicians, and policymakers in the formulation of plans including education, enhanced diagnostics, and access to effective treatment is crucial. Ultimately, through a better understanding of these complex interactions, the health system will be in a position to effectively combat the emerging tide of colon disorders while addressing the primary challenge of AMR globally (Murray et al., 2022; Silva et al., 2020).

References

1. Abdelmoula, N. B., & Abdelmoula, B. (2024). NFS-04. GENETIC COUNSELLING IN A MULTI-TUMOR PREDISPOSITION SYNDROME: A NOVEL FOUR-GENERATION TUNISIAN PEDIGREE. *Neuro-Oncology, 26*(Suppl 4), 0. https://doi.org/10.1093/neuonc/noae064.562(accessed on 15th July 2025).
2. Abegaz, S. B. (2021). Human ABO blood groups and their associations with different diseases. *BioMed Research International, 2021*, 1–9. https://doi.org/10.1155/2021/6629060 (accessed on 15th July 2025).
3. Abu-Elmagd, K., Furukawa, H., Lee, R. G., Rao, et al. (1995). *Outcome analysis of 71 clinical intestinal transplantations.* https://core.ac.uk/download/12205210.pdf (accessed on 15th July 2025).
4. Accarino Garaventa, A. M., Azpiroz Vidaur, F., Bendezú García, Á., Malagelada Benapres, et al. (2017). *Colonic content: Effect of diet, meals, and defecation.* https://core.ac.uk/download/81582130.pdf (accessed on 15th July 2025).
5. P. E. Antoniou, O. Rivera-Romero, M. Karagianni and P. D. Bamidis, "Towards Evidence Based M-Health Application Design in Cancer Patient Healthy Lifestyle Interventions," *2017 IEEE 30th International Symposium on Computer-Based Medical Systems (CBMS)*, Thessaloniki, Greece, 2017, pp. 690-695, doi: 10.1109/CBMS.2017.117.(accessed on 15th July 2025).
6. Barreto, R., Mandili, G., Witzmann, F. A., Novelli, F., Zimmers, T. A., & Bonetto, A. (2016). Cancer and chemotherapy contribute to muscle loss by activating common signaling pathways. *Frontiers in Physiology, 7.* https://doi.org/10.3389/fphys.2016.00472 (accessed on 15th July 2025).
7. Blakely, T., Chen, J., Cormack, D., Cunningham, et al. (2010). *Survival disparities in Indigenous and non-Indigenous New Zealanders with colon cancer: The role of patient comorbidity, treatment and health service factors.* https://core.ac.uk/download/148643017.pdf (accessed on 15th July 2025).
8. Calabrese, E., Dietrich, C. F., Dirks, K., Gilja, et al. (2016). *EFSUMB recommendations and guidelines for gastrointestinal ultrasound – Part 1: Examination techniques and normal findings (Long version).* https://core.ac.uk/download/74321241.pdf (accessed on 15th July 2025).
9. Camargo, S. M. R., Vuille-dit-Bille, R. N., Meier, C., & Verrey, F. (2020). ACE2 and gut amino acid transport. *Clinical Science, 134*, 2823–2833. https://doi.org/10.1042/cs20200477 (accessed on 15th July 2025).
10. Camilleri, M. (1999). *Functional bowel disease: A challenging frontier in gastroenterology.* https://core.ac.uk/download/46601769.pdf (accessed on 15th July 2025).
11. Choi, W., Ko, S., Jung, D., Kim, S. C., Choi, N., Park, J. W., Kim, B. (2024). Therapeutic effects of *Zanthoxyli Pericarpium* on intestinal inflammation and network pharmacological mechanism analysis in a dextran sodium sulfate-induced colitis mouse model. *Nutrients, 16.* https://www.semanticscholar.org/paper/b5c46fd694e8e42b74bd7b18a3c7c1497c9a4471 (accessed on 15th July 2025).
12. Clarke, S. F., Cotter, P. D., Cronin, O., Molloy, et al. (2015). *Exercise and the Microbiota.* https://core.ac.uk/download/45656552.pdf (accessed on 15th July 2025).

13. Colón-Emeric, C. S., McDermott, C., Lee, D. S., & Berry, S. D. (2024). Risk assessment and prevention of falls in older community-dwelling adults: A review. *JAMA.* https://www.semanticscholar.org/paper/b0f06cabae8c5dd08118becac4de418c89fb8a1b (accessed on 15th July 2025).

14. Colon-Soto, J., Vega-Sanabria, B., Cardona-Quiñones, R. A., Balsalobre-Vélez, A., & De Jesus-Rojas, W. (2024). 1184 The leptin puzzle: Decoding genes, morbid obesity, sleep-related disorders and its influence. *SLEEP.* https://www.semanticscholar.org/paper/0cdcdf7fe71b7f6c61fe6af9fcdc204b57bc9b11 (accessed on 15th July 2025).

15. Cryan, J. F., O'Riordan, K. J., Cowan, C. S. M., Sandhu, K. V., Bastiaanssen, T. F. S., Boehme, M., Codagnone, M. G., et al. (2019). The microbiota-gut-brain axis. *Physiological Reviews, 99,* 1877–2013. https://doi.org/10.1152/physrev.00018.2018 (accessed on 15th July 2025).

16. de Vos, W. M., Tilg, H., Van Hul, M., & Cani, P. D. (2022). Gut microbiome and health: Mechanistic insights. *Gut, 71,* 1020–1032. https://doi.org/10.1136/gutjnl-2021-326789 (accessed on 15th July 2025).

17. Denis, F., Le Goff, F., Desbois, M., Gepner, A., Feliciano, G., Silber, D., Zeitoun, J., et al. (2024). Early detection of 5 neurodevelopmental disorders of children and prevention of postnatal depression with a mobile health app: Observational cross-sectional study. *JMIR Public Health and Surveillance, 10.* https://www.semanticscholar.org/paper/f2c51d91258fdcf18c1fcde85169b8c6dbb6f5da (accessed on 15th July 2025).

18. Di Rienzo, A., Marinelli, L., Dimmito, M. P., Toto, E. C., Di Stefano, A., & Cacciatore, I. (2024). Advancements in inflammatory bowel disease management: From traditional treatments to monoclonal antibodies and future drug delivery systems. *Pharmaceutics, 16.* https://www.semanticscholar.org/paper/d3fd21f847e27aa0989ce84aca71edbe12060324 (accessed on 15th July 2025).

19. Dunn, J. C. Y., Hong, S. N., Martín, M. G., Stelzner, et al. (2016). *Concise review: The potential use of intestinal stem cells to treat patients with intestinal failure.* https://core.ac.uk/download/323078733.pdf (accessed on 15th July 2025).

20. Gómez-Peralta, F., Pinés-Corrales, P. J., Santos, E., Cuesta, M., González-Albarrán, O., Azriel, S., Castaño, L., et al. (2025). Autoimmune type 1 diabetes: An early approach appraisal for Spain by the AGORA Diabetes Collaborative Group. *Journal of Clinical Medicine, 14.* https://www.semanticscholar.org/paper/4480f955f8538ea1e0ff8ec0f717dc39fda15690 (accessed on 15th July 2025).

21. González-Castro, A., Fernández-Bañares, F., Zabana, Y., Farago-Pérez, G., Ortega-Barrionuevo, J., Expósito, E., & Guagnozzi, D. (2024). Microscopic colitis and celiac disease: Sharing more than a diagnostic overlap. *Nutrients, 16.* https://www.semanticscholar.org/paper/5a99d419c592adea2a597d64bf4d906baa39377c (accessed on 15th July 2025).

22. Hall, J., Hardiman, K. M., Lee, S. H., Lightner, A. L., Stocchi, L., Paquette, I. M., Steele, S. R., et al. (2020). The American Society of Colon and Rectal Surgeons Clinical Practice Guidelines for the treatment of left-sided colonic diverticulitis. *Diseases of the Colon & Rectum, 63,* 728–747. https://doi.org/10.1097/dcr.0000000000001679 (accessed on 15th July 2025).

23. Hijdra, T., Health Science 2 Department of Sociology and Social University, et al. (2023). The effect of mental disorders in youth on NEET and the mediating role of high school dropout. *The European Journal of Public Health, 33.* https://www.semanticscholar.org/paper/aa08b70ee71f346a0fa5f5ce8555dbe56513e1b0 (accessed on 15th July 2025).

24. Himmerich, H., Herpertz-Dahlmann, B., & Mörkl, S. (2024). Editorial: Biological therapies and eating disorders. *European Eating Disorders Review.* https://www.semanticscholar.org/paper/287a6650e674fcac50e84a43fc621efccc5edc77 (accessed on 15th July 2025).

25. Huang, K., Wu, L., & Yang, Y. (2021). Gut microbiota: An emerging biological diagnostic and treatment approach for gastrointestinal diseases. *JGH Open, 5*, 973–975. https://doi.org/10.1002/jgh3.12659 (accessed on 15th July 2025).

26. Jain, M., Mann, T., Stulić, M., Rao, S., Kirsch, A., Pullirsch, D., Strobl, X., et al. (2018). *RNA* editing of Filamin A pre-*mRNA* regulates vascular contraction and diastolic blood pressure. *The EMBO Journal, 37.* https://doi.org/10.15252/embj.201694813 (accessed on 15th July 2025).

27. Jansone, K., Eichler, A., Fasching, P., Kornhuber, J., Kaiser, A., Millenet, S., Banaschewski, T., et al. (2023). Association of maternal smoking during pregnancy with neurophysiological and ADHD-related outcomes in school-aged children. *International Journal of Environmental Research and Public Health, 20.* https://www.semanticscholar.org/paper/83796f9ba22ed2e9ce2445f37e5cdb6eda09fa19 (accessed on 15th July 2025).

28. Khoury, J. D., Solary, É., Abla, O., Akkari, Y., Alaggio, R., Apperley, J. F., Bejar, R., et al. (2022). The 5th edition of the World Health Organization Classification of Hematolymphoid Tumors: Myeloid and histiocytic/dendritic neoplasms. *Leukemia, 36*, 1703–1719. https://doi.org/10.1038/s41375-022-01613-1 (accessed on 15th July 2025).

29. Kızıloluk, S., & Sert, E. (2022). COVID-CCD-Net: COVID-19 and colon cancer diagnosis system with optimized CNN hyperparameters using gradient-based optimizer. *Medical & Biological Engineering & Computing, 60*, 1595–1612. https://www.semanticscholar.org/paper/be669809d544ce2abe5df3e361537fcb7b08343b (accessed on 15th July 2025).

30. Koumpias, A. M., Schwartzman, D. A., & Fleming, O. (2022). Long-haul COVID: Healthcare utilization and medical expenditures 6 months post-diagnosis. *BMC Health Services Research, 22.* https://www.semanticscholar.org/paper/b9d436545ac3f54c51d8b1f22b016d0db48c0d3c (accessed on 15th July 2025).

31. Larauche, M., Mulak, A., & Taché, Y. (2011). *Stress-related alterations of visceral sensation: Animal models for irritable bowel syndrome study.* https://core.ac.uk/download/323080393.pdf (accessed on 15th July 2025).

32. Lyon, M., & Kacinik, V. (2012). Is there a place for dietary fiber supplements in weight management? *Current Obesity Reports, 1*, 59–67. https://www.semanticscholar.org/paper/4da478b0578e39d349285fbef2f74232a6456b3d (accessed on 15th July 2025).

33. Mao, Q. Q., Xu, X. Y., Cao, S. Y., Gan, R. Y., Corke, H., Beta, T., & Li, H. B. (2019). Bioactive compounds and bioactivities of *Zingiber officinale* Roscoe. *Foods, 8*, 185. https://doi.org/10.3390/foods8060185 (accessed on 15th July 2025).

34. Mauvais-Jarvis, F., Bairey Merz, C. N., Barnes, P. J., Brinton, R. D., Carrero, J. J., DeMeo, D. L., De Vries, G. J., et al. (2020). Sex and gender: Modifiers of health, disease, and medicine. *The Lancet, 396*, 565–582. https://doi.org/10.1016/s0140-6736(20)31561-0 (accessed on 15th July 2025).

35. Moshiree, B., Drossman, D. A., & Shaukat, A. (2023). AGA clinical practice update on evaluation and management of belching, abdominal bloating, and distention: Expert review. *Gastroenterology, 165*, 791–800.e3. https://doi.org/10.1053/j.gastro.2023.04.039 (accessed on 15th July 2025).

36. Murray, C. J. L., Ikuta, K. S., Sharara, F., Swetschinski, L. R., Robles Aguilar, G., Gray, A. P., Han, C., et al. (2022). Global burden of bacterial antimicrobial resistance in 2019: A systematic analysis. *The Lancet, 399*, 629–655. https://doi.org/10.1016/s0140-6736(21)02724-0 (accessed on 15th July 2025).

37. Nazarov, G., Ilyosova, D., Matchanov, A., Zikirullaeva, N., Dilmurod, et al. (2025). Key determinants of investment flow and fiscal health for data-driven policy decisions and information retrieval. *Innovation Science and Technology.* https://www.semanticscholar.org/paper/ca6ce18469cff8b1b3aed5214f65cc017ec22ac6 (accessed on 15th July 2025).

38. Park, K. (2015). The role of low FODMAP diet in the management of irritable bowel syndrome. *Journal of Gastroenterology and Hepatology Research, 4*, 1810–1814. https://www.semanticscholar.org/paper/c4492c7e214a789976304d632a893b64301a2d34 (accessed on 15th July 2025).

39. Pawełczyk, O. (2024). Treatment options of human demodicosis. *Journal of Education, Health and Sport.* https://www.semanticscholar.org/paper/dc811568a65cf42f12ed0352cd0d43e0df9759b7 (accessed on 15th July 2025).

40. Rathi, K. M., Verma, A., & Pingat, P. (2024). Early detection and intervention for Hirschsprung's disease: A key to successful outcomes. *Clinical Medicine Insights. Case Reports, 17.* https://www.semanticscholar.org/paper/d8d1b0e446ec962e700dddfc92511d1df176b514 (accessed on 15th July 2025).

41. Rawla, P., Sunkara, T., & Barsouk, A. (2019). Epidemiology of colorectal cancer: Incidence, mortality, survival, and risk factors. *Gastroenterology Review, 14*, 89–103. https://doi.org/10.5114/pg.2018.81072 (accessed on 15th July 2025).

42. Reichardt, F., Chassaing, B., Ghazi Nezami, B., Li, G., Tabatabavakili, S., Mwangi, S. M., Uppal, K., et al. (2016). Western diet induces colonic nitrergic myenteric neuropathy and dysmotility in mice via saturated fatty acid- and lipopolysaccharide-induced TLR4 signaling. *The Journal of Physiology, 595*, 1831–1846. https://doi.org/10.1113/jp273269 (accessed on 15th July 2025).

43. Rinninella, E., Raoul, P., Cintoni, M., Franceschi, F., Miggiano, G. A. D., Gasbarrini, A., & Mele, M. C. (2019). What is the healthy gut microbiota composition? A changing ecosystem across age, environment, diet, and diseases. *Microorganisms, 7*, 14. https://doi.org/10.3390/microorganisms7010014 (accessed on 15th July 2025).

44. Silva, Y. P., Bernardi, A., & Frozza, R. L. (2020). The role of short-chain fatty acids from gut microbiota in gut-brain communication. *Frontiers in Endocrinology, 11.* https://doi.org/10.3389/fendo.2020.00025 (accessed on 15th July 2025).

45. Vogel, J. D., Felder, S., Bhama, A. R., Hawkins, A. T., Langenfeld, S. J., Shaffer, V., Thorsen, A. J., et al. (2021). The American Society of Colon and Rectal Surgeons Clinical Practice Guidelines for the management of colon cancer. *Diseases of the Colon & Rectum, 65*, 148–177. https://doi.org/10.1097/dcr.0000000000002323 (accessed on 15th July 2025).

46. Watanabe, T., Muro, K., Ajioka, Y., Hashiguchi, Y., Ito, Y., Saito, Y., Hamaguchi, T., et al. (2017). Japanese Society for Cancer of the Colon and Rectum (JSCCR) guidelines 2016 for the treatment of colorectal cancer. *International Journal of Clinical Oncology, 23*, 1–34. https://doi.org/10.1007/s10147-017-1101-6 (accessed on 15th July 2025).

47. You, Y. T., Hardiman, K. M., Bafford, A. C., Poylin, V., Francone, T. D., Davis, K. G., Paquette, I. M., et al. (2020). The American Society of Colon and Rectal Surgeons Clinical Practice Guidelines for the management of rectal cancer. *Diseases of the Colon & Rectum, 63*, 1191–1222. https://doi.org/10.1097/dcr.0000000000001762 (accessed on 15th July 2025).

48. Zezos, P. (2021). Artificial intelligence-assisted endoscopy in ulcerative colitis. *International Journal of Extreme Automation and Connectivity in Healthcare.* https://www.semanticscholar.org/paper/7fbed7c25b2e49c54fd8e13b0f10eba9dac9b1cf (accessed on 15th July 2025).

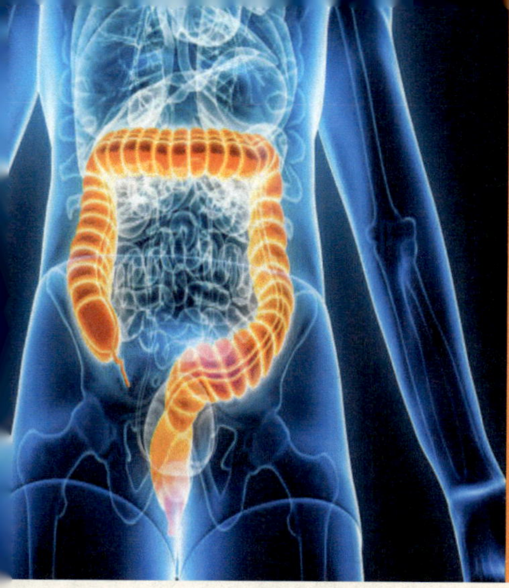

Chapter 7

INFLAMMATORY BOWEL DISEASE (IBD)

Contents

Introduction

The introduction of the topic of inflammatory bowel disease (IBD) is a critical point of departure in understanding the complexity of the chronic condition. Characterized by the presence of two dominant forms, Crohn's disease and ulcerative colitis, IBD is endemic in millions of individuals across the globe, its occurrence in Western countries dramatically escalating. Not only does this complicate an individual's health profile, but it also poses serious concerns for health systems wary of shouldering its financial burden. With many aspects of IBD pathogenesis implicated, including genetic disposition, environmental influences, and immune dysregulation, it is apparent that a multi-faceted approach must be employed in both understanding the nature of and addressing the ramifications. The need for ongoing research, patient education, and effective treatment regimens serves to highlight the nature of building an extensive understanding of IBD. Complicating the issues presented by IBD are also issues of difficulty in effective clinical research, namely with regard to patient recruitment for clinical studies. Research verifies that recruitment has been on the decline, and while reasons for such are poorly understood, one of the primary contributing factors is the rising screen failure (SF) rate for clinical studies. For instance, the primary reasons for SFs include failure to meet certain eligibility criteria set within studies, such as the aggregate modified Mayo score for ulcerative colitis or the Crohn's Disease Activity Index (CDAI) criteria for Crohn's disease trials (Uzzan et al., 2024). Identifying the nature of such problems is critical to developing strategies to enhance recruitment practices in clinical studies, as an awareness of such problems can better inform practices within the context of IBD treatment and research. In addition, patient self-care and caregiver play a key role in chronic disease management, including IBD. As patients fight the day-to-day struggles of IBD, its impact on mental well-being, as well as the emotional burden on caregivers, is significant. Evidence has shown that IBD symptoms can be a contributing factor to higher anxiety and depression levels, significantly impacting the quality of life of patients and caregivers (Napolitano et al., 2024). Through studies of patient self-care and the caregiver role, studies can facilitate holistic management practices, improving overall outcomes. Therefore, these findings not only highlight the significance of self-care in IBD management but also underscore the importance of the involvement of patients and their support networks in treatment interventions (Figure 7.1).

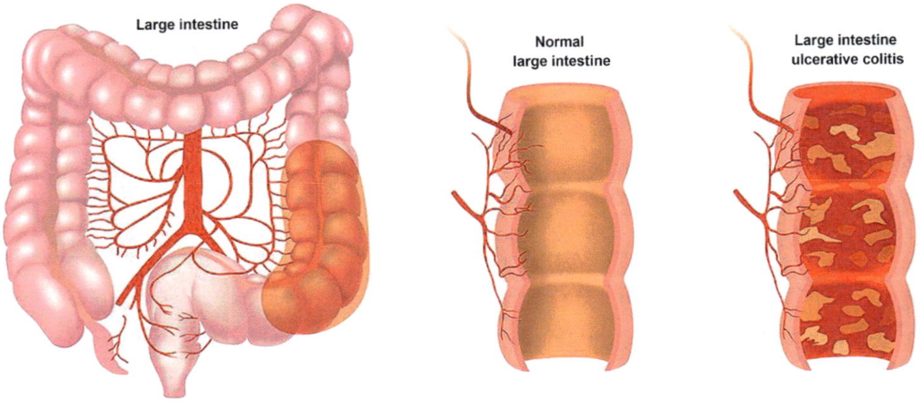

Figure 7.1. Inflammatory bowel disease (IBD).

Source: https://www.cdc.gov/inflammatory-bowel-disease/media/images/2024/06/IBD-UlcerativeColitis-Graphic.jpg.

Definition of Inflammatory Bowel Disease

The Inflammatory Bowel Disease (IBD) is a group of chronic inflammatory gastrointestinal tract disorders, most commonly ulcerative colitis (UC) and Crohn's disease (CD). They all share a commonality of an abnormal immune response to intestinal microbiota, resulting in chronic inflammation and mucosal injury within the gut. Patients present with a range of symptoms, including abdominal pain, diarrhea, weight loss, bleeding per rectum and fatigue, which not only impact physical health but also have a significant impact on quality of life. What is most problematic about IBD is that it is a heterogeneous condition, with variable presentation and sites of disease, which complicates diagnosis and treatment strategy. Appreciation of these nuances is important, as effective management often involves an individualized approach that considers patient factors and disease presentation.

Growing evidence supports the role of diet in the control of symptoms of IBD. Diet is an important consideration for individuals who live with IBD, who are frequently confronted with nutritional deficiencies secondary to malabsorption and increased metabolic demand. Despite growing evidence for a range of dietary treatments, professional guidelines are variable regarding the provision of specific dietary advice to IBD patients. Nutritional therapies , such as the Low-FODMAP diet and Gluten-free diet have gained popularity, with evidence of efficacy in the relief of intestinal symptoms. Importantly, the identification of interactions between diet and gut microbiota can be critical, with evidence to support that some elements of the diet may have anti-inflammatory effects to improve outcomes for IBD patients. As growing research continues to progress, further understanding of the role of diet in the management of IBD will be central to improving patient outcomes, particularly as nutritional considerations are typically not included in standard treatment protocols (Covello et al., 2024). Further, exploration of complementary therapies, such as tea polyphenols, uncovers a novel area of exploration in IBD management. Studies show that tea polyphenols, natural bioactive compounds, are antioxidative and anti-inflammatory in character and can potentially be involved in the regulation of gut well-being. The interaction of these compounds with gut microbiota explains how tea can act as a prebiotic, potentially enhancing populations of beneficial microbes and suppressing populations of pathogens. By continuing to learn how such dietary compounds modulate gut inflammation and contribute to overall well-being, researchers are opening the door to novel dietary strategies in IBD management. As the science matures, the intricate interaction between dietary therapy and IBD pathophysiology will likely be a component of integrated treatment regimens for patients (Xu, 2024).

Importance of Studying IBD

It is essential to understand inflammatory bowel disease (IBD) due to its multifaceted and complex nature beyond gastrointestinal manifestations. IBD constitutes chronic inflammatory disorders, such as Crohn's disease and ulcerative colitis, with far-reaching effects on the quality of life of the patient. The systemic manifestations of IBD, such as abdominal pain, weight loss, and fatigue, have far-reaching effects on a person's functioning and are a cause of emotional distress and depression. Moreover, such conditions may lead to the development of associated comorbidities that complicate patient management. Studies have revealed a strong correlation of IBD with other extra-intestinal disorders, such as immune-mediated disorders, which suggest that disease mechanisms result from complex interactions between genetic susceptibility, environmental influences, and microbial effects. Therefore, although studies on IBD improve our understanding of its pathophysiology, they also shed light on effective treatment and management modalities to improve patient outcomes and quality of life. Additionally, the study of IBD's co-morbidities is significant in the understanding of the disease's broader implications. Recent studies have revealed a high prevalence of associated conditions, such as arthritis, psoriasis, and liver disease, that usually present years before a definitive diagnosis of IBD has been rendered. This association lends importance to early detection and intervention since it has implications on long-term prognosis and management regimens of the affected population. For instance, the identification of patients at risk of developing such conditions as osteoporosis, usually aggravated by IBD-management regimens, enables the clinician to initiate preventive regimens early. Through the study of , such associations, researchers can determine at-risk populations and come up with strategies that treat IBD and its associated co-morbidities, enabling multifaceted care practices that reduce side effects and maximize patient well-being. Also, studies on potential causative infectious pathogens, i.e., cytomegalovirus (CMV), provide insight into important complications in IBD patients. Studies have identified that opportunistic infections exacerbate the symptoms of IBD, making the treatment schedule more complex. For instance, the use of CMV-DNA polymerase chain reaction assays has been found to be more effective in the detection of CMV infection among IBD patients and in the development of antiviral therapy, with high remission rates. This identification of infectious complications warrants the use of cautious diagnosis and targeted therapies, with the ultimate outcome being improved IBD management protocols. With ongoing studies identifying the IBD-infectious agent relationship, evidence-based recommendations can be developed, which can enhance the quality of care and patient outcomes in this patient population. The emphasis on such studies reflects the important role of interdisciplinary research in the elucidation of the complexities of inflammatory bowel disease management.

7.1. Types of Inflammatory Bowel Disease

The clinical presentation of Inflammatory Bowel Disease (IBD) consists primarily of two major types: Crohn's disease (CD) and ulcerative colitis (UC). Crohn's disease can affect any region of the gastrointestinal tract, from the mouth to the anus, and manifests a range of symptoms , such as chronic diarrhea, abdominal cramps, and weight loss. Inflammation in CD is typically transmural, which can cause complications , such as stricture and fistula. Ulcerative colitis, however, is confined to the rectum and colon and tends to manifest contiguous inflammation. Symptoms of UC include bloody diarrhea, urgency, and abdominal cramps. It should be understood to identify the peculiar features of these diseases to diagnose them properly and treat them accordingly, because interventions can be quite different depending on whether a patient presents with CD or UC, thus highlighting the importance of having specific clinical guidelines to treat IBD. New evidence demonstrates the dynamic nature of IBD and suggests that its epidemiology can change over time, impacting the types and prevalence of the disease in the world. Recent studies with the application of advanced statistical techniques demonstrate that regions progress through typified epidemiologic IBD phases, marked by incidence and prevalence rates. For instance, studies demonstrate that North America and parts of Europe have reached advanced phases with high prevalence rates, while most regions in Asia and Latin America are in the early phases with low incidences (Hracs et al., 2024). Such epidemiology statistics assist in better understanding the disease burden, which directs interventions in public health. An understanding of the changing landscape of IBD is necessary for policymakers and clinicians as it facilitates better healthcare resource allocation as well as optimal disease management strategies globally. In addition to CD and UC, new ideas in IBD classification include the identification of unclassified inflammatory bowel diseases that do not fit neatly into either category. Then, in CD, there are several phenotypes with typical clinical, surgical, and radiographic presentations. New studies identify the application of fecal calprotectin (FC) as a cheap, non-invasive biomarker for disease activity monitoring in various phenotypes of pediatric IBD, with a positive correlation with disease activity indices (Plume et al., 2024). This observation suggests that FC monitoring could enhance clinical decision-making as it allows healthcare providers to estimate the degree of inflammation without undue reliance on invasive investigations. By recognizing the spectrum of inflammatory bowel diseases and the application of biomarkers , such as FC in everyday practice, healthcare providers can maximize patient care with treatment being adapted to the type and severity of the disease (Figure 7.2).

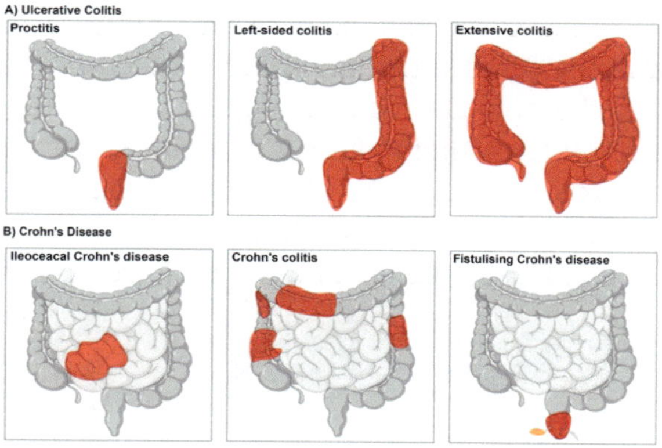

Figure 7.2. Types of inflammatory bowel disease.

Source: https://www.researchgate.net/publication/340986188/figure/fig1/AS:11431281213071184@1702966301726/Different-types-of-Inflammatory-Bowel-diseases-A-Ulcerative-colitis-proctitis.tif.

7.1.1. Crohn's Disease

The clinical presentation of Inflammatory Bowel Disease (IBD) is dominated by two most prevalent variants, i.e., Crohn's disease (CD) and ulcerative colitis (UC). Crohn's disease can affect any region of the gastrointestinal tract, i.e., from the mouth to the anus, and can lead to a wide range of signs that vary from chronic diarrhea, abdominal pain, to weight loss. Inflammation in CD is generally transmural in origin and can lead to complications , such as strictures and fistulas. Ulcerative colitis, on the other hand, is limited to the colon and rectum, wherein it most typically appears as continuous colitis. UC symptoms are dominated by bloody diarrhea, urgency, and crampy abdominal pain. It is essential to identify the distinguishing features of these diseases to conduct an appropriate diagnosis and treatment because interventions would significantly vary depending on whether the patient suffers from CD or UC, and hence the necessity for customized clinical strategies in the management of IBD. Current literature focuses on the dynamic nature of IBD and suggests that its epidemiology can vary with time, which would affect the types and frequencies of the disease across the globe. Recent studies that incorporate the application of sophisticated statistical models confirm that regions can evolve through stipulated epidemiologic phases of IBD, categorized by incidence and prevalence rates. For instance, it is demonstrated that North America and parts of Europe have evolved to advanced stages with high prevalence rates, while parts of Asia and Latin America are in initial stages with low incidences (Hracs et al., 2024). Such epidemiologic information would help understand the disease burden and guiding public health policy. Understanding the evolving IBD landscape is critical to both health workers and policymakers since it permits better healthcare resource allocation and better disease management across various geographic regions. In addition to CD and UC, new IBD classification concepts also include recognition of unclassified inflammatory bowel diseases that do not fit into either of the former. Additionally, in CD, various phenotypes are characterized by variable clinical, surgical, and radiographic presentations. New evidence supports the use of fecal calprotectin (FC) as an easily accessible biomarker in the measurement of disease activity in various phenotypes of pediatric IBD, positively correlating with disease activity scores (Plume et al., 2024). This implies that FC monitoring can be beneficial in enriching clinical decision-making by allowing healthcare professionals to estimate the level of inflammation without necessarily incurring invasive methods. With knowledge of the range of inflammatory bowel diseases and the inclusion of biomarkers , such as FC in routine care, healthcare professionals can improve patient management, with interventions being adjusted to the nature and severity of the disease (Figure 7.3).

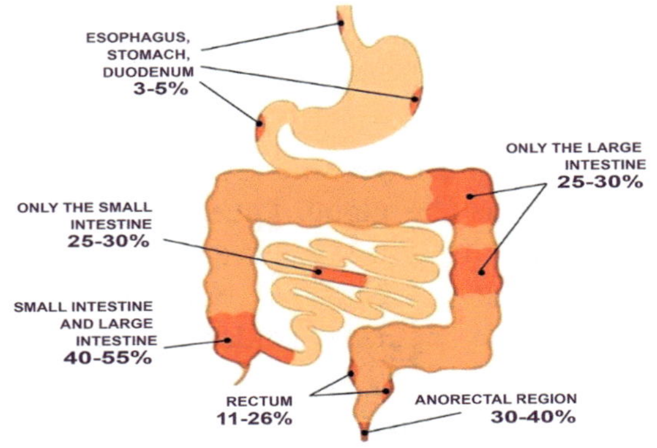

Figure 7.3. Crohn's disease.

Source: https://ecosh.com/wp-content/uploads/sites/3/2021/04/Crohn's_Disease_Infection_Areas_Crohn's_Disease_Prevalence_Infected_Areas_In_Crohn's_Disease.jpg.

7.1.2. Ulcerative Colitis

Ulcerative colitis (UC), an inflammatory bowel disease (IBD), is characterized by chronic inflammation of the mucosa and submucosa of the colon. The disease primarily affects the rectum and colon, causing a range of quality-of-life-related symptoms. Predominant symptoms are abdominal pain, diarrhea, and rectal bleeding, which, if untreated, are accompanied by serious complications like colorectal cancer. The pathogenesis of UC is multifactorial with an interplay of complex factors, including genetic predisposition, immune mechanisms, and environmental factors. The etiological model, which is multifactorial, highlights the need for early and accurate diagnosis due to symptom overlap with other gastrointestinal diseases. Further, the progressive nature of UC necessitates individualized management with consideration of immediate relief of symptoms and long-term maintenance of control of the disease to prevent flares and complications. Ulcerative colitis treatment has evolved dramatically, especially following the advent of sophisticated therapeutic agents. Aminosalicylates and corticosteroids remained the cornerstone of conventional therapy to decrease inflammation and alleviate symptoms. However, the treatment may have an uncertain outcome in all patients, especially in moderate to severe UC. As highlighted in recent literature, the biologic agents anti-tumor necrosis factor (anti-TNF) therapy have become popular, providing a more targeted therapeutic intervention. Further, new agents like Janus kinase (JAK) inhibitors and integrin antagonists have the potential to cause mucosal healing and maintain remission.

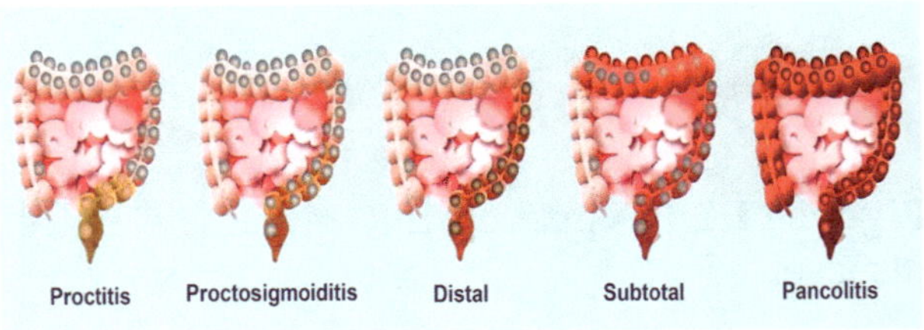

Figure 7.4. Ulcerative colitis

Source: https://www.kaizengastrocare.com/wp-content/uploads/2023/04/Types-of-Ulcerative-Colitis.jpg.

The clinical course of patients is extremely variable based on personal factors, highlighting the importance of individualized treatment regimens for successful management of UC, as highlighted in literature studies in children and adults (Adedara et al., 2024; Bhalla et al., 2025). The psychosocial aspects of living with ulcerative colitis are also central and warrant thorough consideration in treatment plans. Patients usually experience emotional and psychological distress associated with the condition, including anxiety, depression, and social withdrawal. Such complications may worsen the physical symptoms of UC and result in poor adaptation to treatment plans. Holistic management not only offers pharmacologic therapy but also psychological counseling and lifestyle adaptation. Addition of interventions like nutrition therapy, stress coping, and support groups can greatly improve the overall health and well-being and quality of life in UC patients. With continuous research, it is equally important to know the complexities of the physical and mental health complications of ulcerative colitis to develop effective, patient-tailored care interventions (Adedara et al., 2024; Bhalla et al., 2025) (Figure 7.4).

7.1.3. Indeterminate Colitis

Indeterminate Colitis (IC) is a significant diagnostic dilemma within the greater Inflammatory Bowel Disease (IBD) family. IC is characterized by clinical and histological presentations that are not clearly characteristic of either ulcerative colitis or Crohn's disease, with an inherent level of diagnostic imprecision and management complexity. This imprecision, in general, is of specific importance because effective treatment regimens vary significantly for such diseases. IC is not an intermediate diagnosis; rather, it requires diligent clinical observation and monitoring to avoid mismanagement. Additionally, the complexity of IC also requires the clinician's incorporation of individual patient evaluations, as symptoms and disease behavior may vary significantly. Identification of the subtleties of IC may uncover individualized treatment regimens accounting for the patient's specific disease manifestations and responsiveness to therapy. The pathophysiology of Indeterminate Colitis is less clearly defined than that of its counterparts, Crohn's disease and ulcerative colitis. While inflammation of the colonic mucosa is characteristic among IBD subtypes, etiologic factors underlying the development of IC—genetic predispositions and environmental influences—continue to be the focus of research. Emerging literature indicates microbial dysbiosis and immune system dysregulation as possible determinants of IC. In opposition to the more divergent presentations of Crohn's and ulcerative colitis, juxtaposed characteristics of IC may complicate diagnosis and associated therapeutic measures. Clinicians must therefore remain keenly aware of revising diagnoses over time, as affected patients may later present patterns characteristic of the other established categories of IBD, necessitating alteration of treatment strategies. Treatment of Indeterminate Colitis presently borrows extensively from therapy employed in both Crohn's disease and ulcerative colitis, highlighting the necessity for a responsive and adaptive treatment strategy. With IC complexity, treatment is initiated based on current symptoms and severity and not a definitive diagnosis. With advancing science in IBD treatment, new biological therapies , such as anti-tumor necrosis factor (anti-TNF) drugs, are being used more with encouraging efficacy in subtypes of IBD (Bhalla et al., 2025). Concurrently, systematic review of the literature indicates that treatment must be individualized to address the unique needs of IC accordingly. Therefore, more works on long-term outcomes and their response to treatment in Indeterminate Colitis need to be conducted to establish holistic management plans (Adedara et al., 2024). Such specific studies shall allow optimal therapeutic decisions and overall patient quality of life.

7.2. Causes and Risk Factors

The pathogenesis of Inflammatory Bowel Disease (IBD) is still multifactorial and complex, and research is still discovering a variety of potential causative factors. Genetic predisposition is key, with IBD patient first-degree relatives having a much greater risk of developing the disease themselves, indicating a hereditary factor. Immunological responses are also key, with the body's immune response over-reacting to intestinal bacteria. Abnormal provocation of the immune system can induce chronic gastrointestinal inflammation, underlining the pathophysiological complexity of IBD. Other studies have identified factors, such as intestinal dysbiosis, or disrupted balance of the gut microbiota, as factors in IBD development. A high percentage of IBD patients have presented with issues with intestinal flora which can predispose to developing the condition, further underlining how genetic and microbial factors interact in the pathophysiology of IBD (Ekstedt et al., 2024). In addition to genetic and immunological factors, there are also some environmental factors in the risk of developing IBD. Lifestyle factors , such as diet and stress have been studied in relation to disease progression and exacerbation. Western dietary patterns with high fat intake and low fiber intake have been linked to increasing rates of IBD, and diet has been proposed as a possible key factor in gut health and inflammatory processes. Stress has also been proposed as a possible exacerbating factor in those at risk of IBD and may have an impact on immune processes. Tobacco smoking is another risk factor, with smoking being linked to Crohn's disease exacerbation but being seemingly protective against ulcerative colitis. The heterogeneity of such lifestyle-correlated factors illustrates the multifactorial understanding required for IBD etiology and further underscores the necessity of an integrative strategy in risk assessment and management. Another important aspect in the etiology of IBD concerns infectious etiologies and, more specifically, the role of viruses , such as human cytomegalovirus (HCMV). Although typically asymptomatic in most of the population, HCMV is capable of reactivating in immunosuppressive and inflammatory states and causing complications in IBD patients. HCMV reactivation has been linked to severe exacerbation and failure of treatment in affected patients. Authors emphasize the importance of additional research on the relation between CMV and IBD as a risk factor that should be closely monitored during treatment. Understanding the epidemiology and clinical importance of HCMV reactivation can be utilized to create personalized treatment regimens, in particular regarding the administration of immunosuppressive treatments, to reduce potential risks. Further research illustrates how infectious agents interact with genetic and environmental factors in the multifactorial environment of IBD (Sanat et al., 2024) (Figure 7.5).

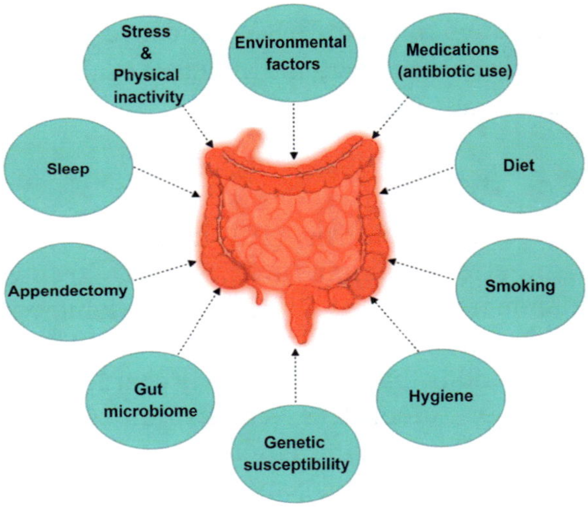

Figure 7.5. Causes and risk factors.

Source: https://www.mdpi.com/jcm/jcm-09-01273/article_deploy/html/images/jcm-09-01273-g006.png.

7.2.1. Genetic Predisposition

The etiology of inflammatory bowel disease (IBD) pathogenesis has come a long way, particularly in elucidating the genetics of predisposition. Genetics contributes significantly to the etiology of IBD, and therefore, patients with a history of the disease in their families are at increased risk. The evidence suggests that genetic susceptibility loci may vary between populations, as evidenced by differences between Asian and Western cohorts of IBD. These particular genetic markers may be utilized to identify persons at risk of developing IBD across different populations, underlining the importance of patient-specific healthcare approaches based on genetic platforms. By investigating the interaction between heredity and the expression of IBD, researchers are beginning to demystify the disease pathogenesis, thereby laying the foundation for more targeted approaches. Furthermore, identification of specific gene variants predisposing to IBD has far-reaching implications for disentangling its etiology. Multiple risk alleles involved in immune mechanisms, microbial interaction, and intestinal barrier integrity have been discovered through research, which all have a central role to play in the etiology of IBD. This genetic information enhances the understanding of an individual's risk of the disease as well as to its pathophysiology. For instance, how certain genes modulate inflammation or react to environmental stimuli may help clarify better how genetic predisposition is translated into disease in the context of lifestyle and dietary exposures, particularly in populations undergoing unprecedented epidemiological transitions, e.g., Asian populations. Large-scale genetic research, thus, informs clinical and public health interventions to control the disease burden. In addition to genetic characterization, the appreciation of environmental contributions is also critical to a complete understanding of IBD. Genetic predisposition is not standalone; rather, it is part of a multifactorial system with environmental determinants like diet, lifestyle, and hygiene contributing significantly to the development and course of disease. The rising incidence of IBD, particularly in regions of rapid urbanization, is a testament to this interaction of genetics and environmental determinants. For instance, traditional diets are being replaced by high-processed food diets, and this is parallel to increasing IBD incidence.

This multifactorial perspective lends merit to the necessity of exploring genetic predisposition in relation to environmental determinants, thereby enabling a holistic approach to the understanding of IBD. Such understanding is significant in the formulation of targeted prevention and treatment interventions to address affected populations (Bhayani et al., 2024; Yeshi et al., 2024).

7.2.2. Environmental Triggers

It is necessary to identify the contribution of environmental stimuli to Inflammatory Bowel Disease (IBD) pathogenesis to delineate preventive and therapeutic strategies. Investigators identified a range of environmental stimuli that may trigger or maintain IBD, including diet, microbial exposure, and stress. The gut microbiome also came into focus because the gut microbiome plays a role in gut well-being and immune modulation. Changes in diet, for instance, have been related to the increased consumption of processed foods, which results in higher IBD rates, suggesting that such diet changes can alter gut flora in negative directions. In addition, evidence suggests that environmental exposures, including toxins and antibiotics, impact microbial balance and make the host susceptible to inflammatory disease, which suggests that environmental and genetic factor interactions warrant extensive investigation (Sandrin et al., 2025). Multiomic analysis has shed light on the way environmental stimuli may interact with genetic predispositions to modulate IBD onset and progression. As an example, differential gene expression patterns in patients suggest that some environmental stresses have the capacity to trigger immune responses to mucosal inflammation. Interactions of exogenous factors with the host's genetic factors increase the complexity of the etiopathogenesis of IBDs. Metabolomics and metatranscriptomics analysis of such interactions allow for the identification of putative biomarkers that have the capacity to serve as markers of disease activity or susceptibility. Inferences of this kind may also allow for the planning of future personalized treatment, optimizing management by individually targeted interventions based on patterns of environmental exposures and genetic profiles. The complexity of such interactions underscores the need for an integrated research platform that takes into account both environmental and biological determinants of IBD (Sandrin et al.,

2025). Furthermore, the exploration of natural products as potential attenuators of the adverse effects of environmental stimuli is a promising future for IBD therapy. For example, recent studies suggest that extracts of marine algae, e.g., Ecklonia cava, exhibit anti-inflammatory activity that can reverse IBD dysbiosis and inflammation. Research demonstrates that pretreatment with Ecklonia cava extract has significantly reduced the severity of colitis in murine models, showing its potential to correct immune dysregulation and restore gut barrier function. By inhibiting some inflammatory pathways, e.g., the NLRP3/NF-κB signaling pathway, these natural products can offer alternative therapeutic options with fewer side effects than conventional treatments. Because IBD is caused by multiple environmental stimuli, the application of such botanical extracts might be a breakthrough in preventive and integrative therapy for this complex disease.

7.2.3. Immune System Dysfunction

The immune response plays a role in maintaining intestinal homeostasis, and immune system dysfunction is a hallmark of IBD pathogenesis. In IBD, the immune response is dysregulated, and there is a response to harmless antigens as well as to the resident microbiota. Dysregulation of immune activation then leads to chronic inflammation, a hallmark of IBD. Studies have confirmed that patients with IBD have cytokine profiles that have elevated levels of pro-inflammatory mediators, which further perpetuate the cycle of inflammation.

As the body's natural defense mechanisms fail, that immune system dysfunction not only exacerbates tissue damage but also leads to complications , such as strictures and fistulas. Characterization of the molecular mechanisms of this immune dysregulation is crucial to the design of targeted therapy that will reverse these dysfunctions and induce remission. Another significant but disruptive effect of immune system dysfunction in IBD is the disruption of the intestinal epithelial barrier. The mucosal layer is a first-line defense against pathogens, preventing passage and modulating the absorption of nutrients and metabolites. When immune responses are dysregulated, the epithelial barrier is compromised, and intestinal permeability or leaky gut is increased. This facilitates the translocation of antigens and bacteria into the lamina propria, eliciting further immune responses and further inflammation. Available therapeutic modalities are primarily directed at controlling this inflammatory process; however, they have a tendency to ignore the importance of restoring the integrity of the epithelial barrier.

As stressed by recent publications, more emphasis should be placed on the mechanisms of barrier dysfunction and the design of new therapies that promote mucosal healing, such as stem cell-based therapies (Kong et al., 2024). The complex interaction between the immune system, gut microbiota, and epithelium presents a broader image of immune dysfunction in IBD. Dysbiosis or perturbation of the gut microbiota has been both an aetiology and a consequence of IBD. Altered microbiome structure may trigger abnormal immune activation, which causes inflammation and further damage to the epithelial barrier. Furthermore, the gut-brain axis presents the potential for immune dysfunction beyond the GI tract to affect overall well-being and health. The interaction of immune function with metabolic functions, as in other chronic diseases, suggests that intervention strategies addressing multiple pathways may be necessary for effective treatment of IBD (Doroszkiewicz et al., 2024). A multi-dimensional view of immune dysfunction may thus be the answer to more integrative treatment strategies, addressing the underlying pathophysiological mechanisms rather than disease manifestations.

7.3. Symptoms and Diagnosis

The IBD workup mandates careful examination of clinical presentation, patient history, and diagnostic studies. The classic symptoms of IBD, including abdominal pain, diarrhea, rectal bleeding, and unintentional weight loss, overlap with other gastrointestinal diseases and, thus, present a diagnostic dilemma. Heterogeneity of symptoms mandates a detailed medical history, including symptom duration and nature, and lifestyle factors , such as diet and stress levels. A complete evaluation leads to a better insight into the patient's condition and directs further diagnostic workup, thus preventing overlooking primary etiologies , such as IBD. Endoscopic evaluation remains one of the cornerstone modalities of IBD diagnosis, with direct visualization of the mucosal surface and evaluation of inflammation and ulceration. Methods like colonoscopy and flexible sigmoidoscopy provide scope to physicians to take biopsies for histopathological correlation, a step in differentiating between the types of IBD, i.e., Crohn's disease and ulcerative colitis. Advances in endoscopy technology are further aiding the detection of stricture and other IBD complications more effectively. As reviewed in literature in the past, the correct differentiation of a gastrointestinal stricture as inflammatory vs. fibrotic is imperative to successful management, as inflammatory strictures are responsive to medical treatment, while fibrostenotic strictures necessitate endoscopic or surgical intervention (Klemm & Feuerstein, 2025). Diagnosis can further be complicated by IBD mimicking diseases, like sexually transmitted diseases , such as lymphogranuloma venereum (LGV). Rectal pain, bleeding, and mucous discharge may present with an initial false diagnosis of IBD, particularly in high-risk groups. Therefore, it is important that clinicians obtain a proper patient history, such as sexual activity, to rule out differential diagnoses. An example case that demonstrated this dilemma demonstrated how a patient, who was treated for hemorrhoids initially, underwent additional endoscopic evaluation with evidence of ulcerations, which was later diagnosed as LGV rather than IBD (Khoury et al., 2025). This demonstrates the importance of possessing an integrated diagnostic process involving symptom evaluation, endoscopy, and patient history in arriving at correct diagnoses and interventions (Figure 7.6).

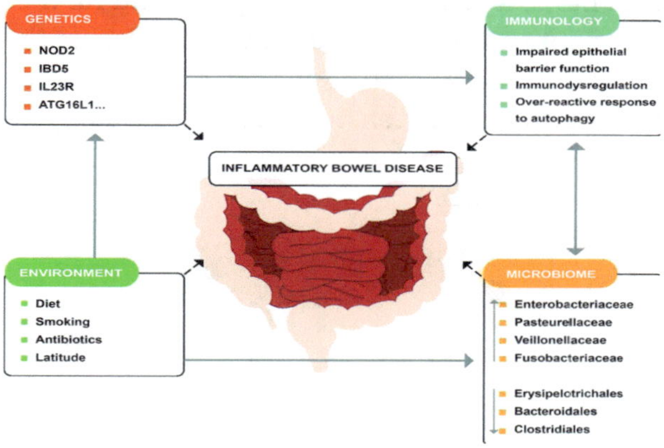

Figure 7.6. Symptoms and diagnosis.

Source: https://www.bmj.com/content/bmj/357/bmj.j2083/F1.large.jpg.

7.3.1. Common Symptoms of IBD

Symptoms of Inflammatory Bowel Disease (IBD), including conditions like Crohn's disease and ulcerative colitis, are debilitating and multifaceted. Chronic diarrhea is one of the most common symptoms, which at times is accompanied by blood or mucus. This symptom is most often the direct consequence of inflammation of the intestines, which compromises the absorptive function of the gut and triggers varying degrees of urgency and frequency that have the tendency to significantly impair daily functioning. This chronic bout of diarrhea is not only annoying but also results in dehydration and malnutrition. Severity and character of these attacks also vary widely from patient to patient, showcasing the individualized character of IBD symptomatology as the disease manifests uniquely in every patient. Abdominal cramping and pain are some of the other prevalent symptoms of IBD. Many patients experience frequent abdominal pain described as cramping or sharp, episodic pain. This is most often a direct consequence of inflammation of the intestines, changes in gut motility, or obstructions in the bowel. This pain may be exacerbated after eating, which may lead patients to avoid food consumption and further contribute to malnutrition. In some cases, the abdominal pain may be preceded or followed by bloating or distension, creating a complex symptomatology that makes it more difficult to live with IBD.

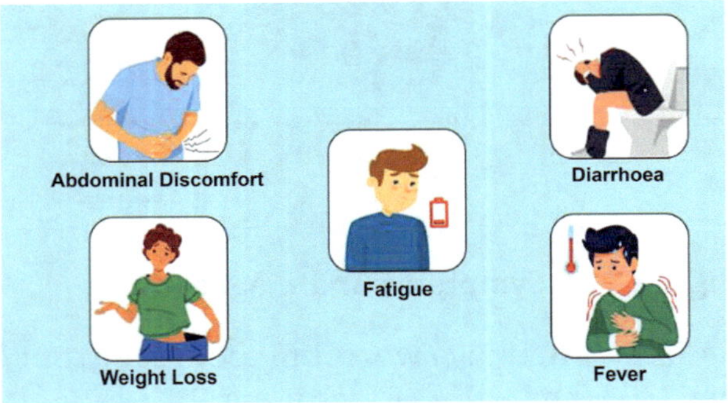

Figure 7.7. Common symptoms of inflammatory bowel disease (IBD).

Source: https://www.hexahealth.com/condition/inflammatory-bowel-disease.

This association between nutrition and symptomatology is a testament to the symbiotic character of the functioning of the digestive tract and the overall health of patients suffering from IBD. Aside from gastrointestinal symptoms, IBD has systemic consequences that can significantly impact quality of life. Fatigue is a frequent complaint in IBD patients, usually a consequence of the body's response to chronic inflammation, malnutrition, or even side effects of medication. It has been shown in research that a substantial percentage of patients have very similar symptoms to those seen in irritable bowel syndrome (IBS), and this suggests that psychological factors may also be playing a role in symptom worsening. Of particular mention are female gender and fatigue as independent variables predictive of increased IBS-like symptom frequency in IBD patients, and this highlights the importance of holistic treatment that will not neglect physical and psychological health (Amaral et al., 2024; Olsen et al., 2024). It is important that this holistic symptomology is employed to devise effective management regimens for each patient (Figure 7.7).

7.3.2. Diagnostic Procedures

The diagnostic process for inflammatory bowel disease (IBD) is based on a holistic approach that combines clinical staging, lab diagnostics, and advanced-technology imaging. Endoscopy is one of the primary methods of IBD diagnosis, a minimally invasive technique that offers direct visualization of the gut. During endoscopy, tissue samples can be obtained through biopsy for histological analysis, which is essential in differentiating between Crohn's disease and ulcerative colitis, the two most common forms of IBD. Endoscopy also offers the ability to monitor disease activity as well as response to treatment, and thus has a vital role in the overall management of IBD. The capacity to assess real-time changes in the mucosal lining enhances the overall diagnostic efficacy and informs subsequent therapeutic regimens. In addition to endoscopy, non-invasive imaging modalities play a fundamental role in the evaluation of IBD, particularly in terms of patient comfort and safety. Ultrasound is increasingly being used due to its non-invasive nature and simplicity of application, making it a great tool for use in everyday clinical practice. Recent studies have centered on the diagnostic efficacy of intestinal ultrasound (IUS) in pediatric ulcerative colitis, showing the potential of real-time assessment of disease activity through the application of multiple scoring systems, including the Milan Ultrasound Criteria. These scoring systems have been shown to have moderate diagnostic sensitivity, making them a valuable alternative in monitoring disease activity while potentially reducing the necessity for invasive procedures. The versatility of ultrasound technology highlights its suitability, particularly in situations where standard endoscopic techniques might be undesirable or unfeasible (Massironi et al., 2025). Laboratory tests, including serological tests and stool tests, supplement the diagnostic arsenal for IBD through the detection of markers for disease, which indicate inflammation. Diagnostic tests like C-reactive protein (CRP) and fecal calprotectin levels provide a report of the gastrointestinal tract's inflammatory status and are useful for diagnosis and follow-up. Although these tests need to be interpreted in the context of clinical presentation, they can be easily used in the outpatient setting, which can also be used to support early intervention strategies. Furthermore, the use of artificial intelligence and machine learning can also improve diagnostic accuracy through better processing of imaging and laboratory results. The use of technology in this manner can result in better diagnostic models that also allow for personalization of treatment regimens and eventually contribute to patient outcomes in the management of IBD (Hong & Baek, 2024).

7.3.3. Differential Diagnosis

Differential diagnosis of Inflammatory Bowel Disease (IBD) is critical to effective clinical management, given that it can mimic the symptoms of other gastrointestinal illnesses. Conditions , such as Irritable Bowel Syndrome (IBS), infection, and cancer of the colon tend to have similar clinical presentations , such as abdominal pain, diarrhea, and weight loss. It is usually difficult to distinguish between these conditions using thorough clinical evaluation and sophisticated diagnostic tools. The application of ultrasound diagnostics, according to the recent literature, enhances the clinician's ability to identify inflammatory and structural abnormalities typical of IBD. The availability, comfort to patients, and reproducibility of ultrasounds allow physicians to quantify disease activity, thus facilitating the possibility of developing a more informed differential diagnosis between IBD and other gastrointestinal conditions inducing analogous presentations (Jenssen et al., 2025). Furthermore, advances in microbiome science have transformed the arena of differential diagnosis of IBD. Clarifying the complexities of gut microbiota not only delineates the pathologic processes of IBD but also enhances differentiation from other gastrointestinal conditions like IBS. Studies using high-resolution next-generation sequencing have characterized distinct microbial signatures associated with IBD, suggesting that shifts in specific bacteria can be employed as diagnostic biomarkers. These findings indicate that gut microbiome quantification could improve the diagnostic sensitivity for distinguishing between IBD and IBS and other disorders by outperforming standard fecal inflammation biomarkers like calprotectin (Ocansey et al., 2023). This quantification capabilities underscore the necessity of integrating microbiome data into the diagnostic criteria for IBD so that it emerges as an earlier and more accurate method of diagnosing this multigenic disorder. Lastly, imaging techniques, such as endoscopic ultrasound and magnetic resonance enterography, are crucial in the differential diagnosis of IBD. The non-invasive techniques are invaluable in offering significant information about the structural integrity of the bowels and the condition of potential complications, such as strictures and abscesses, characteristic features of IBD. By visualizing the intestinal wall and assessing for extraintestinal manifestations, these technologies can greatly assist in differentiating IBD from other inflammatory conditions. Their continuous evolutions, combined with new diagnostic biomarkers becoming available, offer a more complex demarcation of patient presentation, thus further distinguishing IBD from other prevalent gastrointestinal conditions. Therefore, an extensive approach that incorporates clinical evaluation, imaging, and microbiome testing is imperative for accurate diagnosis and an appropriate treatment regimen for suspected cases of IBD (Figure 7.8).

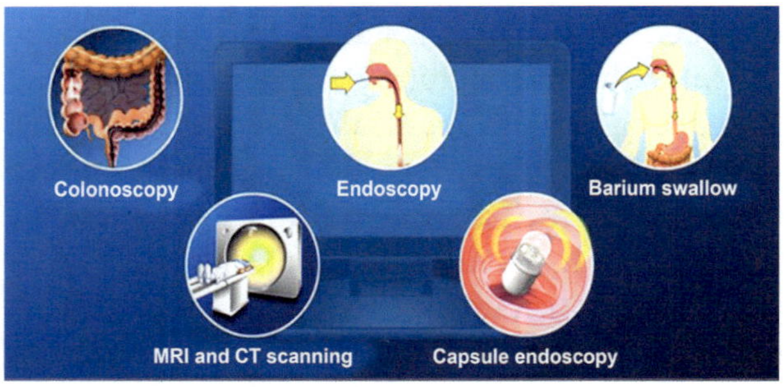

Figure 7.8. Differential diagnosis.

Source: http://www.youandibd.com/en-ibd/view/m101-s3-diagnosing-ibd-slide-show.

7.4. Treatment Options

Adequate management of Inflammatory Bowel Disease (IBD) has significantly improved over the years with advancements in medical science and technology. Traditional therapies like aminosalicylates, corticosteroids and immunomodulators are mostly employed to manage inflammation and induce remission. The chronic nature and complications of IBD necessitate ongoing evaluation of treatment modalities to minimize side effects and improve patients' quality of life. Current studies emphasize significantly the application of personalized medicine, where treatment is targeted towards the individual patient according to their specific condition and reactions to previous therapy. This method enables better precise targeting of treatment to optimize health outcomes, proving that a single model of care may be inadequate in the management of the heterogeneous symptoms and complications of IBD. Another rich area for the treatment of IBD is the creation of novel therapies addressing the disease mechanisms of IBD, i.e., those involving the gut microbiome. Bacteriophages, or viral particles that infect bacteria in a specific way, are a novel therapy in this regard. Since it becomes increasingly evident from research that gut microbiota play a critical role in the pathogenesis and course of IBD, applying bacteriophages for therapeutic purposes has gained considerable attention. These microbial natural controllers not only show host specificity but also can modulate the microbiome in a positive manner. More evidence highlights bacteriophage treatment as a method of enhancing the efficacy of treatment through restoring equilibrium between microbes, thus correcting some of the shortcomings with conventional treatment methods. This new direction is in agreement with present developments, which highlight the association between gut health and symptomology of IBD, as noted in Li et al. (2024). Other present approaches to IBD management also include the application of bile acid modulators, which have a central role to play in both disease onset and symptom management. It has been confirmed by research that bile acid malabsorption can add to chronic diarrhea in IBD patients, resulting in much distress and complications. Management using medications , such as tropifexor has been shown to be effective in enhancing bile acid homeostasis, thereby reducing the symptoms associated with malabsorption. Clinical trials indicate that tropifexor not only increases levels of fibroblast growth factor 19 but also significantly reduces fecal bile acid concentration compared to standard treatments. Such a line of treatment opens new hope for intractable symptom-tormented patients, lighting the path for a means to treat IBD that achieves efficacy with minimal side effects of traditional medications as described in Merza et al. (2024) (Figure 7.9).

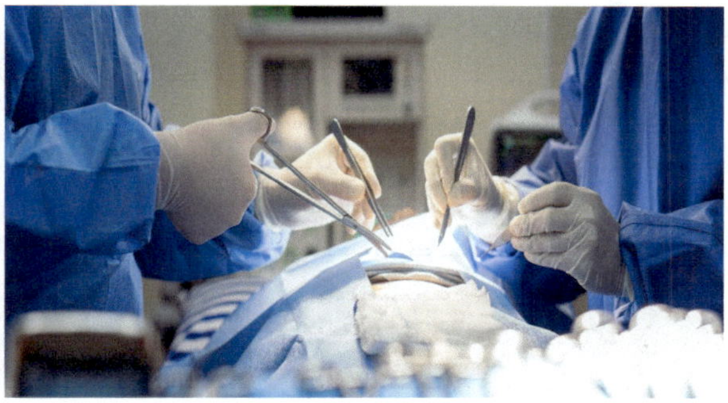

Figure 7.9. Treatment options for inflammatory bowel disease (IBD).

Source: https://assets.children's.com/m/6d01d1bea1276ad7/original/IBD-1200x500.jpg.

7.4.1. Medications

The management of Inflammatory Bowel Disease (IBD) has seen phenomenal evolution with the arrival of targeted therapies that modulate the complexities of this chronic disease. Historically dominated by traditional immunosuppressives, treatment choices are now characterized by the arrival of new therapies, including biologics and small molecule inhibitors. New drug approvals , such as etrasimod, upadacitinib, mirikizumab, and risankizumab are a textbook example, providing disease-specific activity that improves patient outcomes. Such drugs have the intention of minimizing inflammation by inhibiting selective immune response pathways to facilitate an improved treatment plan for Crohn's disease and ulcerative colitis. With changing therapeutic strategies, the focus now is on giving patients timely and adequate therapy to manage their symptoms and enhance their quality of life, a paradigm shift in the treatment of IBD (Mateos et al., 2025). In addition to some of the newer drug classes, Janus kinase (JAK) inhibitors, including tofacitinib, filgotinib, and upadacitinib, have joined the list of valuable drugs in the IBD treatment arsenal. These medications work through immunomodulation, which is dysregulated in IBD patients. JAK inhibitors were shown through studies to markedly reduce inflammation and control flare-up symptoms. With their efficacy, though, have been raised issues of safety risks, notably the formation of malignancies. A critical review of clinical evidence indicates that, as far as concerns go, there is no clear-cut evidence for the risk of cancer in IBD patients because of JAK inhibitors. Evidence is so crucial to alleviating clinicians' and patients' concerns and enabling more informed practice in using these new therapies (Bernardi et al., 2025). As the profile of IBD pharmacotherapy continues to change, research and development in this area are essential to understanding both drug efficacy and safety profiles. The promise of personalized medicine, where treatment regimens are optimized based on genetic markers, underlying disease mechanisms, and patient response, is a promising area for future IBD care. Concurrent with this development are the calls to address the growing costs of biologics and new therapies, which can keep patients from obtaining access to the medicines they require. Policymakers and health care stakeholders must identify ways to reconcile the financial realities with the imperative of providing access to new therapies in a just fashion. As collaborative activities intensify to maximize treatment access and affordability, patients are soon likely to enjoy an enhanced, personalized therapeutic strategy for addressing their IBD (Mateos et al., 2025) (Figure 7.10).

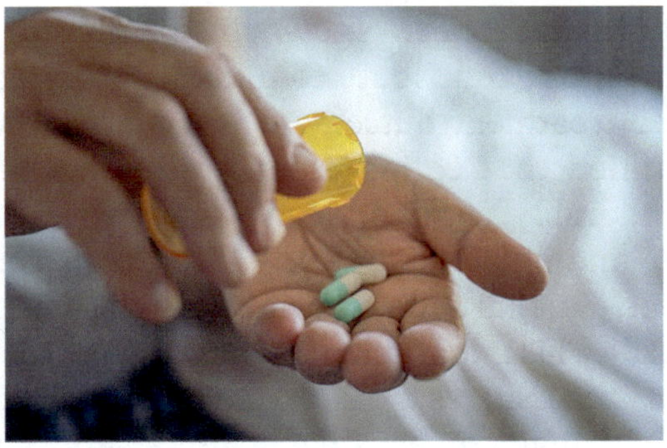

Figure 7.10. Medications.

Source: https://www.verywellhealth.com/thmb/-CMhn3PEuh22U4GfnevOKPoVuVo=/212

5x1411/filters:fill(87E3EF,1)/man-hand-taking-medicine-1029339748-0c4f3f86d5db48b2a28ab193ac92dcf7.jpg.

7.4.2. Dietary Management

In IBD, dietary management is also increasingly being recognized as a major component of overall management. The gut-diet basis relationship between diet and the gut explains why it is so important to tailor nutritional therapies to suit particular patient groups. Many studies have indicated that IBD patients usually have a range of food intolerances, which exacerbate symptoms further and lead to nutritional derangement. Identification of these intolerances and implementation of individualized dietary modification, therefore, can very effectively improve the quality of life in such individuals. Successful treatment requires not only the avoidance of specific foods but also the consideration of supplying patients with the nutrition required for general overall wellness and inflammatory control. Such targeted dietary practice will directly aid in improved symptom management and may aid in improved psychological status by minimizing food choice anxiety and gut reactivity. The rate of eating disorders behavior in patients with gastrointestinal disorders, including IBD, is another challenge for the dietary treatment. Maladaptive eating habits in IBD patients have been shown by studies to be present, but contribute to nutritional loss and shape treatment outcomes. Systematic review identified that eating disordered behavior is considerably common, ranging between 13–55%, and showing a strong interest in young female patients and those having high symptom severity. This important prevalence of disordered eating necessitates the intervention of healthcare professionals to assume a global approach, integrating disordered eating assessment into the broader framework of IBD management. Detection of such behavior will enable clinicians to enact proper dietary intervention and psychological therapy, intervening on both the physical and emotional states of IBD subsequently. Such a multi-disciplinary approach ultimately produces an enhanced management program that focuses on nutritional adequacy alongside behavioral health. There have been encouraging developments in IBD-specific dietary treatments in recent years, particularly in pediatric patients. Exclusive enteral nutrition (EEN), for instance, has been shown to induce remission in pediatric Crohn's Disease, which illustrates the potential of nutritional therapy to lower inflammation and restore gut integrity. That said, it is challenging to adhere to such restrictive diets due to their unvaried nature, and attention must be paid to more blended dietary strategies. More current approaches, including the Crohn's Disease Exclusion Diet, try to balance flexibility with the effort to address the underlying inflammatory mechanisms and nutritional problems. These dietary management regimens emphasize the significant impact that tailored nutritional interventions can have on the overall management of IBD. Lastly, upon integration well, dietary management not only improves symptom control but also enhances the patient's quality of life in managing this chronic illness (Peters et al., 2021; Scarallo & Lionetti, 2021) (Figure 7.11).

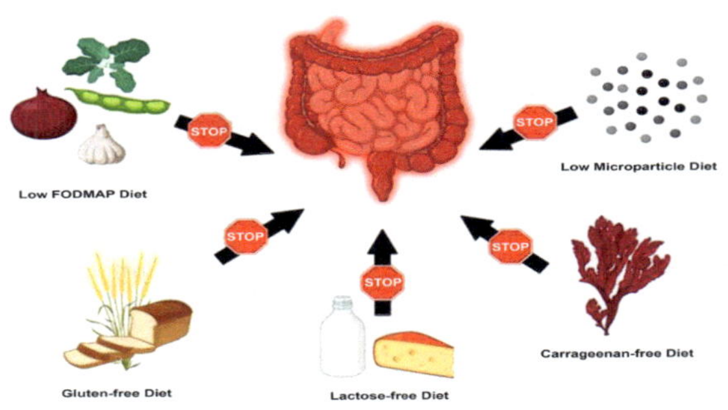

Figure 7.11. Dietary management inflammatory bowel disease (IBD).

Source: https://www.researchgate.net/publication/367346431/figure/fig2/AS:11431281212402124@1702599348905/Elimination-and-Exclusion-Diets-in-IBD.tif.

7.4.3. Surgical Interventions

Surgery is also necessary in the treatment of Inflammatory Bowel Disease (IBD) when medical therapy is not effective or complications have already arisen. Ulcerative colitis and Crohn's disease, the two predominant forms of IBD, can potentially progress to serious complications , such as bowel obstruction, perforation, or malignancy, which necessitate surgery. Surgery involves multifaceted patient evaluation and detailed assessment of disease activity. Surgical options may vary from resection of infected bowel segments or, in the case of ulcerative colitis, colectomy, which may be of curative benefit. However, these are risky procedures and must be balanced against potential gain and the individual patient's situation. The surgical procedure is also tailored to the individual patient, with an emphasis on a multidisciplinary approach by surgeons, gastroenterologists, and nutritionists to enhance outcomes and recover faster (Lamb et al., 2019). The Enhanced Recovery After Surgery (ERAS) program has been put in place as an advisory outline in order to improve perioperative care for patients undergoing colorectal surgery. One such evidence-based approach is a series of enhanced recovery plans designed to decrease complications, shorten hospital stay, and enable patients to return to normal functioning earlier. Preoperative counseling, enhanced nutritional support, and pain control following surgery are all cornerstones of the ERAS® guidelines. By having such structured protocols, surgical teams are able to ensure that patients undergoing procedures for IBD are given care that maximizes their recovery path. The implementation of ERAS® principles is a shift towards patient-focused perioperative care with the ultimate goal being informed consent and shared decision-making. Therefore, patients are incentivized with improved experience and results of surgery for the treatment of IBD and re-emphasizing the requirement for concomitant care modalities (Gustafsson et al., 2018). Postoperative care is also critical to achieve maximum surgical outcomes in patients with IBD. Patients may have numerous complications after surgery, including infection, anastomotic leak, or bowel obstruction. Thus, a total monitoring program should be implemented to address the potential problem at an early stage. Moreover, the inclusion of nutrition support postoperatively is important because most patients with IBD are malnourished due to the inflammatory manifestations of their disease. Multidisciplinary postoperative management is a structured surveillance of such complications by dieticians, nurses, and surgeons acting collectively to develop personalized recovery plans. An integrated system is the bedrock of longitudinal health gains, stressing the fact that operations in IBD should not just focus on optimal short-term surgical results but also must be given priority to provide complete postoperative care to enhance the overall quality of life in patients (Lee et al., 2019) (Figure 7.12).

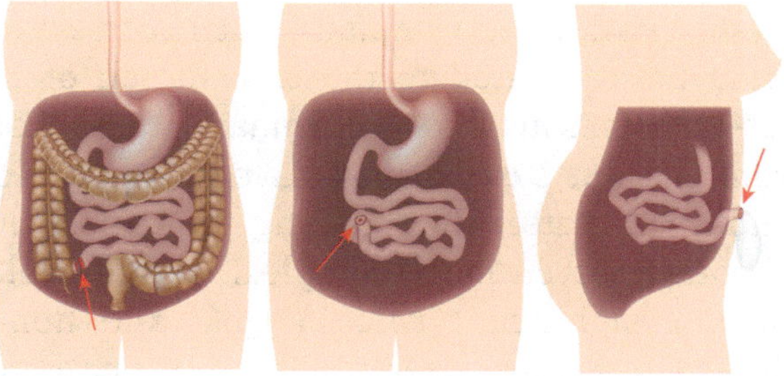

Figure 7.12. Surgical interventions.

Source: https://www.ibdrelief.com/uploads/resizes/proctocolectomy-with-ileostomy-1_c1170x549.jpg.

7.5. Impact on Quality of Life

The impact of inflammatory bowel disease (IBD) on quality of life (QoL) is profound and widespread. Individuals who suffer from this chronic condition often experience extreme physical and emotional distress that undermines their overall well-being. Patients with active IBD have been shown to have substantially lower QoL scores compared to patients in remission, highlighting the relationship between disease activity and psychological health. Besides, a systematic review of 83 separate studies also showed that the same trend occurred: CD patients typically have a poorer QoL than UC patients. Such a striking difference could be attributed to differences in the clinical presentations and complications of each type, hence why the demand for personalized management approaches towards addressing the unique challenges of IBD patients exists (Knowles et al., 2018). In addition, the psychological impact of IBD cannot be minimized. Mental illness and IBD, such as anxiety and depression, are best illustrated when the disease is active. Psychological disturbances have been found to be prevalent in patients with IBD due to possibly the stress related to the handling of a chronic medical condition, as well as the disabling characteristics of its symptoms. Such a correlation could be attributed to the explanation of the gut-brain axis in which inflammatory responses from the gut system may have an impact on emotional states, thus making the experience of patients even more complex. Mental health plays a significant role in QoL, and hence medical personnel need to screen IBD patients' psychological distress regularly to enable timely intervention and improve their general health status (Abautret-Daly et al., 2017). Improvement interventions in QoL among patients with IBD have been encouraging, suggesting that active management can achieve significant improvements. Literature indicates that effective management of IBD symptoms, combined with psychological therapy, can lead to significant gains in patients' quality of life in the long term. For instance, the implementation of lifestyle modifications, diet change, and psychological counseling can address the issues stemming from this condition. Further, encouraging patient engagement in self-management and education regarding their disease can enable patients to become responsible actors in their health journey. By further encouraging an integrative approach that addresses both physical and mental welfare, the healthcare industry can significantly improve the QoL of patients with IBD, motivating them to withstand their chronic disease with resilience and increased sense of self-efficacy (Knowles et al., 2018) (Figure 7.13).

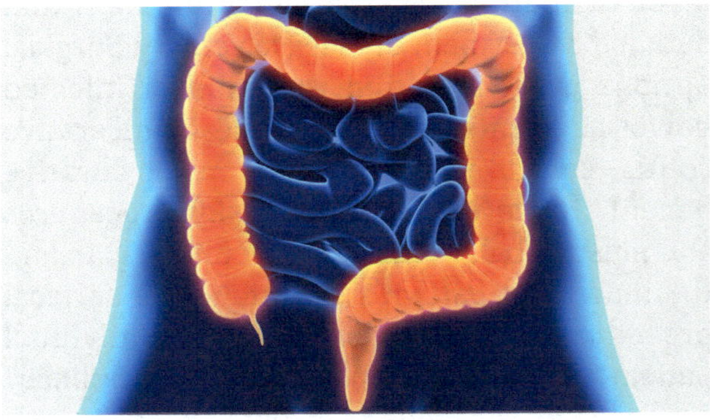

Figure 7.13. Impact on quality of life.

Source: https://children'sgimd.com/wp-content/uploads/2015/07/inflammatory-bowel-disease-1.png.

7.5.1. Physical Health Implications

Inflammatory Bowel Disease (IBD) has profound impacts on physical health, expressing itself through a variety of gastrointestinal symptoms that can potentially alter an individual's quality of life. Most common symptoms include abdominal pain, diarrhea, and rectal bleeding, which can lead to nutritional deficiencies due to malabsorption. Such symptoms, besides hindering everyday living, have the capability to establish a vicious cycle of tension and depression among affected individuals. The data from the Global Burden of Diseases, Injuries, and Risk Factors Study indicate the increasing prevalence of IBD, which was 6.8 million in 2017 globally, identifying the need for effective health care strategies to offset these physical health results (Alatab et al., 2019). In addition, the amplified prevalence of IBD places a significant financial burden on the healthcare system in terms of increased hospital visits, prolonged treatment requirements, and specialized services. Aside from direct intestinal issues, IBD is also implicated in systemic complications that further compromise bodily health. Inflammatory processes can lead to extraintestinal manifestations in other bodily organs like the skin, eyes, and joints, complicating the disease overall. Additionally, chronic inflammation characteristic of IBD can disrupt the body's immune response, leading to increased susceptibility to infection and disease. The microbiota-gut-brain axis demonstrates how gut function is linked to neurological and psychological well-being, and emerging research is postulating that gut dysbiosis might exacerbate mental illness in IBD patients (Cryan et al., 2019). Management of these interconnected axes of physical and psychological health is necessary for comprehensive patient care, addressing a multidisciplinary approach with both gastrointestinal and psychological treatment. The long-term physical health implications of IBD go beyond acute symptomatology, affecting the overall health status and life expectancy of patients. As the increasing burden of disability-adjusted life-years (DALYs) attributed to IBD in the last decades is mirrored by the doubling of years lived with disability (YLDs) from 1990 to 2017, it is vital to recognize the long-term impacts of this disease (Alatab et al., 2019). These can be reversed by lifestyle modifications and advances in medical treatment; patient adherence and availability of optimal care are, in fact, the most significant. A proactive approach incorporating diet control, compliance with medication, and strict observation has the possibility of allowing patients to gain better control over their disease. The inclusion of such strategies not only aids in lessening the physical impact of IBD but also in overall improved health and quality of life for individuals suffering from the disease (Figure 7.14).

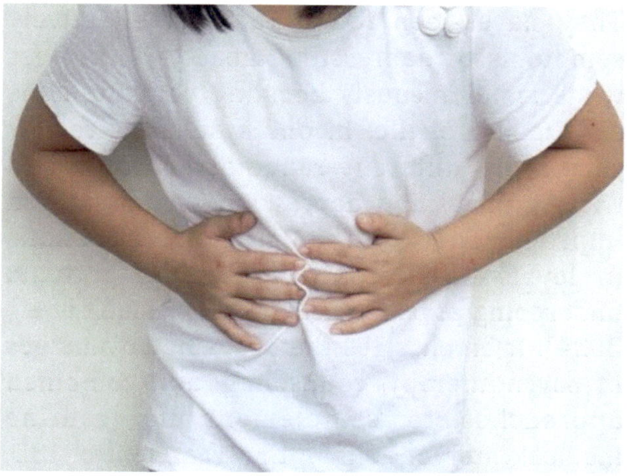

Figure 7.14. Physical health implications.

Source: https://scx1.b-cdn.net/csz/news/800a/2023/cardiovascular-fitness.jpg.

7.5.2. Psychological Effects

The psychological effect of Inflammatory Bowel Disease (IBD) is immense and multifaceted, affecting the patients' mental health to a considerable degree. IBD is often characterized by chronic symptoms , such as abdominal cramping, diarrhea, and fatigue, which can heighten anxiety and depression in patients afflicted with the disease. These psychological burdens not only arise from the physical characteristics of the disease but are also compounded by the stress of having to endure a chronic condition that can strike at random against daily life. Studies also demonstrate that the relationship between the brain and gut still makes this correlation obscure, and therefore, alterations in the microbiota may influence mood and behavior, further underpinning the importance of understanding the psychological implications of IBD (Chen et al., 2025). It is therefore the requirement for comprehensive care approaches that encompass both physical and psychological health that arises in managing IBD. In the last few years, there has been increasing evidence that positive psychological interventions can reduce some of the mental health problems experienced by IBD sufferers.

They have been found to treat effectively symptoms of depression, anxiety, and stress while simultaneously boosting patients' hope and quality of life. In one systematic review comparing different randomized controlled trials, anxiety and depression scores showed improvement, with significant reductions in levels of stress noted among patients undergoing psychological therapy (Liang et al., 2024). It emphasizes the probable advantages of psychotherapy, counseling, and combined approaches to complement the routine medical interventions in the treatment of IBD, emphasizing the importance of psychological health for the betterment of the lives of the patients.

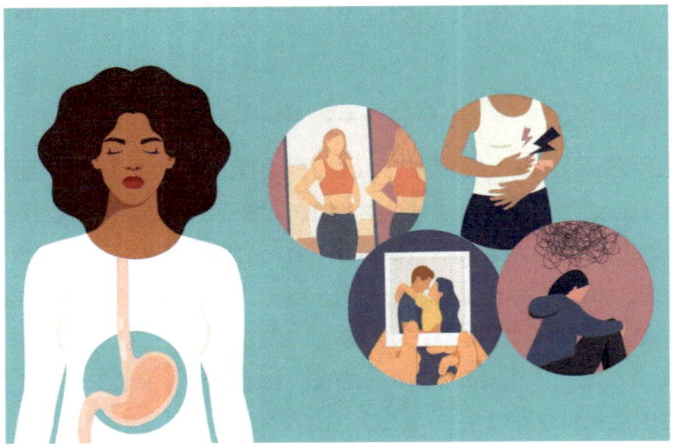

Figure 7.15. Psychological effects.

Source: https://www.healthywomen.org/media-library/social-and-emotional-effects-of-life-with-inflammatory-bowel-disease-ibd.jpg?id=29284084&width=1200&height=800&quality=85&coordinates=131%2C0%2C131%2C0.

Besides, an understanding of the psychological profile of IBD is required for the development of effective treatment strategies. The chronic nature of IBD also poses ongoing psychological concerns that can be responsible for disease progression, as well as symptom severity. For instance, increased psychological stress might interfere with the microbiota-gut-brain axis, producing a cycle that exacerbates inflammation and mental illness (Chen et al., 2025). To balance such effects, medical practitioners are increasingly being prompted to incorporate psychological treatment and care within treatment regimens. By extension, the promotion of a wider approach that integrates mental health services can enhance patient outcomes, effectively alleviating the psychological burden of chronic disease while assisting with overall physical health and well-being (Figure 7.15).

7.5.3. Social and Economic Challenges

The social problems faced by the individuals who are suffering from Inflammatory Bowel Disease (IBD) have a very critical effect, not only on their own health but also on their interpersonal relationships and social interactions. A majority of patients report feeling stigmatized from the disease, in either the form of social withdrawal or the inability to maintain interpersonal relationships. This stigma is further enhanced by the overt and covert signs of the illness, which quite frequently cause embarrassment or fear of being judged by others. Wang et al. (2022) reminds us that patients with an IBD-associated stoma experience a high level of perceived stigma that can prejudice their ability to be integrated into social life. All of these social problems must be tackled to improve the overall quality of IBD patients' lives, and supportive community programs and education must be initiated to establish an atmosphere of acceptability and understanding of this chronic disease. Economically, the cost of IBD is very significant and multifaceted. The financial implications of the illness extend beyond the mere cost of healthcare to include loss of productivity, the need for specialized dietary requirements, and ongoing financial expenses of purchasing necessary equipment, such as ostomy equipment accessories. According to Wang et al. (2022), a majority of the patients lose between 500 to 999 RMB monthly purchasing these supplies, which represents the economic impact the chronic illness can cause. Aside from the direct costs, patients also suffer from indirect financial impacts through loss of employment or lost working hours caused by flare-ups and hospitalization. This economic impact tends to exacerbate the psychological burden of suffering from IBD, with the two reinforcing each other in a vicious cycle that proves challenging to overcome and self-manage. Policymakers should take these economic issues into account when creating healthcare policies designed to assist patients who have IBD. Support systems will play an important role in preventing the social and economic issues associated with IBD. More education and awareness among healthcare providers and the public in general regarding IBD can result in more acceptance and less stigmatization. Further, community support groups offer patients a crucial platform for sharing experience and coping strategies, given that 91% of online peer support group participants felt that such resources made a significant contribution to disease management (Wang et al., 2022). Besides, interventions aimed at raising awareness among patients about self-management and available resources can empower people to handle their condition more effectively, ultimately leading to social engagement and economic benefits. In the process of developing means of improving the living conditions of patients with IBD, there is a need to keep emphasizing education, financial support, and acceptance as part of an overall care package.

7.6. Current Research and Advances

Recent advances in knowledge about the role of the gut microbiota have shed light on the complexity involved in Inflammatory Bowel Disease (IBD). The gut microbiota, an active microecosystem of microbes that populate the intestinal tract, is now not viewed as an abiotic factor but rather as a critical modulator in host health. Changes to this microbial community, known as dysbiosis, have been associated with various diseases, including IBD. Research has demonstrated that changes in gut microbiota can influence immune function and metabolic processes, thus influencing the pathogenesis and course of IBD. The use of high-end molecular tools , such as metagenomics and metabolomics, has unlocked insights into these interactions more extensively, allowing scientists to identify certain microbial communities that are likely protective or causative of IBD. Furthermore, research is currently underway to look at the therapeutic application of modulating gut microbiota as a form of therapy for IBD. Probiotics, prebiotics, and fecal microbiota transplantation (FMT) are being explored for their ability to restore a normal balance of microbes and inhibit inflammatory reactions. Initial clinical trials have been promising, with some evidence that such treatments can enhance the quality of life in patients and lead to remission in a proportion of patients. Also, explaining how metabolites from gut bacteria, such as SCFAs, affect immune signaling and gut integrity is deciphering molecular mechanisms that can be targeted for therapeutic benefit. Such advances are generating interest in the development of microbiota-directed therapies as adjunctive therapies to traditional medications used to manage IBD (Tsung-Lee et al., 2023). Technological advances are also impacting IBD monitoring and management. Artificial intelligence (AI) and machine learning algorithms are being applied to change how clinicians analyze patient data. AI is able to identify patterns and predict disease flares by prospecting large databases of data. In addition, the use of mobile health tools allows patients to track their symptoms, diets, and medication, facilitating an active response to their condition. These new tools not only empower the patient but also provide clinician's with valuable information to inform treatment. With ongoing advances in such research, the convergence of AI and digital health technology promises to advance the general care of IBD (Tsung-Lee et al., 2023) (Figure 7.16).

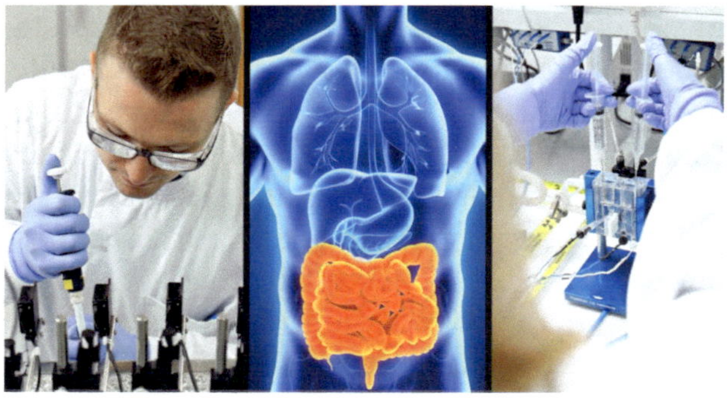

Figure 7.16. Current research and advances.

Source: https://www.reprocell.com/hs-fs/hubfs/IBD%20trio.png?width=951&name=IBD%20trio.png.

7.6.1. New Treatment Modalities

The treatment paradigm for inflammatory bowel disease (IBD) has evolved dramatically in recent years due to the necessity of possessing more powerful and targeted therapies. One of the most dramatic developments is novel classes of drugs , such as sphingosine-1-phosphate (S1P) modulators and interleukin-23 (IL-23) inhibitors. These treatments offer a new approach to the management of IBD through the targeting of the underlying immune dysregulation that characterizes the disease. S1P modulators, for example, work by regulating the traffic of lymphocytes, i.e., essentially suppressing inflammatory responses. IL-23 inhibitors work on separate cytokine pathways that maintain gut inflammation. This shift to targeted therapy is a milestone for the treatment of IBD, as it allows for more individualized therapy for patients with separate disease phenotypes and responsiveness to treatment. In addition to S1P modulators and IL-23 antagonists, immunomodulatory therapy is another major field in the treatment of IBD. The clinical studies on drugs like ozanimod and etrasimod have been recently assessed for safety and efficacy and have had favorable results for both short- and long-term management of IBD. These agents have demonstrated the ability to induce remission in patients with moderate to severe illness and have had favorable safety profiles. Further, their mechanism of action promises to reduce dependency on systemic corticosteroids as well as diminish side effects associated with long-term steroid use. Through ongoing research endeavors to optimize these therapeutic approaches, the aim is to possess a robust armamentarium of therapies to meet the diverse demands of IBD patients (Lenti et al., 2025). Emerging treatment strategies also involve important consideration of safety and long-term effectiveness. The use of biologics and new immunomodulatory drugs also raises questions of efficacy and cancer risk, particularly in high-risk populations , such as individuals with existing malignancies. Experimental data have reported conflicting outcomes on low risk in patients treated with biologics for cancer progression, but significant data gaps remain. As outlined in recent reviews, there is a need to determine the potential impact of these therapies on cancer progression (Lenti et al., 2025). Lastly, the integration of new treatment modalities into practice needs to be balanced in a fair assessment of their risk versus benefit, along with an appreciation and dedication to patient-specific treatment plans based on patient-specific variables and the dynamic nature of IBD therapeutics (Lenti et al., 2025).

7.6.2. Genetic Research

The intricate dynamics between genetic elements and Inflammatory Bowel Disease (IBD) have precipitated extensive research activity aimed at deciphering the intricacies of the disorder. Genetic predisposition is a causative element in IBD, as evidenced by studies that reveal the disease to be heritable. It is thus crucial to characterize unique genetic markers associated with IBD for pathophysiology insight and in the development of targeted therapies. Genetic research has enabled the identification of numerous loci common to both Crohn's disease and ulcerative colitis, two of the dominant forms of IBD. The continued investigation into genomic data has not only illuminated the genetic landscape of IBD but has also started debates around personalized medicine, wherein patient-specific genomic data could impact disease management strategies and treatment modalities, paving the way for more efficacious interventions. Recent studies have also expanded the concept of genetic correlations between IBD and other conditions, a concept of great theoretical importance to comorbidities. As a matter of fact, studies exist to demonstrate a robust genetic correlation between IBD and ocular conditions , such as iridocyclitis (IC), with common pathways leading to both diseases. A precise analysis of genome-wide association studies (GWAS) has revealed shared genetic architectures and specific genes, including IL23R and GPR35, which are applicable to both IBD and IC. This identification demonstrates the importance of finding , such associations in genetic research as they have the ability to guide clinical strategies towards personalized management of multifactorial diseases to which IBD patients are prone. Greater understanding of these correlations ultimately energizes debate surrounding productive management of IBD and associated disorders. Beyond identification of association alone, however, potential uses of genetic investigation are poised to expand to therapeutic development. Investigation of the phenolic acids, for example, demonstrates how components of diet may be synergistically coordinated with genetic profiles in alleviation of IBD symptoms. These compounds possess antioxidant and anti-inflammatory activities, which suggest that they would serve as adjuncts for the therapy of IBD. Ongoing studies on the determination of mechanisms by which these phenolic acids and their derivatives can enhance intestinal well-being are the signature of the adaptive nature of therapeutic protocols based on genetic information. Hence, with advances in genetic research, they open a twofold possibility: not only to deepen our understanding of the etiology of IBDs but also to facilitate the development of newer nutritional therapies aimed at more effectively modulating patient conditions, an upbeat prediction regarding the future of IBD management (Liao et al., 2024; Lu et al., 2024) (Figure 7.14).

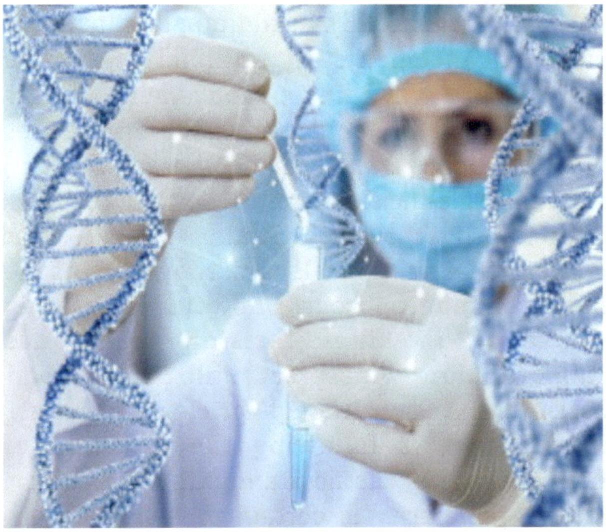

Figure 7.17. Genetic research.

Source: https://pediatrics.queensu.ca/sites/pediatrics/files/gbb-uploads/Untitled%20design%20(14)-abe1r5.png.

7.6.3. Future Directions in IBD Management

With increasing knowledge on Inflammatory Bowel Disease (IBD), several new diet interventions have the potential to enhance patient management. Current studies underscore the significant role nutritional therapy has to offer in addition to standard pharmacotherapy. Exclusive Enteral Nutrition (EEN) has proved to be a first-line treatment in children with Crohn's Disease (CD), while Partial Enteral Nutrition (PEN) and the Crohn's Disease Exclusion Diet (CDED) are increasingly established as successful therapies for adults. Aside from offering a possible remission, these treatments also encourage greater compliance than more conventional approaches. Furthermore, whole food-based diets, i.e., the Mediterranean Diet and new low-FODMAP strategies, have preliminary evidence of modifying inflammatory pathways and symptoms. Person-centred nutrition plans in the future will become the cornerstone in multi-disciplinary care pathways to unlock the full therapeutic potential of diet therapy in IBD (Barberio et al., 2025). In addition to nutritional care, advancements in minimally invasive surgery are a leading advancement in IBD management. Previously invasive procedures are now being transformed by technologies , such as single-incision laparoscopy and robotics, with improved results. Studies indicate that conventional multiport laparoscopy remains the most common approach; however, increasing efficiency in single-incision techniques supports more widespread utilization. Robot-assisted surgery, although pricier and longer in duration, is following the direction of future surgery exactness and patient recovery. Future popularity is certain to increase with improved training and reduced costs. In the long term, integration of minimally invasive methods in IBD management will not only optimize surgery outcomes but also allow better control of disease and patient quality of life (Rathod et al., 2024). Finally, the field of IBD management is poised to undergo revolutionary growth through the integration of personalized medicine. Genetic and microbiome studies are transforming traditional models of treatment through a focus on individualized reactions to therapy. This approach has vast potential for individualizing drugs and nutritional therapies to meet the unique physiological needs of each patient. As more disease and treatment response biomarkers approach the market, care plans will be individualized by clinicians. In addition, advances in telemedicine and digital health technologies will enable monitoring and access to specialty care in real time. These advances enable an active disease management that is needed in the management of the fluctuating nature of IBD. Through the emphasis on personalization in therapeutic strategies, future directions in the management of IBD can lead to improved patient outcomes and a more directed solution for the management of this multifactorial disorder.

A CLOSER LOOK

MOBILE HEALTH TOOLS:

Mobile health tools—often referred to as mHealth—have rapidly become integral to modern healthcare delivery. These tools include smartphone applications, wearable devices, SMS-based health reminders, remote monitoring systems, and telehealth platforms. A closer look at mobile health tools reveals their transformative potential in improving access to care, enhancing patient engagement, and supporting real-time data collection, particularly in settings where resources or healthcare personnel are limited. One of the major strengths of mobile health tools lies in their ability to empower patients. Apps designed for chronic disease management allow individuals to track blood glucose, blood pressure, medication adherence, physical activity, and dietary habits. These tools offer personalized feedback, alerts, and educational content, helping users understand their conditions and make timely adjustments. For many patients, especially those managing long-term illnesses such as diabetes, asthma, or hypertension, mHealth interventions foster better self-management and can reduce hospital visits.

Wearable devices add another layer of functionality by monitoring physiological indicators such as heart rate, sleep patterns, oxygen saturation, and activity levels. When integrated with healthcare systems, these data streams allow clinicians to track trends over time and identify early warning signs of deterioration. Remote patient monitoring has proven particularly valuable for older adults, post-surgical patients, and individuals living in rural or underserved areas.

Mobile health tools have also strengthened communication and continuity of care. Telehealth platforms and secure messaging systems allow patients to consult providers without traveling, reducing barriers related to distance, mobility, and cost. SMS-based programs have demonstrated success in improving vaccination adherence, prenatal care attendance, and medication compliance—especially in low-resource environments. In public health, mobile tools support disease surveillance, contact tracing, and rapid dissemination of information during outbreaks or emergencies. Health workers can collect field data using mobile devices, improving accuracy and reducing delays associated with paper-based systems. This capability is especially valuable during epidemics, natural disasters, or humanitarian crises.

Despite their benefits, mobile health tools face challenges. Data privacy, digital literacy, and unequal access to technology can limit their reach. Additionally, not all health apps are evidence-based, and quality varies widely. Ensuring regulatory oversight, integrating mHealth tools into existing healthcare frameworks, and addressing disparities in connectivity are essential for maximizing impact.

Overall, mobile health tools offer powerful opportunities to enhance healthcare delivery, support patient autonomy, and strengthen health systems. A closer look shows that when thoughtfully implemented, they can significantly improve health outcomes across diverse populations.

SUMMARY

The final part of an Inflammatory Bowel Disease (IBD) essay is to summarize the complexities of the disease and identify how it has a crucial impact on patients and the healthcare system. The rising incidence of both Crohn's disease and ulcerative colitis lends an imperative for the proper understanding of the disease mechanisms, clinical management, and the economic impact. Existing evidence has argued that the cost of IBD patients' care has increased significantly over the past few years, with the main drivers being treatment expenses, healthcare utilization, and overall disease influence on the patient's health and productivity. This mounting financial burden highlights the sharp need for innovative interventions that are able to effectively counteract these problems alongside the enhancement of the quality of life for IBD patients (Park et al., 2019). In addition to this, recent studies have shed light on the potential application of probiotics in controlling IBD. The evidence of their usefulness has been mixed, being beneficial in some environments, particularly for ulcerative colitis, but inconclusive in Crohn's disease. The findings showed that some probiotics, such as VSL #3, might contribute positively to remission in patients with active ulcerative colitis. However, the lack of a uniform advantage highlights the necessity for further studies to establish more specifically the role of microbiota in IBD and that of probiotics in comparison with other treatments. Therefore, increased understanding of such interventions can pave the way for precision medicine approaches addressing the unique needs of each patient, enhancing clinical outcomes and possibly reducing disease management expenditure (Derwa et al., 2017). In summary, the multifaceted nature of Inflammatory Bowel Disease reveals the necessary intersections of pathophysiology, treatment choice, and economic cost. The rising healthcare costs of IBD necessitate an urgent call to action to improve the provision of care and cost-effectiveness. Bridging the gap in treatment approaches, including exploring the use of probiotics and other emerging therapies, can contribute significantly to shifting the practice for the management of IBD. As our knowledge about this intricate set of diseases advances, it is essential that researchers, clinicians, and policymakers act together to evolve holistic and patient-focused care strategies, ultimately improving the quality of life for patients suffering from these chronic inflammatory conditions. The journey to better management of IBD continues, illuminating the need for ongoing research and development in the healthcare sector (Park et al., 2019).

In comprehending the complexities of Inflammatory Bowel Disease (IBD), it is important to consider the multifactorial etiology of the disease in terms of genetic, environmental, and microbial etiologies. Recent investigations have stressed the essential role of the gut microbiota in the pathogenesis and etiology of IBD. The relationship between microbial communities and host physiology requires advanced analytical methods to account for these associations. For instance, the publication of MaAsLin 2, a robust analytical software program employed to examine microbial community traits in various environmental and dietary metadata, facilitates improved etiology understanding of IBD. This method's ability to process vast amounts of data while maintaining false discovery rates in check positions it as a critical tool in today's research towards the characterization of microbial landscape in IBD, with potential to translate into therapeutic interventions based on these microbial alterations (Mallick et al., 2021). Additionally, identification of specific biomarkers and pathways altered by IBD has been an emphasis in recent years. Understanding the biochemical and immunologic mechanisms of IBD can become better diagnostics and treatment. For example, changing the expression of angiotensin-converting enzyme 2 (ACE2) has been researched for its functions in more non-specific pathologies as well as in IBD. There are many comorbidities and drugs that impact the regulation of ACE2 to either increase or reduce inflammation. Correspondingly, the identification of ACE2's involvement in the disease process illustrates a therapeutic promise bright spot. As research unfolds and continues to make clear the intricate interaction between the immune system and gut microbiome, clinicians may gain valuable insights that are translated into more effective management of patients with IBD (Bourgonje et al., 2020). As IBD research has evolved, multi-omics techniques are now more critical to building a comprehensive understanding of the condition. Advanced technology means genetic, transcriptomic, and metabolomic profiles can be investigated in tandem, and researchers now have the capacity to follow the dynamic interactions of the gut microbiota and how these influence inflammation. This conjoined approach not only prioritizes the underlying biological mechanisms but also aids in deciding patient-specific therapy, and thus precision medicine is a viable target in treating IBD. With continued research into the complex relationships between diet, microbiota, and immune response, the research community can create new knowledge with the potential for groundbreaking therapy and improved patient outcomes for the treatment of Inflammatory Bowel Disease (Mallick et al., 2021).

References

1. Abautret-Daly, Á., Dempsey, E., Parra-Blanco, A., Medina, C., Harkin, A. (2017). Gut–brain actions underlying comorbid anxiety and depression associated with inflammatory bowel disease. *Acta Neuropsychiatrica, 30*, 275–296. https://doi.org/10.1017/neu.2017.3 (accessed on 15th July 2025).
2. Alatab, S., Sepanlou, S. G., Ikuta, K. S., Vahedi, H., Bisignano, C., Safiri, S., Sadeghi, A., et al. (2019). The global, regional, and national burden of inflammatory bowel disease in 195 countries and territories, 1990–2017: A systematic analysis for the Global Burden of Disease Study 2017. *The Lancet. Gastroenterology & Hepatology, 5*, 17–30. https://doi.org/10.1016/s2468-1253(19)30333-4 (accessed on 15th July 2025).
3. Amaral, A. R., Rentas, M. F., Rosa, T. C. T., Pereira, T. A. E., Marchi, P. H., Teixeira, F., Roberti Filho, F. O., et al. (2024). Microbiota in mild inflammatory bowel disease (IBD) can be modulated by beta-glucans and mannanoligosaccharides: A randomized, double-blinded study in dogs. *Veterinary Sciences, 11.* https://www.semanticscholar.org/paper/47f13d6a767c7b2341d9f25e474be10bbf2eb07e (accessed on 15th July 2025).
4. Barberio, B., Bertin, L., Facchin, S., Bonazzi, E., Cusano, S., Romanelli, G., Francini Pesenti, F., et al. (2025). Dietary interventions and oral nutritional supplementation in inflammatory bowel disease: Current evidence and future directions. *Nutrients, 17.* https://www.semanticscholar.org/paper/0b284ab9cc9df6d435ce25e617009e9f0c15a109 (accessed on 15th July 2025).
5. Bernardi, F., Faggiani, I., Parigi, T., Zilli, A., Allocca, M., Furfaro, F., Peyrin-Biroulet, L., et al. (2025). JAK inhibitors and risk of cancer in IBD patients. *Cancers, 17.* https://www.semanticscholar.org/paper/2a5658f66526eda4389d0640a0814f4de7b85b36 (accessed on 15th July 2025).
6. Bhalla, A., Shahi, A., Maity, M., Safa, F., Srividya, V., Clementina, R., Anugu, G. R., et al. (2025). Inflammatory bowel disease in children: Current diagnosis and treatment strategies. *Cureus, 17.* https://www.semanticscholar.org/paper/02451bde4fcdc19edde1ca8a00985bc66e797ebc (accessed on 15th July 2025).
7. Bhayani, P., Natarajan, K., & Coelho-Prabhu, N. (2024). Rising incidence of inflammatory bowel disease in the Asian subcontinent—An exploration of causative factors. *Gastrointestinal Disorders.* https://www.semanticscholar.org/paper/c3b34ddacdbb2f809e8fa60dd9e43c7e806b0815 (accessed on 15th July 2025).
8. Bourgonje, A. R., Abdulle, A. E., Timens, W., Hillebrands, J.-L., Navis, G., Gordijn, S. J., Bolling, M. C., et al. (2020). Angiotensin-converting enzyme 2 (*ACE2*), *SARS-CoV-2* and the pathophysiology of coronavirus disease 2019 (*COVID-19*). *The Journal of Pathology, 251*, 228–248. https://doi.org/10.1002/path.5471 (accessed on 15th July 2025).
9. Caballero Mateos, A. M., Cañadas de la Fuente, G. A., Gros, B. (2025). Paradigm shift in inflammatory bowel disease management: Precision medicine, artificial intelligence, and emerging therapies. *Journal of Clinical Medicine, 14.* https://www.semanticscholar.org/paper/f43bf43733ce7a6d747328b942fb9cba57b1aa0c (accessed on 15th July 2025).
10. Chen, Y., Chen, X., Lin, S., Huang, S., Li, L., Hong, M., Li, J., et al. (2025). Effects of psychological stress on inflammatory bowel disease via affecting the microbiota–gut–brain axis. *Chinese Medical Journal, 138*, 664–677. https://www.semanticscholar.org/paper/07c5859bcac98ce4954c2aae0bfb955a52463828 (accessed on 15th July 2025).

11. Covello, C., Becherucci, G., Scaldaferri, F., Laterza, L., Gasbarrini, A., & Mentella, M. C. (2024). Popular diets and nutritional assessment in the management of irritable bowel syndrome in inflammatory bowel disease: An overview of current evidence. *Polish Archives of Internal Medicine.* https://www.semanticscholar.org/paper/3d36be2b1ebe143d9f2d6340101c9006233d5240 (accessed on 15th July 2025).

12. Cryan, J. F., O'Riordan, K. J., Cowan, C. S. M., Sandhu, K. V., Bastiaanssen, T. F. S., Boehme, M., Codagnone, M. G., et al. (2019). The microbiota-gut-brain axis. *Physiological Reviews, 99,* 1877–2013. https://doi.org/10.1152/physrev.00018.2018 (accessed on 15th July 2025).

13. de Vos, W. M., Tilg, H., Van Hul, M., & Cani, P. D. (2022). Gut microbiome and health: Mechanistic insights. *Gut, 71,* 1020–1032. https://doi.org/10.1136/gutjnl-2021-326789 (accessed on 15th July 2025).

14. Derwa, Y., Gracie, D. J., Hamlin, P. J., & Ford, A. C. (2017). Systematic review with meta-analysis: The efficacy of probiotics in inflammatory bowel disease. *Alimentary Pharmacology & Therapeutics, 46,* 389–400. https://doi.org/10.1111/apt.14203 (accessed on 15th July 2025).

15. Doroszkiewicz, J., Mroczko, J., Winkel, I., Mroczko, B. (2024). Metabolic and immune system dysregulation: Unraveling the connections between Alzheimer's disease, diabetes, inflammatory bowel diseases, and rheumatoid arthritis. *Journal of Clinical Medicine, 13.* https://www.semanticscholar.org/paper/0aff59786dfa0924e01c8c9f6907fb6387a9d60d (accessed on 15th July 2025).

16. Ebert, A., Elmahdi, R., Poulsen, G., Bogsted, M., Verstockt, B., Lees, C., Jess, T. (2024). P1167 Inflammatory bowel disease: A phenome-wide pre- and post-diagnostic association study. *Journal of Crohn's and Colitis.* https://www.semanticscholar.org/paper/505b5b5f6d7eb504441dfdf506f169b6a029b5d4 (accessed on 15th July 2025).

17. Ekstedt, N., Jamioł-Milc, D., Pieczyńska, J. (2024). Importance of gut microbiota in patients with inflammatory bowel disease. *Nutrients, 16.* https://www.semanticscholar.org/paper/fc1c21f5c097499853a714a06304b977d8662175 (accessed on 15th July 2025).

18. Hong, S., & Baek, D. (2024). Diagnostic procedures for inflammatory bowel disease: Laboratory, endoscopy, pathology, imaging, and beyond. *Diagnostics, 14.* https://www.semanticscholar.org/paper/7d8abb62c26ec51ded6f041150a52fd2471d677f (accessed on 15th July 2025).

19. Hracs, L., Windsor, J., Gorospe, J., Buie, M., Quan, J., Caplan, L., Markovinović, A., et al. (2024). Machine learning classification of the epidemiologic stages of inflammatory bowel disease across geography and time. *Gastroenterology.* https://www.semanticscholar.org/paper/b457a8e69c01854ce0eb4a73afea291fd8902e31 (accessed on 15th July 2025).

20. Jenssen, C., Petersen, F., Höpfner, M., Nürnberg, D., Strobel, D., Vogelpohl, J., Dietrich, C. (2025). Why and when are activity scores and advanced ultrasound techniques needed in inflammatory bowel disease (IBD)? *Medical Ultrasonography.* https://www.semanticscholar.org/paper/0437291720023f76304bebb85a156c6cbefab72b (accessed on 15th July 2025).

21. Khoury, K. M., Jradi, A., Karam, K., Fiani, E. (2025). Lymphogranuloma venereum proctosigmoiditis misdiagnosed as inflammatory bowel disease: A case report. *World Journal of Clinical Cases, 13.* https://www.semanticscholar.org/paper/5934c7b2b18d64da8bab0b58168eec286239f509 (accessed on 15th July 2025).

22. Kim, Y.-M., Kim, H.-Y., Jang, J.-T., & Hong, S. (2023). Preventive effect of *Ecklonia cava* extract on DSS-induced colitis by elevating intestinal barrier function and improving

pathogenic inflammation. *Molecules, 28.* https://www.semanticscholar.org/paper/d6d5bf0f27ae4b2265eb1956f567fe063299634e (accessed on 15th July 2025).

23. Klemm, N. K., & Feuerstein, J. (2025). A practical guide to dilating inflammatory bowel disease strictures. *Expert Review of Gastroenterology & Hepatology, 19*, 377–387. https://www.semanticscholar.org/paper/60dc8c3778e64b2ce6f8f652629f7d594fb4e983 (accessed on 15th July 2025).
24. Knowles, S. R., Keefer, L., Wilding, H., Hewitt, C., Graff, L. A., & Mikocka-Walus, A. (2018). Quality of life in inflammatory bowel disease: A systematic review and meta-analyses—Part II. *Inflammatory Bowel Diseases, 24*, 966–976. https://doi.org/10.1093/ibd/izy015 (accessed on 15th July 2025).
25. Kong, C., Yang, M. F., Yue, N.-n., Zhang, Y., Tian, C., Wei, D., Shi, R., et al. (2024). Restore intestinal barrier integrity: An approach for inflammatory bowel disease therapy. *Journal of Inflammation Research, 17*, 5389–5413. https://www.semanticscholar.org/paper/90bc5f236dd5f444c300c403dcbdabe5096db01c (accessed on 15th July 2025).
26. Lamb, C. A., Kennedy, N. A., Raine, T., Hendy, P., Smith, P. J., Limdi, J. K., Hayee, B., et al. (2019). British Society of Gastroenterology consensus guidelines on the management of inflammatory bowel disease in adults. *Gut, 68*, s1–s106. https://doi.org/10.1136/gutjnl-2019-318484 (accessed on 15th July 2025).
27. Lee, T.-C., Staller, K., Botoman, V., Pathipati, M. P., Varma, S., & Kuo, B. (2023). ChatGPT answers common patient questions about colonoscopy. *Gastroenterology, 165*, 509–511.e7. https://doi.org/10.1053/j.gastro.2023.04.033 (accessed on 15th July 2025).
28. Lenti, M. V., Santacroce, G., Di Sabatino, A. (2025). Rethinking the use of biologics in inflammatory bowel disease patients with malignancy: Insights from the treatment of immune checkpoint inhibitor-induced colitis. *Inflammatory Bowel Diseases.* https://www.semanticscholar.org/paper/91f08fd2d759ce390a6b2534a61056aab577315a (accessed on 15th July 2025).
29. Li, Y., Li, X.-M., Duan, H.-Y., Yang, K.-D., & Ye, J.-F. (2024). Advances and optimization strategies in bacteriophage therapy for treating inflammatory bowel disease. *Frontiers in Immunology, 15.* https://www.semanticscholar.org/paper/c5b3953ea122c9857a641daaa3902fa7ad60ef99 (accessed on 15th July 2025).
30. Liang, Y., Li, Y., & Zhou, M. (2024). Effects of positive psychological interventions on psychological outcomes, quality of life, and inflammation biomarkers in inflammatory bowel disease patients. *Gastroenterology Nursing, 47*, 455–466. https://www.semanticscholar.org/paper/520835feea06897eb42f2f988e560e75fe44c01c (accessed on 15th July 2025).
31. Liao, W., Luo, Q., Zhang, L., Wang, H., Ge, W., Wang, J., & Zuo, Z. (2024). Genetic overlap between inflammatory bowel disease and iridocyclitis: Insights from a genome-wide association study in a European population. *BMC Genomic Data, 25.* https://www.semanticscholar.org/paper/9564a0140a8d63047c2b64360ab1c9eedf9d7e72 (accessed on 15th July 2025).
32. Lightner, A. L., Vogel, J. D., Carmichael, J. C., Keller, D. S., Shah, S. A., Mahadevan, U., Kane, S. V., et al. (2020). The American Society of Colon and Rectal Surgeons Clinical Practice Guidelines for the surgical management of Crohn's disease. *Diseases of the Colon & Rectum, 63*, 1028–1052. https://doi.org/10.1097/dcr.0000000000001716 (accessed on 15th July 2025).

33. Lu, Y., & Han, X. (2024). Therapeutic implications of phenolic acids for ameliorating inflammatory bowel disease. *Nutrients, 16.* https://www.semanticscholar.org/paper/150ce6a53b830f0974c8d66df7953ffdb72d75fe (accessed on 15th July 2025).

34. Mallick, H., Rahnavard, A., McIver, L. J., Ma, S., Zhang, Y., Nguyen, L. H., Tickle, T. L., et al. (2021). Multivariable association discovery in population-scale meta-omics studies. *PLoS Computational Biology, 17*, e1009442–e1009442. https://doi.org/10.1371/journal.pcbi.1009442 (accessed on 15th July 2025).

35. Massironi, S., Furfaro, F., Bencardino, S., Allocca, M., & Danese, S. (2024). Immunity in digestive diseases: New drugs for inflammatory bowel disease treatment—Insights from Phase II and III trials. *Journal of Gastroenterology, 59*, 761–787. https://www.semanticscholar.org/paper/530215fa50c4656387daab872190c6c1807f76c6 (accessed on 15th July 2025).

36. Massironi, S., Mulinacci, G., Zuin, G., Pirola, L., Mancini, F., Carzaniga, V., Zucchini, N., et al. (2025). P0483 Assessment of disease activity in pediatric inflammatory bowel disease using intestinal ultrasound: A comparative diagnostic analysis. *Journal of Crohn's and Colitis.* https://www.semanticscholar.org/paper/d4e133faa21d85873049f4783efc1de8522cdca3 (accessed on 15th July 2025).

37. Merza, N., Saab, O., Nawras, Y., Abdulhussein, R., Elmoursi, A., Daddoo, L., Yaqoob, Z., et al. (2024). Evaluation of alternative treatment strategies for bile acid malabsorption in inflammatory bowel disease patients: A network meta-analysis. *Journal of Clinical Medicine Research, 16*, 33–45. https://www.semanticscholar.org/paper/9d5f5f274d3912470872e20a7dd3d1229317e204 (accessed on 15th July 2025).

38. Napolitano, D., Vellone, E., Iovino, P., Scaldaferri, F., Cocchieri, A. (2024). Self-care in patients affected by inflammatory bowel disease and caregiver contribution to self-care (IBD-SELF): A protocol for a longitudinal observational study. *BMJ Open Gastroenterology, 11.* https://www.semanticscholar.org/paper/37f16bf1b80f3fcd73dfa4f363c3e4bc9b34a204 (accessed on 15th July 2025).

39. Ocansey, D. K. W., Hang, S., Yuan, X., Qian, H., Zhou, M., Olovo, C. V., Zhang, X., et al. (2023). The diagnostic and prognostic potential of gut bacteria in inflammatory bowel disease. *Gut Microbes, 15.* https://www.semanticscholar.org/paper/1117c9d7781918f8cf867887a1f14a1b0ef317c4 (accessed on 15th July 2025).

40. Olsen, B., Opheim, R., Kristensen, V., Høivik, M., Lund, C., Aabrekk, T. B., Johansen, I., et al. (2024). P1147 Symptoms of irritable bowel syndrome are common in patients in remission from inflammatory bowel disease: Results from an observational population-based cohort study in Norway. *Journal of Crohn's and Colitis.* https://www.semanticscholar.org/paper/c1de012104d9604b4d7880c5d9031d4f5a7a530f (accessed on 15th July 2025).

41. Ozdemir, B., Atay, A., Kayhan, M. A., Ozin, Y., Gokce, D., Altunsoy, A., Guner, R. (2023). Tissue quantitative RT–PCR test for diagnostic significance of cytomegalovirus infection in patients with inflammatory bowel disease and treatment response. *Medicine, 102.* https://www.semanticscholar.org/paper/0a70a961d077f4b63645639433da87bd9a31709b (accessed on 15th July 2025).

42. Park, K. T., Ehrlich, O., Allen, J. I., Meadows, P., Szigethy, E., Henrichsen, K., Kim, S. C., et al. (2019). The cost of inflammatory bowel disease: An initiative from the Crohn's & Colitis Foundation. *Inflammatory Bowel Diseases, 26*, 1–10. https://doi.org/10.1093/ibd/izz104 (accessed on 15th July 2025).

43. Peters, J. E., Basnayake, C., Hebbard, G., Salzberg, M., & Kamm, M. A. (2021). Prevalence of disordered eating in adults with gastrointestinal disorders: A systematic review. *Neurogastroenterology & Motility, 34.* https://doi.org/10.1111/nmo.14278 (accessed on 15th July 2025).

44. Plume, J., De, A., Mutalib, M. (2024). Assessing the correlation between fecal calprotectin, blood markers and disease activity in pediatric inflammatory bowel disease. *Annals of Gastroenterology, 37*, 436–441. https://www.semanticscholar.org/paper/e807a90f643016e86601921f8fd8d9cea4d0bfcb (accessed on 15th July 2025).

45. Ramiro, S., Nikiphorou, E., Sepriano, A., Ortolan, A., Webers, C., Baraliakos, X., Landewé, R., et al. (2022). ASAS-EULAR recommendations for the management of axial spondyloarthritis: 2022 update. *Annals of the Rheumatic Diseases, 82*, 19–34. https://doi.org/10.1136/ard-2022-223296 (accessed on 15th July 2025).

46. Rathod, S., Kumar, N., Matiz, G. D., Biju, S., Girgis, P., Sabu, N., Mumtaz, H., et al. (2024). The role of minimally invasive surgery in the management of inflammatory bowel disease: Current trends and future directions. *Cureus, 16.* https://www.semanticscholar.org/paper/6d5ba5e6ea18160d9e7e2cf2eb480cca466bafa5 (accessed on 15th July 2025).

47. Robinson, P. C., Richards, D., Tanner, H., & Feldmann, M. (2020). Accumulating evidence suggests anti-TNF therapy needs to be given trial priority in COVID-19 treatment. *The Lancet Rheumatology, 2*, e653–e655. https://doi.org/10.1016/s2665-9913(20)30309-x (accessed on 15th July 2025).

48. Sanat, Z. M., Siami, Z., Alatab, S., Vahedi, H., & Fanni, Z. (2024). Cytomegalovirus infection in adult patients with inflammatory bowel disease: A literature review. *Archives of Iranian Medicine, 27*, 277–286. https://www.semanticscholar.org/paper/49c096e47e1d90f39eb1bc75b5c4f0341fc52a9a (accessed on 15th July 2025).

49. Sandrin, T. R., Pasternak, B. A., Jurutka, P. W., Buss, K., Gu, H., DeSantis, A. H., & Coker, K. M. (2025). A multiomics-based analysis of the fecal microbiome of pediatric inflammatory bowel disease (IBD) patients reveals potential disease-specific features more effectively than microbiome community composition sequence data. *Gastroenterology.* https://www.semanticscholar.org/paper/fa9d78132f0fec9c9e566ba73c6943ffff9a2111 (accessed on 15th July 2025).

50. Scarallo, L., Lionetti, P. (2021). Dietary management in pediatric patients with Crohn's disease. *Nutrients, 13*, 1611–1611. https://doi.org/10.3390/nu13051611 (accessed on 15th July 2025).

51. Uzzan, M., Georgiev, G., Peyrin-Biroulet, L., Bouhnik, Y., Narula, N., Jairath, V., Ungaro, R. C., et al. (2024). Screen failures and causes in inflammatory bowel disease randomized controlled trials: A study of 16,913 screened patients. *Inflammatory Bowel Diseases.* https://www.semanticscholar.org/paper/705a2ca5933873065ba7072e313955bf0579a0b5 (accessed on 15th July 2025).

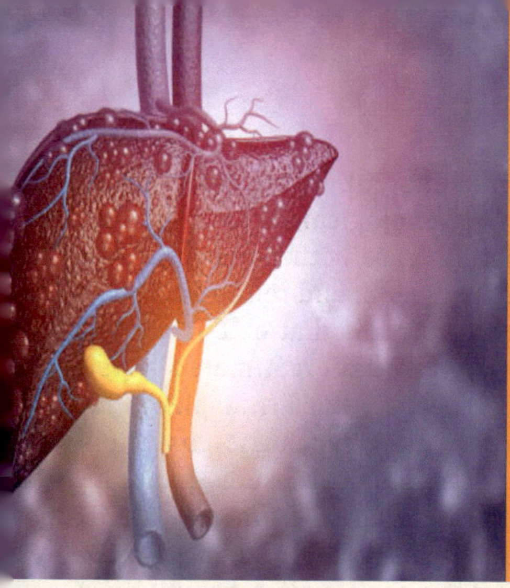

Chapter 8
LIVER DISORDERS

Contents

Introduction

Liver disease encompasses a broad range of conditions that impact liver structure and function, and profoundly influence general health and well-being. These diseases may occur due to many etiologies, and are characterized by viral infections, genetic causes, autoimmune disease, and lifestyle factors , such as alcohol consumption and obesity. Liver function is crucial in various physiological processes, including metabolism, detoxification, and the production of vital proteins, and thus its normal function is essential to help maintain overall good health. It is crucial to know the various liver diseases because early detection and treatment can help to avoid the onset of other complications , such as liver failure or hepatocellular carcinoma. In the last couple of decades, the situation of liver transplantation has evolved with an emphasis on post-transplant quality of life (QoL) as a main outcome measure. According to research, QoL significantly improves after liver transplantation, especially within the first year, when it holds stable or slightly decreases afterwards. This is based on a variety of factors, varying from physical well-being to psychological status and socio-demographic characteristics , such as employment and marital status. The acknowledgment of psychological factors, coupled with physical rehabilitation, highlights the integrative process of patient care within the context of hepatology. Therefore, addressing QoL has the potential to guide future research and refine guidelines for patient management of liver disease to ensure holistic treatment protocols that extend beyond survival. In addition, psychiatric disorders constitute a crucial yet often underestimated aspect of the management of liver disease, particularly in the setting of orthotopic liver transplantation (OLT). Research indicates that up to 22.7% of OLT recipients experience psychiatric conditions that can adversely affect health-related quality of life (HRQOL). Psychological issues, including posttraumatic stress disorder (PTSD) and major depressive disorder, can arise from the intense clinical experiences surrounding transplantation. These conditions are linked to a decline in cognitive performance and perceptions of social support, further exacerbating the challenges faced by these patients. Understanding psychiatric morbidity effects on HRQOL is essential in medical practice as it allows the design of intervention strategies capable of improving psychological as well as physical outcomes in liver disease patients (Bilzer et al., 2002; Onghena et al., 2016).

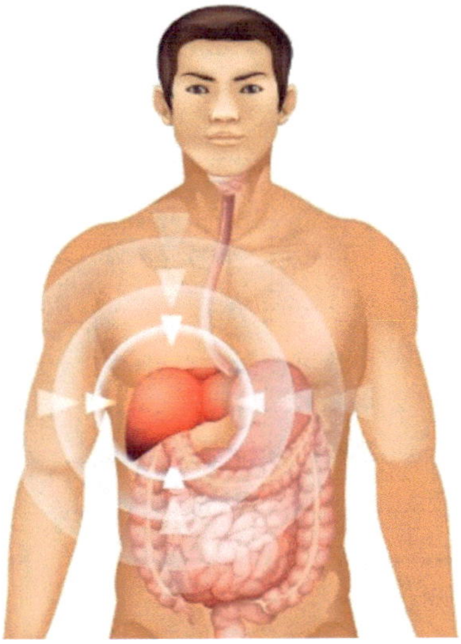

Figure 8.1 Liver disorders.

Source: https://lirp.cdn-website.com/69c0b277/dms3rep/multi/opt/liver+related+diseases+name+list-640w.jpg.

Definition of Liver Disorders

Liver disease is a heterogeneous condition encompassing a large spectrum of conditions affecting the liver's structure and function, producing a significant public health problem across the globe. Liver diseases can range from benign conditions , such as fatty liver, to dangerous conditions , such as cirrhosis and liver cancer. The liver plays a central role in various metabolic activities , such as detoxification, protein synthesis, and the production of biochemicals necessary for digestion. When the liver is involved, it can result in systemic effects that impact overall health. It is necessary to learn the definition of liver disorders to enable early diagnosis and effective management, as the majority of liver diseases are latent until they reach advanced stages. An accurate understanding of these conditions thus results in favorable outcomes for patients and enhances preventive healthcare strategies. The classification of liver illnesses is primarily into two broad divisions: acute and chronic. Acute liver diseases can arise suddenly, usually due to viral infection, toxic consumption, or drug overdose, and result in rapid liver failure if not promptly treated. Chronic liver diseases are a long time in the making, usually as a consequence of continued alcohol consumption, viral hepatitis, or alcoholic fatty liver disease. Chronic illnesses, such as cirrhosis, are defined by irreversible scarring and damage of the liver cells that lead to reduced liver function and increased risk of complications, such as hepatic encephalopathy and liver cancer. One of the salient features of chronic liver disease is that it can exacerbate other illnesses. For instance, chronic obstructive pulmonary disease (COPD) patients are at a heightened risk of complications arising from the liver, as evidenced by studies that confirmed a strong correlation between COPD and other types of cancers, including liver cancer (Chung-Ho et al., 2017). Furthermore, recent research underscores the importance of dietary habits and the health of the liver, more importantly, the consumption of added sugars. Excessive sugar consumption has been found to be associated with various pathologies, including hepatic alterations and the development of non-alcoholic fatty liver disease. This association underlines the necessity of taking into account dietary impact in the evaluation of liver disease. In addition to its association with liver disease, excessive sugar intake has been linked with components of metabolic syndrome , such as obesity and cardiovascular disease, which also make liver conditions complex. Measures of control to reduce sugar consumption are needed to mitigate these risks. Thus, the address of the definition of liver diseases should also encompass familiarity with lifestyle determinants, in this case, diet, because such determinants play a significant role in the occurrence and prognosis of liver diseases (Cabezas-Zabala et al., 2016).

Importance of Liver Health

The liver plays a key role in overall health by virtue of its multifunctional nature, including metabolism, detoxification, and energy storage. The vital organ is responsible for metabolizing food nutrients into essential substances and regulating the level of chemicals in the bloodstream. It decomposes proteins, carbohydrates, and fats and impacts weight and energy. In addition, the liver detoxifies by metabolizing the waste materials and toxins so that they can be eliminated through bile or urine. Given these crucial roles, liver function is a necessity; compromised liver function can lead to severe systemic disorders. Moreover, liver diseases, such as cirrhosis and hepatitis, not only disturb local liver function but also introduce complications that affect other organ systems, highlighting the necessity of preventive measures to maintain liver integrity and prevent disorders apt to arise from its dysfunctions (Lai et al., 2021). Preventive care interventions and lifestyle changes are essential strategies to ensure liver wellness. Some of these behaviors include a diet rich in fruits, vegetables, and whole grains that can avert non-alcoholic fatty liver disease (NAFLD) and other chronic liver ailments. Physical exercise is also a key element in strengthening the liver since it helps to regulate weight and enhance hepatic metabolism. Further, avoiding excessive alcohol consumption and the use of hepatotoxic drugs are paramount in preventing liver injury. Routine medical check-ups, including liver function tests and viral hepatitis screenings, are equally important for the early diagnosis of potential liver issues. Awareness and education among individuals about the determinants of liver health can facilitate healthier lifestyle habits and thus reduce the prevalence of liver disorders in the general population as a whole (Ghany & Morgan, 2019). In recognizing the significance of liver health, there is a need to tackle the social determinants that affect the incidence of and outcomes in liver disease. They are socioeconomic status, access to healthcare, and environmental factors, and these interrelate to generate inequalities in health in affected populations. Individuals from disadvantaged socioeconomic groups can be prevented from accessing a healthy diet, healthcare services, and knowledge on liver disease prevention. Thus, targeted public health initiatives aimed at improving awareness and access to preventive care services are necessary. Collaboration with community organizations to give information about the topic of liver health and encourage healthy, resilient living can bridge the access gap in health. Moreover, integrating liver health awareness into broader public health programs will not only enhance individual health but also contribute to a healthier population in general, with interconnectedness of other health issues and the necessity to maintain optimal liver function (Lai et al., 2021) (Figure 8.2).

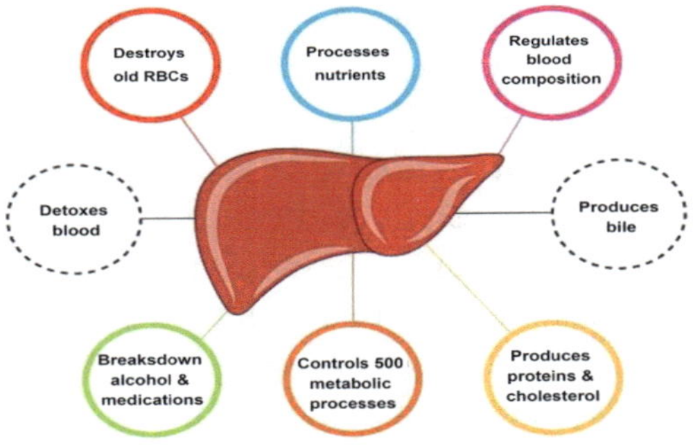

Figure 8.2. Importance of liver health.

Source: https://qph.cf2.quoracdn.net/main-qimg-8c2c9200a1c9564ef2cd5d054a960bec-lq.

8.1. Anatomy and Function of the Liver

The liver, an essential organ of the human body, performs many important functions that are crucial in maintaining overall health. Anatomically, it is positioned in the upper right quadrant of the abdomen below the diaphragm and consists of a complex structure involving lobes, hepatocytes, bile ducts, and blood vessels. The liver consists of two major lobes, the right and left lobes, which are further divided into lobules—tiny functional units consisting of hepatocytes grouped about central veins. This structure maximizes the work of blood entering from the gut via the portal vein to enable the liver to perform its function of metabolism, detoxification, and synthesis of proteins and biochemicals required for digestion and other body processes. Functionally, the liver has an essential role in numerous biochemical processes, including metabolism, detoxification, and bile secretion. The liver maintains glucose levels by storing excess glucose as glycogen, which can be reversed when glucose is needed. The liver metabolizes lipids, produces cholesterol, and detoxifies ammonia, a protein metabolic product that is toxic, into urea, which is excreted by the kidneys. Bile secretion, a digestive juice that emulsifies fats and facilitates the absorption of nutrients, is another indication of the variety of functions of the liver. The balance that is maintained by the liver is very crucial; any derangement in its functioning can lead to life-threatening conditions, emphasizing the importance of being aware of the anatomy and physiology of the liver with reference to liver disease. Furthermore, liver functionality is largely dependent on age, lifestyle, and pre-existing conditions. It has also been discovered that certain chronic diseases, such as obesity and liver disease, can significantly impair the liver's ability to perform as required, leading to complications , such as cirrhosis or liver failure. Particularly, the evidence demonstrates a correlation between liver failure and other illnesses , such as cardiovascular disease and diabetes, thereby pointing toward the liver's critical function in maintaining metabolic homeostasis. In addition, as specified in some research studies, the health-related quality of life (HRQoL) of patients suffering from chronic liver disease may be adversely affected, while decreased scores have been mentioned in physical and mental health domains (Deana et al., 2023). Thus, both identification of liver ailments and prescription of proper treatment strategies rely heavily on understanding the anatomy and physiology of the liver (Brito-Zerón et al., 2021) (Figure 8.3).

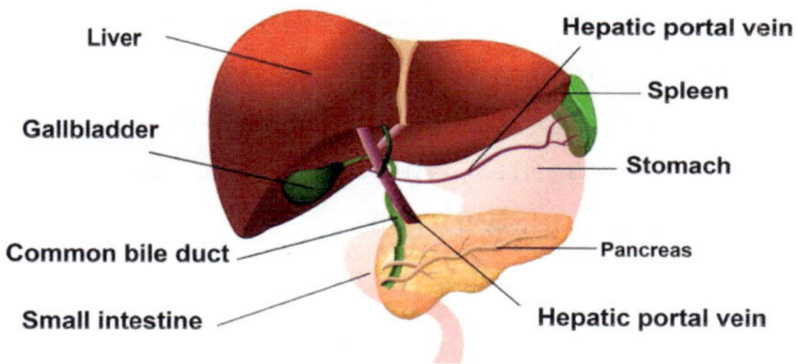

Figure 8.3 Anatomy and function of the liver.

Source: https://media.geeksforgeeks.org/wp-content/uploads/20231213114717/Liver.png.

8.1.1. Location and Size of the Liver

The liver, the largest solid organ in the human body, is strategically located in the right upper region of the abdomen, below the diaphragm and above the stomach. The liver is also shielded by the rib cage, so it is never subjected to any external injury. The weight of the liver, which normally weighs around 1.5 kilograms in an adult, allows it to perform several important functions, including detoxification, protein synthesis, and the production of biochemicals for digestion. Its anatomical structure consists of two major lobes, the right lobe and the smaller left lobe, and other functional segments according to Couinaud's classification system. This classification becomes of particular significance in the clinical scenario, particularly in liver surgery, with bearings in the context of the decision to perform surgical procedures in the event of liver illnesses, such as hepatocellular carcinoma (HCC), which may develop in any of these segments of anatomy (Floc L'h et al., 2025). Aside from its size and location, the liver's association with major blood vessels contributes to its significance in health and disease. The hepatic artery supplies oxygenated blood, while the portal vein supplies nutrient-rich blood from the gastrointestinal system. The intricate bile duct system of the liver gives the facility to secrete bile, which plays a critical role in fat digestion. The relative positioning of the liver with respect to the inferior vena cava is significant during surgery, particularly in the case of HCC, where vascular invasion complicates the treatment strategy. The understanding of these anatomical relationships allows clinicians to devise improved methods to treat liver pathology. Knowledge of this information, especially for risky procedures like vascular resections, influences postoperative results and survival levels in patients with severe liver pathology (Kolokolnikov et al., 2025).

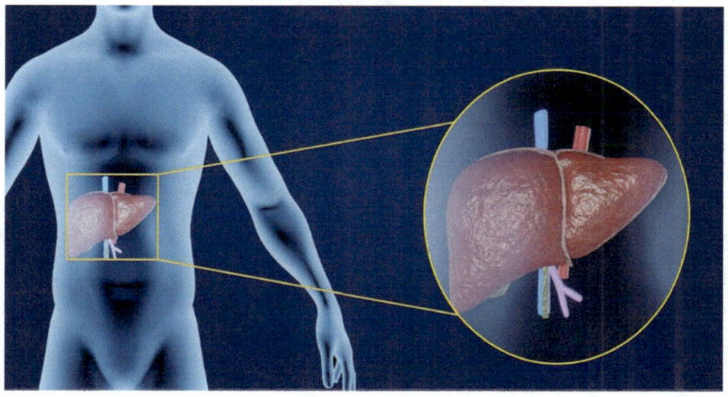

Figure 8.4. Location and size of the liver.

Source: https://i.ytimg.com/vi/U6-U1sfSiBU/maxresdefault.jpg.

Also, the physiological ramifications of liver size and position are significant when taking into consideration liver pathology. An enlarged liver may be a sign of cirrhosis or fatty liver disease that impacts the liver's function. On the other hand, changes in position due to liver enlargement or associated tumors may lead to compression of adjacent structures and cause pain and discomfort, as well as further complications. Tumors like hepatocellular carcinoma also have variations in their location within the liver, which in turn has immediate consequences for the treatment and outcome. Knowledge of liver architecture is vital to enable appropriate diagnosis and treatment of liver disease. As more advances in liver technology continue to occur, newer imaging modalities like MRI additionally increase our ability to assess liver size and status so as to treat liver disease better (Floc L'h et al., 2025) (Figure 8.4).

8.1.2. Key Functions of the Liver

The liver plays a middle role in metabolism, and it serves as a central point for the regulation and breakdown of nutrients. Its primary task involves the disintegration of glucose into glycogen, which is reserved for usage if future energy demands arise. Glycogenolysis and gluconeogenesis maintain the blood glucose level of the body steady, which is crucial for normal cell functioning. Moreover, the liver metabolizes lipids and proteins, yielding crucial components , such as cholesterol and albumin. Through its coordinated pathways, the liver not only facilitates the storage of energy but also regulates fat metabolism, avoiding its associated complications , such as fatty liver disease, an illness that can have serious effects on liver health and function. Hence, interruption of metabolic functions can lead to the development of life-threatening liver diseases, highlighting the paramount importance of liver function to the general metabolic homeostasis. In addition to metabolic regulation, the liver is also an essential detoxification organ that removes toxic substances from the bloodstream. This detoxifying process enables the liver to metabolize drugs, alcohol, and metabolic byproducts of metabolism into their non-toxic metabolites, which are eventually excreted via urine or bile. The liver is also involved in the detoxification and metabolism of toxic substances, something that can be utilized with conditions affecting the liver , such as cirrhosis, when the toxin's ability for detoxification is grossly compromised. The liver's ability to detoxify is important not just to individual health, but also to the body's systemic response to toxic agents in the environment. An abnormal detoxification process will worsen the liver damage and result in a condition that further compromises liver function, highlighting the importance of ensuring liver health through lifestyle modifications and interventions. Furthermore, the liver is responsible for synthesizing and regulating important proteins like clotting factors and digestive enzymes. It produces coagulation proteins to facilitate blood clotting and is thus directly implicated in the process of hemostasis.

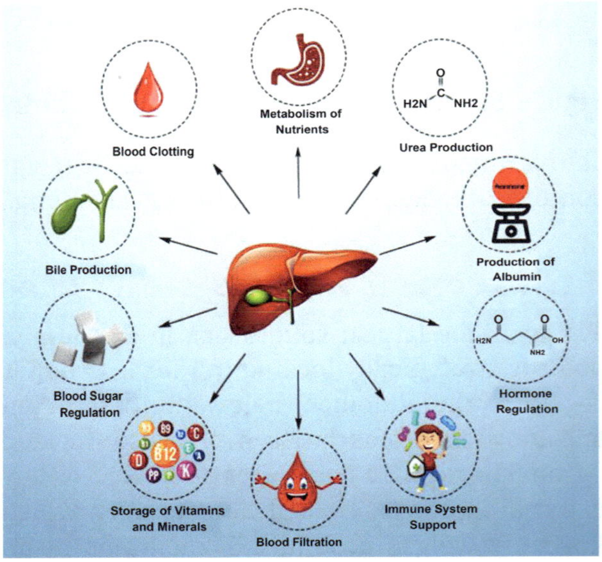

Figure 8.5. Key functions of the liver.

Source: https://clinicone.com.np/wp-content/uploads/2025/04/list-of-10-functions-of-the-liver.png.

The liver also secretes bile, which plays an important role in the emulsification and absorption of dietary fats. Liver functional impairment could lead to a cascade of illnesses like bleeding disorders and malabsorption syndromes, further making the clinical presentation of liver disease even more complex. For instance, patients with cirrhosis of the liver not only have a coagulation defect but also an impaired absorption of nutrients, leading to a complex set of symptoms that complicates treatment. Therefore, the multifunctional processes of synthesis and regulation of the liver are important not only for the well-being of humans but also for the causation and therapy of liver-associated disorders, which underscores its role as a critical organ of human physiology.

8.1.3. Role of the Liver in Metabolism

The liver is an essential organ that plays a key role in maintaining metabolic homeostasis as a focal point for many biochemical reactions that play a vital role in energy balance. It regulates the metabolism of carbohydrates, fats, and proteins to match the energy needs of the body. For instance, during fasting, the liver carries out gluconeogenesis, which is the process of producing glucose from non-carbohydrate precursors to offer a constant level of energy to tissues, particularly the brain. Secondly, the liver is critical in fatty acid metabolism, where it not only stores triglycerides but also produces ketone bodies during prolonged fasting situations. Dysfunctions in such metabolic processes can be the cause of diseases like non-alcoholic fatty liver disease (NAFLD), where improper accumulation of lipids may further exacerbate hepatic injury and lead to serious complications, which accentuates the liver's central role in metabolic well-being (Rinella et al., 2023). In addition, the liver is very much involved in lipid metabolism, wherein not only the breakdown and synthesis of lipids but also plasma lipid levels play a crucial role under its regulation, as well as cholesterol homeostasis. Under normal state, the liver secretes very-low-density lipoproteins (VLDL) to transport triglycerides and cholesterol from the liver to peripheral tissues. This balance is disrupted in dyslipidemias, where lipid concentrations are modified to induce cardiovascular and liver diseases , such as steatosis. Systemic disturbances , such as insulin resistance and obesity, influence the liver's capacity for lipoprotein synthesis and metabolism tremendously. Such conditions enhance inflammation and alter metabolic pathways, and the outcome is the development of conditions like NAFLD, whose prevalence has significantly risen, particularly among individuals with metabolic syndrome (Lai et al., 2021). Besides carbohydrate and lipid metabolism, the liver is the organ responsible for the metabolism of amino acids, acting as a site for deamination and transamination of amino acids. This activity plays a crucial role in non-essential amino acid synthesis and nitrogen balance in the body. The liver's capacity to convert ammonia, a metabolically poisonous protein metabolism byproduct, into urea for excretion is a measure of its detoxifying function. These metabolic processes are disturbed in conditions like cirrhosis, however, leading to the accumulation of poisonous metabolites and nutritional imbalance. This can exacerbate underlying conditions and greatly affect outcomes in patients. The knowledge of the liver's complex role in metabolism is therefore central in the management and treatment of different liver ailments (Rinella et al., 2023).

8.2. Common Liver Disorders

A broad recognition of the prevalent liver diseases confirms the complexity of their aetiology and the necessity of treating them early. Non-alcoholic fatty liver disease (NAFLD) and alcoholic liver disease are the two most prevalent conditions that are major public health issues. NAFLD, with the deposition of excess fat in liver cells without excessive alcohol consumption, has been associated with metabolic syndrome and is on the cusp of becoming a global -preeminent cause of liver dysfunction. One of the key contributors to the pathogenesis of NAFLD is the interaction between dietary habits and intestinal microbiota, where dysbiosis would potentially lead to enhanced inflammation and injury to the liver. The extremely high prevalence of NAFLD is compounded by escalating rates of obesity and physical inactivity, requiring multi-faceted intervention in the management of underlying causes (Liu et al., 2025). Another major liver disease is hepatitis, which can be caused by viral infections, autoimmune conditions, or exposure to toxins. The most frequently discussed forms are hepatitis A, B, and C, each having distinct modes of transmission and medical impacts. Hepatitis C and B pose significant threats that often become chronic illnesses and liver cirrhosis, with their acceleration of hepatocellular carcinoma development. The implications of chronic infection of hepatitis reach far beyond the overall health of an individual, touching broader healthcare systems due to long-term monitoring and treatment requirements. Proper assessment of social determinants of health (SDoH) among affected populations signifies racial and ethnic disparities and how economic instability and the availability of healthcare exacerbate outcomes.

The analysis of such variations is essential to the development of more equitable treatment models for hepatitis patients (Rubaye et al., 2025). In addition to viral hepatitis, environmental external toxins , such as acrylamide and nanoplastics, cause liver disease. These toxins have been reported to be harmful to the liver. They have been found to produce toxic effects on the liver. The co-localization of these toxins has been reported to cause severe liver metabolic disorders and damage in recent studies, which highlights the importance of research in the gut-liver axis. Specifically, experiments demonstrate that acrylamide and polystyrene nanoplastic synergistic toxicity causes greater injury to the liver than single exposure. This finding supports the need for public health programs to minimize exposure to such toxins and promote education on dietary and environmental factors in relation to liver health. Thorough policy and educational strategies will be important in mitigating the burden of liver disease among both patients and healthcare systems (Liu et al., 2025) (Figure 8.6).

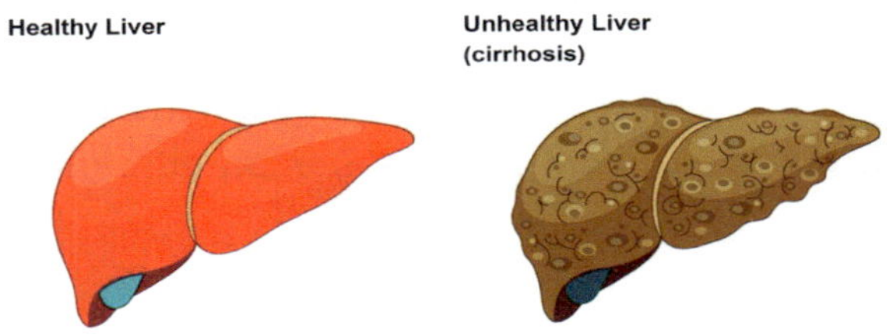

Figure 8.6. Common liver disorders.

Source: https://i0.wp.com/post.healthline.com/wp-content/uploads/2021/11/1684500-Liver-Problems-and-Their-Causes.png?w=1155&h=1436.

8.2.1. Hepatitis (A, B, C)

Hepatitis A, B, and C are significant liver diseases, each due to a distinct virus that affects liver function in a dissimilar manner. Hepatitis A virus (HAV) is an RNA virus that most commonly is spread by the fecal-oral route, frequently secondary to contaminated water or food. This form of hepatitis is typically acute and self-limited but can cause significant morbidity in certain populations, particularly in patients with pre-existing liver disease. Opposed to this are Hepatitis B virus (HBV), a DNA virus transmitted through contact with infected body fluids, i.e., during birth, sexual contact, or needle sharing. HBV chronic infection is an etiologic factor for fatal liver disease, including cirrhosis and hepatocellular carcinoma. Vaccination and surveillance programs are significant factors in public health interventions that are engaged in the prevention of hepatitis A and B, and show the role of education and prevention in the regulation of liver health (Rinella et al., 2023). Hepatitis C virus (HCV) significantly complicates liver disease pathophysiology as it is primarily transmitted through contact with blood. The opioid abuse epidemic has produced a rising number of HCV infections, particularly among young injectors of drugs. HCV infection can lead to severe liver disease, including cirrhosis and liver cancer, but it often is unsuspected until late in the course. Treatment advances over the last few years have transformed the management of HCV, with DAAs yielding greater than 95% cure rates in most patients. This success emphasizes the importance of ongoing screening and the presence of treatment as core components of public health initiatives committed to eliminating HCV as a public health issue (Ghany & Morgan, 2019). The growing, improved understanding of these viral hepatitis diseases is critical to informing effective clinical models and interventions in health policy. Briefly, the differential characteristics of hepatitis A, B, and C demonstrate the complexity of hepatitis as an epidemiologic problem and its significance in liver pathology. Although hepatitis A is often interrupted with complete recovery after the acute attack, hepatitis B and C require constant vigilance and surveillance due to their chronicity and serious health consequences. Better hepatitis A and B vaccination approaches, along with regular screening of hepatitis C, are critical interventions that have the potential to decrease the burden of these diseases. Continued research into hepatitis transmission, prevention, and treatment is important to guide public health policy and to improve outcomes for individuals with viral hepatitis-related liver diseases, thereby further advancing our understanding of liver health in the setting of chronic disease (Rinella et al., 2023).

8.2.2. Fatty Liver Disease

Fatty liver disease, also known as hepatic steatosis, is characterized by the pathological accumulation of fat in liver cells. Fatty liver disease has gained significant attention due to its rising prevalence, particularly in affluent populations where lifestyle elements , such as diet and physical inactivity, are the main causative factors for its onset. Fatty liver disease comes in two predominant forms: alcoholic fatty liver disease (AFLD) and nonalcoholic fatty liver disease (NAFLD). While AFLD is associated with alcohol excess, NAFLD is associated with metabolic aberrations, for example, obesity and diabetes. The two are differentiated by significant distinctions to make an accurate diagnosis and treatment. Physical examinations typically reveal elevated liver enzymes, and imaging examinations, for example, ultrasound, assist in the confirmation of diagnosis. With growing public education, awareness of the risk factors and consequences of fatty liver disease has become increasingly vital for public health interventions. Fatty liver disease has an impact extending beyond the liver, as recent discoveries demonstrate its connection with general systemic disease. Patients with fatty liver disease are also at a higher risk of contracting type 2 diabetes, hypertension, cardiovascular disease, and some types of liver disease, such as cirrhosis and hepatocellular carcinoma. The metabolic condition of NAFLD, which is estimated to affect about 25% of the population worldwide, especially necessitates risk stratification as well as the early intervention of preventive mechanisms against additional health complications. A study by Qu and Li highlights the urgent necessity for non-invasive diagnostic modalities to optimize risk estimation and treatment monitoring. These modalities seek to recognize individuals at increased risk of liver-related morbidity, optimizing patient management and outcomes. Thus, tackling these co-related health issues is pivotal in reducing the combined burden of fatty liver disease on the healthcare system. Therapies for fatty liver disease are primarily lifestyle modifications and, in some cases, pharmacotherapy. Although there are no drugs specifically approved for use in NAFLD, therapy with weight loss, diet, and physical activity plays a key role in reversing the status of liver steatosis and in promoting metabolic function. Clinical practices support interventions that lead to 7% to 10% weight loss since studies have found that this level of weight loss has been able to achieve remarkable changes in liver histology. Wadhawan (2025) also establishes new, upcoming therapeutic techniques, including the use of farnesoid X receptor agonists and peroxisome proliferator-activated receptor agonists as desirable targets for treatment. Clinical knowledge gaps, though, hinder optimal patient care; therefore, standardized guidelines and monitoring systems should be developed. Multidisciplinary health professional collaboration has been necessary in addressing the numerous issues raised by fatty liver disease, with the hope of improving patient outcomes across populations (Figure 8.7).

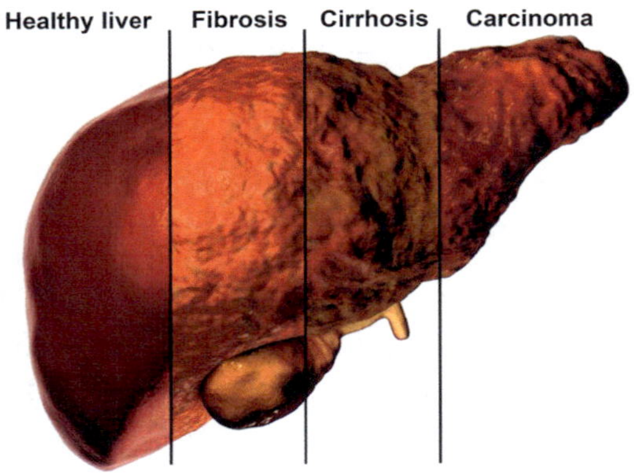

Figure 8.7. Fatty liver disease.

Source: https://scmsc.com/wp-content/uploads/2023/03/stages-of-liver-disease.jpg.

8.2.3. Cirrhosis

Cirrhosis is a chronic liver illness in which liver tissue is increasingly replaced by scar tissue, ultimately leading to liver impairment and derangement of blood circulation. There can be more than one etiology of cirrhosis, including chronic alcohol use, viral hepatitis, and non-alcoholic steatohepatitis. As the underlying liver damage continues, the functional ability of the liver to perform its critical functions decreases, causing a multifaceted set of complications , such as jaundice, ascites, and hepatic encephalopathy. Furthermore, the asymptomatic presentation of the initial phases of liver diseases causes a delay in detection, contributing to the growing prevalence of cirrhosis. The challenges reflect the need for awareness and prevention in the identification of risk groups, particularly with regard to the alarming statistics regarding liver disease among children, where intervention early on can significantly influence outcomes during adulthood (Della Corte et al., 2016). Treatment of cirrhosis is most commonly reliant on the complications and evolution of its status, such as the risk of portal hypertension. Portal hypertension occurs when there is an increase in blood pressure within the portal venous system due to obstructed blood flow, which is usually secondary to cirrhosis. Portal hypertension clinical presentation of patients with cirrhosis can occur as esophageal varices with a risk of significant bleeding. Literature indicates that variceal development is different among various patients who have different underlying liver diseases. Interestingly, non-cirrhotic individuals have a more aggressive progression to varices at risk of hemorrhage than those with well-established cirrhosis, suggesting that individualized strategies of management are necessary to meet the specific requirements of these patients (Gioia et al., 2018). Early diagnosis and treatment cannot be emphasized too much because advanced cirrhosis will eventually cause liver failure or hepatocellular carcinoma. Regular monitoring of liver function and appropriate screening for complications are integral components of the management of patients with cirrhosis. Further, ongoing research into the pathophysiological processes of cirrhosis and its complications has yielded potential areas for future therapeutic targets. The advancement in pediatric liver disease knowledge also implies the complexity of cirrhosis treatment, as some of the least apparent conditions may begin in childhood and progress unremarked into adulthood, thus reasserting the need for a life-course approach to liver health (Della Corte et al., 2016). Having these issues sorted out, healthcare providers are able to improve the impact of cirrhosis and patient outcomes.

8.3. Causes of Liver Disorders

The pathogenesis of liver diseases is multifactorial and increasingly so and is heavily influenced by lifestyle and environmental factors combined with genetic predisposition. Diseases like chronic hepatitis B virus (CHB), chronic hepatitis C virus (CHC) infections, and nonalcoholic fatty liver disease (NAFLD) dominate chronic liver disease (CLD). With the rising global rates of obesity, NAFLD has emerged as the leading cause of liver dysfunction, affecting an estimated 1.2 billion patients globally. The evolution from uncomplicated steatosis to NASH, and further to cirrhosis and hepatocellular carcinoma, highlights the need for early screening and treatment in at-risk populations. These are the Middle East and North Africa, in which both viral hepatitis and NAFLD have specific effects, indicating the way in which liver disease epidemiology is influenced by sociodemographic determinants (Younossi et al., 2023). Alcohol-induced liver disease (ALD) is another of the leading causes of liver disease that is inexorably linked to alcohol drinking patterns characteristic of various populations. The model that computes nearly half of all deaths due to liver disease attributable to alcohol consumption attests to the seriousness of this public health issue. Notably, Eastern European and Central Asian nations report appallingly high levels of ALD, with systemic diagnostic challenges rendering reliable estimation of disease prevalence problematic. In contrast to viral infections that may be absolutely confirmed using serological assays, ALD diagnosis also depends on self-reported alcohol consumption, leading to inconsistencies in data. The wider implications of ALD on health systems are apparent since it adds to mortality and disability-adjusted life years (DALYs), making preventative efforts a pressing need as well as strengthened public health interventions (Lai et al., 2021). Additionally, emerging studies emphasize the interconnection between liver diseases and overlapping conditions , such as obesity, diabetes, and cardiovascular disease. Systemic inflammation of liver disease complicates these relationships by making overall health status worse and contributing to the vicious cycle of chronic disease. Worthily, the rising incidence of metabolic syndrome necessitates coordinated action by health providers to cure these overlapping health maladies. This multi-component approach should include interventions in lifestyle, targeted therapies, and health education to reduce the incidence of liver disorders. Given the ever-growing burden of liver disease, understanding the interaction between these causative factors is of highest priority for developing useful treatment methods and health strategies for mitigating their effects globally (Younossi et al., 2023) (Figure 8.8).

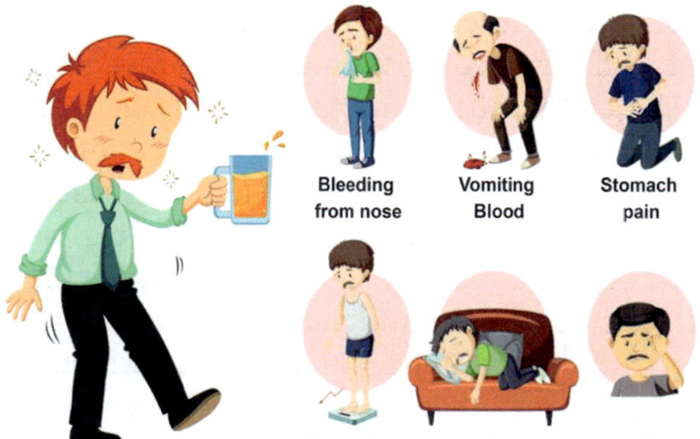

Figure 8.8. Causes of liver disorders.

Source: https://drramchandrasoni.in/wp-content/uploads/2022/05/Liver-disease-Symptoms-scaled.jpg.

8.3.1. Viral Infections

The relationship between viral infection and liver disease is profound and intricate, because numerous viruses have been found to produce direct liver damage. Of particular interest among these viruses are the types A, B, C, D, and E of the hepatitis viruses, which are well-known causative agents of acute and chronic liver disease, in hepatitis B, C and D, leading to cirrhosis and hepatocellular carcinoma. These viruses induce hepatocellular damage by mechanisms involving direct cytopathic effects, immune-mediated liver damage, and interference with cellular metabolism. The clinical course of viral hepatitis may vary from asymptomatic infection to fulminant liver failure, which may be augmented by associated conditions like alcohol use or other liver disease. Moreover, the occurrence of viral infection during epidemics and pandemics, such as has been observed with SARS-CoV-2, has focused attention on the ability of different pathogens to affect liver function and disease modulation, and therefore emphasizes the necessity for careful evaluation of liver function in the setting of viral outbreaks. In recent years, there has been evidence of how viral infection leads to mitochondrial collapse and its significance for liver health. Mitochondrial integrity is critical in cell metabolism and energy production, and its destruction could hasten liver diseases. A case study, for instance, revealed that a child with COVID-19 suffered from acute liver failure related to mitochondrial genetic disorders superimposed on viral infection. The induction of stress responses by viral replication can interfere with normal mitochondrial functions and metabolic processes in hepatocytes, which in turn enhance liver injury and failure. As noted through various reports, the interplay between viral infections and inborn metabolic weaknesses highlights the importance of incorporating genetic factors in evaluation of patients with liver diseases associated with viral etiologies, particularly in children where genetic vulnerability can remain asymptomatic until ushered into the clinical context (Suroviakov et al., 2025). Moreover, the hepatotoxic potential of drugs that are applied to treat or reduce the symptoms of viral infections must also be remembered. Medications like fosfomycin, while mainly used to treat urinary tract infections, have presented cases of drug-induced liver injury (DILI). A report of a 73-year-old female patient disclosed acute liver damage within days of receiving fosfomycin, highlighting that even tolerable drugs can present threats to the health of the liver during viral infections. Risk identification and reduction are most important in such patients with underlying liver disease or when they are put on antiviral therapy. Increased suspicion of the hepatotoxicity potential of drugs, along with close observation of patients, is very important to managing the viral infections themselves as well as the secondary effects of these on liver function (Ribeiro et al., 2024). This approach ultimately aims to optimize patient outcomes by means of early treatment and an integrated understanding of the complex dynamics between viral pathogenesis, liver function, and therapeutic regulation.

8.3.2. Alcohol Consumption

The relationship between alcohol consumption and liver disease has long been recognized, with abuse being a prime cause of most liver abnormalities. After being ingested, approximately 90% of alcohol is metabolized within the liver, with the majority being reduced to acetaldehyde, a toxic metabolite that is detrimental to the liver. Chronic consumption can lead to cumulative liver damage, presenting as conditions , such as fatty liver, steatosis, and ultimately cirrhosis. The World Health Organization (WHO) has estimated that 20% of alcohol-related deaths are caused by liver cirrhosis, which points to the extent of the issue. More specifically, chronic excessive alcohol drinking initiates oxidative stress, which exacerbates liver inflammation and fibrosis, further deranging liver functions and enhancing the potential for liver cancer. These consequences accentuate the pressing need for addressing alcohol consumption as a vital aspect of public health and liver disease prevention (Toropova et al., 2025). Another significant fact regarding alcohol consumption is that it is associated with cognitive impairment and neurodegenerative changes, particularly in terms of liver condition. Long-term ethanol use has been seen to initiate oxidative damage not just in the liver but also in the neurological system. Studies have discovered that neurodegenerative conditions, like advanced dementia, can be caused by chronic alcoholism due to oxidative stress initiated within neural tissues. This connection is brought out by research that proposes other modes of therapy, such as the use of Lophanthus chinensis extract, that might effectively reverse such oxidative damage.

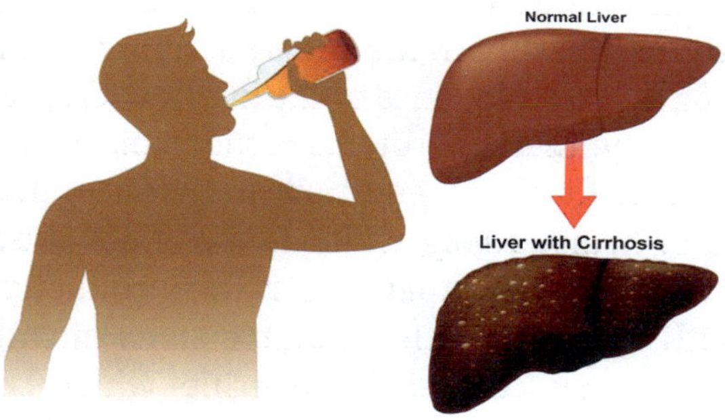

Figure 8.9. Alcohol consumption.

Source: https://www.apollohospitals.com/sites/default/files/2025-02/shutterstock_794599600-scaled.jpg.

Therefore, alcohol's cognitive effects necessitate an integrated understanding of its position in liver health and functionality, calling for a multidisciplinary management of treatment and prevention of liver disorders (Toropova et al., 2025). Besides, the social effects of alcohol consumption are rooted deep in society and reach far beyond individual health. Alcohol is a factor in nearly 200 illnesses and a leading causative factor for numerous social illnesses, including accidents and alcohol illnesses. The massive scale of alcohol morbidity and mortality calls for public education and increased awareness of the risks of even moderate consumption. Moderate drinking is not found to lower the risk of mortality, as opposed to popular myths regarding alcohol as a harmless social lubricant. By the provision of a clearer understanding of alcohol's health-damaging effects, particularly concerning liver disease, society will be able to better contend with alcohol use as a public health concern, eventually leading to minimizing its damaging effects on populations at large (Caputo et al., 2024) (Figure 8.9).

8.3.3. Obesity and Metabolic Syndrome

The prevalence of obesity and metabolic syndrome has already crossed alarming levels around the globe, with significant implications for the liver. Obesity is closely associated with the development of nonalcoholic fatty liver disease (NAFLD), a condition characterized by the excessive deposition of fat in the liver, not from alcohol consumption. Notably, metabolic syndrome, which is an aggregate of risk factors , such as hypertension, dyslipidemia, and insulin resistance, typically precedes the onset of liver disease. The interconnectedness of the conditions highlights the need for early diagnosis and targeted treatment to restrict liver damage. Evidence indicates that individuals with metabolic syndrome are at a substantially increased risk of NAFLD, which is an indicator of the need for a public health strategy focusing on the management of obesity and metabolic derangement to preserve liver health and general health (Usama et al., 2025). The pathways through which pathophysiology connects obesity and metabolic syndrome with liver diseases are complex inflammatory pathways. Increased adiposity encourages a pro-inflammatory trend within adipose tissue, a polarization towards M1 macrophage. This influences the release of pro-inflammatory adipokines and cytokines, which not only maintain systemic inflammation but also perpetuate the worsening of insulin resistance and metabolic syndrome (Varra et al., 2024). Therefore, these inflammatory mechanisms drive the progression of NAFLD and secondary liver injury. It is necessary to fully understand these mechanisms to develop efficient intervention methods. Physicians and scientists should give utmost importance to investigating the connections between obesity, metabolic syndrome, and liver disease to make therapies available that treat the causes of these connected diseases rather than their symptoms. Obesity and metabolic syndrome in the setting of liver disease are best managed by a multidisciplinary approach consisting of lifestyle modification, medical therapy, and community intervention. The first priority is to implement lifestyle modification, such as improved diets and exercise, which have been shown to significantly enhance insulin sensitivity and promote weight loss. Additionally, medication for the pharmacological management of metabolic syndrome comorbidities can minimize their harmful effects on the liver (Usama et al., 2025). However, this response to the interventions might vary among individuals, and this is why personalized treatment methods are needed. Overall, the development of awareness regarding the interconnection between obesity, metabolic syndrome, and liver disease will allow for appropriate prevention and control interventions, thereby improving health outcomes among the affected populations (Varra et al., 2024).

8.4. Symptoms of Liver Disorders

The clinical presentations of liver disease are often subtle and quite nonspecific, depending on the nature of the pathology. The presenting symptoms can be non-specific fatigue, weakness, and malaise that are readily attributable to other minor medical illnesses. With progressive deterioration of the liver, symptoms may advance to more classical presentations , such as jaundice, characterized by a yellow discoloration of the eyes and other skin surfaces. This condition comes about due to the inability of the liver to break down bilirubin, which, consequently, starts to accumulate in the blood. Interestingly, presentation could also manifest as alterations in appetite, unexplained weight loss, or abdominal pain, forming the basis for the importance of sensitivity and prompt medical evaluation upon such presentation. Such presentations are critical signs of an underlying liver disease that must be evaluated early enough before disease progression. Aside from jaundice, several other indications can be proof of the presence of liver conditions. Abdominal distension, or ascites, usually occurs because of increased pressure in the veins surrounding the liver or as a consequence of the liver's decreased ability to synthesize proteins responsible for the balance of fluids. In addition, individuals may bleed or bruise easily, which is the effect of the liver's decreased capacity for the production of clotting factors. Other notable signs include pale stools and dark-colored urine, which can provide clinicians with an indication of liver function and potential blockages in the biliary system. Carefully, these signs should not be underrated since they may indicate severe dysfunction of the liver that requires immediate attention to avoid potential complications , such as liver failure or other severe hepatic disease. Interestingly, chronic liver diseases like thalassemia influence the prevalence of liver symptoms. The patient, in severe forms of thalassemia, will have enlarged organs due to iron accumulation from frequent transfusion of blood, hence swelling of the abdomen and weakness are more common (Bhandari et al., 2025). Furthermore, the disease can lead to liver-related complications, like infection or cirrhosis of the liver, where scarring of the liver tissue occurs. Furthermore, the way in which disorders relate shows the function of thorough diagnosis and monitoring. As indicated in studies on stroke victims, knowing how various bodily factors—, such as platelet count, affect other diseases is able to enhance general patient care (Zarmehri et al., 2020). This intricate relationship emphasizes the need for thorough checkups in order to determine the presence and magnitude of liver disorders (Figure 8.10).

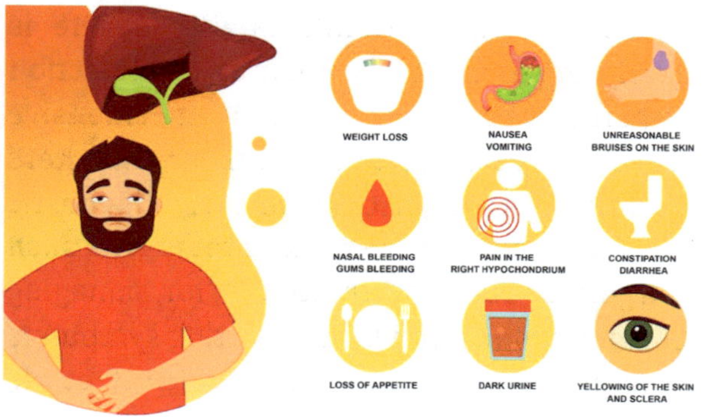

Figure 8.10. Symptoms of liver disorders.

Source: https://family-intervention.com/wp-content/uploads/2016/10/GettyImages-1126803220.jpg.

8.4.1. Jaundice

Jaundice is frequently a symptom of underlying liver failure, characterized by the accumulation of bilirubin in the blood. Bilirubin is a yellow pigment produced from the degradation of hemoglobin in red blood cells. Under normal conditions, the liver can metabolize this bilirubin into a water-soluble compound that can be excreted. However, upon impairment of the liver function by conditions , such as hepatitis, cirrhosis, or obstruction of the bile ducts, bilirubin levels can rise to result in yellow pigmentation of the skin and sclera. The symptom is one of clinical importance, prompting liver status investigation, particularly in children, where liver disease presentation varies and can go undetected for years. Diagnosis of jaundice is not merely the measurement of bilirubin but also the identification of the etiology of the liver disease. Jaundice can be due to various reasons in pre-hepatic, hepatic, and post-hepatic situations. Pre-hepatic jaundice is due to increased hemolysis, which results in the elevation of unconjugated bilirubin. Hepatic jaundice, which can be found in hepatitis or alcohol-induced liver disease, tends to cause elevated conjugated and unconjugated bilirubin. Post-hepatic jaundice results from biliary tract obstructions, which are most commonly caused by gallstones or tumors that interfere with the bile. Understanding these mechanisms is of the greatest significance because accurate diagnosis will have a great bearing on treatment modalities, which can enhance patient outcomes and address the systemic manifestations of liver disease concerning jaundice and overall health (Della Corte et al., 2016). Since the interaction between jaundice and liver disease is multifactorial, the therapy employed is highly determined by the etiology. For instance, antiviral drugs can be used in treating infectious hepatitis, while immunosuppression is possible for autoimmune diseases. If biliary obstruction is part of the picture, then surgery may be considered to evacuate the obstruction. Along with that, management of chronic liver conditions that predispose individuals to jaundice may involve lifestyle modification and constant monitoring of liver status. As more is studied about the pathogenesis of liver disease, furthering our understanding of its symptoms, like jaundice, remains important. Pediatric liver disease has been highlighted more in recent times, as with the necessity of more comprehensive care among this vulnerable population (Ionova et al., 2018). Such intervention may greatly enhance the quality of life for those who suffer from such disabling conditions.

8.4.2. Abdominal Pain and Swelling

Abdominal pain and distension are common presenting features of a range of liver diseases , such as hepatitis, cirrhosis, and liver cancer. The liver plays a significant role in metabolism, detoxification, and synthesis of essential proteins and hence injury to it may manifest in the form of severe physical symptoms. Pain is characteristically referred to the right upper quadrant of the abdomen, where the liver is situated, in the form of a dull ache or a feeling of vague discomfort. This sensation may result from inflammation, distension secondary to the accumulation of fluid, or increased intraperitoneal pressure. Of great interest, ascites or abdominal distension is secondary to fluid buildup in the peritoneal cavity and is frequently secondary to portal hypertension and liver disease. These symptoms should be observed for because they can lead to severe complications if the underlying liver disease is not treated. Cirrhosis, a progressive scarring and chronic disease of the liver associated with impaired liver function, is the most common cause of abdominal pain and bloating. Decreased function results as the tissue of the liver becomes hardened and fibrotic, and symptoms produced warn of complications , such as portal hypertension or liver failure. Blood stasis results in elevated pressure in the hepatic veins, which stimulates the formation of ascites, painful and uncomfortable for patients. The ascites can also make the patients more susceptible to infection, like spontaneous bacterial peritonitis, which aggravates the health of the patients. Research indicates that efficient management practices in use, like dietary modifications and medication, can curb symptoms of pain and abdominal swelling among patients with cirrhosis, although early diagnosis and treatment are crucial to achieve the best outcomes. Reference from multi-disciplinary methods may provide insight into improved symptom control and liver health in general (Puzanov et al., 2017). Liver cancer, a life-threatening situation, is yet another major cause of abdominal pain and bloating. Gradual symptoms , such as chronic pain in the abdomen and a growing belly due to ascites or enlargement of the liver, are experienced by the patient. The enlargement of the tumors may press on neighboring organs and tissues, giving rise to a sensation of fullness and a sense of intense discomfort.

Moreover, as the liver fails, the body will no longer be able to clear waste products effectively, resulting in additional problems like jaundice and metabolic derangements. When combined with ascites, the patient's quality of life is severely impaired. Thus, their early detection is imperative because it may indicate extensive disease progression. The healthcare workers have to put greater priority on early diagnostic tests and schedule case-specific therapies, such as surgery or palliative treatment, for managing liver cancer, which can be debilitating symptoms and improving patient outcomes (Butt et al., 2017) (Figure 8.11).

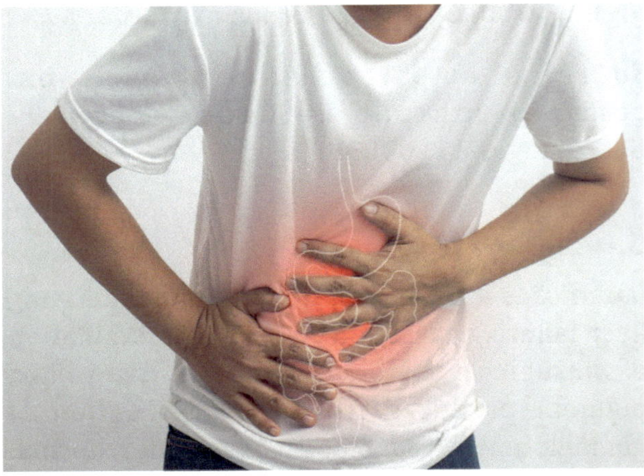

Figure 8.11. Abdominal pain and swelling.

Source: https://lh7-us.googleusercontent.com/f3fF177bNIkPNECW2GDahZ3fMLzF-KTLb-QJjenuoeuTN52wbGViINGO09V0ONZVa0WvLCN1pWefFQdP7kCoiTzOH_zOvO7HfJsT0lwpTn4l8mM9O3-eM8hTGiHv94cbelPqKgI_rKTM.

8.4.3. Fatigue and Weakness

Chronic weakness and fatigue are most prevalent in patients who have liver disease, with extensive quality of life implications. The liver is responsible for the metabolism, and any dysfunction in its operation will lead to energy loss, which manifests as fatigue and generalized weakness. In patients with liver diseases, hepatitis or cirrhosis, compromised liver function to detoxify, synthesize proteins, and produce energy significantly affects the body's general endurance. Besides, toxic metabolite accumulation, due to impaired hepatic clearance, increases the sense of tiredness. This symptom is also commonly worsened by the psychological distress of chronic illness, as depression and anxiety will further contribute to physical fatigue and lower levels of motivation to do normal activities, ultimately creating a cycle of perpetuation fatigue. The physiological basis of fatigue in liver disease is multifactorial and complex. One of the main contributors is the alteration in systemic energy metabolism, which may be induced by both liver disease and secondary conditions like muscle wasting. Liver disease is able to repress the production of the substrates needed that are essential for energy production, as well as substrate utilization by the body. In cirrhosis patients, for instance, hepatic albumin production is decreased, resulting in muscle atrophy and weakness. Moreover, the central nervous system is also adversely affected by the neurotoxic action of ammonia accumulation that could lead to hepatic encephalopathy, a disease that further worsens fatigue and cognitive impairment. Explanation of such mechanisms underlies the importance of devising specific interventions that would alleviate fatigue with liver disease. Recent research highlights the significance of fatigue management as part of the overall management of liver disease. Current treatment options remain directed primarily toward correcting the underlying liver dysfunction, yet increasingly, there is recognition that an overall approach must include addressing fatigue as a standalone entity. Non-pharmacological treatments , such as exercise regimens and diet therapy, have also been found helpful in alleviating patients' subjective complaints of fatigue and enhancing their energy status. Exercise in particular is recognized to reverse muscle weakness and metabolic disease, hence potentially reversing some of the fatigue seen in liver diseases. Thus, a multimodal strategy involving medical management combined with lifestyle modification may constitute an optimal solution for managing incapacitating weakness and fatigue signs in this category of patients.

8.5. Diagnosis of Liver Disorders

Diagnosis for liver disease needs to be an integrated process involving both clinical evaluation and advanced diagnostic methods. Liver dysfunction can be caused by many diseases, including viral hepatitis, alcoholic liver disease, and fatty liver disease; hence, a comprehensive diagnostic protocol must be used by medical professionals. Routine procedures commonly include serological tests that measure the level of liver enzymes and markers of inflammation. But limitations of such strategies, such as cost and accessibility, require scientists to look for new diagnostic avenues. Leverage of machine learning has been a new alternative that could unjam diagnostic processes and enhance precision, particularly among vulnerable groups. Optimization of the feature selection process has helped researchers improve the predictive power of these models, as shown in recent studies involving the diagnosis of liver disease (Altawati et al., 2025). Imaging modalities are significant in the diagnosis of liver disease as well, offering non-invasive methods for the evaluation of liver pathology. Techniques , such as elastography, computed tomography (CT), and ultrasonography are increasingly being utilized to detect diffuse liver parenchymal diseases, characterized by extensive tissue involvement with potential severe health complications. Studies at Maharani Laxmi Bai Medical College found that Fibroscan and ultrasound provide precise diagnostic capabilities with fewer patient complications than invasive methods , such as liver biopsies. The technologies enable clinicians to quantify liver stiffness and tissue composition in real-time, which is important for early diagnosis and efficient disease management. Utilization of these imaging techniques not only enables early diagnosis but also continuous monitoring of liver diseases, thus improving overall patient outcomes (Chaurasia et al., 2024). Effective diagnosis of liver disease often relies on the synergy of laboratory tests, imaging studies, and, if required, advanced computational methods. The value of early identification cannot be overstated; early diagnosis allows treatment regimens to be instituted that can halt the progression of disease and improve prognosis. More sophisticated techniques, such as machine learning algorithms used in predictive analytics, can help clinicians make decisions that are informed by data and sound analysis of the data. Synoptic reporting of non-invasive imaging modalities is an added level of precision that can allow clinicians to comprehend liver health with greater acuity. This multifactorial diagnostic approach to liver diseases not only enhances the validity of measurements but also tries to limit the effect of liver disorders through anticipatory treatment planning and management (Chaurasia et al., 2024; Altawati et al., 2025).

8.5.1. Blood Tests and Liver Function Tests

Liver function tests and blood tests are required diagnostic procedures in diagnosing and managing liver disease. Liver function is assessed on the basis of a series of blood tests that measure levels of liver enzymes, proteins, and other substances the liver secretes. High levels of enzymes , such as alanine aminotransferase (ALT) and aspartate aminotransferase (AST) will usually indicate inflammation or liver injury, often due to conditions , such as hepatitis or fatty liver. Bilirubin is also monitored because elevated bilirubin is recognized to induce jaundice, which is a feature of liver disease. Identification of such biomarkers is significant so that clinicians may tailor treatment plans accordingly and monitor disease progression, ultimately leading to the prevention of advanced liver complications resulting from delayed diagnoses. Providing even more importance to blood tests, liver function tests can yield significant information about a patient's overall state of health. The tests evaluate liver function to metabolize medications and produce proteins, providing cues for such conditions as cirrhosis or cancer of the liver. As an example, the prothrombin time (PT) test evaluates blood clotting capacity, which reflects the ability of the liver to produce clotting factors. An abnormally high PT can reflect severe liver impairment. Levels of serum albumin also provide an estimation of the liver's capacity to produce proteins. Low albumin levels do not just indicate liver failure but may also cause conditions like ascites or edema. Therefore, frequent monitoring through these tests plays a critical part in the management of liver disease overall and may assist healthcare practitioners in predicting imminent worsening of liver function. The application of sophisticated technology , such as machine learning through blood tests, can possibly identify liver disease. Recent studies identify the potential of algorithms to quickly scan blood samples and identify critical parameters that would otherwise go undetected under standard tests. To illustrate, research has proven that certain indicators, such as beta-2 microglobulin and red blood cell distribution width, are predictors for various liver ailments, thus allowing interventions early on. This is particularly pertinent in pediatric populations where early diagnosis of conditions like neonatal jaundice is crucial; courts have documented up to a 20% decline in severe jaundice rates after intensified screening practices were made available (Pavithra et al., 2024). These developments accentuate the demands for blood and liver function tests in the early diagnosis and the evolving nature of diagnostics in the management of liver diseases, ultimately tending towards better patient outcomes (Zhang et al., 2025) (Figure 8.12).

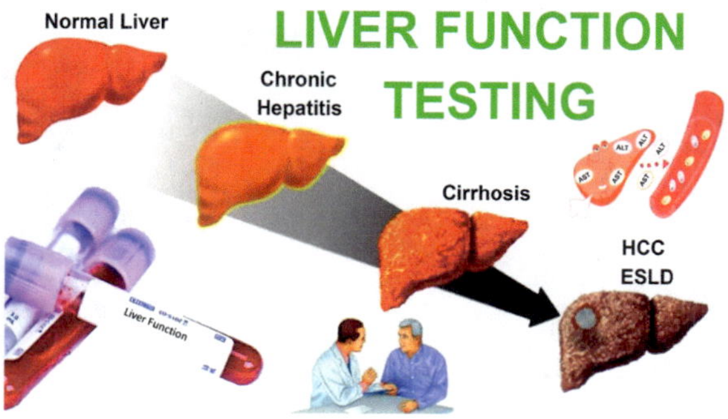

Figure 8.12. Blood tests and liver function tests.

Source: https://fattyliverguide.com/wp-content/uploads/2019/07/Liver-Function-Tests.jpg.

8.5.2. Imaging Studies (Ultrasound, CT, MRI)

Imaging tests are the cornerstone of diagnosing and treating liver disease, particularly in the evaluation of lesions and other liver abnormalities. The primary modalities—ultrasound, computed tomography (CT), and magnetic resonance imaging (MRI)—provide complementary advantages in sensitivity, specificity, and applicability to most clinical contexts. Ultrasound is generally the first imaging modality of choice, giving cost-effective and non-invasive initial assessment in liver cirrhosis patients. Due to its ability to detect the presence of fluid and liver morphology, it is a crucial instrument for ascertaining the progression of disease. However, limitations , such as operator dependence and reduced resolution with smaller lesions require support imaging modalities , such as CT and MRI for further evaluation of suspected liver disease, particularly where cirrhosis is suspected (Yi-Lee et al., 2021). CT and MRI offer better diagnostic functions, particularly in characterizing the characteristics of liver tumors. For instance, multiphasic CT is especially effective for HCC diagnosis.

The imaging features of HCC, such as nonrim arterial phase hyperenhancement (APHE) and washout on portal venous phases, form the basis for result interpretation in the Liver Imaging Reporting and Data System (LI-RADS) paradigm (Yi-Lee et al., 2021). The system provides a structured approach to establishing the likelihood of malignancy so that timely and appropriate therapeutic intervention can be initiated. MRI, on the other hand, is useful when contrast agents used in CT are toxic due to renal failure or in pregnant women. Further, functional MRI techniques , such as diffusion-weighted imaging, can provide information about subtleties in tissue characteristics necessary for differentiation of various liver lesions. The integration of imaging investigations into clinical algorithms not only aids in diagnosis but also enhances the accuracy of liver disease management planning. High-resolution imaging enables measurement of tumor size, local extension, and potential metastases, which are crucial determinants of management plans. Imaging investigations can also help differentiate benign from malignant lesions, thus reducing invasive procedures , such as liver biopsies. With the progress of imaging technology, the scope of novel directions, such as liquid biopsies and better imaging agents, can further optimize non-invasive evaluation of liver disease. Research and development of imaging modalities are thus essential to upgrade the diagnostic scenario of liver disease and provide the best possible treatment to the patient.

8.5.3. Liver Biopsy

The liver biopsy is a critical investigative procedure performed to assess various conditions of the liver, particularly when the etiology is uncertain following non-invasive investigations. By obtaining a tissue specimen from the liver, the doctor is able to obtain vital histopathological information useful in the diagnosis of conditions , such as cirrhosis, hepatitis, and liver tumors. When a liver biopsy is conducted, the histological architecture of the liver is examined so that special abnormalities can be recognized and help in treatment planning. Most notably, its utility is acknowledged when non-invasive studies fail to offer full answers, and thus the biopsy stands as an absolute tool within the liver pathology diagnosis kit (Lorenza et al., 2022). Although of diagnostic value, liver biopsy is not without danger. In a comprehensive report on 261 patients undergoing percutaneous liver biopsy (PLB), complications were noted, but only occasionally. Among the patients being evaluated, mostly with pain or minor hemorrhage, significant complications were few, and no deaths were reported (Androutsakos et al., 2023). This is a testament to the procedure's safety when performed by experienced operators and a reflection of the persistence of its validity in the clinical environment. A prudent consideration of the risks and benefits, however, should be the foundation of the decision to undergo a liver biopsy because there might be contraindications for the procedure. Against the backdrop of advancing diagnostic technologies, the liver biopsy remains a key investigation, particularly in instances that have remained refractory to earlier assessment. Though non-invasive methods , such as transient hepatic elastography and biomarker panels, have the potential to replace it, they are not globally available, specifically in complex cases (Lorenza et al., 2022). For instance, imaging techniques' sensitivity and specificity cannot suffice in the diagnosis of liver disease that needs histological confirmation. Thus, the liver biopsy remains a necessary procedure for doctors to provide accurate diagnoses that inform personalized treatment plans, illustrating the value of this invasive procedure in certain clinical contexts (Androutsakos et al., 2023) (Figure 8.13).

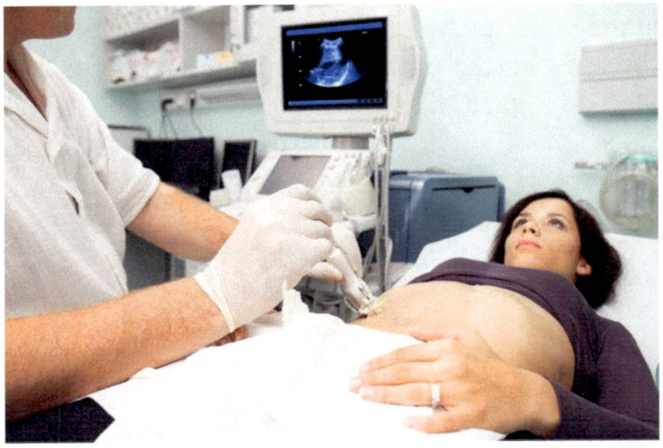

Figure 8.13. Liver biopsy.

Source: https://www.gpddc.com/wp-content/uploads/2019/08/iStock-185093873.jpg.

8.6. Treatment Options for Liver Disorders

Liver disorders are an extensive range of diseases, like viral hepatitis, non-alcoholic fatty liver disease (NAFLD), and cirrhosis, that all require specific treatment methods. Underlying it is lifestyle modification in the form of diet and exercise, the latter of which plays an important role in the management of NAFLD and liver disease due to obesity. Weight control can significantly prevent hepatic fat accumulation and enhance liver function. Bariatric surgery thus emerges as an option in severe obesity, proving to be effective in the improvement of liver and metabolic parameters. Further therapeutic options are also offered by the addition of pharmacological therapies, including glucagon-like peptide-1 (GLP-1) agonists semaglutide and liraglutide. These medications not only assist in weight control but also address the pathophysiology of liver disorders directly, highlighting the need for a multidisciplinary treatment strategy for these disorders (Yang et al., 2022). In more advanced cases of liver disorders, particularly cirrhosis, treatment regimens are more complex, with a requirement for close monitoring of coagulopathy and bleeding risks. The advanced nature of this is indicated by the observation that both thrombosis and bleeding may occur simultaneously in vascular liver diseases. The American Association for the Study of Liver Diseases (AASLD) has provided guidelines on how to handle such risks, observing that patients with cirrhosis will have alterations in their hemostatic systems and hence may present with a tendency to bleed as well as acquire thrombotic complications. More advanced testing technologies, such as rotational thromboelastometry (ROTEM) or thromboelastography (TEG), are capable of more accurately measuring hemostatic balance in such patients and allow clinicians to implement appropriate periprocedure management protocols (Northup et al., 2020). Lastly, effective management is dependent on tailoring care to the individual factors of each patient's disease state. Other than the learning of lifestyle and medical management, interventional therapies also play an important role in the management of liver diseases. Therapies , such as endoscopic variceal ligation and transjugular intrahepatic portosystemic shunt (TIPS) have become routine therapy for controlling portal hypertension and its complications. Radiofrequency ablation and transarterial chemoembolization are useful localized therapies that improve survival in patients with primary liver cancers. Furthermore, the newer advancements in targeted therapies and immunotherapies for liver cancer also hold potential for future treatment options, underscoring the necessity for ongoing research. The integration of multiple modes of treatment, from lifestyle change and pharmacotherapy to more elaborate procedural treatments, through the establishment of a synergistic therapeutic environment creates a multidimensional approach to the multifaceted issues of liver disease while attempting to expand patient outcomes and overall liver well-being (Yang et al., 2022) (Figure 8.14).

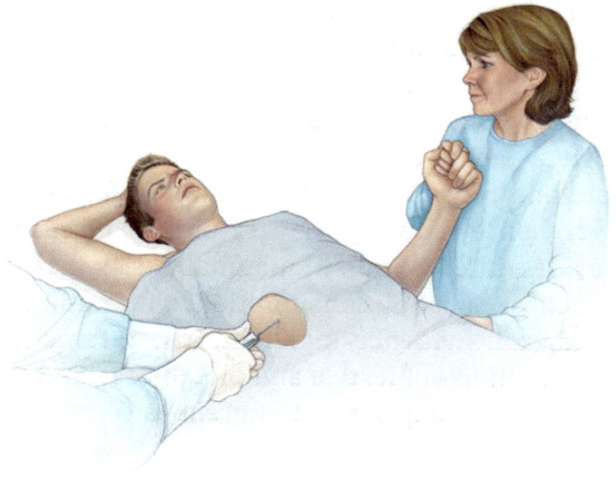

Figure 8.14. Treatment options for liver disorders.

Source: https://www.mayoclinic.org/-/media/kcms/gbs/patient-consumer/images/2013/11/15/17/39/ca00083_-ds00097_-ds00373_-ds00398_-ds00411_-ds00577_-ds00638_-ds00676_-ds00785_-ds00918_-my00088_-ds00811_-my00949_im04144_mcdc7_liver_biopsythu_jpg.jpg.

8.6.1. Lifestyle Changes and Dietary Modifications

Dietary changes and lifestyle changes are crucial parameters in liver disease prevention and cure. There is mounting evidence that unhealthy food habits, including excessive consumption of saturated fats, processed foods, and sugars, play a predominant role in the genesis of liver diseases , such as NAFLD and hepatitis. These illnesses are especially exacerbated by metabolic syndrome and obesity, which may be caused by sedentary lifestyles and poor eating habits. The shift from traditional diets to Westernized dietary styles has been associated with greater liver-related morbidity, pinpointing the need for nutritional education and improved food environments to offset such threats. By moving towards a more balanced diet of whole foods, fruits, vegetables, and lean protein, individuals can potentially reduce their susceptibility to liver disease and promote overall liver health. Lifestyle modification comes even further than dietary modification; it involves exercise, stress management, and regular health checkups. A regular exercise regime can enhance metabolic rate and reduce the accumulation of fat in the liver, hence reducing the risk of liver diseases. Besides, intervention in modifiable risk factors , such as alcohol consumption and smoking, is crucial. Evidence highlights the interactive contribution of lifestyle and diet in accelerating liver disease, implying a comprehensive strategy for effective management.

The European Society of Cardiology (ESC) guidelines emphasize individual responsibility to make appropriate decisions based on the latest available evidence to facilitate clinical practice in patient management. Adherence to these guidelines can improve patient health outcomes to a considerable extent when it comes to liver wellness and overall lifestyle. Beyond this, sensitivity to the role that socioeconomic determinants of lifestyles play in decisions is critical when understanding the prevalence of liver diseases. Economic disparities have a tendency to dictate healthy food availability and physical activity choices, compounding complexity around liver disease prevention. Societies that have food deserts, areas with poor access to healthy and affordable food, are particularly vulnerable to the consequences of unhealthy diets. As outlined in recent statistics on gastrointestinal malignancies, lifestyle modifications have a direct correlation with chronic conditions, such as liver diseases. Thus, a holistic approach that unites diet, physical activity, and socio-economic settings is central in simplifying liver health concerns. Interventions to support community-based interventions can enable people to make well-informed choices, which would in the long run lower the prevalence of liver disorder among specified groups (Visseren et al., 2021; Jardim et al., 2023).

8.6.2. Medications and Antiviral Therapies

The treatment milieu of chronic liver illnesses, particularly those concomitant with viral hepatitis, has been transformed by advances in drugs and antiviral therapies. Previously, the treatment of hepatitis C virus (HCV) relied extensively on interferon-based regimens, which were associated with side effects and questionable efficacy. New all-oral antiviral regimens are bringing in an era of more patient-friendly practices with improved tolerability and effectiveness. These new regimens are not only shorter in duration but also simplify the administration, providing a paradigm shift in managing the therapy of chronic HCV by healthcare providers. With such treatments becoming better, more efficient screening and diagnosis methods are needed to ensure that timely treatment becomes the norm of the day rather than an exception in the treatment of viral infection-associated liver diseases to ultimately enhance patient outcomes (Afdhal et al., 2013). With improvements in antiviral medications, combined strategies for screening and early intervention have become totally imperative, particularly among high-risk populations. Homeless patients, for example, have a distinctive profile with issues that complicate access to HCV testing and treatment. Absence of health insurance, stigma around HCV, and absence of proper health infrastructure are some of the obstacles to effective management in this group. Research has identified societal, system, and individual-level barriers to be overcome to increase accessibility of HCV care in homeless shelters. Stakeholder feedback during the development of a universal HCV screening protocol confirms broad consensus regarding the need to expand testing programs within such affected populations. Therefore, merging antiviral treatment with outreach and education targeted towards these populations is necessary to meet the healthcare disparities seen among at-risk populations for liver disease (Fokuo et al., 2020). In addition, the effectiveness of antiviral therapy depends on breaking barriers to treatment completion and compliance. Solutions must extend beyond the medications; solutions must engage the social determinants of health that influence patient engagement. For instance, those with substance use disorders comorbidities will have additional barriers to their ability to access HCV treatment, complicating their recovery trajectory. Addressing these complexities requires a multifaceted approach, incorporating social services alongside medical treatment to support patients holistically. Providers must foster partnerships with social service organizations to work collaboratively towards facilitating access to care. With the advancement of treatment options, it is essential to enable patients to successfully navigate through the health system to ensure long-term success with the treatment of viral infection-related liver diseases and overall public health outcomes (Afdhal et al., 2013; Fokuo et al., 2020) (Figure 8.15).

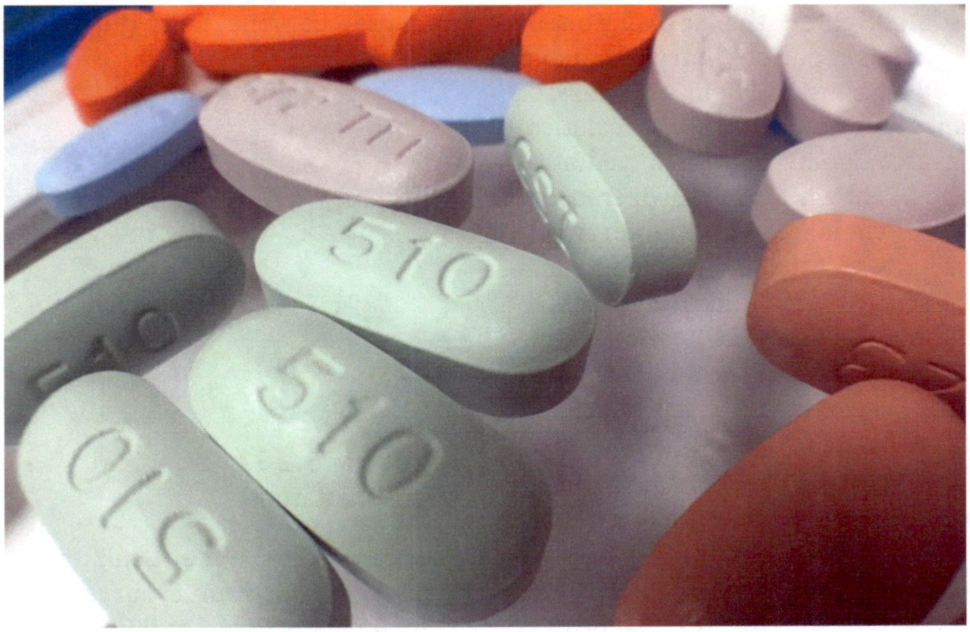

Figure 8.15. Medications and antiviral therapies.

Source: https://cdn.britannica.com/57/215757-050-FE54D0A6/Variety-antiretroviral-drugs-HIV-infection-treatment.jpg.

8.6.3. Surgical Interventions (Transplantation)

In liver disease, surgical therapy in the form of liver transplant is a cornerstone of the treatment of end-stage liver disease. These surgeries have intrinsic complexities that are brought into focus by the requirement of careful pre-operative evaluation and selection of candidates. Sick individuals with chronic illnesses who bear liver diseases have loss of hepatocellular function that leads to complications , such as cholestasis, which has a telling effect on their quality of life. Transplantation not only represents an absolute treatment in such patients, but also necessitates multi-disciplinary cooperation between hepatologists, transplant surgeons, and anesthesiologists. Such collaboration is necessary in optimizing outcomes and dealing with potential postoperative complications, including the risk of biliary obstruction, which remains a common issue post-transplant. These dynamics are necessary to understand to optimize surgical success rates and patient survival. Complications in the postoperative period due to liver transplantation can be very difficult, as far as biliary and vascular integrity is concerned. Their usual rates of complications often determine the indication for the need for more surgical or intervention-related procedures. For instance, research has highlighted the application of percutaneous transhepatic biliary drainage (PTCD) as an effective method of management of post-transplant biliary complications. Technical success at an astonishing 93.3% in pediatric patients has been shown for PTCD, decreasing the occurrence of cholangitis and requirement for surgical re-intervention in the long term (Pape et al., 2025). All these minimally invasive procedures not only enhance the post-operative safety profile but also improve graft function as a whole, thereby preventing the risks associated with conventional surgical revision. Living-donor liver transplantation (LDLT) has increasingly been perceived as a good therapeutic solution for recipients with advanced liver disease. With complications following transplantation, including vascular or biliary stricture, intervention becomes unavoidable. Minimally invasive image-guided interventions , such as PTBD and venoplasty, have been demonstrated to be good alternative solutions to surgical revision. Evidence shows that such intervention brings about acute clinical and biochemical improvement while confirming the resolution of complications on follow-up imaging (Bright et al., 2025). The incorporation of interventional radiology in the post-transplant care continuum is a demonstration of the evolving landscape of liver disease management. It emphasizes the movement toward techniques that not only minimize the risks of re-exploration but also enhance patient outcomes in a patient group who frequently present with challenging post-operative complications (Figure 8.16).

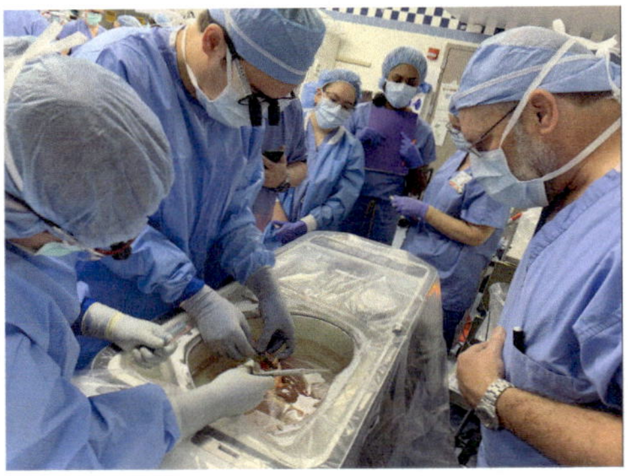

Figure 8.16. Surgical interventions (transplantation).

Source: https://meduc.azurewebsites.net/images/default-source/surgery/img_0008.jpg?Status=Master&sfvrsn=97a57af1_1.

CLOSER LOOK

ALCOHOL-RELATED DEATHS:

Alcohol-related deaths represent a significant and preventable global public health burden. A closer look reveals that these deaths arise not only from long-term physiological damage but also from acute toxic effects, risky behaviors, and social determinants that shape alcohol use patterns. Because alcohol is widely available and culturally accepted in many societies, its harms are often underestimated despite its substantial impact on morbidity and mortality. Alcohol contributes to death through several primary pathways. Chronic heavy drinking leads to progressive organ damage, particularly in the liver, where conditions such as alcoholic hepatitis, cirrhosis, and hepatocellular carcinoma can develop. Cardiovascular complications—including cardiomyopathy, arrhythmias, and hypertension-related events—also increase with prolonged excessive consumption. Long-term alcohol use weakens the immune system, raising susceptibility to infections like pneumonia and tuberculosis, which may become fatal in vulnerable populations.

Equally significant are acute alcohol-related deaths, which include alcohol poisoning, injuries, and accidents. Impaired judgment and slowed reaction time under the influence of alcohol contribute to motor vehicle crashes, falls, drownings, and workplace injuries. Alcohol also plays a major role in violent incidents, including homicide and suicide. In younger age groups, these unintentional injuries account for a large proportion of alcohol-related fatalities. Psychosocial factors often amplify these risks. Individuals facing economic hardship, trauma, mental health disorders, or unstable housing may be disproportionately affected by alcohol misuse. Communities with limited access to healthcare, social support, or treatment services experience higher rates of preventable deaths, highlighting the strong influence of social determinants. In some regions, harmful drinking patterns such as binge drinking intensify the risk of both acute and chronic consequences.

Prevention strategies to reduce alcohol-related deaths rely on public health interventions, policy approaches, and clinical support. Evidence-based policies include regulating alcohol pricing, restricting marketing, enforcing age limits, and limiting outlet density. Screening and brief interventions in healthcare settings can identify at-risk individuals early, guiding them toward counseling or treatment. For people with alcohol use disorder, medications such as naltrexone or acamprosate, combined with behavioral therapies, improve outcomes and reduce the likelihood of fatal complications.

Public education is equally important. Raising awareness about the dangers of binge drinking, impaired driving, and polysubstance use can shift societal norms and reduce harm. Community programs that address underlying stressors—such as unemployment, mental health needs, or social isolation—also play a crucial role.

Alcohol-related deaths shows that they are largely preventable through coordinated, multisector efforts. Addressing both individual behaviors and structural factors is essential for reducing the profound health and social impact of harmful alcohol use.

SUMMARY

In coming up with the conclusion of liver disease analysis, it is evident that the earlier the detection and management, the better placed it is in preventing the otherwise catastrophic consequences of these diseases. The complexity of liver diseases, running across a wide spectrum of diseases , such as non-alcoholic fatty liver disease (NAFLD) and liver cirrhosis, requires a holistic treatment and management plan. The use of classical and modern therapeutic strategies, such as the use of remedies like Ling Gui Zhu Gan Decoction, as evidenced by recent studies, shows the significance of adapting treatment protocols to the specific needs and responses of individual patients (Lu et al., 2025). With the continuous development of healthcare, it is necessary that research advancements play a role in influencing therapeutic guidelines, creating a situation of continuous learning and adjustment in clinical practice. Furthermore, the resemblance between metabolic syndromes and liver diseases points to the dependency of physiological systems on one another and the need for giving holistic treatment centered on the liver alongside associated metabolic pathways. For instance, patients with lipodystrophies exhibit serious metabolic derangement that in turn can exacerbate liver disease, thereby complicating the treatment process (Kńska et al., 2025). A thorough strategy that is responsive to these complexities has the capacity to enhance patient outcomes significantly. Prioritization of interdisciplinary collaboration between hepatologists, endocrinologists, and primary care physicians within the healthcare system will enable it to generate targeted interventions that are responsive to the multifactorial etiology of liver disease. While planning future research studies, there is a need to prioritize topics that will fill existing knowledge gaps related to the pathophysiology and management of liver disease. Investment in intensive clinical trials and new therapies will pave the way for improved therapy choices. The findings on Ling Gui Zhu Gan Decoction are well-argued as proof of a requirement for ongoing research into herbal and integrative medicine in hepatology (Lu et al., 2025). Moreover, overcoming challenges in diagnosing and treating rare diseases like lipodystrophies will allow for more effective care and prevention of patients (Kńska et al., 2025). Through collaborative effort and a proactive approach, the medical community can upgrade the quality of patient care for those suffering from liver disease, ultimately reducing the effects of these diseases on people and society at large.

Liver disease is a complex process with a long list of complications from a multitude of causes, all contributing to the loss of liver function. Cirrhosis and fatty liver are two such chronic diseases that contribute significantly to morbidity and mortality worldwide. The etiologies vary from infectious causes, i.e., hepatitis B and C virus infection, to alcohol consumption and obesity. It is necessary to know the pathophysiology of these conditions so that early intervention and management can be initiated. The liver's complex function in metabolism, detoxification, and synthesis gives the impetus that any liver disorder can have implications elsewhere in the body and hence treatment must be holistic so that both the liver disease and its health implications at large are addressed. Recent advances in the management of liver disease speak volumes about the use of individualized therapy. As an example, recent debates question the efficacy of liver resection compared to percutaneous thermal ablation for smaller tumors measuring less than three centimeters. Both of these treatments are viable options but require meticulous patient selection depending on tumor location and resultant risks. Subcapsular tumors, which present higher surgical difficulties, generally need liver resection because of fears about obtaining sufficient safety margins. Imaging technologies and AI-based approaches are also revolutionizing the landscape through more focused facilitation during thermal ablation, which can help enhance patient outcomes. These developments imply the dynamic nature of treatment techniques in the context of liver disease (Tombesi et al., 2025). Additionally, novel studies shed light on the molecular mechanisms of liver pathology, which indicate that genetic and immune processes may have crucial roles in disease initiation and treatment response. Exercise and sleep deprivation studies show that physiological stressors regulate liver function and can worsen disease. Discovery of key genes involved in such stressors has the potential to unveil novel therapeutic avenues for liver disease. For example, gene expression studies propose that specific biomarkers can enable early diagnosis and targeted therapy for liver disease, as in the case of other areas of health biology (Chen et al., 2025). Such an integrative research focus emphasizes the need for multidisciplinary measures in addressing liver disorders while emphasizing the importance of early detection and patient-specific therapy options.

References

1. Afdhal, N. H., Zeuzem, S., Schooley, R. T., Thomas, D. L., Ward, J. W., Litwin, A. H., Razavi, H., Castera, L., Poynard, T., Muir, A., Mehta, S. H., Dee, L., Graham, C., Church, D. R., Talal, A. H., Sulkowski, M. S., Jacobson, I. M., & New Paradigm of HCV Therapy Meeting Participants (2013). The new paradigm of hepatitis C therapy: integration of oral therapies into best practices. *Journal of viral hepatitis*, *20*(11), 745–760. https://doi.org/10.1111/jvh.12173(accessed on 16th July 2025).

2. Al Rubaye, M. Z., Zafar, S. N., Loconte, N., Owusu-Brackett, N., Venkatesh, M., Stalter, L. N., Ali, M. M., et al. (2025). Comparative analysis of racial disparities in social determinants of health among patients with GI cancer in the All of Us dataset. *Journal of Clinical Oncology.* https://www.semanticscholar.org/paper/3789a4b6028301efac06b934de0fa68c5f586612 (accessed on 16th July 2025).

3. Della Corte, C., Mosca, A., Vania, A., Alterio, A., Alisi, A., & Nobili, V. (2016). Pediatric liver diseases: current challenges and future perspectives. *Expert review of gastroenterology & hepatology*, *10*(2), 255–265. https://doi.org/10.1586/17474124.2016.1129274(accessed on 16th July 2025).

4. W. A. A. Altawati, L. A. B. Mohammed and M. A. E. Abdalla, "Leveraging the Machine Learning Techniques for Diagnosing Liver Diseases," *2025 1st International Conference on Computational Intelligence Approaches and Applications (ICCIAA)*, Amman, Jordan, 2025, pp. 1-5, doi: 10.1109/ICCIAA65327.2025.11013022.(accessed on 16th July 2025).

5. Fokuo, J. K., Masson, C. L., Anderson, A., Powell, J., Bush, D., Ricco, M., Zevin, B., Ayala, C., & Khalili, M. (2020). Recommendations for Implementing Hepatitis C Virus Care in Homeless Shelters: The Stakeholder Perspective. *Hepatology communications*, *4*(5), 646–656. https://doi.org/10.1002/hep4.1492 (accessed on 16th July 2025).

6. Androutsakos, T., Dimitriadis, K., Revenas, K., Vergadis, C., Papadakis, D. D., Sakellariou, S., Vallilas, C., et al. (2023). Liver biopsy: To do or not to do – A single-center study. *Digestive Diseases, 41*, 913–921. https://www.semanticscholar.org/paper/9798a391755323224210dc0d269e21bc36f0a9af (accessed on 16th July 2025).

7. Gioia, S., Nardelli, S., Pasquale, C., Pentassuglio, I., Nicoletti, V., Aprile, F., Merli, M., & Riggio, O. (2018). Natural history of patients with non cirrhotic portal hypertension: Comparison with patients with compensated cirrhosis. *Digestive and liver disease : official journal of the Italian Society of Gastroenterology and the Italian Association for the Study of the Liver*, *50*(8), 839–844. https://doi.org/10.1016/j.dld.2018.01.132 (accessed on 16th July 2025).

8. Onghena, L., Develtere, W., Poppe, C., Geerts, A., Troisi, R., Vanlander, A., Berrevoet, F., Rogiers, X., Van Vlierberghe, H., & Verhelst, X. (2016). Quality of life after liver transplantation: State of the art. *World journal of hepatology*, *8*(18), 749–756. https://doi.org/10.4254/wjh.v8.i18.749 (accessed on 16th July 2025).

9. Bhandari, P., Manandhar, L., & Kandel, D. (2025). Thalassemia – Types, risk factors, symptoms, diagnosis and treatment. *The American Journal of Patient Health Info.* https://www.semanticscholar.org/paper/f0bf1b448ca646244890b8263ca3cb5ff8691c99 (accessed on 16th July 2025).

10. Bilzer, M., Ehrentraut, S., Gerbes, A. L., Kapfhammer, et al. (2002). *Psychiatric and psychosocial outcome of orthotopic liver transplantation.* https://core.ac.uk/download/16432271.pdf (accessed on 16th July 2025).

11. Bright, B., Nair, M. M., Moorthy, S., Sreekumar, K. P., Kulkarni, C., & Nazar, P. K. (2025). Life-saving precision: Image-guided interventions transforming outcomes in living-donor liver transplant complications. *Cureus, 17.* https://www.semanticscholar.org/paper/3ab688d8d3b98557c1112bea5dcd9efda71a323d (accessed on 16th July 2025).

12. Brito-Zerón, P., Gracia-Tello, B., Robles, Á., Alguacil, A., Bonet, M., De-Escalante, B., Noblejas-Mosso, A., et al. (2021). Characterization and outcomes of SARS-CoV-2 infection in patients with sarcoidosis. *Viruses, 13.* https://www.semanticscholar.org/paper/8fb2677abf3adda60d272e6edfaaa7bcbaf72b01 (accessed on 16th July 2025).

13. Butt, N. M., Lambert, J., Ali, S., Beer, P., Cross, N. C. P., Duncombe, A., Ewing, J., et al. (2017). Guideline for the investigation and management of eosinophilia. *British Journal of Hematology, 176*, 553–572. https://doi.org/10.1111/bjh.14488 (accessed on 16th July 2025).

14. Cabezas-Zabala, C. C., Hernández-Torres, B. C., & Vargas-Zárate, M. (2016). Sugars added in food: Health effects and global regulation. *Revista de la Facultad de Medicina, 64*, 319–329. https://www.semanticscholar.org/paper/252fea2950a2ff1761f7bfea31125a360a64de39 (accessed on 16th July 2025).

15. Caputo, F., Lungaro, L., Guarino, M., Costanzini, A., Caio, G., Testino, G., & De Giorgio, R. (2024). Alcohol-related diseases: From metabolism to the main effect on the body. *Minerva Medica.* https://www.semanticscholar.org/paper/b88a37c6eb740232cea19ad3b83acd173a2368ae (accessed on 16th July 2025).

16. Chaurasia, R., Sunil, Junior Sunil, & Resident. (2024). Radiological approach for early diagnosis of liver parenchymal disease. *Asian Journal of Medical Sciences.* https://www.semanticscholar.org/paper/a72c63007c468898b556226e29cbb644088a3e8c (accessed on 16th July 2025).

17. Chen, J., Hou, J., Chen, X., Fan, W., & Sun, P. (2025). Identifying key genes for neurobehavioral disorders caused by long-term sleep deprivation. *Current Analytical Chemistry.* https://www.semanticscholar.org/paper/226aaea61497554fdc3e4ec669387aa3c0f2d43c (accessed on 16th July 2025).

18. Deana, C., Vetrugno, L., Cortegiani, A., Mongodi, S., Salve, G., Mangiagalli, M., Boscolo, A., et al. (2023). Quality of life in COVID-related ARDS patients one year after intensive care discharge (Odissea Study): A multicenter observational study. *Journal of Clinical Medicine, 12.* https://www.semanticscholar.org/paper/6cf8ce186af524698be547e7670a190e297fff77 (accessed on 16th July 2025).

19. Donea, L., Cojocariu, C., Sîngeap, A., Gîrleanu, I., & Trifan, A. (2022). Patient with liver disorders: Exploration tools and treatment. *Annals of the Academy of Romanian Scientists Series on Biological Sciences.* https://www.semanticscholar.org/paper/7bda5521e5e71bc9ddbcfb04aaba150602122637 (accessed on 16th July 2025).

20. Ghany, M. G., & Morgan, T. R. (2019). Hepatitis C guidance 2019 update: American Association for the Study of Liver Diseases–Infectious Diseases Society of America recommendations for testing, managing, and treating hepatitis C virus infection. *Hepatology, 71*, 686–721. https://doi.org/10.1002/hep.31060 (accessed on 16th July 2025).

21. Ho, C. H., Chen, Y. C., Wang, J. J., & Liao, K. (2017). Incidence and relative risk for developing cancer among patients with COPD: A nationwide cohort study in Taiwan. *BMJ Open, 7.* https://www.semanticscholar.org/paper/487b3cb555827cfd6165d34cde259ce048c76042 (accessed on 16th July 2025).

22. Ionova, T., Johns, J., Oliva, E. N., Salek, et al. (2018). *Appraisal of patient-reported outcome measures in analogous diseases and recommendations for use in phase II and III clinical trials of pyruvate kinase deficiency.* https://core.ac.uk/download/287581341.pdf (accessed on 16th July 2025).

23. Jardim, S. R., Perrotta de Souza, L. M., & Pereira de Souza, H. S. (2023). The rise of gastrointestinal cancers as a global phenomenon: Unhealthy behavior or progress? *International Journal of Environmental Research and Public Health, 20,* 3640. https://doi.org/10.3390/ijerph20043640 (accessed on 16th July 2025).

24. Kolokolnikov, G., Schmalhofer, M. L., Well, L., Farschtschi, S., Mautner, V. F., Ristow, I., & Werner, R. (2025). *Anatomy-informed deep learning and radiomics for automated neurofibroma segmentation in whole-body MRI.* ArXiv, abs/2502.15424. https://www.semanticscholar.org/paper/a89930d527924ac488893c683fa0d677c26ca738 (accessed on 16th July 2025).

25. Lai, J. C., Tandon, P., Bernal, W., Tapper, E. B., Ekong, U. D., Dasarathy, S., & Carey, E. J. (2021). Malnutrition, frailty, and sarcopenia in patients with cirrhosis: 2021 practice guidance by the American Association for the Study of Liver Diseases. *Hepatology, 74,* 1611–1644. https://doi.org/10.1002/hep.32049 (accessed on 16th July 2025).

26. Le Floc'h, B., Livin, M., Tzedakis, S., Robin, F., Jeddou, H., & Boudjema, K. (2025). Posterior hepatectomy and inferior vena cava graft reconstruction for en bloc resection of a hepatocellular carcinoma: A tribute to Couinaud's liver anatomy description. *Annals of Surgical Oncology.* https://www.semanticscholar.org/paper/e5d0b397e713bd3ba9c9fb1c70e72824ddf5365c (accessed on 16th July 2025).

27. Lee, Y. T., Wang, J. J., Zhu, Y., Agopian, V. G., Tseng, H. R., & Yang, J. D. (2021). Diagnostic criteria and LI-RADS for hepatocellular carcinoma. *Clinical Liver Disease, 17,* 409–413. https://doi.org/10.1002/cld.1075 (accessed on 16th July 2025).

28. Liu, Y., Luo, R., Sun, Z., Zhang, Y., Guo, Y., Chen, Y., Li, L., et al. (2025). Synergistic toxicity of combined exposure to acrylamide and polystyrene nanoplastics on the gut–liver axis in mice. *Biology, 14.* https://www.semanticscholar.org/paper/254bc738667bac5db0ccc6a7ab6c589719f7ef00 (accessed on 16th July 2025).

29. Lu, Y., Nie, L., Yang, X., Zhao, Z., Wang, Y., Wu, Q., Zhou, X. (2025). *Lingguizhugan* decoction in the treatment of non-alcoholic fatty liver disease: A systematic review and meta-analysis. *Endocrine, Metabolic & Immune Disorders Drug Targets.* https://www.semanticscholar.org/paper/b7796c6ca3a73d72cb62a77b26b96444a908237b (accessed on 16th July 2025).

30. Mantle, D., Hargreaves, I. P., Domingo, J. C., & Castro-Marrero, J. (2024). Mitochondrial dysfunction and Coenzyme Q10 supplementation in post-viral fatigue syndrome: An overview. *International Journal of Molecular Sciences, 25.* https://www.semanticscholar.org/paper/a7798b6564b317467635585df20079b00c4e20c2 (accessed on 16th July 2025).

31. Northup, P. G., García-Pagán, J. C., García–Tsao, G., Intagliata, N. M., Superina, R., Roberts, L. N., Lisman, T., et al. (2020). Vascular liver disorders, portal vein thrombosis, and procedural

bleeding in patients with liver disease: 2020 practice guidance by the American Association for the Study of Liver Diseases. *Hepatology, 73*, 366–413. https://doi.org/10.1002/hep.31646 (accessed on 16th July 2025).

32. Panigrahi, B., Pillai, K., Radhakrishnan, D., Rajan, R., & Srivastava, A. (2024). Fatigue in Parkinson's disease—A narrative review. *Annals of Movement Disorders.* https://www.semanticscholar.org/paper/c5a98d330bfbc02dd0e18b28a54dc800338a3790 (accessed on 16th July 2025).

33. Pape, T., Baumann, U., Pfister, E., Vondran, F. W., Richter, N., Dingemann, J., Hunkemöller, A. M., et al. (2025). Clinical outcomes of percutaneous transhepatic biliary drainage in pediatric patients following liver transplantation. *Pediatric Gastroenterology, Hepatology & Nutrition, 28*, 113–123. https://www.semanticscholar.org/paper/1e2fd5fc313859519a34bd82f77661cd14000126 (accessed on 16th July 2025).

34. Pavithra, S., Boomika, V., Rabin, R., Mariya, D. P., & Surya, N. M. (2024). Non-invasive neonatal golden hue detector. *i-manager's Journal on Image Processing.* https://www.semanticscholar.org/paper/f2f6c7bbb3196a785a50ea576eeec76db275c9fe (accessed on 16th July 2025).

35. Puzanov, I., Diab, A., Abdallah, K., Bingham, C. O., Brogdon, C. F., Dadu, R., Hamad, L., et al. (2017). Managing toxicities associated with immune checkpoint inhibitors: Consensus recommendations from the Society for Immunotherapy of Cancer (SITC) Toxicity Management Working Group. *Journal for ImmunoTherapy of Cancer, 5.* https://doi.org/10.1186/s40425-017-0300-z (accessed on 16th July 2025).

36. Ramoni, D., Liberale, L., & Montecucco, F. (2024). Inflammatory biomarkers as cost-effective predictive tools in metabolic dysfunction-associated fatty liver disease. *World Journal of Gastroenterology, 30*, 5086–5091. https://www.semanticscholar.org/paper/cc00b088016b2935f5d7f09d1f2056d42e7a43b9 (accessed on 16th July 2025).

37. Ribeiro, R., Antas, J., Monteiro, A. P., Magalhães, J., Miranda, D., & Cruz, C. (2024). Fosfomycin-induced liver injury: A case report. *Cureus, 16.* https://www.semanticscholar.org/paper/1a9c0622051fd97438c871d69d018967f1938a39 (accessed on 16th July 2025).

38. Rinella, M. E., Neuschwander-Tetri, B. A., Siddiqui, M. S., Abdelmalek, M. F., Caldwell, S. H., Barb, D., Kleiner, D. E., et al. (2023). AASLD practice guidance on the clinical assessment and management of nonalcoholic fatty liver disease. *Hepatology, 77*, 1797–1835. https://doi.org/10.1097/hep.0000000000000323 (accessed on 16th July 2025).

39. Rosińska, K., Janicka, E. J., Skibicka, J. N., Niedźwiedzka, M., & Rosiński, M. (2025). Disorders of adipose tissue and lipodystrophies: Causes, consequences, and treatment perspectives. *Quality in Sport.* https://www.semanticscholar.org/paper/65bb6dd98894ed4e6045649bf419e6f5c754a0c4 (accessed on 16th July 2025).

40. Suroviaková, S., Zoľák, V., Igaz, M., Kršiaková, J., & Bánovčin, P. (2025). COVID-19 infection as a possible trigger for POLG-related mitochondrial disease: A case report. *Cureus, 17.* https://www.semanticscholar.org/paper/7ee12112823dee8b0504778eb48cf1f311a35c0a (accessed on 16th July 2025).

41. Tombesi, P., Cutini, A., Di Vece, F., Grasso, V., Politti, U., Capatti, E., & Sartori, S. (2025). Surgery or percutaneous ablation for liver tumors? The key points are: When, where, and how large. *Cancers, 17.* https://www.semanticscholar.org/paper/214bb196b3569fd963a995208a2652d9b2a83b41 (accessed on 16th July 2025).

42. Toropova, A. A., Razuvaeva, Y., Khaltagarova, E. D., & Olennikov, D. (2025). *Improvement of antioxidant protection and energy production in neurodegenerative processes in the brain caused by long-term alcoholism under the influence of Lophantus chinensis Benth extract.* Сибирский научный медицинский журнал. https://www.semanticscholar.org/paper/c8baaa22b271bb76b4b20d0493970a54cab91750 (accessed on 16th July 2025).

43. Usama, M., Saeed, S., Fatima, R., Ahmad, I., Iqbal, S., Imran, M., & Hameed, F. (2025). Association of lipid profile abnormalities with NAFLD severity in patients with metabolic syndrome. *Physical Education, Health and Social Sciences.* https://www.semanticscholar.org/paper/aec4d20a1f2ab37ac8f2552e56f0ca9958d9e139 (accessed on 16th July 2025).

44. Varra, F., Varras, M., Varra, V., & Theodosis-Nobelos, P. (2024). Molecular and pathophysiological relationship between obesity and chronic inflammation in the manifestation of metabolic dysfunctions and their inflammationmediating treatment options (Review). *Molecular Medicine Reports, 29.* https://www.semanticscholar.org/paper/278c41556edeec2e0975c1afab9cd5c41bfc0e31 (accessed on 16th July 2025).

45. Visseren, F. L. J., Mach, F., Smulders, Y. M., Carballo, D., Koskinas, K. C., Bäck, M., Bénétos, A., et al. (2021). 2021 ESC guidelines on cardiovascular disease prevention in clinical practice. *European Heart Journal, 42*, 3227–3337. https://doi.org/10.1093/eurheartj/ehab484 (accessed on 16th July 2025).

46. Wadhawan, M. (2025). Updates in chronic cholestatic liver diseases: Indian expert recommendations for diagnosing and managing complex cases. *International Journal of Research in Medical Sciences.* https://www.semanticscholar.org/paper/68aee3821f140704a6dbfb5232b719a711536615 (accessed on 16th July 2025).

47. Yang, M., Liu, S., & Zhang, C. (2022). The related metabolic diseases and treatments of obesity. *Healthcare, 10*, 1616. https://doi.org/10.3390/healthcare10091616 (accessed on 16th July 2025).

48. Yang, Y. Q., Meng, F., Liu, X., Zhang, M., Gu, W., Yan, H.-l., Yu, J., et al. (2021). Distinct metabonomic signatures of *Polygoni Multiflori Radix Praeparata* against glucolipid metabolic disorders. *The Journal of Pharmacy and Pharmacology.* https://www.semanticscholar.org/paper/a95f8de57727471f9478d25a65476900b891fe33 (accessed on 16th July 2025).

49. You, Y. T., Hardiman, K. M., Bafford, A. C., Poylin, V., Francone, T. D., Davis, K. G., Paquette, I. M., et al. (2020). The American Society of Colon and Rectal Surgeons clinical practice guidelines for the management of rectal cancer. *Diseases of the Colon & Rectum, 63*, 1191–1222. https://doi.org/10.1097/dcr.0000000000001762 (accessed on 16th July 2025).

50. Younossi, Z. M., Wong, G. L. H., Anstee, Q. M., & Henry, L. (2023). The global burden of liver disease. *Clinical Gastroenterology and Hepatology, 21*, 1978–1991. https://doi.org/10.1016/j.cgh.2023.04.015 (accessed on 16th July 2025).

51. Zarmehri, B., Shahi, B., Rahmani, S., Dehghan Tafti, F., & Foroughian, M. (2020). Association of platelet count and mean platelet volume (MPV) index with types of stroke. *Caspian Journal of Internal Medicine, 11*, 398–402. https://www.semanticscholar.org/paper/768372f81e175aae8fd184f63acaf92613ecdcf1 (accessed on 16th July 2025).

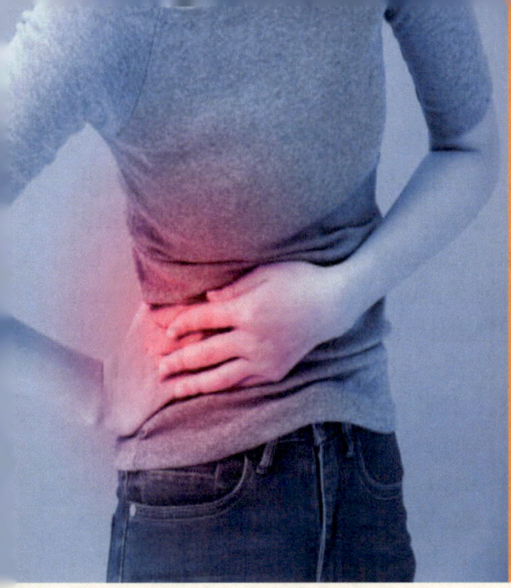

Chapter 9
PANCREATIC DISORDERS

Contents

Introduction

The pancreas is a vital organ that plays a major role in digestion and glucose metabolism and is thus vital for general health. The fact that it has a dual function as an exocrine and endocrine gland means that it has the responsibility to secrete digestive enzymes and hormones, including insulin. If its function is compromised by a host of disorders, patients are likely to develop significant diseases ranging from digestive issues to diabetes. An understanding of such disorders requires an interdisciplinary strategy, combining insights from gastroenterology, endocrinology, and nutrition science. A consideration of pancreatic disorders, their etiology, pathophysiology, and clinical presentation provides the background for a further focus on their impact on patient quality of life and health, and leads to effective management and intervention strategies. In addition, dietary impacts and pancreatic health are hand in hand. Recent literature is placing increasing importance on the dietary role in preventing as well as managing disorders of the pancreas. For example, recent evidence is raising debate on the role of dietary fiber consumption in patients with pancreatic disorders. Although some high fiber diets are helpful in the management of acute pancreatitis by maintaining intestinal barrier homeostasis, other disorders like exocrine pancreatic insufficiency may be worsened by high consumption of fiber due to suppressed activity of pancreatic enzymes. This duality reinforces the necessity of patient-specific nutritional approaches in patients with pancreatic disease at risk or affected, since a compromise between dietary modification and the complexity of pancreatic disease and function. Because of this complex interaction between diet and pancreatic health, further exploration of the mechanisms of such interactions is necessary. For example, recent studies of the non-starch polysaccharides (NSP) reveal their potential impact on digestive efficiency and gut health in a variety of situations, including farm animals , such as pigs. This study emphasizes the broader significance of food components on gastrointestinal function that can presumably have a valid carry-over to human health, specifically of the pancreas. Investigating the significance of these findings for diseases of the pancreas could further enlighten us on effective dietary management that not only abates symptoms but also promotes healing and improves quality of life in those afflicted with such diseases, with significant implications for further research in this critical area of health science (Figure 9.1).

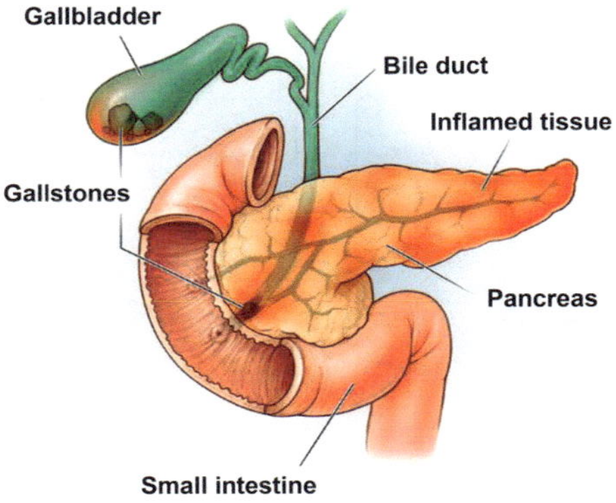

Figure 9.1. Pancreatic disorders.

Source: https://my.clevelandclinic.org/-/scassets/images/org/health/articles/8103-pancreatitis-illustration.

Definition of Pancreatic Disorders

Pancreatic diseases encompass a range of medical ailments that adversely affect the pancreas's structure and function, which is a vital organ in digestion and glucose metabolism. The most common diseases include acute and chronic pancreatitis, pancreatic cancer, and pancreatic insufficiency. Acute pancreatitis includes acute inflammation of the pancreas, usually due to gallstones or excessive alcohol intake. This disease may cause intense abdominal pain and other body-wide complications that need to be addressed by medical professionals as soon as possible. Chronic pancreatitis is a chronic inflammation of the pancreas that results in irreparable damage to pancreatic tissue, leading to long-term health effects, including malabsorption and diabetes. These conditions are interdependent; they can interact with the gut microbiome and influence digestive well-being overall, proving the significance of the pancreas in maintaining homeostasis. Nutritional management of pancreatic diseases reflects a shifting understanding of their complexity. Recent studies have established that dietary management, and particularly fiber intake, possesses therapeutic possibilities in individuals with such diseases. For acute pancreatitis, a prebiotic diet could maintain the integrity of the intestinal barrier and block infection, potentially altering the disease course (Ribichini et al., 2019). Contrariwise, in chronic pancreatitis, excessive dietary fiber can paradoxically lead to increased fecal fat loss due to its inhibition of pancreatic enzyme activity. This duality indicates the need for patient-specific nutritional management with consideration for the character of the pancreatic disease and each patient's physiological adaptation, influencing long-term health states further. In addition, the pathophysiology of pancreatic disorders extends beyond the organ itself, into the broader arena of the brain-gut axis and general well-being. Current evidence suggests that the gut microbiota play a significant role in the regulation of both the pancreas and the central nervous system, particularly in conditions like Parkinson's disease. The implications of this two-way communication refer to the mechanisms whereby dysregulated gut microbiota can feed back to drive the pathophysiology of pancreatic disorders and vice versa (Caputi & Giron, 2018). Illuminating these interconnected associations may generate novel therapeutic avenues that not only regulate pancreatic function but also reverse systemic repercussions stemming from gut health. This integrative strategy stresses that pancreatic disorders should be addressed in the context of a global program for disease prevention and control.

Importance of the Pancreas in the Digestive System

The pancreas is a vital digestive organ of the digestive system and also an exocrine and endocrine organ. As an exocrine organ, the pancreas produces a variety of digestive enzymes, including amylase, lipase, and proteases, which break down carbohydrates, fats, and proteins, respectively. The enzymes are released into the small intestine through the pancreatic duct, which allows efficient digestion and nutrient absorption. This enzymatic function emphasizes the pancreass function to secure nutritional balance within the body. Disruptions in enzyme secretion can lead to severe malabsorption and deficiencies, emphasizing the importance of normal pancreatic function (Rindi et al., 2018). In addition to its digestive functions, the pancreas also regulates blood sugar levels by virtue of its endocrine functions. The islets of Langerhans, clusters of cells in the pancreas, secrete hormones , such as insulin and glucagon, which are responsible for regulating glucose metabolism. Insulin allows cells to take in glucose, while glucagon causes the release of glucose when blood glucose levels are abnormally low. The balance of these hormones is crucial in bringing about homeostasis and preventing metabolic disease. Pancreatic hormonal imbalance could result in ailments , such as diabetes mellitus, which further increases the significance of the pancreas not just in digestion but also in metabolic well-being (Vos et al., 2017). It is even more important to possess a clear understanding of its working and its extension to the digestive system, owing to the condition of pancreatic disorders. Ailments , such as pancreatitis, pancreatic cancer, and endocrine disorders demonstrate the complex and vital function of this organ. Pancreatitis, for instance, may suppress the secretion of enzymes, thus leading to digestive issues and severe stomach pain. Pancreatic cancer also typically presents challenges in its early detection, as its manifestation may mimic other GI conditions. These conditions indicate the significant role of the pancreas in digestion and metabolism and the necessity of ongoing research and clinical monitoring for preserving pancreatic function (Vos et al., 2017; Rindi et al., 2018) (Figure 8.2).

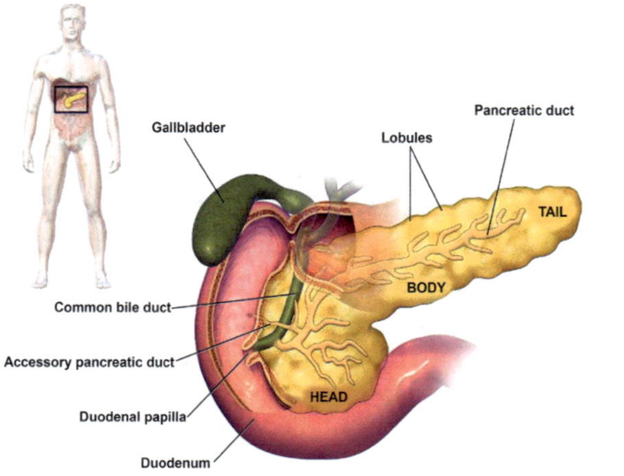

Figure 9.2. Importance of the pancreas in the digestive system.

Source: https://upload.wikimedia.org/wikipedia/commons/7/7e/Blausen_0699_PancreasAnatomy2.png.

9.1. Anatomy and Physiology of the Pancreas

Anatomy of the pancreas reveals a very specialized and very significant organ to the endocrine as well as the digestive system. The pancreas is made up of four distinct regions known as head, body, tail, and uncinate process. The primary function of the pancreas is to release the digestive enzymes like amylase, lipase, and proteases into the small intestine to facilitate the digestion of carbohydrates, fats, and proteins. The pancreas also contains islands of cells referred to as islets of Langerhans that release hormones , such as insulin and glucagon. These play a vital role in maintaining glucose homeostasis in the body. Awareness of the anatomical structure of the pancreas aids in the comprehension of its physiological function as well as the explanation of potential channels for pathology that might be caused by any form of abnormality in its anatomy or physiology. The pancreas's physiology cannot be divorced from its two functions. In its exocrine state, the pancreas releases a mixture of digestive enzymes into the duodenum to assist in the successful digestion of food. This process is strictly controlled by hormonal messages from other organs, including the release of cholecystokinin and secretin that promote the release of enzymes and bile. By contrast, endocrine function controls metabolic processes through the excretion of insulin and glucagon into the circulatory system. These must remain in balance; thus, inability to release insulin can lead to hyperglycemia and ultimately diabetes mellitus. Furthermore, the entwining of these endocrine and exocrine functions makes the pancreatic role in homeostasis and metabolism all the more important and implies the possible effect of pancreatic dysfunction on health. Pancreatic disease can be caused by different etiologic factors and has significant health implications. Pancreatitis, pancreatic carcinoma, and type 2 diabetes mellitus constitute the range of pancreatic disease, all with distinctive anatomical and physiological effects.

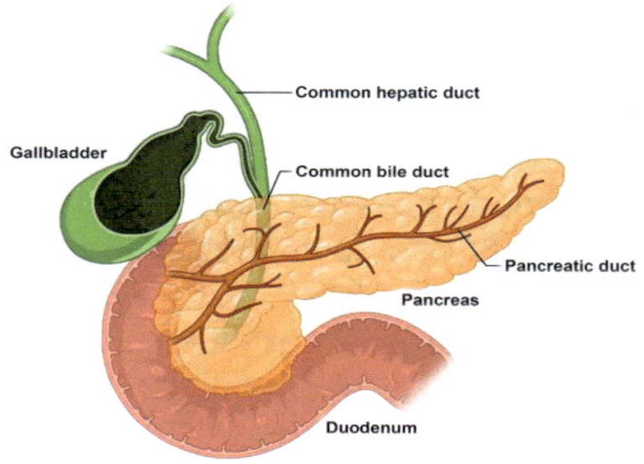

Figure 9.3. Anatomy and physiology of the pancreas.

Source: https://microbenotes.com/wp-content/uploads/2024/04/Pancreas-Anatomy.jpeg.

As discussed before, obesity has a significant effect on pancreatic health, leading to type 2 diabetes mellitus due to increased insulin resistance (Kansra et al., 2021). In addition, vascular supply abnormalities to the pancreas, especially with the portal vein, can lead to impaired regulation of nutrient supply and hormonal balance (Carneiro et al., 2019). Therefore, a comprehensive knowledge of the anatomy and physiology of the pancreas is critical to the development of appropriate prevention and treatment strategies for pancreatic diseases, thus determining patient outcomes and quality of life (Figure 9.3).

9.1.1. Location and Structure of the Pancreas

The pancreas is a vital organ located within the abdomen, running along the back of the stomach. It is bordered on the right side by the duodenum and on the left side by the spleen, making its anatomical location central to digestive function. The pancreas is roughly six to eight inches in length and is further classified into three primary regions: head, body, and tail. The head of the pancreas rests in the curve of the duodenum, where it has a central role in secreting digestive enzymes. The body and tail advance towards the spleen, while the tail is in close anatomical relation with the splenic artery and vein. This specific architecture not only points towards the pancreas's function in digestion but also towards its importance in metabolic control, as it releases hormones that are critical in glucose homeostasis, thus implying its integrated function in human physiology. The pancreas is structurally an exocrine as well as an endocrine gland, which contributes to its function of being multi-functional in the body. The exocrine portion accounts for approximately 98% of the organ mass and is responsible for the secretion of digestive enzymes , such as amylase, lipase, and proteases, which are required to break down carbohydrates, fats, and proteins in the small intestine. The endocrine component consists of clusters of cells that form the islets of Langerhans, which play an important role in hormonal regulation. The islets produce insulin and glucagon, which are needed to regulate blood glucose concentrations. This dual role is central to the explanation of many pancreatic disorders because dysfunction in either the exocrine or endocrine system can yield significant diseases ranging from pancreatitis to diabetes mellitus. The anatomical intricacy of the pancreas lends itself to the integration of these functions and hence, this anatomy is crucial in deciphering pancreatic diseases. Complicating matters further, pancreatic structure and its relationship to adjacent organs significantly engage in the pathophysiology of pancreatic disease.

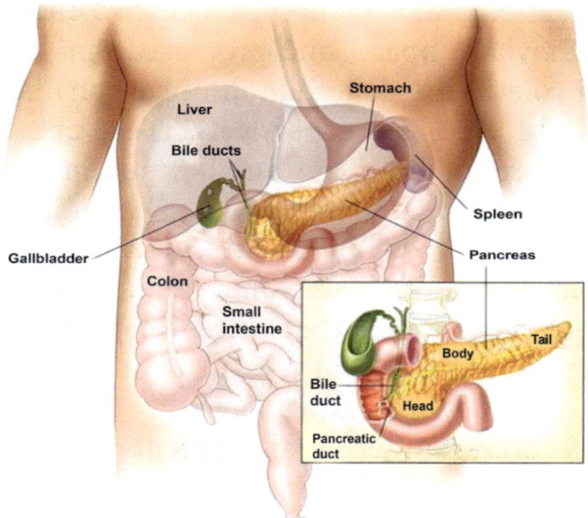

Figure 9.4. Location and structure of the pancreas.

Source: https://healthjade.com/wp-content/uploads/2017/10/pancreas-location.jpg.

Pancreatitis, as illustrated in acute and chronic pancreatitis, can be induced by many etiologic factors like gallstones, alcoholism, and metabolic derangements. Inflammation by whatever origin tends to interfere with the delicate architecture of the pancreas and to have harmful effects on both exocrine and endocrine functions. Chen et al. (2017) indicates the manner in which inflammatory mechanisms in the pancreas have the potential to trigger a cascade of signaling responses that ultimately lead to dysfunction. The complexity of pancreatic structure demands a detailed analysis of the way and reason diseases arise and propagate in this organ. Recognition of the complex relationships between the pancreas and other anatomical structures is central to successful diagnosis and treatment of pancreatic disease (Figure 9.4).

9.1.2. Functions of the Pancreas in Digestion

The pancreas plays a pivotal role in digestion in that it is both an exocrine and an endocrine gland. Its exocrine function is mainly the production and secretion of digestive enzymes like amylase, lipase, and proteases that play a vital role in the degradation of carbohydrates, fats, and proteins, respectively. These enzymes are secreted into the small intestine after food intake, where they are activated and the process of digestion starts. Additionally, the pancreas releases bicarbonate that neutralizes stomach acid so that intestinal enzymes function optimally in a neutral pH. Without these processes, nutrient absorption would be severely hindered, and the person would end up being malnourished and developing related disorders. Malabsorption in instances of defects in pancreatic enzyme production is a phenomenon that is frequently observed in pancreatic disease patients, attesting to the significance of the pancreas in digestive function. Its vital role in the absorption of nutrients is brought out through the complex interaction with the digestive system. In healthy individuals, pancreatic digestive enzymes have an obligatory function to digest food into smaller molecules for effortless absorption by the intestine. In cases where pancreatic function is lost, such as in chronic pancreatitis or pancreatic insufficiency, patients can develop severe digestive disorders. The malabsorption of essential nutrients leads to the signs and symptoms of diarrhea, weight loss, and fat-soluble vitamin deficiency. Not only does this loss of digestive capacity exacerbate the initial conditions, but it also leads to new conditions like malnutrition and impaired immune status, which are crucial for overall health. Hence, the understanding of the role of the pancreas in digestion is extremely important in order to manage various pancreatic disorders effectively. Apart from this, nutrition is also a vital component of the functioning mode of the pancreas, particularly in the context of pancreatic pathology. For instance, dietary fiber intake is reported to influence pancreatic well-being. According to some reports, a prebiotic-enriched diet has been decreasing the rates of complications like pancreatic necrosis and systemic inflammatory response syndrome in acute pancreatitis.

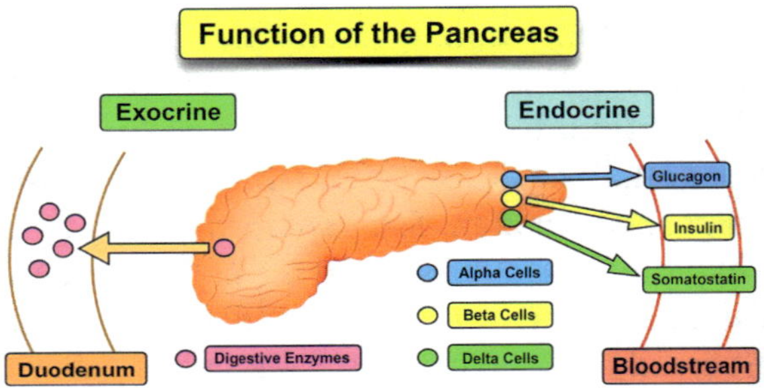

Figure 9.5. Functions of the pancreas in digestion.

Source: https://images.squarespace-cdn.com/content/v1/5e48489da899cd09424943db/3e1b4ea6-b4bd-441d-bbd7-29a8d6e3e1da/pancreas-function-digestive-endocrine-insulin.jpeg.

Conversely, a high-fiber diet may aggravate symptoms in patients with exocrine pancreatic insufficiency because it increases fecal fat excretion due to fiber interference with pancreatic enzyme activity. This complex interaction attests to the need for individualized dietary maneuvers responsive to the specific conditions affecting pancreatic function. As researchers look into the nutritional connections to pancreatic health, nutrition management becomes increasingly significant in both prevention and therapy of pancreatic disease, as it offers patients with balanced care that maintains their gastrointestinal systems (Rémond et al., 2015; Ribichini et al., 2019) (Figure 9.5).

9.1.3. Role of the Pancreas in Blood Sugar Regulation

The pancreas plays a vital role in maintaining glucose homeostasis, which is critical for overall metabolic well-being. The endocrine and exocrine gland located behind the stomach releases digestive enzymes and hormones, mainly insulin and glucagon, that are responsible for regulating blood sugar levels. Insulin, secreted by the beta cells of the islets of Langerhans, promotes the uptake of glucose into the cells and, thereby, lowers blood sugar levels after meals. Conversely, glucagon released by the alpha cells prompts the liver to release glucose that is being stored within it, hence increasing blood glucose levels whenever they fall too low. This minute regulation of insulin and glucagon release is critical in the prevention of hyperglycemia and hypoglycemia states, demonstrating the pancreas's vital role in the control of metabolism. Abnormality in the functioning of the pancreas can potentially lead to dangerous diseases, most prominently observed in diseases like diabetes mellitus. In Type 1 diabetes, the immune system destroys the beta cells, severely restricting insulin production and leading to elevated blood sugar levels. The pancreas is still able to release sufficient insulin in Type 2 diabetes, but the body cells become resistant to it, necessitating more insulin production. Over time, the pancreas can become exhausted, further compromising blood sugar regulation. The effects of pancreatic impairment extend beyond diabetes; research has also determined relationships between pancreatic integrity and other conditions within the body, demonstrating the multidimensional impact of pancreatic disease on metabolic homeostasis and overall health. Yang et al. (2020) demonstrate how pancreatic dysfunction can affect many different metabolic processes, including insulin resistance. Improved understanding of how the pancreas regulates blood glucose will inform treatment strategies for pancreatic diseases. As medical research continues to advance, various interventions that aim to maximize pancreatic function and insulin sensitivity have been explored. Targeted therapies that aim to preserve beta-cell function or augment insulin signaling pathways are prime examples with great promise. In addition, alterations in lifestyle, such as diet and exercise, have also been discovered to influence pancreatic health and consequently, blood glucose control in a positive manner. Emerging studies also investigate the intricate signaling networks that underlie pancreatic function, with potential for novel treatment approaches to diabetes as well as other conditions. As found in Amaravadi et al. (2019), a growing body of research that surfaces illustrates how to affect metabolic pathways intricately related to pancreatic function can provide new therapeutic strategies in treating pancreatic disease and its systemic consequences.

9.2. Types of Pancreatic Disorders

Pancreatic diseases encompass a wide range of disorders, each with distinctive etiologies and clinical manifestations. Among the primary categories are acute and chronic pancreatitis, which are inflammatory conditions of the pancreas. The acute pancreatitis is most commonly due to gallstones or excessive alcohol consumption, leading to intense abdominal pain, vomiting, and potential systemic involvement. Alternatively, there is chronic pancreatitis, an ongoing inflammatory process possibly resulting from repeated episodes of acute pancreatitis, often alcohol or genetic in origin. Chronic pancreatitis can lead to permanent impairment of pancreatic tissue, which has its functionality compromised by the task of producing digestive enzymes and hormones, the ultimate outcome of which is diabetes and malnutrition (Alvaro et al., 2018). Thus, awareness of these acute and chronic presentations is essential for early diagnosis and appropriate treatment of pancreatic disease. Another salient characteristic of pancreatic disease is the development of pancreatic tumors, which can be benign or malignant. The most important malignancy is pancreatic adenocarcinoma, with a poor outcome due to late presentation and aggressive proliferation. This type of cancer tends to be a result of exocrine cells of the pancreas, with most cases predominantly occurring in those with risk factors, including smoking, chronic pancreatitis, or family tendency. Cholangiocarcinoma (CCA), while mostly occurring in bile ducts, also tends to have forms affecting pancreatic function, mainly in its intrahepatic type. Intrahepatic CCA is biologically distinct and requires a fine understanding of its pathogenesis, given that it tends to arise from alternative stem cell niches compared to other pancreatic carcinomas (Alvaro et al., 2018). The complexity of pancreatic tumors provides evidence for specialized screening and novel therapies in the treatment of these conditions. Endocrine pancreatic diseases, such as diabetes mellitus, are also a significant class of pancreatic diseases. Glucose metabolism is mediated by the pancreas through the secretion of insulin and glucagon from the islets of Langerhans. Autoimmune destruction of beta-cells in Type 1 diabetes causes absolute insulin deficiency, while Type 2 diabetes results from insulin resistance accompanied by relative insulin deficiency, often associated with obesity and lifestyle. Interestingly, in more recent studies, the nutritional content may play a vital role in the causation of acute pancreatitis complications, with unsaturated fatty acids (UFAs), particularly monounsaturated fatty acids (MUFAs), influencing disease severity and prognosis (Argüelles-Arias et al., 2020). The relationship between diet and endocrine function will be key in designing successful management regimens for individuals with pancreatic disorders (Figure 9.6).

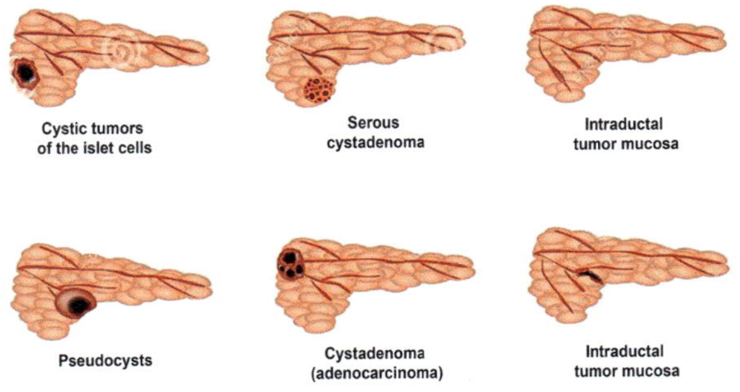

Figure 9.6. Types of pancreatic disorders.

Source: https://thumbs.dreamstime.com/z/types-neoplasms-pancreas-infographics-set-vector-illustration-isolated-background-74056850.jpg.

9.2.1. Acute Pancreatitis

Acute pancreatitis is a serious condition characterized by the acute inflammation of the pancreas and is capable of causing acute abdominal pain, systemic disease, and even death in severe cases. The primary etiologic causes of the disease are gallstones and alcohol consumption and are accountable for the majority of the cases. Pathophysiologic processes of acute pancreatitis involve the premature activation of pancreatic enzymes within the pancreas itself that results in self-digestion and inflammation. When the pancreas is swollen, it may disrupt its usual operations, including digestion and endocrine regulation, emphasizing its very important role in the body's metabolic processes. Treatment of acute pancreatitis is usually successful and requires hospitalization, where patients are provided with supportive therapy, including pain management and intravenous fluids, to alleviate symptoms and allow the organ to recover. This emphasizes the importance of prompt medical intervention in acute pancreatitis to prevent complications and permanent damage from unresolved inflammation (Yrkm, 2024). Depending on the progression of acute pancreatitis, prognosis largely depends on its severity, which can be classified into mild, moderate, and severe forms. Mild acute pancreatitis can spontaneously recover with successful medical management, but necrosis of the pancreas, infection, and multi-organ failure may complicate severe attacks. An early evaluation of the severity of acute pancreatitis is important in order to permit optimal therapy. There have been considerable advancements over the last few years in diagnostic imaging modalities , such as computed tomography (CT) and magnetic resonance imaging (MRI), which have significantly improved our ability to assess the extent of injury to the pancreas and the resulting complications. Moreover, investigations are increasingly focused on the gut microbiota as an influencer of the course of acute pancreatitis. Knowledge of how the complex interplay between microbial communities and pancreatic well-being can help guide future therapeutic strategies towards better recovery and reduced recurrence (Boicean et al., 2024). There are several challenges that still exist with effective management of this multi-factorial disorder, despite the progress in our knowledge and treatment of acute pancreatitis. Factors like nutrition, timing of intervention, and management of pancreatic necrosis must be weighed suitably to optimize patient recovery. Research on individualized medicine interventions like fecal microbiota transplantation (FMT) has gained momentum as a potential course of treatment for the enhancement of disease outcomes in a host of pancreatic disorders, ranging from acute pancreatitis. Through correcting an imbalanced gut microbiome, FMT may lower inflammation and promote pancreatic recovery. However, use of such new therapies must be done with rigorous clinical trials to resolve the ideal practices and long-term effects. As our understanding of acute pancreatitis develops further, an integrated understanding of its mechanisms and effective treatments will be essential to enhance the care of patients and diminish the health burden of this serious health problem (Yrkm, 2024).

9.2.2. Chronic Pancreatitis

Chronic pancreatitis is characterized by ongoing pancreatic tissue injury and irreversible loss of exocrine and endocrine function. Long-term alcohol use, autoimmune conditions, and inherited disorders most frequently lead to it. Worsening abdominal pain, inability to absorb nutrients, and weight loss are the consequences of the inability to secrete digestive enzymes. Over time, the inflammation can also lead to the development of diabetes mellitus type 3c (T3cDM), with pancreatic injury impacting insulin secretion and regulation. For successful management and treatment to occur, it is critical to recognize the connection between chronic pancreatitis and its complications. Studies highlight that chronic pancreatitis significantly impacts a patient's nutritional status, particularly the consumption of dietary fiber. A high-fiber diet, while proposed to normalize the intestinal barrier, can be harmful in patients with exocrine pancreatic insufficiency. This is since a high-fiber diet will clog pancreatic enzymes needed for the digestion and absorption of nutrients. Interestingly, patients who have malabsorption often excrete more fecal fat than is required, which further aggravates their condition. Management of these nutritional restrictions is crucial in the case of chronic pancreatitis and requires an individualized nutritional approach to deal with the metabolic as well as the digestive needs of involved patients (Ribichini et al., 2019). Furthermore, the association between T3cDM and chronic pancreatitis complicates the clinical picture even more. As observed in studies, a large proportion of patients with chronic pancreatitis develop secondary diabetes, primarily as a consequence of the destruction of insulin-secreting beta cells of the pancreas. In a cohort study, investigators have reported high rates of obesity and insulin resistance in patients with chronic pancreatitis, indicating that metabolic derangement is a significant problem in such patients (Diaconu et al., 2018). Thus, physicians should be attentive towards the screening for diabetes and managing its management in combination with chronic pancreatitis treatment. Such a combined process can lead to improved patient outcomes and quality of life (Figure 9.7).

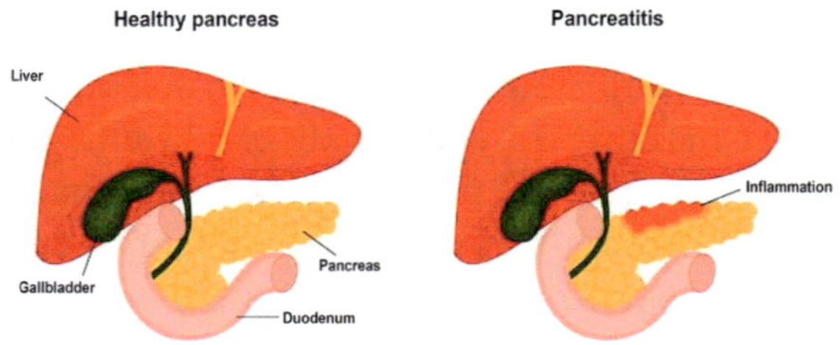

Figure 9.7. Chronic pancreatitis.

Source: https://drrajasekhargastro.com/images/managing-chronic-pancreatitis.jpg.

9.2.3. Pancreatic Cancer

Pancreatic carcinoma, characterized by the malignant growth of cells in the pancreas, is one of the most lethal forms of cancer since it is often diagnosed late and progresses very quickly. The pancreas plays a central function in digestion and insulin release, and cancer in the pancreas disrupts these critical activities, leading to calamitous physiological consequences. Risk factors most associated with pancreatic cancer include age, smoking, obesity, and certain genetic vulnerabilities. Moreover, chronic pancreatitis, especially autoimmune pancreatitis, has been found to be a potential pre-malignant lesion for pancreatic cancer, which highlights the necessity to explain mechanisms behind the two diseases. Identification of such risk factors is crucial in guiding preventive strategies and screening interventions, which may ultimately result in earlier diagnosis and improved survival rates among high-risk subjects for pancreatic cancer. Pancreatic cancer has an indolent clinical course with the onset of symptoms only during the late phases of the disease. Patients can have nonspecific manifestations , such as abdominal pain, jaundice, weight loss, and gastrointestinal disturbance and so may not be easily diagnosed in a timely fashion. The linkage between chronic pancreatitis and pancreatic cancer is particularly important; chronic inflammation and pancreatic tissue injury can provide the basis for neoplastic change. As chronic pancreatitis can also have symptoms overlapping with pancreatic cancer, differential diagnosis is necessary. Moreover, the sensitivity of advanced diagnostic imaging modalities , such as CT and MRI, significantly affects the detection of tumors at an early stage. Multidisciplinary management in such instances is needed, in which oncologists, gastroenterologists, and radiologists collaborate to distinguish between the two ailments and establish good management practices, highlighting the intricacy of pancreatic diseases in a clinical setting.

The therapeutic context for pancreatic cancer remains challenging, largely due to the metastatic potential of the cancers and the relative lack of effectiveness of conventional therapies. Surgical resection, when feasible, is the best hope for cure by long-term survival; regretfully, relatively few patients are diagnosed with localized, potentially resectable disease. Adjuvant and neoadjuvant chemotherapy and radiation are employed for the management of unresectable cases, but these modalities do not generally offer much survival benefit. The introduction of the targeted therapies and immunotherapy, accompanied by an increasingly more clinical trials, is a ray of hope in the fight against pancreatic cancer. Additionally, understanding the connection between chronic pancreatitis and pancreatic cancer is essential as Gallo et al. (2024) suggest the need for improved understanding of autoimmune cancer. Through enhancement of treatment models and improvement of early detection practices, clinicians can facilitate better patient prognosis for this deadly disease, supporting the need for multidisciplinary management suggested in Capurso et al. (2023).

9.3. Causes and Risk Factors

The etiology of pancreatic diseases is complex and often intertwined with lifestyle and genetic predispositions. One strong risk factor is obesity, which has spread globally and contributes to some of the metabolic derangements directly affecting the pancreas. Obesity is associated with inflammation and insulin resistance, which may induce inflammation of the pancreas or pancreatitis. This can cause impaired enzyme secretion, complicating existing diseases , such as pancreatic exocrine insufficiency (PEI). The second reason why PEI complicates patient care is that its own manifestations, weight loss, maldigestion, and steatorrhea, are apt to be confusingly like other complications. Obesity is not only a precipitant of pancreatic disease but also clinically challenging in presenting diagnosis, hence the need for careful evaluation and observation to differentiate underlying conditions. Genetic disorders also contribute to the development of pancreatic disease. Hereditary pancreatitis is just such a condition predisposed by specific genetic mutations, which significantly increase the risk of acute and chronic pancreatitis. Mutations of the PRSS1, SPINK1, and CFTR genes have been associated with such hereditary forms of disease, suggesting direct genetic association with pancreatic dysfunction. Further, family history of pancreatic disease also increases risk, suggesting that genetic susceptibility may result in deleterious pancreatic health over generations. An understanding of such genetic factors is important, especially in recurrent abdominal pain or idiopathic gastrointestinal disease patients, since early diagnosis may be able to prevent more serious pancreatic disease. Introduction of genetic screening into the routine evaluation of high-risk groups may lead to more targeted and effective treatments. Basal diseases like diabetes mellitus add to the risk factors associated with pancreatic disease. The interaction between the exocrine and endocrine functions of the pancreas is multifaceted; diabetes can cause defective exocrine function, with the subsequent development of PEI. Diabetic patients commonly experience gastrointestinal complications, such as malabsorption and dysmotility, which may be contributing factors to the development of symptoms of pancreatic insufficiency. Besides, the correlation between diabetes and obesity represents a vicious cycle where the high incidence of obesity gives rise to the exponential rate of diabetes, increasing the collective burden of pancreatic disease. The interlocking relationships between such ailments represent the need for interconnected strategies that address not only pancreatic wellness but metabolic syndrome in general as well. Because both obesity and diabetes present pancreatic function with unique threats, treatments aimed at managing weight and blood glucose are particularly important. They aid in reducing the risk of pancreatic disease overall.

9.3.1. Genetic Predispositions

Knowing genetic dispositions is very important to grasp the etiology of pancreatic illness, particularly in dogs. Genetic dispositions significantly determine whether one develops illnesses , such as pancreatitis and diabetes mellitus. The German Shepherd Dog (GSD), for instance, is known to have multiple roles, but its diseases, including genetic illnesses, have been of concern to breeders and veterinarians. Population studies have indicated that proper demographic data can enhance breed-specific susceptibility knowledge and guide clinical priorities. Through analysis of the genetic makeup that predisposes certain breeds to pancreatic disease, veterinary medicine can facilitate improved breeding decisions and health outcomes for such animals, resulting in overall welfare and lifespan (O'Neill et al., 2017). When it comes to pancreatic diseases, such as diabetes mellitus, genetic susceptibilities hold the central position in the occurrence and expression of disease. Research has shown that certain breeds, i.e., Yorkshire terriers, are at greater risk of developing diabetes, whereas others, such as GSDs and golden retrievers, have a lower probability. These findings emphasize the importance of genetic factors in determining the incidence of the disease, as well as the prognosis and survival of infected dogs. Quantitative analysis from digital patient records in many practices has provided a standard against which to identify how genetic vulnerabilities interact with other risk factors, such as obesity or co-morbid conditions , such as pancreatitis. This combined approach to establishing genetic predisposition allows for better management plans for specific breeds and specific cases, much appreciated by veterinary clinicians and owners (Brodbelt et al., 2014).

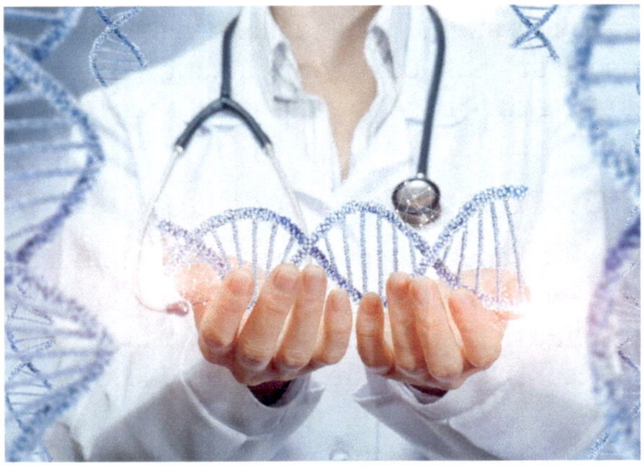

Figure 9.8. Genetic predispositions.

Source: https://centerforfamilymedicine.com/wp-content/uploads/2021/02/center-for-family-medicine-What-Does-It-Mean-To-Have-A-Genetic-Predisposition-Family-History-And-Your-Health.jpg.

Furthermore, the dynamic interaction of genetic predispositions and environmental factors introduces a complex factor to the development of pancreatic disease. For example, neutered male cats, especially in some breeds, have presented with higher risks for diabetes, which implies that hormonal effects must be compounded by genetic factors to complicate health risks. In combination with other comorbidities, including pancreatitis and urinary tract infection, this presents the compound picture of how genetics interact with lifestyle or medical history to define health outcomes. This integrative information facilitates targeted interventions, accentuating the contribution of genetics to susceptibility to pancreatic disease as well as the effectiveness of prevention interventions. By embracing a strategic approach that considers both genetic and environmental components, veterinary practice can extend management protocols and secure better health outcomes for susceptible breeds (Brodbelt et al., 2014) (Figure 9.8).

9.3.2. Lifestyle Factors (Diet, Alcohol Consumption)

Dietary habits play an important role in the causation of pancreatic disorders, particularly pancreatic cancer. A diet high in processed food, red meat, and saturated fats is associated with a strong risk of digestive tract cancers, including the pancreas. Increasing consumption of a Western diet that has high caloric but low nutritional value is a significant factor in the world disease burden of non-communicable diseases. Studies show that individuals on a diet that is rich in fruits, vegetables, whole grains, and healthy fats , such as those contained in fish are at lower risk for pancreatic cancer. This suggests that dietary interventions can serve as probable preventive treatments of pancreatic disorders, particularly among groups that are on a change of diet. Modification of these lifestyle determinants offers a key opportunity to influence disease outcome beneficially and can lead to more efficient public health interventions aimed at reducing instances of pancreatic cancer (Boutayeb & Boutayeb, 2005). Alcohol consumption is another lifestyle determinant with a high correlation with risk for pancreatic disorder. Although moderate drinking has been associated with some medical advantages, heavy alcohol consumption is a significant risk factor for the pathogenesis of pancreatic disease, i.e., pancreatitis and pancreatic cancer. Epidemiologic data indicate an immediate relationship between heavy drinking and inflammatory processes that result in pancreatic damage. Additionally, alcohol interacts synergistically with other lifestyle elements , such as smoking, which enhances the overall risk. It is interesting to note that, while alcohol's effect on the majority of cancers is proven, its link to pancreatic cancer is moderate but frightening. Poor diet and alcohol are likely to increase the risk factor, calling for worldwide lifestyle modification in susceptible subjects for pancreatic conditions (D'Avan et al., 2017). The interplay between diet and alcohol consumption also complicates lifestyle variables in influencing pancreatic function. With changing eating patterns across the globe, the additional increase in intake of high-calorie and low-nutrient foods, in addition to excessive alcohol consumption, gives rise to specific health problems.

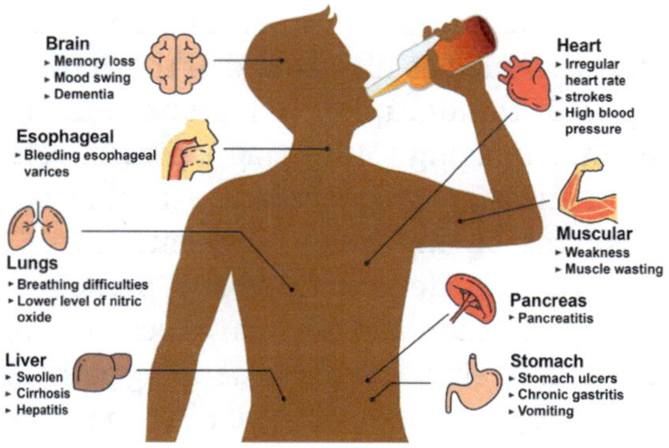

Figure 9.9. Lifestyle factors (diet, alcohol consumption).

Source: https://www.decisionpointcenter.com/images/blog/shutterstock_1027527763.1).jpg.

Such a pattern is likely to lead to obesity, an established risk factor for pancreatic disease as well as other chronic ailments. The transition towards alcohol and processed food is particularly overstated in developing nations, where the twin burden of infectious and non-infectious diseases poses a growing problem. Preventive interventions targeting lifestyle determinants, such as promoting healthy diets and less consumption of alcohol, are essential in reversing risks associated with pancreatic ailments. Through public awareness generation and compliance with improved lifestyles, public health interventions can effectively address the rising incidence of pancreatic diseases, hence minimizing the healthcare burden of such conditions (Boutayeb & Boutayeb, 2005) (Figure 9.9).

9.3.3. Other Medical Conditions (Diabetes, Gallstones)

The reciprocal relationship between pancreatic disorders and diabetes is complex and important. Prolonged pancreatitis, which involves prolonged inflammation of the pancreas, tends to result in diabetes mellitus as a consequence of the injury caused to the insulin-secreting beta cells. Approximately 30% to 50% of chronic pancreatitis patients will eventually develop diabetes, either type 2 or maturity-onset diabetes of the young (MODY) due to specific genetic mutations, such as those in the CEL gene (Molven et al., 2015). The destruction of viable pancreatic tissue compromises the organ's function to produce insulin correctly, resulting in dysfunctional glucose metabolism. Conversely, diabetes is also a risk factor for pancreatic illness, as the derangements of metabolism are likely to make inflammatory processes in the pancreas more severe and trigger a vicious cycle leading to worse complications and increased likelihood of acute or chronic pancreatitis. Gallstones are also an important risk factor for pancreatic disease, particularly acute pancreatitis. About 30% of acute pancreatitis results from choledocholithiasis, with gallstones obstructing the pancreatic duct and exerting intraductal pressure that leads to inflammation. Migration of gallstones might result in obstruction that interferes with the passage of pancreatic enzymes into the intestine, and they are retained and lead to injury of pancreatic tissue (Kiraly et al., 2008). Interestingly, management of gallstone pancreatitis involves extraction of the obstructing stones in the ducts to alleviate symptoms and prevent recurrent inflammation or potentially necrosis of pancreatic tissue. Untimely treatment of gallstones predisposes to the development of severe acute pancreatitis and resultant chronic diseases, emphasizing the importance of early treatment and comprehensive management of gallbladder disease in pancreatic disease patients.

The development of diabetes as a complication of pancreatic disease underlines the fine balance between metabolic health and glandular function. Atypical antipsychotic medications, such as clozapine and olanzapine, have been linked with the induction of acute pancreatitis, particularly in patients predisposed to metabolic illness , such as hyperglycemia and type 2 diabetes (Kiraly et al., 2008).

While less frequently affected, there have also been instances of pancreatitis occurring in patients who have been placed on newer medications, like aripiprazole, invalidating the hypothesis that newer drugs do not exert rigorous metabolic effects. Hyperlipasemia, while typically an indicator of pancreatitis, may complicate diagnosis when medication impinges upon glucose metabolism. The shared mechanisms for drug-induced pancreatitis and underlying conditions like diabetes demand careful monitoring of patients for complications involving the pancreas because there have to be definite differential diagnoses to manage their care properly. Hence, knowledge of these interdependent medical conditions is crucial in improving patient outcomes in patients with disorders of the pancreas.

9.4. Symptoms and Diagnosis

Diagnosis of pancreatic illness is often initiated by careful analysis of the symptoms, which are often variable and subtle. Abdominal pain, weight loss, and gastrointestinal upset worsening over time are also seen in patients. Steatorrhea resulting from malabsorption because the pancreas is unable to secrete adequate enzymes, for example, is a cause of chronic pancreatitis. Diagnosis is difficult due to the tremendous overlap with other gastrointestinal illnesses. Of particular importance is that since the symptoms can be very broad across individuals, a detailed medical history and careful physical examination become crucial in eliminating the conditions of interest. Diagnosticians should be aware of the possibility of other causes, i.e., SIBO, which has been reported in a high percentage of chronic pancreatitis patients, indicating an increased complexity of diagnosis and management (Capurso et al., 2016). Diagnostic imaging plays a key role in the diagnosis of pancreatic disease, adding to the initial clinical evaluation. Imaging modalities , such as ultrasound of the abdomen, computed tomography (CT), and magnetic resonance imaging (MRI) play a pivotal role in the visualization of pancreatic structures and assessment of any likely abnormalities. The modalities can demonstrate the presence of detection of pancreatic necrosis, calcification, or cysts and thus elucidate the underlying pathology. Endoscopic procedures can also be used to assess and obtain tissue samples where necessary. The use of the fecal elastase-1 test emerges as a potent approach to the diagnosis of pancreatic exocrine insufficiency (PEI), which is a common condition in the aftermath of pancreatic illness or interventions. By quantification of pancreatic enzyme concentration in stool, it is also possible to safely establish the functional capability of the pancreas, enabling early and appropriate interventions in individuals with confirmed PEI or indicative findings (Vujasinovic et al., 2017).

Finally, the radiological diagnosis of pancreatic diseases extends beyond symptom detection and imaging techniques. Multidisciplinary management with nutrition monitoring is necessary, particularly in the surgery-treated patients and those with chronic gastrointestinal symptoms. In the case of post-bariatric surgery, as is obvious, maldigestion and malabsorption syndrome can have symptoms masquerading as pancreatic insufficiency with challenging differential diagnoses.

Therefore, it is of utmost importance that all such patients are monitored closely for such complications with serious consideration of the therapeutic regimens that would be appropriate. The treatment includes pancreatic enzyme replacement therapy, which aims to normalize nutritional deficiencies and improve the quality of life in such patients. Therefore, early diagnosis and ongoing management of symptoms remain important in accurately diagnosing and treating pancreatic disorders, underlining the importance of a multi-disciplinary healthcare strategy (Figure 9.10).

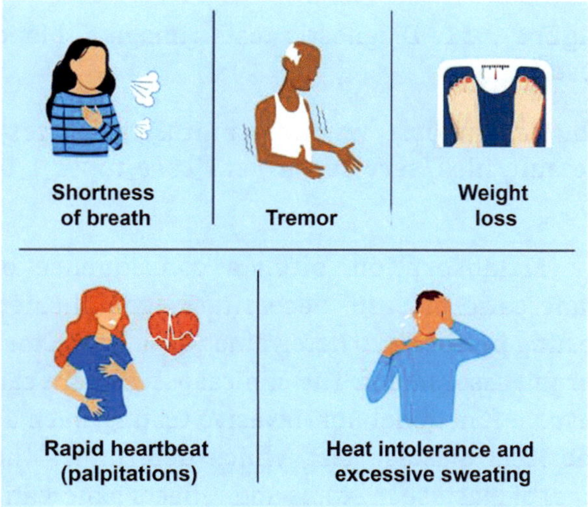

Figure 9.10. Symptoms and diagnosis.

Source: https://my.clevelandclinic.org/-/scassets/images/org/health/articles/15244-graves-disease.

9.4.1. Common Symptoms of Pancreatic Disorders

The signs of pancreatitis can have a significant impact on the patient's quality of life, with an extremely complex combination of gastrointestinal and systemic symptoms. The most common symptom is abdominal pain, a characteristic being a sharp, persistent ache that can radiate to the back. Pain may be worsened by the ingestion of food, particularly fatty food, and helps to highlight the pancreas's digestive and metabolic role. Additionally, the majority of patients also develop weight loss with usual or increased appetite, which is accounted for by malabsorption secondary to impaired production of digestive enzymes. This disruption leads to deficiencies in nutrients, further exacerbating the physiological effects of the disease. Clinically, such symptoms are significant indicators for physicians, suggesting the need for further diagnostic studies to determine the reasons for pancreatic dysfunction. Furthermore, pancreatic patients typically report symptoms of change in digestive function, for example, steatorrhea or diarrhea as smelly, greasy stools. The symptom follows malabsorption of fats due to the inability to produce enough enzymes, indicative of exocrine pancreatic insufficiency. This is thus accompanied by bloating, abdominal discomfort, flatulence, and postprandial pain, factors that cause significant impairment of daily life and overall health. Such gastrointestinal disturbances have to be treated with care, sometimes calling for dietary modification or enzyme replacement to dampen the disturbances while improving nutritional absorption. Such common gastrointestinal symptoms are important not just because they contribute to the clinical picture of pancreatic disorders but also because they have a determining role in therapy aimed at improving patients' digestion and quality of life. In addition to gastrointestinal manifestations, systemic presentations can also occur in patients with pancreatic disease, complicating clinical assessment and management. For instance, metabolic derangement can lead to the development of diabetes, particularly in chronic pancreatitis, where insulin production is compromised. This can result in polydipsia, polyuria, and unintentional weight loss, necessitating blood glucose assessment and even insulin therapy. Furthermore, patients will often present with fatigue and generalized weakness, typically exacerbated by nutritional deficiencies secondary to defective absorption. These systemic signs may be underemphasized but are of key significance in the detection of the more extensive effects of pancreatic disease on the body. The intricacy of such symptoms demonstrates the requirement of a wholistic approach to diagnosis and management, to ensure that all aspects of a patient's health are examined in the context of pancreatic disease.

9.4.2. Diagnostic Tests (Imaging, Blood Tests)

The accurate diagnosis of pancreatic illnesses largely relies on the application of a combination of imaging techniques and laboratory tests from blood specimens. Imaging equipment, including ultrasonography, computed tomography (CT), and magnetic resonance imaging (MRI), plays a critical role in acquiring images of the pancreas anatomy and identifying structural pathology. The imaging techniques could be employed for verifying conditions , such as pancreatitis, pancreatic tumors, or cysts, which may not be detected through physical examinations. For instance, a CT scan can exhibit inflammation, necrosis, or abscessation, whereas an MRI can show detailed images of soft tissue anatomy and enable improved diagnosis of pancreatic cancer. All these non-invasive imaging methods play a significant role in understanding the extent of disease and complications related to it and ultimately result in directing the treatment modalities and prognosis. At the same time as imaging tests, blood tests are crucial in the evaluation of pancreatic disease, especially in the assessment of pancreatic function and the identification of disease markers. Serum amylase and lipase levels are commonly tested for acute pancreatitis diagnosis, as these enzymes characteristically rise with pancreatic inflammation. Blood tests to determine glucose and insulin levels are also used to diagnose exocrine pancreatic insufficiency or diabetes, both usual sequelae of chronic pancreatic disease. In addition, laboratory evaluation for the presence of specific antibodies or genetic mutations can diagnose hereditary pancreatitis or autoimmune pancreatitis. Combine blood tests with imaging to maximize diagnostic yield and stratify patients for intervention, such as surgery or endocrine management.

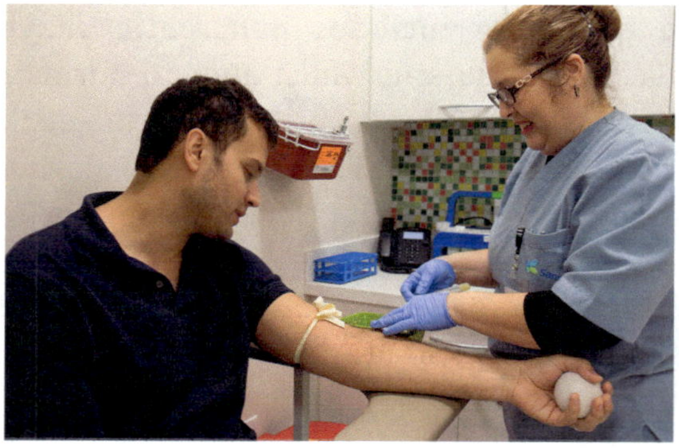

Figure 9.11. Diagnostic tests (imaging, blood tests).

Source: https://www.mysanitas.com/sites/default/files/services/urgent_care_topic_1_0.jpg.

Malabsorption, often a consequence of pancreatic disease, necessitates complicated testing protocols to determine causative factors for full assessment. The clinical assessment can involve functional non-invasive testing, such as the fecal elastase test, which determines the level of elastase in stools and reflects pancreatic exocrine function. If malabsorption is established or suspected, further imaging and endoscopy might be required to assess the small intestine and perform biopsies as appropriate. This may be particularly so for conditions like cystic fibrosis or exocrine pancreatic insufficiency (EPI), where nutrient absorption is compromised. Early identification of malabsorption can lead to effective nutritional support measures on time, which are particularly important in the complete management of these pancreatic conditions. Through the coordinated use of imaging and blood work, health professionals can formulate integrated treatment regimens based on the individual needs of the patients with pancreatic diseases, hence improving their effectiveness of care and results (Lenti et al., 2025) (Figure 9.11).

9.4.3. Importance of Early Detection

The value of early detection in pancreatic disease cannot be overstated, particularly in the context of the notoriously poor prognosis of pancreatic cancer. Early diagnosis is critical since it profoundly affects treatment modalities and outcomes. Non-specific or even missing symptoms in early PDAC render regular screening vital, particularly in those who are at high risk. Genetic risk factors, such as some inherited mutations, have been discovered to enhance the risk of pancreatic cancer. For instance, research revealed an association between immune regulator gene IDO2 loss-of-function single nucleotide polymorphisms and higher familial pancreatic cancer risk, highlighting a potential window for early genetic screening and interventions for care (Brody et al., 2018). With that, active surveillance and awareness may lead to earlier diagnosis and better survival in patients with pancreatic diseases. Furthermore, advances in technological tools for diagnosis have underlined the importance of serologic and genetic markers in early detection, especially for pancreatic disease. Early research indicates that quantifying certain biomarkers is able to enhance the accuracy of diagnoses and make it feasible to detect individuals at heightened risk for diseases like pancreatic cancer. Their presence may also direct clinicians as to the likelihood of progressing towards more aggressive types (Altorjay et al., 2007). For instance, an understanding of the genetic mutations that are involved in familial pancreatic cancer may result in more targeted screening among high-risk individuals and, therefore, ultimately, earlier intervention.

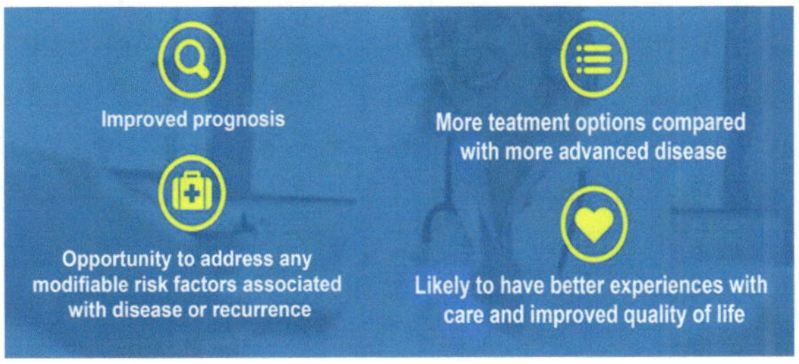

Figure 9.12. Importance of early detection.

Source: https://www.cxbladder.com/assets/Uploads/Benefits-of-Early-Detection.png.

This underscores the need for systematic screening guidelines incorporating genetic and serologic markers in standard practice among populations at risk. In addition to encouraging early diagnosis, early detection proves useful to guide treatment regimens and improve the general quality of patients' lives. Early detection of pancreatic disease enables clinicians to use less invasive treatment techniques, hence preserving patients' health as well as preventing complications. In pancreatitis or early-stage pancreatic cancer patients, early intervention will stop disease progression and prevent serious complications. Moreover, successful early detection procedures can stimulate ongoing investigations on novel therapeutic approaches, resulting in a proactive treatment strategy for pancreatic diseases. Overall, the integration of early screening measures within healthcare systems, especially for genetically high-risk individuals, is crucial in order to enhance outcomes and create a guide to more effectively treat pancreatic illnesses (Figure 9.12).

9.5. Treatment Options

Pancreatic diseases are managed by a multidisciplinary approach, taking into account both the pathological background and symptomatic presentation of the disease. Dietary modifications play an important role, particularly in the management of diseases , such as acute pancreatitis and exocrine pancreatic insufficiency. Clinical evidence supports the hypothesis that a diet fortified with prebiotics is capable of significantly reducing complications of acute pancreatitis, i.e., the occurrence of pancreatic necrosis and systemic inflammatory response syndrome. This dietary treatment appears to regulate the intestinal barrier homeostasis, hence lowering infection risk.

However, in exocrine pancreatic insufficiency patients, diets rich in fiber have paradoxically been linked with adverse effects, including increased fecal fat excretion due to inhibition of pancreatic enzymes by fiber. Proper balancing of food composition is thus important in achieving maximum treatment benefits in pancreatic disorder patients (Ribichini et al., 2019). Pharmacotherapies are another important element of the management of pancreatic disease, and especially of chronic pancreatitis. Among several treatment models, treatment of diabetes mellitus type 3c (T3cDM)–secondary diabetes resulting from pancreatic damage – has attracted increasing attention. The complication contributes to chronic pancreatitis and requires an individualized approach, taking into account both endocrine and exocrine insufficiency of the pancreas. Insulin therapy may be needed in patients with T3cDM, since the majority of post-acute pancreatitis patients experience insulin resistance accompanied by hyperglycemia. Additional research is necessary to fully understand this pathology, maximize diagnostic approaches, and enhance therapeutic interventions. Therefore, clinicians must be vigilant in managing blood glucose and also in adjusting treatment plans accordingly to prevent secondary complications of diabetes in conjunction with pancreatic disease (Diaconu et al., 2018). Finally, surgical procedures can also be an appropriate choice in some cases of pancreatic disease, particularly for patients with chronic pancreatitis that is resistant to conservative treatments. Surgical procedures , such as the Whipple procedure or pancreaticoduodenectomy can be necessary in cases of pancreatic cancer or gross structural deformity.

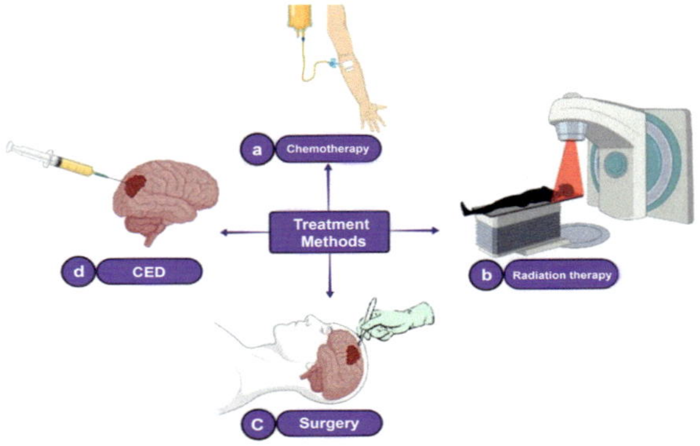

Figure 9.13. Treatment options.

Source: https://www.researchgate.net/publication/365317240/figure/fig1/AS:11431281096661553@1668226281968/Different-treatment-strategies-of-brain-tumors-In-chemotherapy-the-drug-solution-is.png.

These treatments not only serve the aim of palliating obstructive symptoms but also offer an opportunity for curative therapy when indicated. The choice of surgical treatment should be made following extensive imaging investigations and multidisciplinary evaluation, considering , such aspects as the patient's overall health status and preference. In addition to surgical treatments, ongoing monitoring and lifestyle adjustments remain integral components of effective long-term treatment strategies for patients suffering from pancreatic illness to guarantee an integrated treatment approach (Ribichini et al., 2019) (Figure 9.13).

9.5.1. Medical Management (Medications, Enzyme Replacement)

The management of pancreatic illnesses is often centered on the use of drugs and enzyme replacement therapy. In pancreatic insufficiency, deficiency in the pancreas to secrete sufficient digestive enzymes—enzyme replacement therapy is a cornerstone of treatment. Products containing lipase, amylase, and protease facilitate nutrient digestion and absorption, significantly improving patients' quality of life. These therapies are significant because malabsorption can cause severe nutritional deficiencies, weight loss, and overall ill health. Moreover, dosing needs to be watched in a careful manner since patients may react differently to enzyme supplementation, so tailor-made treatment protocols need to be developed to optimize therapeutic response while avoiding complications that are secondary to inadequate digestion. Drugs also have a significant role to play in the management of pancreatic diseases, particularly for diseases , such as pancreatitis or pancreatic cancer. Nonsteroidal anti-inflammatory drugs (NSAIDs) and opioids are used in the management of pain associated with such diseases. More complicated situations, including pancreatic neuroendocrine tumors, are managed using targeted therapies or chemotherapy agents in a bid to manage tumor growth and increase survival. Each treatment method must be developed based on the patient's clinical profile, considering comorbidities as well as the type of pancreatic disorder. In this situation, current research comprises ongoing searches for new drugs possessing the promise to exhibit greater efficacy along with fewer side effects, thus improving the therapeutic situation in the event of pancreatic disease patients (Focal Spot, Fall/Winter 2010/2011). Moreover, continuous advances in medical management prove a better understanding of pancreatic diseases and their systemic impact. Incorporation of extensive care models that encompass dietary modification, psychosocial treatment, and patient education can enhance overall treatment effectiveness. For instance, patient education on self-management of the condition using lifestyle changes and proper compliance with medication will maximize the success of treatment. Specific nutrition and dietetic counseling may be necessary, particularly for exocrine pancreatic insufficiency that requires significant alterations to meet their nutritional needs. Treating both the medical and holistic aspects of care will enable healthcare professionals to provide a more integrated means of managing pancreatic disorders and hence gain enhanced clinical outcomes and improve patients' long-term quality of life (Benvenga et al., 2017) (Figure 9.14).

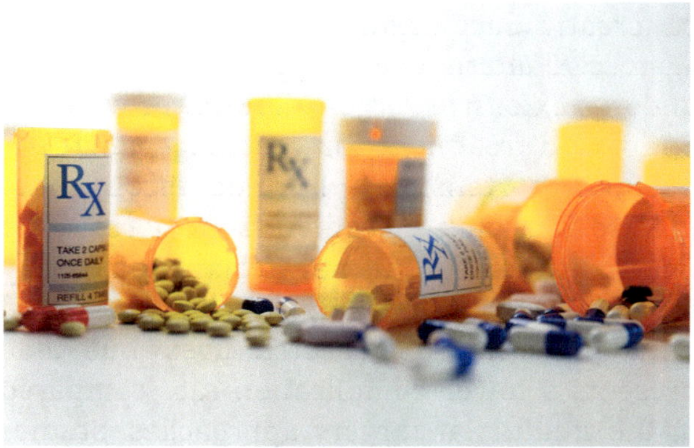

Figure 9.14. Medical management (medications, enzyme replacement).

Source: https://fthmb.tqn.com/aoQI0eDVyzLJsHofOkiqr6X9iL0=/5184x3456/filters:fill(87E3EF,1)/prescription-pills-164478117-58b229bd5f9b58604699ca58.jpg.

9.5.2. Surgical Interventions (Whipple Procedure, Drainage)

Surgical intervention plays a key role in the management of pancreatic conditions, particularly in pancreatic cancer and chronic pancreatitis. Whipple procedure or pancreatoduodenectomy is the most common surgical intervention for the resection of tumors in the head of the pancreas. This complex operation involves the removal of the head of the pancreas, the duodenum, a portion of the bile duct, and sometimes the gallbladder, followed by reconstruction of the gastrointestinal tract. While the Whipple operation can extend survival times and improve the quality of life for the majority of patients, it does possess significant postoperative complications like delayed gastric emptying, infections, and pancreatic fistulas. Because of its complexity, patient selection is most critical, and preoperative optimization will enhance surgical outcomes as well as minimize adverse effects from this intervention. Except for the Whipple operation, there are multiple techniques of drainage employed when stone formation or malignancies are the cause of pancreatic duct obstruction. Endoscopic ultrasonography-guided pancreatic duct drainage (EUS-PD) is a less aggressive alternative for patients who cannot undergo extensive surgery. EUS-PD provides an option for treatment for reducing pancreatic ductal hypertension syndrome through the precise insertion of catheters with real-time imaging guidance. This new technique not only resolves the severe complications associated with pancreatic duct strictures but also presents a lower complication rate compared to the traditional surgery approaches. Studies in literature have indicated that EUS-PD is extremely effective in symptom palliation for malignant obstructions and chronic pancreatitis and thus can be regarded as an effective intervention in pancreatic pathology (Wang et al., 2025). Another innovation of the endoscopic method is combined procedures, i.e., endoscopic ultrasound-guided hepaticogastrostomy, which can be employed in association with EUS-PD for the overall management of stones in the biliary and pancreatic ducts. The modality of the combined approach provides evidence for the ability of endoscopic interventions to manage multiple complications of pancreatic disorder treatments during a single sitting. The use of newer technologies, including artificial intelligence-guided interventions and newer imaging modalities, has enhanced the efficacy and precision of such interventions. Challenges continue to exist, such as anatomical issues and the development of pancreatitis or fistula following the intervention. Close observation therapy and the development of standardized protocols are important to optimize results and make sure that these new therapies attain their therapeutic potential (Nagai et al., 2022).

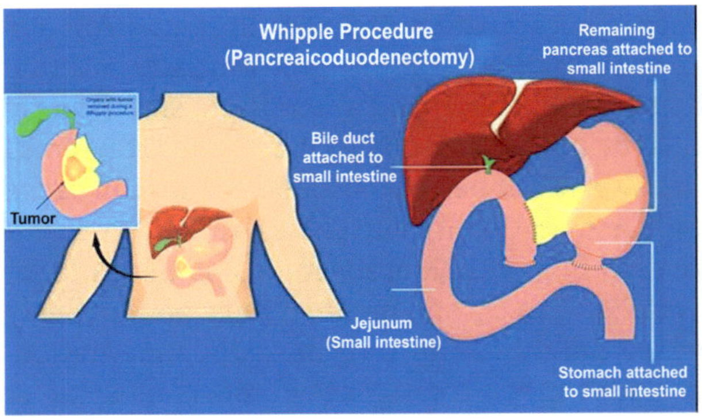

Figure 9.15. Surgical interventions (Whipple procedure, drainage).

Source: https://www.medicoverhospitals.in/images/surgery-cost/whipple-surgery-procedure.webp.

9.5.3. Lifestyle Modifications (Dietary Changes, Exercise)

In the treatment of pancreatic disorders, dietary modifications and a reduction in the level of lifestyle, i.e., increased physical activity, become central components of effective management regimens. A balanced diet rich in whole grains, fruits, vegetables, and healthy fats is critical in promoting pancreatic health and overall metabolic function. Dietary modification can also alleviate symptoms and reduce the risk of pancreatic disorder complications. For example, research on patients with diseases like diabetes shows that diets rich in fiber, such as the Mediterranean diet, can enhance the production of short-chain fatty acids (SCFA), which have a correlation with improved metabolic and immune function. Such dietary practices would thus prove to be a beneficial adjunct therapy, targeting inflammation and metabolic risk of pancreatic impairment, resulting in better health outcomes (Cadenhead et al., 2017). Exercise also has a significant part to play in the management of pancreatic disease, as an adjunct to diet to optimize patient well-being. Blood glucose levels can be stabilized, insulin sensitivity enhanced, and metabolic conditions improved using physical activity. The combined actions of exercise and diet can reverse the consequences of obesity and type II diabetes, both significant factors influencing pancreatic health. Even though other studies establish that lifestyle interventions can lead to fewer complications in patients with diseases like gestational diabetes, the efficacy of exercise alone is not clear. For instance, evidence attests that lifestyle interventions likely reduce risks but inadvertently may add to some complications, e.g., labor induction, in some cases (Alsweiler et al., 2018). Therefore, it is crucial to incorporate exercise wisely into an individualized treatment plan for those with pancreatic disorders. The addition of dietary adjustment and exercise to the treatment regimen for pancreatic disorders not only provides a holistic approach towards management but also promotes patient empowerment through self-management. Patient education about the roles of nutrition and exercise enhances an active management approach to the condition, leading to higher compliance and, potentially, better health status. But these must be addressed with consideration for individual circumstances, e.g., prior health status and individual preferences. With the continued growth of research in this area, the role of lifestyle changes will likely become more settled, moving towards individualized intervention. Finally, these changes can be crucial agents for reducing the burden of pancreatic diseases, promoting longevity and quality of life (Cadenhead et al., 2017).

9.6. Complications of Pancreatic Disorders

Pancreatic disease complications may significantly impact patient health and the success of treatment. One of the most significant complications is exocrine pancreatic insufficiency, in which the pancreas fails to secrete sufficient digestive enzymes. This can lead to steatorrhea, diarrhea, and weight loss owing to malabsorption of food. Management of this complication typically involves enzyme replacement therapy and dietary adjustment. However, it has been established by studies that incorporating dietary fiber into the diet can affect pancreatic function. In acute pancreatitis, a dietary fiber-supplemented diet has been associated with improved results through improved intestinal barrier stability and reduced rates of infection (Ribichini et al., 2019). High-fiber diets, however, exacerbate diseases of exocrine insufficiency due to their ability to impair pancreatic enzyme functions, complicating nutritional management in such patients (Ribichini et al., 2019). Hence, it is vital to understand the bimodal function of dietary fiber to optimize therapeutic measures in pancreatic disease. Another serious complication of pancreatic disease is the development of choledochal cysts. Congenital malformations of the biliary tree can lead to severe pancreatobiliary pathology in the form of cholangitis and pancreatitis. Abnormal bile duct morphology makes people susceptible to infection and inflammation, which can become a reason for further impairment of pancreatic function. Patients with choledochal cysts typically present with abdominal pain, jaundice, and recurrent pancreatitis that could result in intense diagnostic examinations like imaging studies. Moreover, the potential for cholangiocarcinoma with choledochal cysts has long-term care and treatment planning implications for individuals (Koncoro & Wibawa, 2012). Effective management includes the treatment of complications when they occur and planning for potential surgeries to expect in order to prevent complications. Furthermore, complications of pancreatic illnesses may also occur outside the gastrointestinal spectrum, to the systemic spectrum. Chronic pancreatitis patients, for instance, risk diabetes mellitus due to impairment of the insulin-secreting cells of the pancreas.

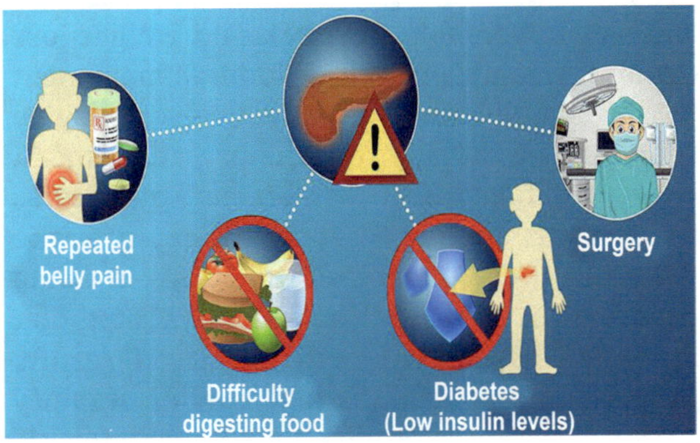

Figure 9.16. Complications of pancreatic disorders.

Source: https://www.animatedpancreaspatient.com/en-pancreas/content.ashx?file=app07/slides/ch16_slide_08.jpg.

This endocrine dysfunction would complicate patient care because it might require that patients monitor blood glucose levels and make significant lifestyle adjustments beyond their management of pancreatic symptoms. Moreover, the acute pancreatitis systemic inflammatory response syndrome can further advance to multi-organ failure, which is a drastic threat to patient survival. Such complications necessitate an integrated, multidisciplinary approach to patient management, addressing both the root pancreatic disorder and its broader effect on overall well-being. It is hence important that medical practitioners are cognizant of potential complications to administer timely and effective interventions in treating pancreatic disorders (Figure 9.16).

9.6.1. Impact on Digestion and Nutrient Absorption

The pancreas plays a critical function in digestion and nutrient absorption by secreting digestive enzymes necessary for macronutrient breakdown. Pancreatic digestive enzymes , such as lipase, amylase, and proteases, are secreted into the small bowel and catalyze fat, carbohydrate, and protein hydrolysis, respectively. An impairment of pancreatic enzyme production, typically noted in disorders of the pancreas like chronic pancreatitis or cystic fibrosis, can have an adverse impact on this process. For instance, aberrant secretion of lipase leads to fat malabsorption and, consequently, steatorrhea, weight loss, and fat-soluble vitamin deficiencies. On enzymatic impairment, the body cannot absorb vital nutrients from food, which consequently affects overall health, energy, and metabolic processes (Omer & Chiodi, 2024). Moreover, the net effect of impaired pancreatic function is not just restricted to macronutrient digestion but extends to the absorption of vital micronutrients as well. The pancreas's failure to secrete adequate amounts of digestive enzymes disrupts the emulsification and digestion of fats, which in turn has a cascading effect on fat-soluble vitamins A, D, E, and K absorption. These vitamins play a central role in many physiological processes , such as vision, bone mineralization, immune function, and antioxidative defense. Consequently, patients with pancreatic disorders usually experience deficiencies in the form of various clinical signs and symptoms, like bone discomfort, impaired immune function, or visual impairment. Pancreatic activity and nutrient absorption interaction highlights the need for proper management to enhance digestive ability in affected individuals (Nkurunziza, 2024). Lastly, the overall implications of enzyme deficiencies on digestive health represent an essential aspect of managing pancreatic disorders. Patients often also present with malabsorption as well as gastrointestinal distress, bloating, and diarrhea that can be socially and psychologically disabling.

Nutrition therapy and replacement with enzymes are part of treatment and can be utilized to alleviate symptoms through the reconstitution of digestive processes. Maximization of nutrient intake via individualized diets and supplementation can allow the healthcare team to improve the quality of life in patients with pancreatic disease. Further research is essential to look into new therapies that enhance the availability of digestive enzymes and allow improved absorption of nutrients, ultimately resulting in improved health conditions for such debilitating disease patients (Omer & Chiodi, 2024).

9.6.2. Risk of Diabetes Development

The ability to acquire diabetes, and especially type 2 diabetes mellitus, is a directly correlated to the multifactorial interaction of environmental and lifestyle factors that are harmful to the function of the pancreas. The pancreas plays a significant role in insulin production, which is a hormone critical for maintaining blood sugar levels. Exposure to harmful chemicals and a diet of processed foods have been identified as primary reasons for pancreatic dysfunction that leads to insulin resistance and disturbed glucose metabolism. Highly advanced risk assessment methodologies, also referred to as New Approach Methodologies (NAMs), have thus emerged to effectively measure these effects. NAMs that include high-throughput screening and modeling at the computational level can define the way such toxic exposures compromise the health of the pancreas, ultimately risking diabetes and other metabolic diseases (Ge, 2025). Such an argument highlights environmental risk reduction and health promotion through healthy dietary practices as a means of reducing the incidence of diabetes.Gestational diabetes mellitus (GDM) provides a classic illustration of the way pancreatic diseases develop in at-risk populations, particularly during pregnancy. GDM is characterized by glucose intolerance acquired during pregnancy attributed predominantly to either pancreatic β-cell impairment or insulin resistance (Volkova et al., 2023). Identification of risk factors for GDM is vital in enabling early intervention and control. Research indicates that heterogeneous demographic and lifestyle factors cross-react to establish the risk for the onset of GDM, including maternal age, weight, and physical activity levels. Identification of these risk factors allows for customization of preventive interventions, ultimately improving fetal and maternal health outcomes. Furthermore, addressing these factors increases visibility regarding the broader implications of pancreatic function and diabetes risk, emphasizing early screening and active management among pregnant women and making it a crucial component for reducing long-term diabetes rates.

The increased prevalence of diabetes calls for an integrated approach towards decreasing its risk through public health interventions and large-scale awareness generation campaigns. Strategies need to focus on generating awareness regarding the relationship between food lifestyle, exposure to environmental pollutants, and well-being. Healthy lifestyle practices , such as regular physical activity, adequate diet, and safety habits against hazardous substance exposure, can decrease the risk of diabetes occurrence considerably. Moreover, government health regulations governing environmental toxins can be used to address one of the fundamental causes of malfunctioning pancreatic activity. By applying data acquired through advanced research techniques like NAMs, policymakers can design improved risk assessment tools that inform clinical practice and public health measures. Therefore, improving the understanding of predisposing factors to diabetes will facilitate effective prevention and management practices that will lead to a reduction in the burden of diabetes among people and society in general (Ge, 2025) (Figure 9.17).

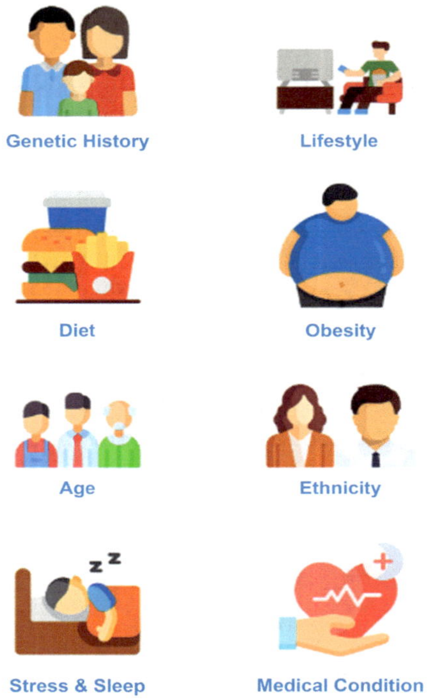

Figure 9.17. Risk of diabetes development.

Source: https://www.fitterfly.com/blog/wp-content/uploads/2024/01/Risk-Factors-for-Diabetes.webp.

9.6.3. Potential for Chronic Pain and Quality of Life Issues

The quality of life is usually impaired through the suffering of chronic pain in patients with pancreatic diseases, particularly those with pancreatic cancer or pancreatitis. Chronic pain can significantly impair the quality of an individual's life by inducing emotional distress, social isolation, and loss of functional capacity. The mechanism by which pancreatic disease culminates in chronic pain is multifactorial, with direct inflammatory processes, nerve damage, and pain perception. While pharmacologic management can be helpful in some patients for a limited period of time, the chronic nature of the disease in so many cases necessitates a more comprehensive pain control regimen to manage discomfort and enhance overall quality of life. An integrative care model for these patients, as proposed in related literature, emphasizes the importance of addressing both psychological and physical health to gain long-term improvements in pain control and daily function (Golovacheva et al., 2025). Furthermore, the impact of chronic pain on quality of life can be long-term and beyond immediate physical effects. Patients with pancreatic illnesses often present with concomitant psychiatric issues, namely anxiety and depression, that intensify pain and general misery. It has been shown through research that graded absence from work can result in beneficial effects on health via the preservation of work engagement, highlighting the linked status of physical health, work-life balance, and well-being (Sanatkar et al., 2025). Employers and physicians need to take an active role in providing these patients through the promotion of adjustments at the workplace and availability of resources for graduated returns to work. In so doing, they not only provide relief for the patients' pain but also give them a sense of fulfillment and social membership, which are crucial to prolonged quality of life in protracted illness. Lastly, in managing the risk of chronic pain in cases involving pancreatic disorders, an integrated plan of care considering both the biological and psychosocial components of the patient's experience is needed. Informing patients regarding their conditions and highlighting the importance of lifestyle modifications can help develop a sense of control over the management of their health outcomes. Integrative therapy, including kinesiotherapy and counseling, is well-positioned to make a meaningful impact on pain relief interventions, which emphasize the need as a whole to treat the individual, rather than the disease (Golovacheva et al., 2025). By giving thorough treatment that acknowledges the uncertainty of chronic pain and its impact on quality of life, physicians can better the physical state of their patients as well as their social and emotional standing, ultimately leading to an improved prognosis in the case of pancreatic ailments.

CLOSER LOOK

FECAL MICROBIOTA TRANSPLANTATION (FMT):

Fecal microbiota transplantation (FMT) is an innovative therapeutic approach that involves transferring processed stool from a healthy donor into the gastrointestinal tract of a recipient. Its primary goal is to restore a balanced and diverse gut microbiome. A closer look at FMT reveals its remarkable effectiveness for certain conditions, its expanding research applications, and the important safety and regulatory considerations that accompany its use.

FMT has gained the most clinical acceptance for treating recurrent or refractory *Clostridioides difficile* infections (CDI). In these cases, repeated antibiotic treatments disrupt the gut flora, allowing *C. difficile* to thrive and cause severe, persistent diarrhea. Restoring gut microbial diversity through FMT has been shown to cure up to 85–90% of recurrent cases in many studies, making it one of the most successful microbiome-based interventions in modern medicine. By reintroducing beneficial bacteria, FMT helps re-establish colonization resistance, suppressing *C. difficile* and restoring intestinal health.

Beyond CDI, interest in FMT is growing across a wide range of conditions. Research is exploring its potential role in treating inflammatory bowel disease (IBD), irritable bowel syndrome, metabolic disorders such as obesity and type 2 diabetes, and even neurological and psychiatric conditions via the gut–brain axis. While findings are promising, results have been mixed, and FMT is not yet considered standard therapy for these conditions. Differences in donor profiles, preparation techniques, and patient factors contribute to variability in outcomes. Safety remains an essential consideration. Although FMT is generally well tolerated, risks include transmission of infectious agents, alterations in immune function, and unpredictable changes in the microbiome. To minimize these risks, donors undergo rigorous screening for pathogens, antibiotic resistance genes, and underlying health issues. Regulatory agencies have increasingly emphasized standardized protocols to ensure the quality, purity, and traceability of transplanted material. Advances in manufacturing—such as freeze-dried capsules and standardized microbial consortia—aim to improve safety and consistency.

SUMMARY

In viewing the intricate terrain of pancreatic disease, it is clear that the consequences reach far into the system, impacting numerous systemic functions and causing great health problems. At the heart of this is the interdependence of pancreatic function and corresponding metabolic activities. The beta cell dysregulation, particularly in diseases , such as diabetes, accentuates the probability of co-morbidities, such as obesity and hypertension, which increase the risk of these diseases. Further, studies on impaired cerebrovascular function reveal how the deterioration in pancreatic function carries cascades through cardiovascular function, illustrating the vicious cycle wherein an impaired system impinges negatively on another. This interconnectedness underscores the vital importance of a multidisciplinary approach to understanding and treating pancreatic disease with an eye not just on the pancreas, but on the broader metabolic system in which it exists, as illustrated by the studies introduced in previous sections of this essay. Moreover, the evolving focus of the study of biomarkers , such as nesfatin-1 opens new lines of inquiry into further advancing our understanding of pancreatic disease. With the findings indicating that nesfatin-1 levels are related to pancreatic beta-cell function, the image is now clearer as to how carbohydrate metabolism and insulin regulation are controlled. It is possible that these findings may pave the way for new therapeutic methods that would be capable of controlling, or even more ideally, preventing the metabolic imbalances characteristic of pancreatic pathology. But as pointed out by recent studies, the varied effects of nesfatin-1 also reflect the multi-factorial processes of pancreatic disorders and point to the need for a more detailed investigation to define its role more distinctly. So, continued research of such biomarkers in larger, more diverse populations can be of benefit to offer valuable information to assist in tailoring interventions and improving overall patient outcomes, indicative of the necessity of continued research in this critical field of medicine. In general, the therapy of pancreatic pathologies encompasses a full understanding of their system-based implications and mechanisms. The intricate interdependence between the function of the pancreas and metabolic health ensures that treatment schemes on a single factor will necessarily prove incomplete. As we conclude this part, it is essential to advocate for combined research studies that do not just consider the pancreas but also the broader metabolic environment in which it functions. This approach might entail investigating other functions of biomarkers and finding possible therapeutic targets, such as those discussed in more recent studies. The need for comprehensive approaches grows increasingly imperative as diabetes incidence continues to grow globally, again confirming the need for continued research and interdisciplinarity. Lastly, enhancing our awareness of pancreatic diseases is important to limiting their impacts and enhancing the quality of life of patients, resulting in informed interventions and a better future outcome rate in public health in general.

Pancreatic diseases constitute a grave health concern, encompassing a range of conditions affecting the organ's functionality and overall health. Among these, cystic fibrosis (CF) has emerged as a significant area of concern following the drastic implications it has on the pancreas and other organs. The link between CF and pancreatic disease is lent by the mutation of the CFTR gene that leads to aberrant secretion of bicarbonate. Recent studies cite the role of specific CFTR variants in pancreatitis, proving that even non-characteristic CF mutations can lead to pancreatic dysfunction. As an example, the identification of CFTRBD variants R117H and L997F proves that these mutations have a specific effect on changing the channels' permeability and conductance, which is indicative of their role in pancreatic integrity (LaRusch et al., 2014). Such a recognition is utilized to make the case for ongoing studies in genetic susceptibility to pancreatic disease.

In addition to genetic susceptibility, the impact of age on pancreatic function is most important. With aging, progressive alterations in gastrointestinal function can cause malnutrition, yet another confounding factor in pancreatic health. The older gastrointestinal tract experiences mechanical and chemical changes with food processing, which convert to impaired nutrient absorption, thus incurring damage on the aging population (Rémond et al., 2015). Such impaired absorption further worsens underlying pancreatic pathologies or even creates new ones. Age signs, such as decreased enzyme secretion and altered digestive kinetics, can hinder the pancreas's ability to work effectively in controlling digestive processes, precipitating a peak of concurrence between aging alterations and pancreatic function. Thus, control of malnutrition in the elderly is necessary in order to preserve pancreatic function and overall well-being. Lastly, current evidence suggests the intricate interaction among pancreatic illness, diet, and genetic susceptibility. There exists a more generally recognized association between certain CFTR mutations and a number of clinical conditions, including rhinosinusitis and male infertility, that are beyond the pancreas. The identification of CFTRBD variants also emphasizes the universal relevance of genetic mutations to organ systems with bicarbonate secretion, indicating the need for integrated therapy. Furthermore, integrating nutritional interventions that are specifically targeted to the pancreatic patient's own unique nutritional requirements can improve the outcome. It is crucial to understand how these genetic and nutritional elements interact to create appropriate care strategies for pancreatic wellness. Ultimately, continued research is required to elucidate these complex interactions and to direct clinical practices for maximizing patient treatment.

References

1. Ackah, J. A., Li, X., Zeng, H., & Chen, X. (2025). Imaging-validated correlates and implications of the pathophysiologic mechanisms of ageing-related cerebral large artery and small vessel diseases: A systematic review and meta-analysis. *Behavioral and Brain Functions: BBF, 21.* https://www.semanticscholar.org/paper/c2e8acd37ad64da0f5e593a4f9768e8c9d9a0662 (accessed on 16th July 2025).
2. O'Neill, D. G., Coulson, N. R., Church, D. B., & Brodbelt, D. C. (2017). Demography and disorders of German Shepherd Dogs under primary veterinary care in the UK. *Canine genetics and epidemiology*, *4*, 7. https://doi.org/10.1186/s40575-017-0046-4(accessed on 16th July 2025).
3. LaRusch, J., Jung, J., General, I. J., Lewis, M. D., Park, H. W., Brand, R. E., Gelrud, A., Anderson, M. A., Banks, P. A., Conwell, D., Lawrence, C., Romagnuolo, J., Baillie, J., Alkaade, S., Cote, G., Gardner, T. B., Amann, S. T., Slivka, A., Sandhu, B., Aloe, A., ... North American Pancreatitis Study Group (2014). Mechanisms of CFTR functional variants that impair regulated bicarbonate permeation and increase risk for pancreatitis but not for cystic fibrosis. *PLoS genetics*, *10*(7), e1004376. https://doi.org/10.1371/journal.pgen.1004376(accessed on 16th July 2025).
4. Alsweiler, J., Brown, J., Crowther, C. A., Downie, et al. (2018). *Treatments for women with gestational diabetes mellitus: An overview of Cochrane systematic reviews.* https://core.ac.uk/download/187724799.pdf (accessed on 16th July 2025).
5. Altorjay, I., Lakatos, P. L., Norman, G. L., Papp, et al. (2007). *Utility of serological markers in inflammatory bowel diseases: Gadget or magic?* https://core.ac.uk/download/11855932.pdf (accessed on 16th July 2025).
6. Alvaro, D., Bragazzi, M. C., Cardinale, V., Carpino, et al. (2018). *Intrahepatic cholangiocarcinoma: Review and update.* https://core.ac.uk/download/159269704.pdf (accessed on 16th July 2025).
7. Amaravadi, R. K., Kimmelman, A. C., & Debnath, J. (2019). Targeting autophagy in cancer: Recent advances and future directions. *Cancer Discovery, 9*, 1167–1181. https://doi.org/10.1158/2159-8290.cd-19-0292 (accessed on 16th July 2025).
8. Aminoff, S., Onyeka, I., Ødegaard, M., Simonsen, C., Lagerberg, T., Andreassen, O., Romm, K. L., et al. (2022). Lifetime and point prevalence of psychotic symptoms in adults with bipolar disorders: A systematic review and meta-analysis. *Psychological Medicine, 52*, 2413–2425. https://www.semanticscholar.org/paper/10ada4ef9caa4a9ef991423911118ab0d698f8a4 (accessed on 16th July 2025).
9. Argüelles-Arias, A. M., Balza-Lareu, N., Bertoletti, F., Bodenlle-Bello, et al. (2020). *Dietary fat patterns and outcomes in acute pancreatitis in Spain.* https://core.ac.uk/download/322903821.pdf (accessed on 16th July 2025).
10. Vujasinovic, M., Valente, R., Thorell, A., Rutkowski, W., Haas, S. L., Arnelo, U., Martin, L., & Löhr, J. M. (2017). Pancreatic Exocrine Insufficiency after Bariatric Surgery. *Nutrients*, *9*(11), 1241. https://doi.org/10.3390/nu9111241(accessed on 16th July 2025).
11. Ribichini, E., Stigliano, S., Rossi, S., Zaccari, P., Sacchi, M. C., Bruno, G., Badiali, D., & Severi, C. (2019). Role of Fibre in Nutritional Management of Pancreatic Diseases. *Nutrients*, *11*(9), 2219. https://doi.org/10.3390/nu11092219 (accessed on 16th July 2025).

12. Benvenga, S., Centanni, M., & Sachmechi, I. (2017). *Diagnosis and management of treatment-refractory hypothyroidism: An expert consensus report.* https://core.ac.uk/download/188829705.pdf (accessed on 16th July 2025).

13. Boicean, A., Ichim, C., Todor, S. B., Anderco, P., & Popa, M. L. (2024). The importance of microbiota and fecal microbiota transplantation in pancreatic disorders. *Diagnostics, 14.* https://www.semanticscholar.org/paper/9a03699fe3d3a211402ae23016468f77c71e74c7 (accessed on 16th July 2025).

14. Rémond, D., Shahar, D. R., Gille, D., Pinto, P., Kachal, J., Peyron, M. A., Dos Santos, C. N., Walther, B., Bordoni, A., Dupont, D., Tomás-Cobos, L., & Vergères, G. (2015). Understanding the gastrointestinal tract of the elderly to develop dietary solutions that prevent malnutrition. *Oncotarget, 6*(16), 13858–13898. https://doi.org/10.18632/oncotarget.4030 (accessed on 16th July 2025).

15. Boutayeb, A., & Boutayeb, S. (2005). The burden of non communicable diseases in developing countries. *International journal for equity in health, 4*(1), 2. https://doi.org/10.1186/1475-9276-4-2(accessed on 16th July 2025).

16. Brodbelt, D. C., Church, D. B., Mattin, M. J., McGreevy, et al. (2014). *An epidemiological study of diabetes mellitus in dogs attending first opinion practice in the UK.* https://core.ac.uk/download/36777545.pdf (accessed on 16th July 2025).

17. Brody, J., Cozzitorto, J. A., Goetz, A., Lavu, et al. (2018). *A sub-type of familial pancreatic cancer: Evidence and implications of loss-of-function polymorphisms in indoleamine-2,3-dioxygenase-2.* https://core.ac.uk/download/155271751.pdf (accessed on 16th July 2025).

18. Cadenhead, K. S., Depp, C., Joseph, J., Schmid-Schönbein, et al. (2017). *Modified Mediterranean diet for enrichment of short chain fatty acids: Potential adjunctive therapeutic to target immune and metabolic dysfunction in schizophrenia?* https://core.ac.uk/download/287622216.pdf (accessed on 16th July 2025).

19. Capurso, G., Tacelli, M., Vanella, G., Ponz de Leon Pisani, R., Dell'anna, G., Abati, M., Mele, R., et al. (2023). Managing complications of chronic pancreatitis: A guide for the gastroenterologist. *Expert Review of Gastroenterology & Hepatology, 17,* 1267–1283. https://www.semanticscholar.org/paper/04af0c8dbb98e4ba3525431762d7c853847e80b8 (accessed on 16th July 2025).

20. Caputi, V., & Giron, M. C. (2018). Microbiome-Gut-Brain Axis and Toll-Like Receptors in Parkinson's Disease. *International journal of molecular sciences, 19*(6), 1689. https://doi.org/10.3390/ijms19061689(accessed on 16th July 2025).

21. Carneiro, C., Brito, J., Bilreiro, C., Barros, M. H., Bahia, C., Santiago, I., & Caseiro-Alves, F. (2019). All about portal vein: A pictorial display to anatomy, variants and physiopathology. *Insights into Imaging, 10.* https://doi.org/10.1186/s13244-019-0716-8 (accessed on 16th July 2025).

22. Chen, L., Deng, H., Cui, H., Fang, J., Zuo, Z., Deng, J., Li, Y., et al. (2017). Inflammatory responses and inflammation-associated diseases in organs. *Oncotarget, 9,* 7204–7218. https://doi.org/10.18632/oncotarget.23208 (accessed on 16th July 2025).

23. D'Avanzo, B., Ferraroni, M., Franceschi, S., Negri, et al. (2017). *Socioeconomic indicators, tobacco and alcohol in the aetiology of digestive tract neoplasms.* https://core.ac.uk/download/85221748.pdf (accessed on 16th July 2025).

24. Diaconu, C. C., Diculescu, M., Ditu, G., Hainarosie, et al. (2018). *Pancreatogenic type 3C diabetes.* https://core.ac.uk/download/216809675.pdf (accessed on 16th July 2025).

25. Gallo, C., Dispinzieri, G., Zucchini, N., Invernizzi, P., & Massironi, S. (2024). Autoimmune pancreatitis: Cornerstones and future perspectives. *World Journal of Gastroenterology, 30,* 817–832. https://www.semanticscholar.org/paper/73374ba9537da687b5f775e585572edd83f24dec (accessed on 16th July 2025).

26. Ge, Y. (2025). Integrating new approach methodologies to address environmental pancreatic toxicity and metabolic disorders. *Biology, 14.* https://www.semanticscholar.org/paper/6be62c2ef0519240067aa472e5993a89b1688572 (accessed on 16th July 2025).

27. Golovacheva, A. A., & Tabeeva, G. R. (2025). Chronic non-specific low back pain in combination with tension-type headache, issues of therapy optimization. *Neurology, Neuropsychiatry, Psychosomatics.* https://www.semanticscholar.org/paper/9a94486378e71621c309b95c53585b5fc07f9637 (accessed on 16th July 2025).

28. Capurso, G., Signoretti, M., Archibugi, L., Stigliano, S., & Delle Fave, G. (2016). Systematic review and meta-analysis: Small intestinal bacterial overgrowth in chronic pancreatitis. *United European gastroenterology journal, 4*(5), 697–705. https://doi.org/10.1177/2050640616630117(accessed on 16th July 2025).

29. Högberg, A. (2003). *Cereal Non-Starch Polysaccharides in Pig Diets.* https://core.ac.uk/download/11694626.pdf (accessed on 16th July 2025).

30. Kansra, A. R., Lakkunarajah, S., & Jay, M. S. (2021). Childhood and adolescent obesity: A review. *Frontiers in Pediatrics, 8.* https://doi.org/10.3389/fped.2020.581461 (accessed on 16th July 2025).

31. Keller, J. N., & Uranga, R. M. (2019). *The Complex Interactions Between Obesity, Metabolism and the Brain.* https://core.ac.uk/download/287882287.pdf (accessed on 16th July 2025).

32. Kiraly, B., & Gunning, K. (2008). A case of pancreatitis associated with aripiprazole in the absence of hyperglycemia. *Primary Care Companion to the Journal of Clinical Psychiatry, 10*(6), 484–485. https://www.semanticscholar.org/paper/e3b05c77e284bad6e56398d28db3d0e158ec01ee (accessed on 16th July 2025).

33. Koncoro, H., & Wibawa, I. D. (2012). *Acute Pancreatitis as a Complication of Choledochal Cyst.* https://media.neliti.com/media/publications/63839-EN-acute-pancreatitis-as-a-complication-of.pdf (accessed on 16th July 2025).

34. Lenti, M. V., Hammer, H., Tachecí, I., Burgos, R., Schneider, S., Foteini, A., Derovs, A., et al. (2025). European consensus on malabsorption—UEG & SIGE, LGA, SPG, SRGH, CGS, ESPCG, EAGEN, ESPEN, and ESPGHAN. Part 1: Definitions, clinical phenotypes, and diagnostic testing for malabsorption. *United European Gastroenterology Journal, 13,* 599–613. https://www.semanticscholar.org/paper/2b9809b57f7b28fb9b95a582a3addd564bf3b5e8 (accessed on 16th July 2025).

35. Molven, A., Njølstad, P., & Weiss, F. (2015). Lipase gene fusion: A new route to chronic pancreatitis. *Oncotarget, 6,* 30443–30444. https://www.semanticscholar.org/paper/9c6d56256e0a8757a05db080d209a02518c80037 (accessed on 16th July 2025).

36. Focal Spot, Fall/Winter 2010/2011. Bernard Becker Medical Library Archives. Washington University School of Medicine, Saint Louis, Missouri(accessed on 16th July 2025).

37. Nagai, K., Itoi, T., Mukai, S., Tsuchiya, T., Ishii, K., Tonozuka, R., Matsunami, Y., et al. (2022). Single-session endoscopic ultrasound-guided hepaticogastrostomy and pancreatic duct drainage for concomitant biliary and pancreatic duct stones in a patient with a surgically altered anatomy. *Journal of Hepato-Biliary-Pancreatic Sciences, 29.* https://www.semanticscholar.org/paper/49fbef11110092c9da335f46b7c7909316cb6a13 (accessed on 16th July 2025).

38. Nkurunziza, B. K. (2024). Unveiling the wonders of animal digestion: A comprehensive exploration. *Newport International Journal of Scientific and Experimental Sciences.* https://www.semanticscholar.org/paper/c808107d7cdf63458a5f69d0b2e576d506f841b5 (accessed on 16th July 2025).

39. Omer, E. M., & Chiodi, C. (2024). Fat digestion and absorption: Normal physiology and pathophysiology of malabsorption, including diagnostic testing. *Nutrition in Clinical Practice, 39*(Suppl 1), S6–S16. https://www.semanticscholar.org/paper/882cef7e35add45ada9330232b2de93728ed23c9 (accessed on 16th July 2025).

40. Pacella, K. A. C., Richson, B. N., Short, N. A., Bottera, A., Irish, L. A., Perko, V. L., & Forbush, K. (2024). Using item response theory to identify key symptoms of insomnia in a sample of university students with probable eating disorders. *Eating and Weight Disorders, 29.* https://www.semanticscholar.org/paper/136fc2b0e59387d869201f00cedde3df5ef3a06d (accessed on 16th July 2025).

41. Rindi, G., Klimstra, D. S., Abedi-Ardekani, B., Sylvia, L., Bosman, F. T., Brambilla, É., Busam, K. J., et al. (2018). A common classification framework for neuroendocrine neoplasms: An International Agency for Research on Cancer (IARC) and World Health Organization (WHO) expert consensus proposal. *Modern Pathology, 31*, 1770–1786. https://doi.org/10.1038/s41379-018-0110-y (accessed on 16th July 2025).

42. Sanatkar, S., Stevelink, S. A. M., Aars, N., Bardal, I., Brandseth, O. L., Brinchmann, B., & Mykletun, A. (2025). Health consequences of graded, full, and no sickness absence among workers with musculoskeletal disorders: Health profiles and six-months symptom changes. *BMC Musculoskeletal Disorders, 26.* https://www.semanticscholar.org/paper/aa03d4473e31d5cfdf60666476c3290efbdf983d (accessed on 16th July 2025).

43. Vizir, M., Zhelezniakova, N., Prosolenko, K., Molodan, V. I., & Goptsii, O. (2024). Nesfatin-1 and pancreatic β-cells in hypertension with abdominal obesity: Implications for dysglycemia. *Ukrainian Therapeutical Journal.* https://www.semanticscholar.org/paper/40bb355d7550d79a2bf71120e759e0ca7322a082 (accessed on 16th July 2025).

44. Volkova, N. I., Davidenko, I., Sorokina, J., Degtyareva, J., & Kovalenko, V. (2023). THU317 Study of risk factors for the development of various subtypes of gestational diabetes mellitus. *Journal of the Endocrine Society, 7.* https://www.semanticscholar.org/paper/f215ee323a498134208828c7db975f066802885d (accessed on 16th July 2025).

45. Vos, T., Abajobir, A. A., Abate, K. H., Abbafati, C., Abbas, K., Abd-Allah, F., Abdulkader, R. S., et al. (2017). Global, regional, and national incidence, prevalence, and years lived with disability for 328 diseases and injuries for 195 countries, 1990–2016: A systematic analysis for the Global Burden of Disease Study 2016. *The Lancet, 390*, 1211–1259. https://doi.org/10.1016/s0140-6736(17)32154-2 (accessed on 16th July 2025).

46. Wang, S. Y., Zhao, S. Q., Wang, S. P., Zhang, Y., Sun, S. Y., & Wang, S. (2025). Endoscopic ultrasound-guided pancreatic duct drainage: Progress and future outlook. *World Journal of Gastrointestinal Surgery, 17.* https://www.semanticscholar.org/paper/d7689e80c47f24c659c071cdac027e3b520b6edc (accessed on 16th July 2025).

47. Yang, L., Shi, P., Zhao, G., Xu, J., Peng, W., Zhang, J., Zhang, G., et al. (2020). Targeting cancer stem cell pathways for cancer therapy. *Signal Transduction and Targeted Therapy, 5.* https://doi.org/10.1038/s41392-020-0110-5 (accessed on 16th July 2025).

48. Yrkm, S. (2024). Understanding pancreatic disorders: Acute and chronic pancreatitis, pancreatic cancer and diabetes: A mini-review on a few of the most common pancreatic disorders. *Annals of Pancreatic Disorders and Treatment.* https://www.semanticscholar.org/paper/a7f885f278aa046c513630e4b89671fc2ef37b94 (accessed on 16th July 2025).

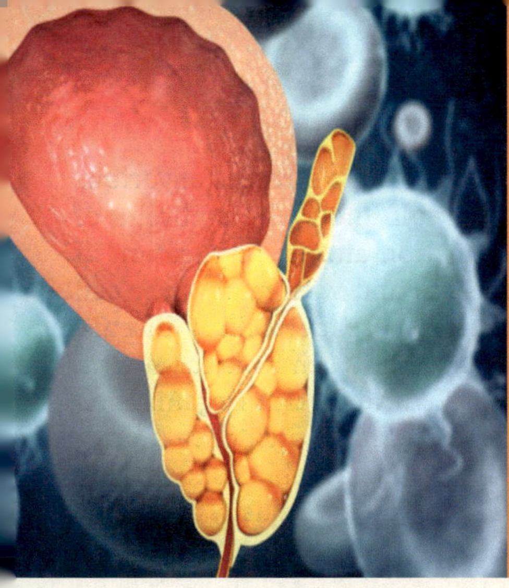

Chapter 10
GALLBLADDER AND BILIARY TRACT DISORDERS

Contents

Introduction

The biliary tree and gallbladder are central to the digestive system and its functioning in terms of storing and transporting bile, a fluid required for fat digestion and fat absorption. Deviations from this system can lead to many disorders that significantly impact a human being's health and well-being. They may be in the form of gallstones, cholangitis, or biliary atresia, each with specific signs and complications. An understanding of the gallbladder and biliary tract anatomy and physiology is key to understanding how these conditions develop and progress. In addition, the pathophysiology of the conditions has become a growing focus for interest in clinical practice and investigation, indicating a demand for an improvement in our knowledge regarding gallbladder and biliary tract health. At the forefront of gallbladder and biliary tract disease research is the role of cholangiocytes, bile duct-lining epithelial cells. Not only are these cells important for the formation of bile, but also important for modulating bile volume and composition. In healthy physiological conditions, cholangiocytes are involved in the overall maintenance of biliary health; however, when subjected to stresses of various types, they can adapt pathologically to cause conditions all of which fall under the umbrella of cholangiopathy. This refers to the sophistication of cholangiocyte function and its implication in conditions of disease, since they are involved in inflammatory processes and with many liver cell types. Hence, learning about these cells gives significant data about the broader biliary disease and its treatment. The incidence of gallbladder and biliary tract disease has risen in tandem with obesity across the globe, and it constitutes a public health crisis. The World Health Organization has characterized obesity as a global epidemic, with a remarkable increase in incidence among children and adults (Kyrou et al., 2010). This trend is accountable for a considerable contribution to the prevalence of concomitant diseases, including gallstones and choledocholithiasis, as weight excess has been linked to altering the saturation and bile composition, thus promoting disorder risk development. As obesity rates continue to increase and with it the resultant health-associated issues, prevention and therapeutic strategies directed toward gallbladder and biliary tract disorders become long overdue to be explored. This calls for an interdisciplinary approach that incorporates epidemiological, clinical, and educational perspectives to address these prevalent health disorders in an effective manner (Figure 10.1).

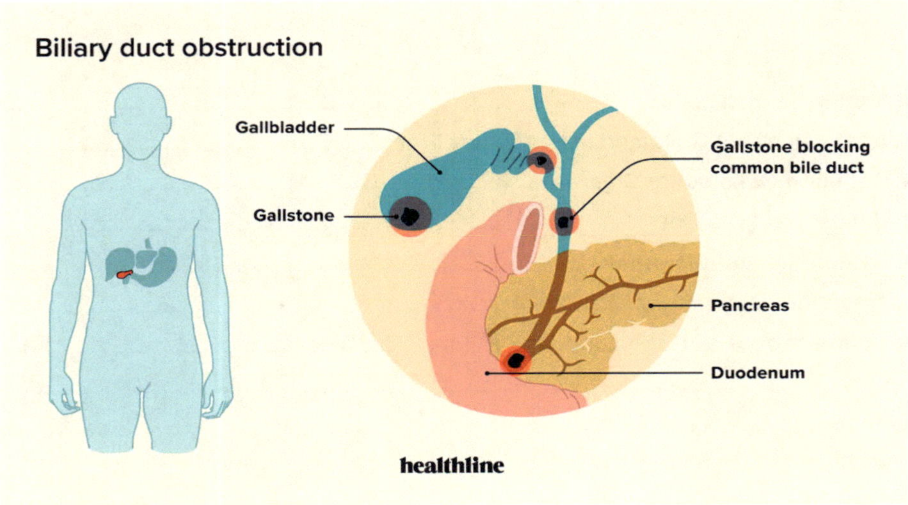

Figure 10.1. Gallbladder and biliary tract disorders.

Source: https://post.healthline.com/wp-content/uploads/2022/01/1827269-Biliary-Duct-Obstruction.png.

Definition of Gallbladder and Biliary Tract Disorders

Gallbladder and biliary tract diseases are worth understanding to appreciate the subtleties of gastrointestinal wellness. The gallbladder, a tiny organ beneath the liver, plays a crucial role in the digestive process in that it concentrates and stores bile, which helps in the emulsification of fats. Gallbladder disorders are diseases , such as gallstones, cholecystitis, and gallbladder cancer. Gallstones, which are hardened gallstones of varying sizes that are formed from the digestive fluid, can be quite painful and cause inflammation. Cholecystitis, or inflammation of the gallbladder, may occur due to obstruction caused by gallstones and is likely to require surgery. Also, the prevalence of cancers like gallbladder cancer highlights the necessity for proper perception and early detection, particularly given that the cancers have been proven to be aggressive and are hard to detect early, as seen in recent research on biliary tract cancers (Yarchoan et al., 2020). The biliary tree is a collection of ducts that drain the liver's bile into the small intestine and plays a key role in digestion. Diseases of the system can significantly affect overall health. This is true for primary sclerosing cholangitis (PSC), which is a disease characterized by chronic inflammation and fibrosis of the bile ducts, leading to bile duct obstruction and potential liver damage. In addition, cholangiocarcinoma, a bile duct cancer, is a cancer that poses major diagnostic problems because it is usually asymptomatic in the early phases, so it presents late in its course when it is hard to cure.

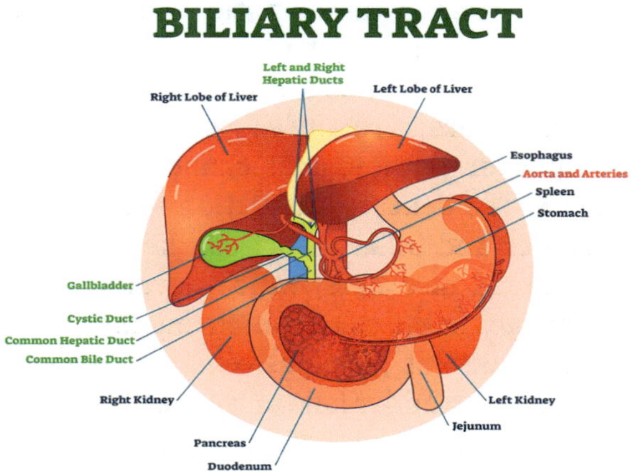

Figure 10.2. Gallbladder and biliary tract disorders (detailed picture).

Source: https://img.lb.wbmdstatic.com/vim/live/webmd/consumer_assets/site_images/article_thumbnails/BigBead/hida_scan_bigbead/1800x1200_hida_scan_bigbead.jpg.

The relationship between obesity, inflammation, and cancers of the biliary tracts is also under question, highlighting the involvement of metabolic factors in the aetiology of these conditions, as indicated by studies that linked various biomarkers to increased cancer risk (Aleksandrova et al., 2014). Effective management of gallbladder and biliary tract diseases requires a multidisciplinary approach combining diagnostics, treatment, and research. Doctors usually classify these diseases through imaging techniques, such as ultrasonography and magnetic resonance cholangiopancreatography (MRCP). The treatments range from dietary to surgical interventions like laparoscopic cholecystectomy for gallbladder-related issues. For architectural biliary tract diseases or malignancy, complicated therapy like endoscopic treatment or chemotherapy can be used. The intricacy of their management again underscores the need for continued research and technological advancements in treatment regimens, particularly in light of new findings on immunotherapy for conditions like cancers of the biliary tree, thus opening up channels towards improved patient outcomes and survival rates (Yarchoan et al., 2020) (Figure 10.2).

Importance of Understanding These Disorders

The importance of knowing gallbladder and biliary tract diseases goes beyond simple medical information; it has very significant implications for patient care and healthcare procedures. Gallbladder and biliary tract disorders can result in severe complications like infection, obstruction of the biliary tract, and even liver injury if not diagnosed immediately and properly. Bacterial infection, for instance, has been identified as one of the major causes of the causation of such disorders, with studies showing that many patients show bacterial colonization in the bile cultures in diagnostic workups. The observation underscores the importance of identifying the microbiological component, as this could direct management and decrease the prevalence of polymicrobial infection complicating gallbladder disease (Alebouyeh et al., 2016). Therefore, an extension of our understanding of these conditions is essential for the development of more efficient treatment strategies and improved patient care. In addition, examination of the immunobiology of the cholangiocytes, bile duct lining cells, can yield important information regarding the pathogenesis of biliary disease. The cholangiocytes play central roles in bile production and control as they respond to stimuli that will lead to proliferation or cell death. The biliary system's dual function emphasizes the intricacy of the system and its vulnerability to pathology. Cholangiocyte dysfunction can precipitate severe inflammatory reactions that promote cholangiopathy, which can progress to end-stage liver disease necessitating transplantation (Yarchoan et al., 2020). It is critical to understand how these cells function in disease and health to untangle not only the pathophysiologic mechanisms of biliary tract disease but also to guide potential therapeutic maneuvers. Such information ultimately improves patient quality of life by delivering timely and targeted treatment strategies. Lastly, public health issues must be considered when treating gallbladder and biliary tract disease. Comprehensive information regarding the risk factors, clinical features, and complications of the conditions enables medical professionals to develop targeted preventive interventions and education programs. Effective treatment of the diseases, particularly among groups with high risks, includes collaborative intervention of community health education for lifestyle modification, dietary practices, and early diagnostic approaches. Moreover, this information encourages interprofessional communication among medical professionals, scientists, and public health professionals to create a comprehensive prevention and treatment plan. As the healthcare systems invest more emphasis on patient-centric care, the understanding of gallbladder and biliary tract disease complexities is crucial in enhancing overall health and reducing the cost of healthcare use of complex disease states.

10.1. Anatomy of the Gallbladder and Biliary Tract

Gallbladder and biliary tract are a well-evolved anatomical and functional system required for digestion and metabolism process. Gallbladder is a pear-shaped sac lying beneath the liver and serves as a reservoir for bile, a liver secretion that promotes emulsification and absorption of dietary fat. The biliary tree is made up of a number of various components, which include the hepatic ducts, common bile duct, and cystic duct, to channel bile from the liver to the duodenum. On the intake of food, the gallbladder goes into a state of contraction and secretes bile into the small intestine, where it performs its critical function during the digestion of nutrients. Understanding the anatomy of this system is essential in the identification of most of the disorders that can affect it, as dysfunctions are normally caused by structural anomalies or pathological changes in these elements. The delicate interaction between the gallbladder and biliary tract can be disrupted by numerous disorders, which normally stem from changes in the composition and in the flow of bile. Conditions , such as biliary dyskinesia, where the gallbladder fails to contract normally, may lead to abnormal secretion of bile, which presents as abdominal pain and gastrointestinal disturbances. These functional derangements are linked to obstruction of bile outflow, typically by lithogenic bile—a type of bile that promotes gallstone formation (Shulpekova et al., 2024). In addition, recurrent inflammation of the biliary tract can result from the inspissation of lithogenic bile and lead to secondary consequences , such as cholecystitis or cholangitis. Understanding these associations while addressing gallbladder and biliary tract illness is important because they are informative about their pathophysiology and treatment. New evidence has indicated the probable impact of pharmacologic therapy on the biliary tree health, particularly for diabetes drugs. For one, in accordance with a study of the side effects of glucagon-like peptide-1 receptor agonists (GLP-1 RAs) and dipeptidyl peptidase-4 (DPP-4) inhibitors, notable risks have been linked with biliary disease, in addition to their known benefit in glycemic regulation (He et al., 2025). The established connection, especially with some of the drugs like sitagliptin and liraglutide, requires that clinicians be wary of the side effects of such drugs on the health of biliary structures. This knowledge necessitates constant monitoring and evaluation of pharmacological treatments, particularly in predisposed patients prone to gallbladder and biliary tract disease. Understanding , such associations carries the discussion beyond the anatomical into implications of treatment modalities that have the potential to greatly influence the production of bile and its flow, in turn impacting patients' gastrointestinal well-being (Figure 10.3).

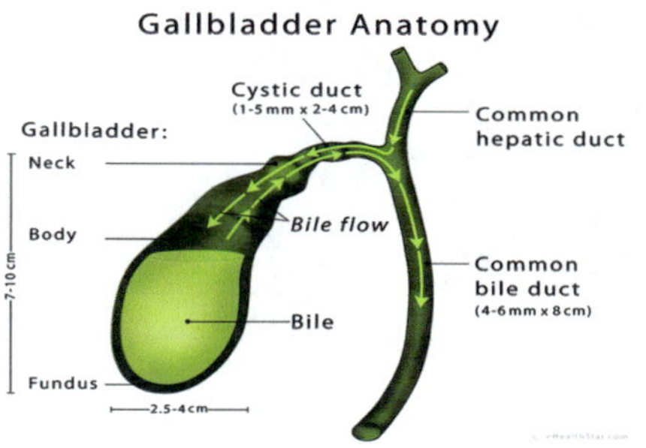

Figure 10.3. Anatomy of the gallbladder and biliary tract.

Source: https://www.ehealthstar.com/wp-content/uploads/2014/12/Gallbladder-Anatomy-15.jpg.

10.1.1. Description of the Gallbladder's Structure

The gallbladder is pear-shaped and small, located below the liver and is a vital component of the digestive system. The gallbladder is anatomically made up of a few key components: the fundus, body, and neck. The fundus is the anterior rounded projection and the body is the major storage of bile. The gallbladder is suspended by the neck to the cystic duct, and the cystic duct ultimately leads to the common bile duct. This intricate association allows for the regulation of the release of bile into the duodenum to aid in the emulsification of fats and the absorption of fat-soluble vitamins. The mucosal lining of the gallbladders is lined with simple columnar epithelium and richly supplied with folds, known as rugae, that increase its surface area and allow it to concentrate bile by absorption of water and electrolytes. The physiological structure of the gallbladder its structure is highly specialized to allow it to perform its primary function of storing and concentrating bile. The three layers constituting the gallbladder wall are the mucosa, muscularis, and serosa. The muscularis layer contains smooth muscle cells that contract in response to hormonal stimuli, namely cholecystokinin, to permit the release of bile into the intestines. This is a significant process that makes bile available at all times whenever fatty food comes near the digestive system. The outermost layer, the serosa, consists of visceral peritoneum, so that the gallbladder is supported in the abdominal cavity, yet is structurally intact and provided with passages of continuity with nearby organs and tissues. Furthermore, the anatomical location and structural make-up of the gallbladder largely determine the susceptibility to a variety of disorders. Because of its relatively secluded location and functional demand, the gallbladder has the potential to develop gallstones, a hardened substance buildup composed of cholesterol or bilirubin. The buildup is capable of blocking bile flow, precipitating disease like cholecystitis or pancreatitis. Also, because of its high concentration abilities, it may become susceptible to inflammation and malfunction, highlighting the need for a well-functioning gallbladder in keeping the overall digestive system healthy. An understanding of the structural intricacies of the gallbladder will help clinicians diagnose and treat biliary tract diseases effectively, allowing early action to prevent complications due to gallbladder dysfunction (Fitzmaurice et al., 2019; Murray et al., 2022).

10.1.2. Function of the Biliary Tract

The biliary system plays a key role within the body for digestion, primarily by emulsifying and absorbing fat. This well-regulated system consists of the gallbladder, bile ducts, and liver and functions to create and transport bile. Bile, a multi-protein fluid composed of bile salts, cholesterol, and bilirubin, is generated in the liver and stored in the gallbladder. When fatty foods are eaten, the gallbladder contracts, pushing out bile through the bile ducts into the small intestine. This spitting breaks down the fats into smaller particles so that lipase enzymes secreted by the pancreas can take effect. Without effective bile formation and secretion, the body cannot digest fats in the diet, leading to malabsorption and ensuing nutritional deficiencies. In addition to aiding in the digestion of fat, the biliary system accomplishes the elimination of metabolic waste products. Bile also serves as a vehicle for the elimination of bilirubin, the end product of hemoglobin breakdown, and the excess cholesterol. The liver detoxifies the blood and produces bile that isolates the waste products. Any break in the process, caused by biliary tract disease , such as cholestasis or bile duct obstruction, can lead to the production of poisonous substances in the blood, which can cause jaundice and increased cholesterol levels. In addition, these diseases have the potential to cause more severe hepatic ailments and systemic disorders of health. It is, therefore, essential to understand the role of the biliary tract in both digestion and the general equilibrium of metabolism. Apart from digestion, the role of the biliary tract also encompasses its antimicrobial functions that are essential to the maintenance of gut health. The bile's composition has bile acids with intrinsic antimicrobial properties that aid in the control of the proliferation of disease-causing bacteria within the small intestine. This protective function is particularly significant with the gut microbiota in a delicate equilibrium needed for nutrient acquisition and immunity. Biliary tract dysfunction, as in gallbladder disease or bile duct trauma, may have a modifying influence upon bile composition with a subsequent potential for dysbiosis, an imbalance within the gut microbiome. Such imbalances have been linked to various gastrointestinal diseases and may contribute to existing illness. Lastly, the complex function of the biliary tracts further confirms its significance in not just digestive wellbeing but also in prevention against systemic disease, and is worthy of further study and explanation in comparison with gallbladder and biliary tract disease (Figure 10.4).

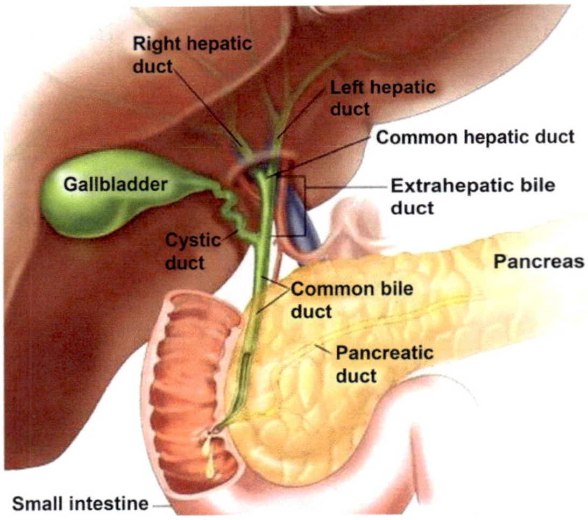

Figure 10.4. Function of the biliary tract.

Source: https://cdn.medizzy.com/D22WUAizrx5I4n_a3TQg3QHWSoY=/680x576/img/posts/f56ac2f7-11e1-4f09-aac2-f711e1cf0900.

10.1.3. Relationship Between the Gallbladder and Liver

The connection of the gallbladder to the liver is in the digestion process, particularly in the emulsification and absorption of dietary fats. The liver secretes bile into the bile ducts, a fluid composed of bile salts, cholesterol, and bilirubin, to emulsify fats during digestion. The bile is then transported by the bile ducts into the gallbladder, where it is stored and concentrated before its use in digestion. When ingested, food, particularly fatty foods, causes relaxation of the gallbladder and the release of bile into the small intestine for lipid emulsification. This collaboration aims to highlight the gallbladder's role as a reservoir with the improvement of the supply of bile, an activity that is crucial for effective digestion and nutrient absorption, and which highlights the mutualism between these two organs toward digestive health and prevention of disorders of bile production and storage. Dysfunction of either the liver or the gallbladder can lead to severe biliary tract disease with a detrimental effect on health. Gallstones can obstruct b and lead to cholecystitis or pancreatitis, while liver disease , such as cirrhosis, can compromise bile secretion. Both of them can lead to elevated levels of bilirubin in the blood, which leads to jaundice and potential complications during digestion. The intricate interrelation thus acts as a double-edged sword; while the gallbladder serves to store and discharge bile, its disease can exacerbate liver illness, and conversely. Such interactions must be realized to diagnose and treat biliary tract disorders, indicating a general approach in medical assessment and intervention methods designed to address gallbladder and liver health in all their complexity. Current studies have emphasized the existence of the microbiota in the biliary tract, shedding light on the composition and physiology of the human bile microbiome. Research indicates that healthy gallbladders are inhabited by separate bacterial populations that are significantly dissimilar from those of individuals with gallbladder pathology, such as cholelithiasis. The variations in the populations of bacteria can influence bile composition and, subsequently, gallbladder and liver well-being. For instance, modification of bile by microbiota can impact gallstone risk and the course of liver disease, suggesting a critical interaction between microbial health and hepatobiliary function. This new region emphasizes the importance not only of knowing the physiological and anatomical interrelationship of these organs but also the biotic factors that may be implicated in their general functioning and susceptibility to disorder, as seen through recent research into the role of bile microbiotas (Molinero et al., 2019) (Figure 10.5).

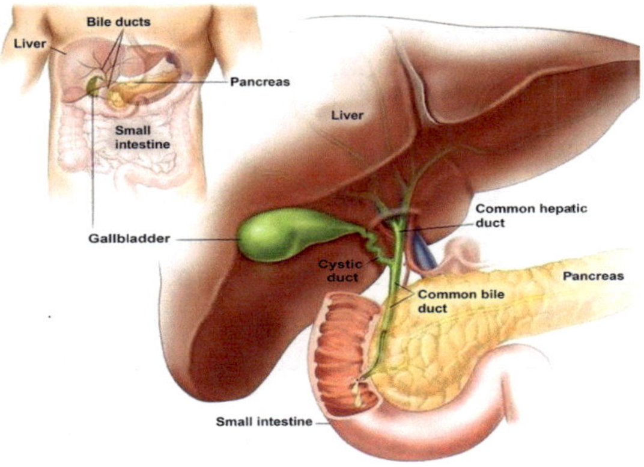

Figure 10.5. Relationship between the gallbladder and liver.

Source: https://external-content.duckduckgo.com/iu/?u=https%3A%2F%2Fwww.researchgate.net%2Fprofile%2FJiayan-Yan-2%2Fpost%2FHow_do_you_understand_the_relationship_between_gallbladder_and_liver%2Fattachment%2F5c87501fcfe4a7299494e2a3%2FAS%3A735514554552322%25401552371743525%2Fimage%2Fc8c66cfb9d6fc7c3b5f983d4c69c6f15_r.jpg&f=1&nofb=1&ipt=a942f70c31be3356207d3855f34161f4b908772d0f789900afab74a2c4726ac4.

10.2. Common Gallbladder Disorders

The gallbladder is a key organ of the biliary apparatus whose principal function is store and concentrate bile secreted by the liver. Cholelithiasis, or gallstones, is one of the most common gallbladder diseases among the usual ones. Gallstones can be formed in the event of the disruption of the composition of the materials that comprise bile and leading to crystallization. Patients typically present with features , such as biliary colic, painful bile pathway obstruction. In severe situations, infections , such as inflammation of the gallbladder, known as cholecystitis, may develop. This may require surgical intervention in the form of a laparoscopic cholecystectomy. By complete comprehension of gallstone pathogenesis, risk factors, and management, physicians are able to properly care for patients with this common but serious disease of the gallbladder and biliary tree. Another critical gallbladder disease is acute cholecystitis, an infection most commonly caused by cystic duct obstruction by gallstones. The disease classically consists of abdominal pain, fever, and vomiting. Untreated acute cholecystitis can lead to gallbladder perforation that significantly increases morbidity and mortality. Diagnosis is usually made by imaging tests like ultrasound or computed tomography, that would reveal evidence of gallstones and inflammation. Intravenous antibiotics and surgical removal of the gallbladder are the usual treatments. It is necessary for clinicians to diagnose the early signs and symptoms of acute cholecystitis to ensure early treatment and prevent severe complications of the disease. Cholangiocarcinoma is a complex and more harmful carcinoma associated with the gallbladder, derived from the bile ducts. It is a carcinoma characterized by its initial phase and late onset, and thus challenging to diagnose and treat. Risk factors in cholangiocarcinoma include chronic inflammation of the biliary tract secondary to disease , such as primary sclerosing cholangitis or choledocholithiasis, with additional risk factors , such as infection by liver fluke in endemic regions. In fact, cholangiocarcinoma is one of the characteristics to be heterogeneous, a term utilized in current research proposing interaction between environmental and genetic predisposition to complicate disease formation. Cholangiocarcinoma remains a negative condition with a devastating prognosis despite the advances in the surgical treatment and chemotherapeutic targeting, for which an attempt must still be made to develop more effective appropriate diagnostic and treatment techniques for the better therapeutic outcome of gallbladder and biliary tract diseases (Khan et al., 2019; Brindley et al., 2021) (Figure 10.6).

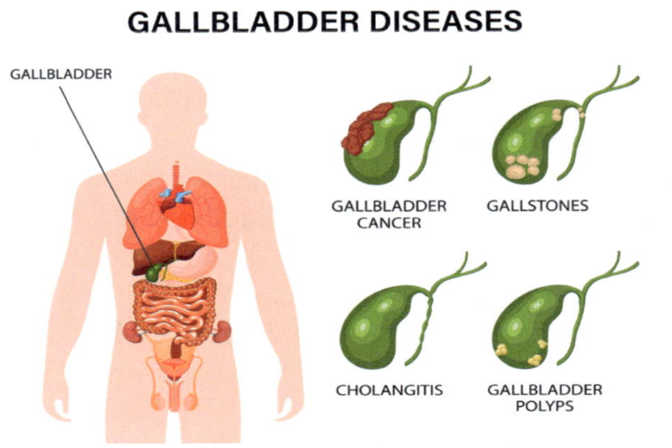

Figure 10.6. Common gallbladder disorders.

Source: https://static.vecteezy.com/system/resources/previews/046/425/963/large_2x/gallbladder-diseases-infographics-gallstone-disease-cancer-acute-cholecystitis-cholangitis-or-polyps-of-the-digestive-system-problems-with-the-biliary-tract-illustration-vector.jpg.

10.2.1. Cholelithiasis (Gallstones)

Cholelithiasis, or gallstones, is a universal affliction that haunts a significant portion of the population, particularly in Western countries. The substance that crystallizes in bile, from which these solid particles are derived, can vary in size and composition. Gallstones are classically classified into two types: cholesterol stones, yellow-green in color and composed mainly of hard cholesterol, and pigment stones, darker in appearance and due to the deposition of excess bilirubin. Gallstone pathogenesis may be understood based on an imbalance in bile composition due to bile stasis or an inflammatory change in the gallbladder. Although cholestasis and its consequences occur in the vast majority of individuals without any symptoms at all, the gallstones can complicate as cholecystitis, acute pancreatitis, or indeed cholangitis, and hence it is imperative to consider this condition against the background of general gallbladder and biliary tract disease. Diagnosis of cholelithiasis often involves imaging tests, with the most common initial modality being ultrasound due to its non-invasive nature and effectiveness in visualization of gallstones. In situations where the diagnosis remains uncertain, other imaging tests , such as magnetic resonance cholangiopancreatography (MRCP) or computed tomographic (CT) scans, may be utilized. Clinical manifestation of gallstones can include biliary colic as recurring abdominal pain, often after meals with high fat content. If obstructed, the gallbladder may get inflamed and cholecystitis will ensue, which presents with increased pain, fever, and jaundice. Understanding pathophysiology and diagnostic strategies for cholelithiasis will be important in early intervention and management that avoids future complications of the disease. Treatment of cholelithiasis is diverse and depends upon the severity of symptoms and complications. While asymptomatic gallstones will not require treatment, symptomatic gallstones will typically require therapeutic management, most typically in the form of laparoscopic cholecystectomy. The minimally invasive removal of the gallbladder has reduced recovery periods and less pain after surgery compared to conventional surgery. Drugs , such as ursodeoxycholic acid may dissolve cholesterol gallstones in certain instances, but this is not an established method due to variation in success rates. Moreover, mounting evidence indicates that conditions , such as intrahepatic cholestasis of pregnancy are capable of influencing the function and functioning of the gallbladder and promoting gallstone formation, confirming close interconnections between various biliary tract illnesses (Williamson & Geenes, 2014). Therefore, correct knowledge regarding the aetiology and management of cholelithiasis is crucial for effective management of the patients (Tenner et al., 2013) (Figure 10.7).

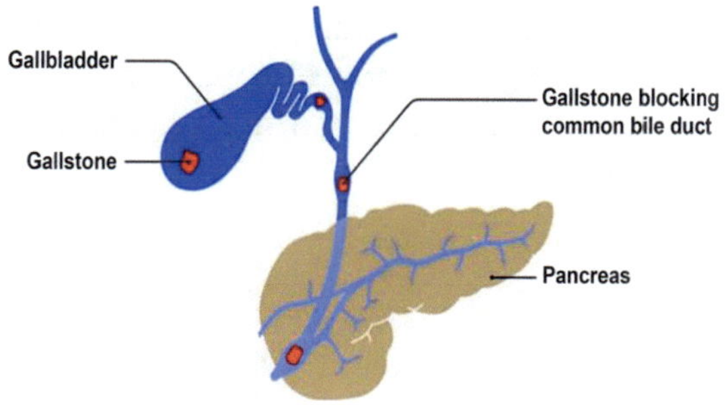

Figure 10.7. Cholelithiasis, commonly known as gallstones.

Source: https://dims.healthgrades.com/dims3/MMH/597e3a1/2147483647/strip/true/crop/1024x600+0+0/resize/800x469!/quality/75/?url=https%3A%2F%2Fucmscdn.healthgrades.com%2F98%2F28%2F2b8770038831c1430407077e72ca%2F349-cholelithiasis-gallstones-1296x760-body-copy-1024x600.jpg.

10.2.2. Cholecystitis (Inflammation of the Gallbladder)

Cholecystitis, or gallbladder inflammation, is typically the consequence of obstructive phenomena caused by gallstones. The obstruction leads to bile stasis, which initiates inflammation and, in rare cases, infection. Symptoms are typically accompanied by a high level of abdominal pain, typically centered over the right upper quadrant, often accompanied by nausea, vomiting, and even fever. Inflammatory response will most probably result in complications , such as perforation or abscess, which will elevate the clinical situation to one that is life-threatening. Imaging with diagnostic equipment, mainly ultrasound, is significant in assessing gallbladder wall thickening and gallstone formation, which is a sign of active inflammation. The clinical presentation and potential complications highlight the need for early diagnosis and treatment, emphasizing the importance of putting cholecystitis in context with gallbladder and biliary tract illness. Therapy of cholecystitis is primarily surgical since the ultimate therapy is cholecystectomy, the operative removal of the gallbladder. The procedure can be performed laparoscopically or openly, depending on the degree of inflammation and the general health of the patients.

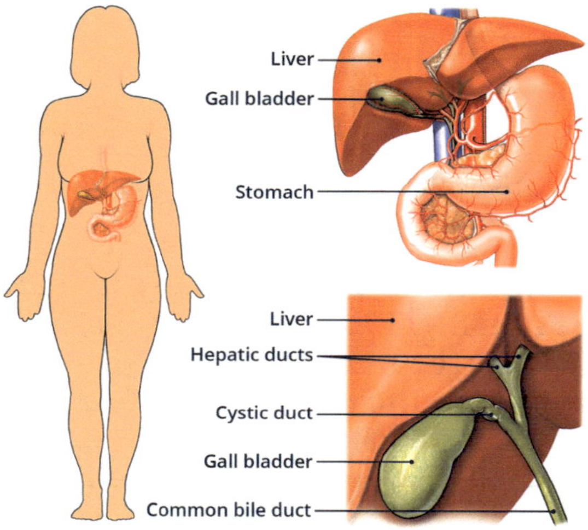

Figure 10.8. Cholecystitis (inflammation of the gallbladder).

Source: https://media.healthdirect.org.au/images/inline/original/cholecystitis-gallbladder-inflammation-78027b.png.

Laparoscopic cholecystectomy is preferred in most cases for its minimally invasive nature, having less postoperative pain and quicker recovery. Preoperative intervention may include antibiotic treatment to avoid the complication of bacterial infection. Conservative therapy with intravenous fluids and antibiotics would be for those patients with severe comorbidity who are poor surgical risks. However, this will not solve the core issue, which, in this case, points to surgery for patients with established cholecystitis to avoid recurrence and associated complications. Secondly, prevention of cholecystitis implies catering to risk factors underlying gallstone formation. These may include obesity, rapid weight loss, and certain food habits, which may result in gallstone pathology. Weight control by incremental dietary modification and increased physical activity will significantly reduce the incidence of gallstones and, consequently, cholecystitis. In addition, elucidation of the environmental and genetic etiology of gallbladder disease can aid in the design of preventive interventions. Although some risk factors, such as gender and age, cannot be modified, education regarding how these possible lifestyle changes may be achieved can enable individuals to engage in preventive practices in their own health care. In combination, awareness and preventive practice outside of cholecystitis can decrease the broader spectrum of gallbladder and biliary disease (Figure 10.8).

10.2.3. Gallbladder Cancer

The identification of gallbladder cancer (GBC) as a vital health issue calls for thorough knowledge of its etiology, and in this regard, the role of microbial communities of the biliary tract. Recent research suggests that there is a strong linkage between bacterial infection and biliary tract disease, and that the occurrence of bacteria , such as Escherichia coli in bile specimens may predispose to gallbladder cancer. Particularly, E. coli has been shown to be involved in inflammatory pathways that potentially lead to malignant transformations of the gallbladder epithelium. As infection levels increase in bile, the likelihood of becoming GBC also increases. Polymicrobial infections have also been reported extensively in gallbladder stone patients and obstructive patients of the common bile duct, hinting at microbial dysbiosis being an etiological factor in the development of this malignancy (Alebouyeh et al., 2016). Aside from bacterial influences, interactions of the bile microbiota form a critical component in terms of gallbladder cancer risk and progression. In an analysis of a patient cohort presenting with various pancreatic and biliary tract diseases, E. coli, Klebsiella pneumoniae, and Pseudomonas aeruginosa were prevalent species associated with poor outcomes, such as GBC. The findings showed that certain strains were potential markers of adverse survival, underlining the need for more research linking bile composition and cancer prognosis. Modulation of the microbiome of the bile may not only be involved in inflammatory mechanisms but may also directly affect the carcinogenic potential in the biliary epithelium (Di Carlo et al., 2019).

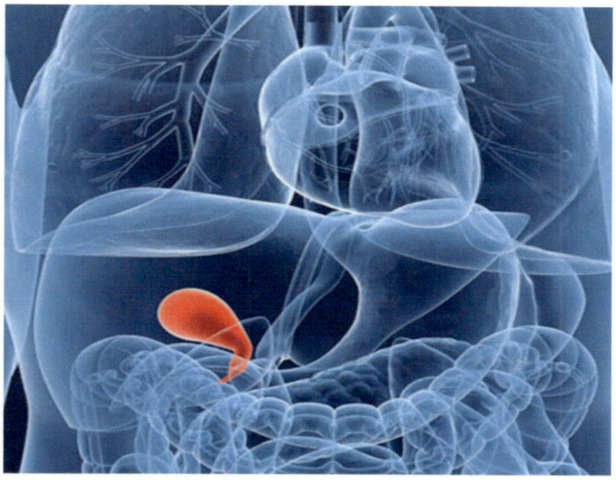

Figure 10.9. Gallbladder cancer.

Source: https://www.omicsgroup.org/articles-admin/disease-images/gallbladder-cancer-48798.jpg.

Thus, understanding the microbiota of bile can provide hints at prevention and treatment for gallbladder cancer. Because of the intricate connection between gallbladder cancer and biliary tract disease, one needs to adopt an interdisciplinary method in clinical management. Bile microbiota could offer a therapeutic avenue to counter the risk of gallbladder cancer by monitoring and regulating the microbiota. Interventions for bacterial infections have the potential to be capable of enhancing patient outcomes, especially among patients who have high resistance rates against the most commonly used antibiotics. By treating the causative microbes of the conditions and implementing strict infection controls, healthcare providers are capable of enhancing the overall prognosis among gallbladder and biliary tract disease patients. As it becomes clear with evidence that how microbiota of the bile is complex, the integration of microbiological testing in clinical assessment as a routine procedure could become unavoidable while preventing and treating gallbladder cancer (Alebouyeh et al., 2016; Di Carlo et al., 2019) (Figure 10.9).

10.3. Biliary Tract Disorders

Diseases of the biliary tract are a collection of diseases affecting the biliary apparatus, including the gallbladder, bile ducts, and allied structures. Disorders tend to affect seriously due to the intimate relationship between the pancreatic and biliary apparatus. For instance, biliary pancreatitis results if bile regurgitates into the pancreatic duct due to biliodoudenal hypertension; premature activation of the pancreatic enzymes under such a condition enhances bile duct complications. Organic and functional conditions lead to biliary hypertension, resulting in multiple clinical presentations. The functional disorders may be attributed to gallbladder or bile duct dysmotility, while organic conditions are presented by biliary sludge and choledocholithiasis, which may result in impaired regular bile movement, ultimately exacerbating pancreatic dysfunction. A clear understanding of these factors is required to design effective treatment regimens for biliary tract disorders (Ferfetska et al., 2024). Prevalence of gallstone disease, a significant feature of disorders of the biliary tract, is a significant public health problem in all segments of society. The figures are not surprising, with over 2.5 million cholecystectomies performed each year globally, pointing out the surgical significance of gallstone complications. Among gallstone complications, choledocholithiasis can lead to severe implications , such as mechanical jaundice and necessitate early surgical treatment. In a fascinating twist, Bouveret syndrome, a rare complication of chronic gallstone disease, illustrates the intricacy of biliary pathophysiology. Bouveret syndrome presents with inflammation and fistula formation between the duodenum and gallbladder, leading to bowel obstruction. Although it is rare, it is not always easy to diagnose due to nonspecific symptoms and the patient possessing the typical comorbidity. Early diagnosis and treatment are critical since the rate of mortality after surgery for these conditions may be horrifyingly high compared to other gastrointestinal obstructions (Khomenko et al., 2021).

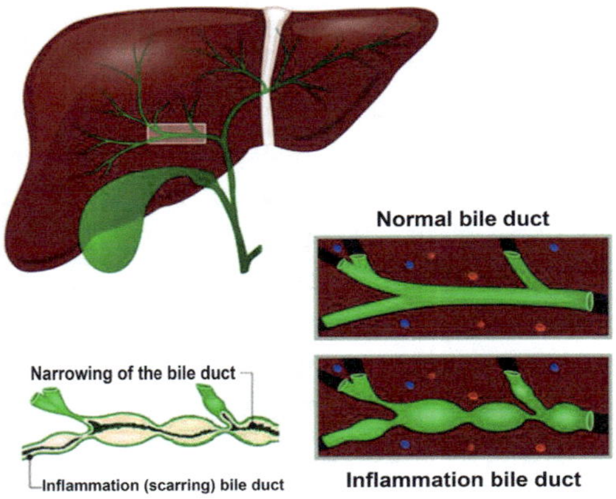

Figure 10.10. Biliary tract disorders.

Source: https://external-content.duckduckgo.com/iu/?u=https%3A%2F%2Fchblob.icloudhospital.com%2Fthumbnailcontainer%2F4-1-5c03cc50-cff2-4f06-95d5-fb0c4fbc34bb.jpg&f=1&nofb=1&ipt=8bc243d7a4cc352b9a57037b857d6f6188499daece8299c1ae38088fc3f1b689.

Therapeutic methods that prove effective for biliary tract diseases must be multidimensional and resolve both the acute and chronic phases of these conditions. Pharmacotherapy is an important element, particularly in managing functional disorders of motility of the biliary tract. Use of antispasmodics and choleretic agents has also found favor, with considerable therapeutic benefits in the management of symptoms. Ursodeoxycholic acid is also becoming well known for its use to enhance symptoms of biliary and chronic pancreatitis disease. Surgical intervention, particularly laparoscopic techniques, has transformed biliary surgery by offering minimally invasive techniques for intricate conditions. Despite advances in imaging modalities , such as CT and MRI, early diagnosis is challenging, especially with rare presentations , such as Bouveret syndrome. Hence, an integrated approach that combines surgical, medicinal, and diagnostic progress is vital to treat biliary tract disease and improve patient outcomes (Khomenko et al., 2021; Ferfetska et al., 2024) (Figure 10.10).

10.3.1. Biliary Obstruction

Obstruction of the bile is a problem of major clinical significance and is a central component of biliary tract and gallbladder disease. Obstruction is comprised of obstruction of bile flow by numerous causes, including strictures, tumors, and gallstones. Characteristic signs of biliary obstruction include jaundice, pain in the abdomen, and pruritus, resulting from the accumulation of bile acids and bilirubin. The condition can lead to serious complications, such as acute cholangitis, due to bacterial infection of the bile ducts, and acute liver failure if it is not treated early. Recognition of the complex interaction between these conditions and the need for early intervention is paramount to the improvement of patient outcomes in clinical practice, especially in the context of the overall increasing incidence of gastrointestinal diseases in populations reported in recent estimates of the economic burden of such conditions in Europe (Rose et al., 2022). Treatment for biliary obstruction often needs a multidisciplinary approach, particularly if options for therapy are to be addressed. Endoscopic intervention, including endoscopic retrograde cholangiopancreatography (ERCP), is usually the first treatment for obstructed relief caused by stricture or gallstones. ERCP is not successful in some instances, however, where other methods , such as percutaneous transhepatic biliary drainage (PTBD) or endoscopic ultrasound-guided biliary drainage (EUS-BD), are used (Merwe et al., 2021). The choice of technique also depends on the site and nature of the obstruction, the overall health of the patients, and the competency of the medical staff. These advances in therapeutic intervention emphasize the necessity of continued research and refinement of techniques to further enhance the effectiveness and safety of the management of biliary obstruction.

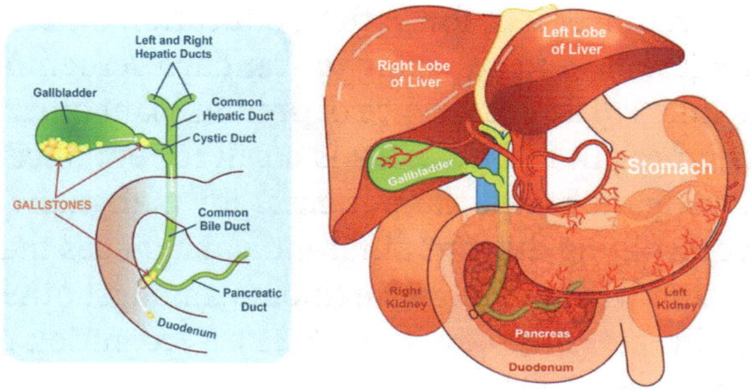

Figure 10.11. Biliary obstruction.

Source: https://d33ljpvc0tflz5.cloudfront.net/dims3/MMH/1342809/2147483647/strip/true/crop/4741x2489+36+0/resize/1200x630!/quality/75/?url=https:%2F%2Fd26ua9paks4zq.cloudfront.net%2Fdd%2F56%2F3bd13fb34c58b51b1b39024e2693%2Fgettyimages-962930900.jpg.

The implications of biliary obstruction extend beyond the immediate clinical significance; they have significant economic implications. The healthcare cost associated with treatment and diagnosis of complications that result as a consequence of biliary obstruction, such as hospital stay for cholangitis or further surgery, is largely responsible for the burden of gastrointestinal diseases (Rose et al., 2022). Furthermore, the social burden of biliary disease tends to occur in the form of lost productivity due to chronic health complications among affected patients, affirming equal research funding needs and policy-specific healthcare initiatives. Striking against the risk factors for biliary obstruction through preventive interventions, such as promoting healthy lifestyle habits and public health promotion of gallbladder well-being, will temper the rising occurrence of these conditions and improve population health outcomes (Figure 10.11).

10.3.2. Cholangiitis (Infection of the Bile Duct)

Cholangiitis, inflammation of the bile ducts caused by infection, is a major problem in the overall category of gallbladder and biliary tract disease. It typically results from bacterial infections, most commonly due to obstructions , such as gallstones, strictures, or tumors. The pathologic consequence of cholangiitis can be disastrous and leads to acute infection with the classic triad of fever, jaundice, and abdominal pain. The risk for systemic involvement requires early diagnosis and management, as cholangiitis not treated could lead to sepsis and notably affect mortality. With the continued increase in gallstone disease, the pathophysiology of cholangiitis and its effective prevention remain important for gastroenterologists to understand. The diagnostic workup for cholangiitis usually consists of clinical evaluation, laboratory studies, and imaging tests. Laboratory results are usually positive for elevated liver enzymes and bilirubin, which are indicative of cholestasis and liver impairment. Imaging procedures , such as ultrasound, computerized tomography, or magnetic resonance cholangiopancreatography are crucial for depicting bile duct obstruction and provide necessary information in the planning of treatment. Notably, identification of the cause of biliary obstruction is significant because it would be extremely variable between patients. For instance, in functional or organic biliary pancreatitis, the treatment would be quite different and the need to have individualized treatment plans in order to accommodate the unique circumstances for each patient and prevent repeated cholangiitis attacks would be extremely crucial (Ferfetska et al., 2024). Treatment of cholangiitis focuses nearly exclusively on the resolution of infection and secondary obstruction of the bile. Antibiotic therapy remains a cornerstone of initial treatment, with agents selected based on the presumed pathogen susceptibility. For situations in which obstruction is identified, procedures , such as ERCP are performed in hopes of unblocking obstructions and promoting bile drainage. In addition, enhanced interventional radiology services have also provided alternative ways of addressing complicated scenarios in which conventional approaches would be insufficient. As highlighted in recent literature, the relationship between cholangiitis and conditions , such as vanishing bile duct syndrome indicates the multifactorial causality of biliary disease, necessitating multimodal treatment. Lastly, the synergy of medical and surgical strategies is crucial in maximizing patient outcomes and minimizing the high risks of cholangiitis (Sukhija et al., 2024).

10.3.3. Primary Sclerosing Cholangitis

The subtleties of primary sclerosing cholangitis (PSC) are critical to the understanding of gallbladder and biliary tract disease. PSC is an idiopathic, chronic liver disease with bile duct inflammation and fibrosis that eventually leads to liver damage and cirrhosis. The disease usually manifests as cholestatic abnormalities of liver enzymes that are potentially identified by imaging techniques , such as magnetic resonance cholangiography (MRC). Diagnosis depends on the identification of characteristic cholangiographic features, which put PSC into a specific category of biliary illness. PSC is traditionally linked to inflammatory bowel disease (IBD), ulcerative colitis in particular, so that i) 80% of those diagnosed with PSC are also diagnosed with IBD. The interaction of the two conditions emphasizes the need for ongoing research into their shared pathophysiology and the genetic basis of their incidence and outcome. As PSC progresses, patients carry a high risk for the development of malignancies, such as cholangiocarcinoma and gallbladder carcinoma. The increased risk makes PSC not only a disabling illness but one with potentially fatal complications. Regime monitoring for cholangiocarcinoma thus forms part of the care for PSC patients, including imaging studies every six to twelve months to detect any malignancies at an early stage. There is also a high requirement for patient education on self-monitoring and adhering to standard screening regimens. The occurrence of predominant biliary strictures in PSC patients is a call for enhanced investigation into the potential for malignancy, necessitating diligent differential diagnoses that present with cholangiocarcinoma amongst other conditions (Brindley et al., 2021). Recognition of such risks underscores the necessity for ongoing monitoring and novel therapeutic interventions in the treatment of PSC patients. While there is no approved pharmacological treatment yet for PSC, the control of the manifestations and complications of the disease is still important. Liver transplantation is far and away the optimal therapy for individuals with advanced PSC, as it can recover liver function and, in some cases, also alleviate symptoms secondary to chronic cholestasis. Interestingly, though, despite the favorable outcomes that have been attributed to transplantation, there has been a reported post-surgical recurrence rate of approximately 20%, highlighting the need for tight long-term follow-up. Research into novel treatment approaches continues to be on the agenda, with new therapies being tested for their efficacy against

PSC and its complications. With progressing research, new treatments may improve the suffering of patients with this challenging disease, showcasing the changing character of gallbladder and biliary tract illnesses (Brindley et al., 2021) (Figure 10.12).

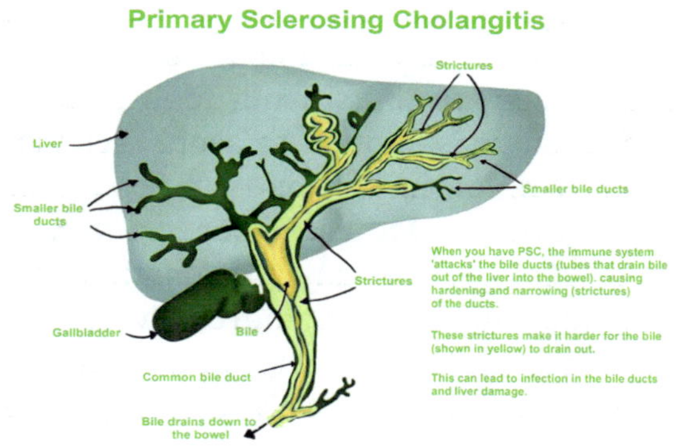

Figure 10.12. Primary sclerosing cholangitis.

Source: https://publish.uwo.ca/~tandrew6/images/PSC.jpg.

10.4. Symptoms and Diagnosis

The clinical presentation of gallbladder and biliary tract disease is usually diverse and often significantly different in each patient. Common presentations are intermittent or constant right upper quadrant pain. This is typically exacerbated after fatty meals due to the impaired gallbladder's contracted efficiency. The patient might also present with nausea and vomiting, characteristics that create diagnostic confusion. Jaundice, yellow discoloration of the skin and eyes, may be a feature if bile duct obstruction is present, highlighting the significance of proper clinical assessment. In a congenital anomaly , such as gallbladder duplication, the presentation is usually uncommon and may confuse even experienced clinicians, highlighting the usefulness of a thorough diagnostic workup (Sharipov et al., 2022). The diagnostic evaluation of biliary tract and gallbladder illness is a combination of clinical examination and sophisticated imaging procedures. The doctor can start off with an intensive patient history and clinical examination, which can provide significant information regarding the pathology. This is followed by imaging modalities , such as abdominal ultrasound, computed tomography (CT), and magnetic resonance cholangiopancreatography (MRCP), which then image the gallbladder and biliary tract in order to detect stones, strictures, or anatomical abnormalities. Routine imaging methods will, at times, miss subtle congenital abnormalities and therefore require further exploration. Correct diagnosis takes precedence because it will determine management strategies, e.g., potential surgical interventions or non-surgical therapies. Increasing evidence suggests that awareness of functional disorders of the gastrointestinal tract can enhance diagnosis accuracy, and thus improve patient outcomes (Minushkin et al., 2020). Early diagnosis is also critical to the effective management of gallbladder and biliary diseases. Delay or misdiagnosis can lead to enormous morbidity and thus early recognition of clinical signs that may signal underlying pathologies is essential. For instance, the challenge in diagnosing duplication of the gallbladder, particularly when associated with other biliary tree anomalies, can be daunting even to seasoned medical practitioners. With the adoption of an interdisciplinary approach that entails input from gastroenterology, surgery, and radiology, diagnostic precision can be significantly enhanced. Recent studies have shown that resolution of biliary dysfunction through focused interventions has been high, implying that early detection of symptoms will ensure improved treatment outcomes. Thus, offer ongoing education to healthcare providers on the varied presentation of such disorders to improve diagnosis and treatment accuracy (Sharipov et al., 2022) (Figure 10.13).

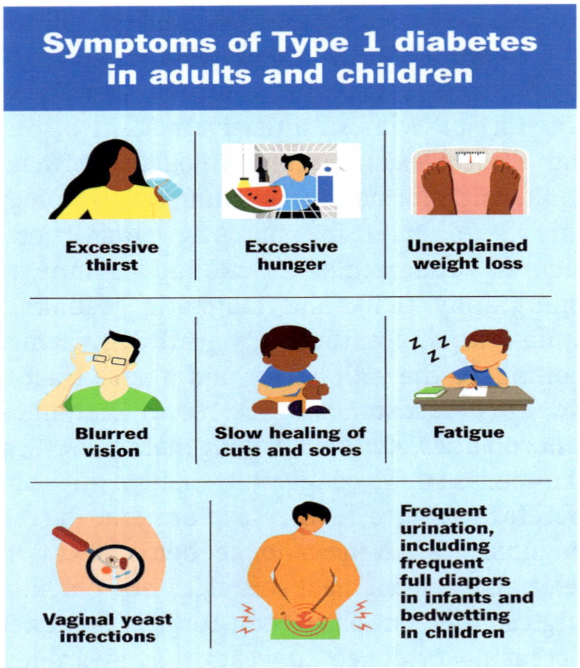

Figure 10.13. Symptoms and diagnosis.

Source: https://my.clevelandclinic.org/-/scassets/images/org/health/articles/21500-type-1-diabetes.

10.4.1. Common Symptoms Associated with Gallbladder Disorders

The presentation of gallbladder disease is diverse, typically simulating the pathophysiology of the disease. One of the most frequent presentations is pain in the upper right quadrant or mid-abdomen. The pain is often sudden and stabbing and has been referred to as a gallbladder attack, particularly following the ingestion of fatty food. Subsequent nausea and vomiting usually occur following this discomfort, as signs of the body's adverse reaction to gastrointestinal disturbances. The aforementioned symptoms are also precursors to underlying issues , such as gallstones or inflammation, wherein diagnostic workup is also needed to identify the underlying cause. In severe cases, jaundice, a symptom that presents as yellowish discoloration of the skin and eyes, may appear, which could be a sign of possible bile flow obstruction by gallbladder dysfunction (Dai et al., 2025). In addition to the more severe symptoms, chronic gallbladder disease may lead to a recurrence of gastrointestinal disturbances. Dyspepsia, bloating, gas, and postprandial fullness are common symptoms that patients report. These can have a detrimental impact on quality of life, and most patients avoid food factors or reduce food consumption to avoid recurrence, possibly with an impact on nutritional status. Chronic course of these disorders can also lead to cholecystitis, an inflammation of the gallbladder itself. It is more severe in its symptoms, including fever and acute pain within the abdomen, typically requiring surgery. Thus, recognition of such common symptoms is essential in early diagnosis and appropriate management of gallbladder disease, which can include lifestyle changes or surgical intervention , such as cholecystectomy, to alleviate recurrent symptomatology and prevent complications (Anderson et al., 2025). As gallbladder disease progresses, patients also start to experience systemic symptoms that reflect the broader impact of biliary tract dysfunction on overall health. These may include fatigue, weight loss, and altered appetite, which are, in turn, typically difficult to correlate directly with gallbladder dysfunction without further research. In addition, bile duct blockage or inflammation for a prolonged period of time can lead to bile salt malabsorption, resulting in diarrhea or steatorrhea, fatty stools that float and are difficult to flush. These symptoms necessitate proper assessment, for example, imaging studies and lab workup, in order to come up with an effective treatment plan. Identification of these varied symptoms is crucial in gallbladder disease management in order to prevent the development of more severe conditions and optimize patient care outcomes (Dai et al., 2025) (Figure 10.14).

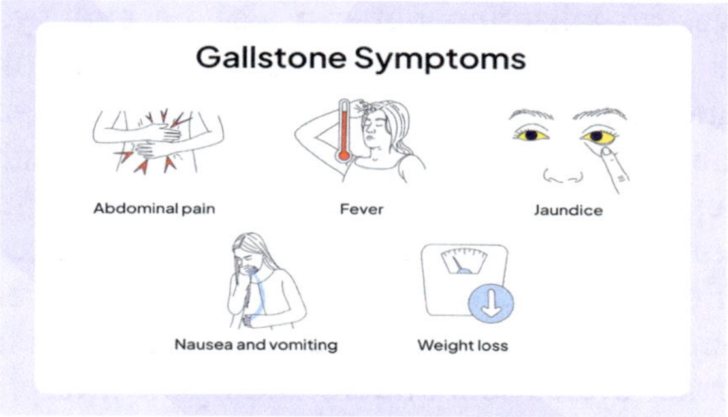

Figure 10.14. Common symptoms associated with gallbladder disorders.

Source: https://www.health.com/thmb/6N1Usj4aZjjYDhcCGdL_WBiPm7s=/1500x0/filters:no_upscale():max_bytes(150000):strip_icc()/Health-Gallstones-Symptoms-23a10c25696e4715afa0e34b35a33ef2.jpg.

10.4.2. Diagnostic Imaging Techniques

Diagnostic imaging modalities play a significant role in the evaluation of gallbladder and biliary tract disease, with accurate diagnosis and staging of the disease. Among the most frequently utilized modalities, ultrasound is frequently the initial imaging test due to its non-invasive nature and effectiveness in the determination of gallbladder abnormality, such as cholelithiasis and gallbladder wall thickening. High-frequency ultrasonic waves create real-time images, enabling physicians to view the anatomy and any pathological changes. However, ultrasound may be limited in the detailed assessment of intra- and extrahepatic bile ducts. Hence, it is often combined with other more advanced imaging modalities to assess suspected biliary tract disease in depth. Computed tomography (CT) and magnetic resonance imaging (MRI) are now necessary adjuncts in diagnosing more complex biliary diseases. CT scanning shows cross-sectional views that assist in focal lesions and local tumor involvement, so it is a crucial component of biliary cancer staging. MRI, particularly magnetic resonance cholangiopancreatography (MRCP), excels at bile duct anatomy and pathologies, e.g., strictures or malignancies. The precision of MRI in defining the extent of disease renders it an excellent method to assess cholangiocarcinoma, as depicted in existing literature (Yakub et al., 2025).

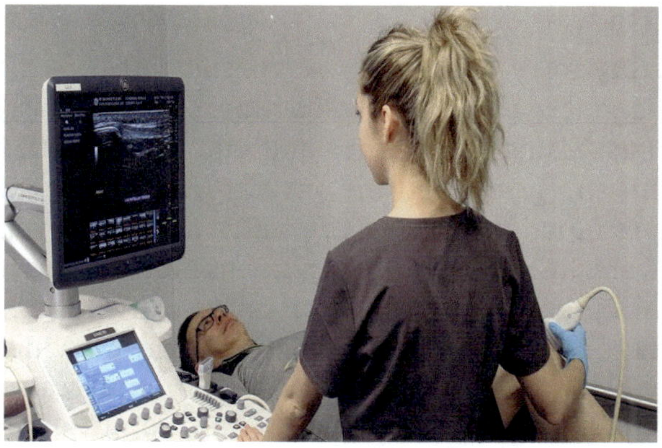

Figure 10.15. Diagnostic imaging techniques.

Source: https://www.recomind.net/wp-content/uploads/2023/05/diagnostic-imaging-systems-875x528.jpg.

The imaging modalities not only augment diagnostic precision but also assist clinicians in making appropriate therapeutic choices. With improvements in diagnostic techniques, endoscopic modalities , such as endoscopic ultrasound (EUS) and endoscopic retrograde cholangiopancreatography (ERCP) have come under consideration because of the potential for both visualization and intervention in a single step. EUS is particularly well-suited to assess extrahepatic biliary anatomy and can also be employed to direct fine-needle aspiration in the suspected malignancy, with optimal diagnostic yield. Conversely, ERCP is both therapeutic and diagnostic as it has the advantage of being able to provide direct visualization of bile ducts, alongside offering the provision of being able to perform interventions , such as stone extraction or stent placement. Nevertheless, while these endoscopic interventions hold merit, their limitations underscore the need for multimodal evaluation of the biliary system as a focus on integrative diagnostic strategies becomes paramount in ensuring optimal care of patients (Lee et al., 2024) (Figure 10.15).

10.4.3. Laboratory Tests for Biliary Tract Disorders

Laboratory tests play a crucial role in the diagnosis of biliary tract illness, particularly in assessing gallbladder and bile duct function and integrity. Routine investigations include liver function tests (LFTs), which measure levels of enzymes , such as alanine aminotransferase (ALT), aspartate aminotransferase (AST), and alkaline phosphatase (ALP). These enzymes rise with biliary obstruction or cholestasis, suggesting possible underlying conditions , such as cholecystitis or choledocholithiasis. Besides, direct and indirect bilirubin are critical indicators of bile flow and liver processing capacity. Accordingly, if bilirubin test results are abnormal, jaundice due to impaired bile excretion because of gallstones or biliary strictures may be suggested. Other specialized studies contribute to the sensitivity of diagnosis of diseases of the biliary tract. The time-honored example is the measurement of serum amylase and lipase levels, which may be appropriate in the context of pancreatitis, perhaps secondary to biliary disease. For conditions specifically involving gallbladder disease, blood cultures will identify infections caused by bacteria that are obstructing biliary outflow. Imaging studies, while technically not laboratory tests, are often combined with those studies. For instance, ultrasound can image gallstones or biliary dilatation without invading the body and, when combined with lab findings, provide an overall picture. Such diagnostic tests enable the clinician to determine the type of intervention needed, be it surgical or medicinal. In some situations, more invasive procedures may be necessitated, for instance, ERCP. This not only gives visualization but can also be employed for therapeutic procedures, such as stone removal. Following such interventions, follow-up laboratory parameters are crucial in determining the efficacy of treatment and identifying complications. Intra- or post-procedure LFTs can reflect improvement in liver function, whereas continued abnormalities can imply the need for further evaluation. Understanding the interplay between laboratory and imaging diagnostics is central to effective management of biliary tract disorders, pointing to the importance of complete testing in avoiding complications and guiding treatment streams.

10.5. Treatment Options

Gallbladder and biliary tract disease treatment varies greatly with the diagnosed conditions and degree. In gallstones, the most common treatment is cholecystectomy or removal of the gallbladder. Cholecystectomy can be performed laparoscopically, which is advantageous in having better recovery rates and fewer complications compared to open surgery. Non-invasive methods, such as endoscopic retrograde cholangiopancreatography (ERCP), are employed for the evacuation of stones obstructing the bile duct. Further, patients with chronic biliary colic or gallstone complications may eventually have to be subjected to cholecystectomy to prevent frequent attacks. It is important to realize the character of the disorder while selecting the appropriate type of treatment modality that improves patient safety and efficacy in recovery. For autoimmune-related biliary disorders, including primary biliary cholangitis and primary sclerosing cholangitis, the treatment plan should be extensive. These conditions lead to chronic inflammation and cirrhosis if left untreated. Treatment may include the administration of immunosuppressive medications and corticosteroids to suppress immune function.

The advances in imaging technologies, such as MRI and MR cholangiopancreatography, allow early detection and follow-up of these autoimmune disorders, thus enhancing the efficacy of the treatment protocol selected (Anderson et al., 2025). Imaging procedures are needed for follow-up to assess response to treatment and detect potential complications, thus enhancing long-term outcomes in patients suffering from such disorders. For cancer of the biliary tract, the treatment process relies predominantly on the site and extent of the malignancy.

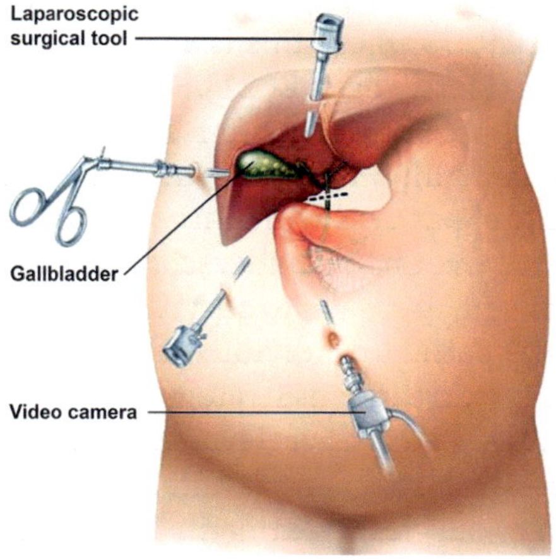

Figure 10.16. Treatment options.

Source: https://assets.mayoclinic.org/content/dam/media/en/images/2023/02/09/laparoscopic-cholecystectomy.jpg.

Surgical resection remains the final treatment for early-stage tumors; however, delayed presentation usually impairs treatment and limits surgical treatment (Liu et al., 2024). For unresectable tumors, chemotherapy regimens, i.e., gemcitabine with cisplatin, are the first-line treatments used. The need for second-line therapies remains a gap; hence, ongoing research into the molecular pathways that cause these malignancies has potential for possible targeted therapy, which brings new hope for the advanced biliary cancers. Awareness of such therapeutic intervention gives a wider approach in the management of gallbladder and biliary tract diseases, which eventually supports patient prognosis (Figure 10.16).

10.5.1. Medical Management and Lifestyle Changes

Effective medical management of gallbladder and biliary tract disease relies on a comprehensive understanding of the involved pathophysiology and appropriate balancing of therapeutic modalities. Diagnosis first employs newer imaging studies like computed tomography (CT) and magnetic resonance imaging (MRI) for the critical evaluation of gallbladder disease. These imaging modalities also help in the identification of structural abnormalities, as well as help differentiate between benign and malignancies, thereby guiding the future management plan. The capability of these tools to provide high-resolution images is critical in managing diseases , such as gallstones and cholangitis, emphasizing the necessity for clear diagnosis to plan the management. With the application of recent advances in imaging, the severity of the condition can be better ascertained and an individualized plan of management can be designed that can involve surgery, pharmacotherapy, or lifestyle changes to optimize patient outcomes (Pivsaeva et al., 2025). Even for adding lifestyle changes to the plan of management, the latter remains essential for gallbladder and biliary tract disease, too. Dietary modification is the foundation of avoiding aggravation of such conditions. For instance, consumption of a low saturated fat and high fiber diet can prevent the development of gallstones and restrict the development of biliary sludge. Daily physical activity could also correct gallbladder function and help control weight, which is important in light of the link between gallbladder disease and obesity. All such lifestyle interventions not only attempt to alleviate symptoms but also attempt to cure recurrent attacks. Patients are encouraged to drink well and to take foods rich in vitamins and antioxidants to support overall biliary health, thus supporting a worldwide approach to the treatment of these conditions (Shcherbynina, 2024). Pharmacologic therapy can also complement lifestyle changes through effects aimed at pathophysiologic abnormalities while stimulating gallbladder function. One of the promising techniques is the use of hepatocomplex preparations like Holoplant®-Tau, which includes natural extracts and substances well known for their hepatoprotective effect. The complex has been found to be effective against functional disorders of the biliary system and in maintaining liver function, hence providing relief from symptoms of gallbladder disease. Clinical experience shows that such integrated treatment can minimize the necessity of violent surgical interventions and cure symptoms, improving patients' living standards. As a rule, the integration of medical treatment and lifestyle modification not only corrects an acute disease but also prepares the patient with tools to manage gallbladder and biliary tract pathology in the long term (Shcherbynina, 2024).

10.5.2. Surgical Interventions (e.g., Cholecystectomy)

Surgical intervention plays a central part in the management of gallbladder and biliary tract disease, and cholecystectomy is the most frequent surgical operation. Cholecystectomy, or surgical removal of the gallbladder, primarily addresses disease of gallstones (cholelithiasis) and inflammation of the gallbladder (cholecystitis). Evolution in the techniques of surgery has had significant effects in improving patients' outcomes, particularly with the advent of laparoscopic techniques, which cause less postoperative pain, shorter hospital stay, and less scarring compared to open surgery. Laparoscopic cholecystectomy, being a minimally invasive surgery, has become an established gold standard in the treatment of symptomatic gallbladder disease. While this operation has a favorable prognosis, success relies on the patient's selection since age, comorbidities, and severity of biliary disease may characterize risks and complications of surgery. The cholecystectomy is done, but in more complex cases, other surgeries are being used when patients present with Biliary obstruction or malignancy. Techniques , such as endoscopic retrograde cholangiopancreatography (ERCP) and endoscopic ultrasound-guided biliary drainage (EUS-BD) are now accepted as good methods of management of biliary pathology. EUS-BD, for instance, has become an acceptable alternative following a failed ERCP for malignant distal biliary obstruction, particularly in high-volume centers where this is a well-established technique (Merwe et al., 2021). Such management not only improves obstructive symptoms but is also centrally involved in the palliative treatment of patients with unresectable tumors. Alternative treatments underscore the need for a personalized approach to surgical management in that the patient's individual clinical situation should direct treatment strategy. The physiology of bile acids and their relevance to gallbladder disease has also been paralleled by altering the plan of surgical treatment. Recent research clarifies the role of bile acids in many metabolic processes and their actions on conditions , such as non-alcoholic steatohepatitis (NASH) and primary biliary cholangitis (PBC) (Perino et al., 2020). Based on these findings, regulation of bile acid signaling could provide therapeutic options apart from surgery for gallbladder disease. Surgeons and gastroenterologists should therefore be informed of new findings regarding the metabolism of bile acids while preparing for surgery. As therapeutic drugs with action on bile acid receptors are being discovered and created, the integration of these advances in the field of medicine with surgical techniques might enhance overall treatment protocols for patients with gallbladder and biliary tract disease, which can be translated into improved clinical outcomes and quality of life (Figure 10.17).

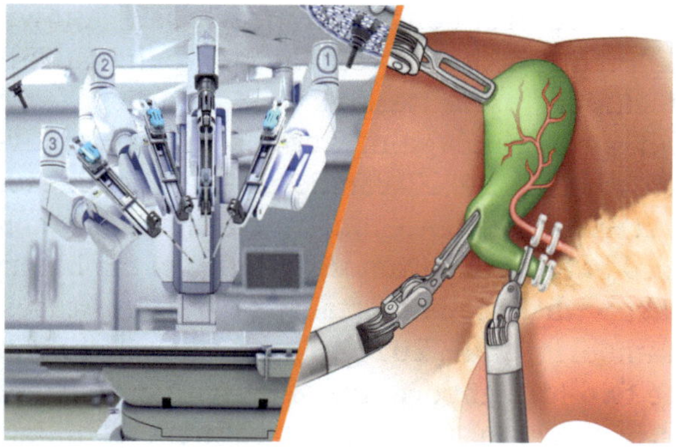

Figure 10.17. Surgical interventions (e.g., cholecystectomy).

Source: https://surgmedia.com/wp-content/uploads/2021/04/2177-robotic-cholecystectomy.jpg.

10.5.3. Emerging Therapies and Research

The new developments in endoscopic treatment of gallbladder and biliary disease highlight the need for new therapies that confront the increasing challenge of these conditions. Recent studies highlight the position of endoscopic techniques, namely endoscopic ultrasonography-guided biliary drainage (EUS-BD), which has some advantages over standard percutaneous approaches following failed endoscopic ERCP. This operation is recognized for reducing the risk of complications, therefore being a significant alternative to malignant distal biliary obstruction where local expertise exists (Merwe et al., 2021). Moreover, as over 300 million people are estimated to have gastrointestinal disorders, the research community is called upon to address therapeutic practices that possess a high potential to improve patient outcomes and minimize the economic burden of the disease (Merwe et al., 2021). Advances in the technology of interventional endoscopy also signify a step towards individualized medicine in the treatment of gallbladder and biliary disease. Techniques , such as EUS-GE and rendezvous EUS procedures for pancreatic duct drainage have emerged as viable options for selected patient groups, especially those who do not qualify for surgical intervention (Merwe et al., 2021). Not only are these easy to manage, but they reduce the need for re-intervention, highlighting the groundbreaking potential of minimally invasive intervention. More importantly, the ongoing discovery of lifestyle determinants and their relationship with gastrointestinal disorders emphasizes preventive approaches and lifestyle modifications as absolutely central to patient management (Merwe et al., 2021). The complete integration of these findings into clinical management can result in improved management regimens that have a direct effect on the unique issues raised by gallbladder and biliary diseases.

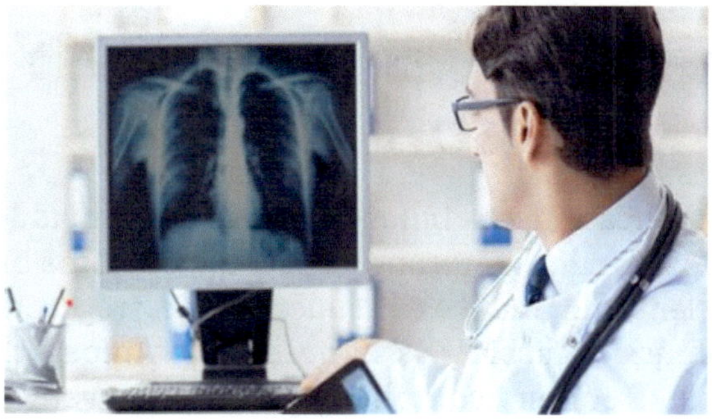

Figure 10.18. Emerging therapies and research.

Source: https://external-content.duckduckgo.com/iu/?u=https%3A%2F%2Ftse4.mm.bing.net%2Ft h%3Fid%3DOIP.qcRdXtfBz5 2ayDFbaPa8BgHaD4%26r%3D0%26pid%3DApi&f=1&ipt=ab89d5c63da542ddb0b74 143eb79ae30519fe50320d0876b433c41fc2a899396.

With continually emerging research uncovering therapeutic gaps, the boost in funding for under-studied conditions , such as alcohol-induced liver disease and irritable bowel syndrome, is of utmost importance. The tremendous health burden brought about by gastrointestinal disorders upon the healthcare system necessitates a realignment of priorities in research since emerging evidence presents evidence of a shortage of adequate resources directed towards effective prevention and treatment measures (Rose et al., 2022). Initiatives like the UEG White Book 2 aim to shine light on these discrepancies, fostering more research with increased intersectoral cooperation between policymakers and health actors (Rose et al., 2022). By funding research according to the unique needs established in the field of digestive health, we can build a more solid foundation that encourages genuine advancement and equitable patient care in the field of gallbladder and biliary tract disease (Figure 10.18).

10.6. Complications of Gallbladder and Biliary Tract Disorders

Complications of biliary tract and gallbladder diseases can significantly affect the outcome of a patient, and thus a clear understanding regarding potential morbidities is necessary. Among the most frequent complications of intervention or surgery in the biliary tract is bile leak or obstruction, particularly in patients subjected to orthotopic liver transplantation (OLT). In a review of 393 OLT procedures, biliary tract complications (BTC) were noted to represent a high rate of graft loss and patient mortality and were referenced in 52 cases (13.2%) as failures of bile duct reconstruction, reported as leakage and obstruction. These complications can have disastrous effects, including direct responsibility for five deaths among patients (9.6%), and highlighting the importance of close surgical technique and postoperative monitoring to manage potential leaks (Lerut et al., 1987). Another serious complication that arises in association with gallbladder and biliary disease is bacterial cholangitis, a cholangitis infection that is sometimes accompanied by cholecystitis. Studies indicate that the conditions are more frequent than previously known, highlighting the importance of being aware of clinical presentations like jaundice, fever, and abdominal pain. Actually, retrospective investigation in 27 canine cases of diagnosed bacterial cholangitis illustrated that nearly one third of them experienced rupture of the biliary tract with serious mortality (4 out of 8 cases) (Tamborini et al., 2016). This finding highlights the two-fold importance of early diagnosis and early intervention in the treatment of biliary tract infections in order to prevent serious sequelae that can cause significant morbidity or mortality.

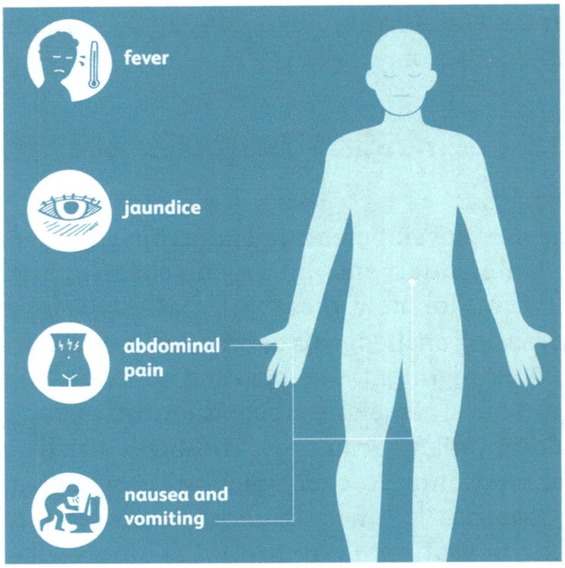

Figure 10.19. Complications of gallbladder and biliary tract disorders.

Source: https://www.verywellhealth.com/thmb/atb5u_sWKsNhXOXlRbcox3Nrffs=/1500x1000/filters:no_upscale():max_bytes(150000):strip_icc()/gallbladder-disease-symptoms-5aec9a54a18d9e0037100eab.png.

Patients undergoing treatment for gallbladder or biliary tract illness must be informed about the dangers of all types of interventions, most notably as regards the material used for biliary reconstruction and the possibility of postoperative complications.

Surgical technique complications, in the guise of duct-to-duct repairs, can be responsible for causing those like hepatic artery thrombosis (HAT), described as the Achilles heel of OLT. The HAT and/or recurrent bile leakage configurations can lead to fulminant hepatic necrosis or delayed bile leakage, emphasizing the crucial need for earlier diagnosis and intervention to prevent risks in graft failure and associated sepsis (Lerut et al., 1987). Furthermore, synoptic comprehension of these complications illustrates the interconnectedness of the anatomy of the biliary system in that successful treatment rests on a highly integrated approach to surgical planning and meticulous postoperative care for the best patient results (Figure 10.19).

10.6.1. Potential Complications from Untreated Disorders

The undiagnosed gallbladder and biliary tract disease may lead to various complications that gravely impair an individual's overall health. Among the most threatening is the development of acute cholecystitis, an inflammation of the gallbladder due to obstruction of the bile ducts, most often caused by gallstones. If this condition is left untreated, it may cause gallbladder perforation and peritonitis, a severe and life-threatening infection of the abdomen. The combined effect of these complications necessitates urgent medical intervention, particularly since they have the potential to quickly deteriorate, resulting in systemic complications , such as sepsis, which has extremely high morbidity and mortality if not addressed promptly. Awareness of these potential consequences underscores the importance of managing gallbladder and biliary tract diseases before they develop into more complicated health crises. Uncontrolled biliary tract diseases can also trigger subsequent cascades of metabolic complications, particularly malabsorption and nutritional deficiency. Conditions , such as chronic bile duct obstruction hinder bile flow, leading to reduced fat digestion and Vitamin K absorption, and in turn cause coagulopathy and susceptibility to bleeding. Patients also get malnourished and lose weight since they cannot absorb nutrients. With chronic gallbladder and biliary disease, secondary complications , such as osteoporosis also become a possibility due to extensive malabsorption of primary nutrients including calcium and vitamin D. This is an intricate function in compromising health that emphasizes the integrated nature of the biliary apparatus with overall metabolic activity and reinforces the importance of early diagnosis and treatment of gallbladder pathologies to prevent progressive complications from nutritional deficiencies.

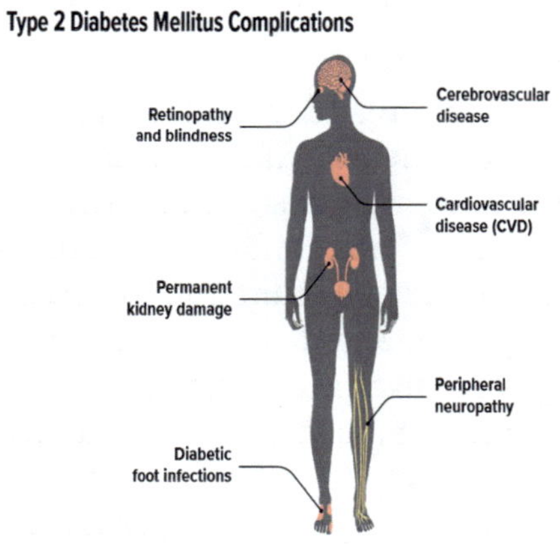

Figure 10.20. Potential complications from untreated disorders.

Source: https://post.medicalnewstoday.com/wp-content/uploads/sites/3/2022/01/1552759-Type-2-Diabetes-Mellitus-Complications_Header-Body_1296x728.png.

The late effects of untreated biliary and gallbladder disorders can also include the development of cholangiocarcinoma, which is a severe but uncommon malignancy of the biliary epithelial cells. Inflammatory chronic bile duct disease secondary to recurrent infection and obstruction has long been recognized as a predisposing cause for such cancers. Studies have demonstrated that patients with untreated biliary tract disorders constitute a population at risk for malignant transformation due to ongoing cellular injury. The risk of cholangiocarcinoma, therefore, necessitates ongoing monitoring and control of biliary tract disease to avoid malignancy development. Given that healthcare workers seek to design integrated treatment plans, the importance of treating acute and chronic conditions in the biliary system cannot be overstated since they can become serious health threats that diminish the quality of life and lifespan of sufferers (Figure 10.20).

10.6.2. Impact on Overall Health and Quality of Life

The impact of gallbladder and biliary tract illness on global health and well-being and quality of life is tremendous, since such illness often leads to severe discomfort in the body and disablement for normal functioning. Patients are frequently tormented by such complaints as recurring pain, distension, and compromised digestive function that can affect their ability to perform ordinary activities. This distress is not just physical but also psychological, as it induces anxiety and social withdrawal, creating a cycle that exacerbates physical and psychological conditions. The presence of these disorders leads to augmented healthcare utilization through repeated physician consultations, diagnostics, and potentially surgical interventions, all with a tendency to be substantial in cost burden on the patients as well as the healthcare systems and eventually contributing towards the overall quality of life. The cross-talk between gallbladder disease and comorbidities , such as obesity, diabetes, and cardiovascular disease, contributes significantly to exacerbating illness states. Obesity disorders are known to predispose an individual towards gallbladder disease, and conversely, gallbladder disease makes the diagnosis and treatment of obesity and metabolic syndromes difficult. For instance, the American Diabetes Association advises that patients who are obese tend to experience diabetes control difficulties, further increased by gallbladder illnesses. The intricate interactions among these connected conditions result in a suboptimal overall quality of life because patients cannot manage multiple illnesses with different treatment protocols and lifestyle changes. Thus, the management of such disorders must be an integrated approach to address not only the basic disorder but also any associated health condition. Also, the psychological aspect of living with gallbladder and biliary tract disorders cannot be overstated. Chronic pain and dietary restriction can frustrate an individual, make them feel helpless and depressed. They may also experience less social contact by avoiding situations where the choice of food is bad or where discomfort is heightened. Social avoidance then results in a smaller support system, and that influences the level of mental health and quality of life. Psychological treatment of the disorders, in addition to physical and lifestyle factors, is important. The Global Burden of Disease Study findings indicate that efficient management of comorbid conditions in most cases is predisposed to improve physical and mental well-being, and therefore an integrated intervention is required to improve quality of life in gallbladder and biliary tract disease patients (Davies et al., 2018; Roth et al., 2018).

10.6.3. Long-Term Management and Follow-Up Care

Long-term care and follow-up treatment of patients with gallbladder and biliary tract diseases are the key factors in enhancing the quality of life and outcome of the patients. After the first treatment, including surgery or palliative therapy, regular checks will guarantee the observation of healing processes and the detection of potential complications. Regular follow-up visits enable clinicians to check on the effectiveness of the treatment and modify management strategies as patients' needs evolve. Furthermore, uniform follow-up procedures will also identify recurrences of cancers of the biliary tracts or complications related to procedures, like stenting-induced bile duct complications, enabling prompt intervention. Observational follow-up of patients with Percutaneous Transhepatic Biliary Drainage (PTBD) emphasizes the importance of assessing long-term quality of life. The findings indicate significant improvements in global health status, physical, emotional, cognitive, and social well-being over the first three months after the procedure. The decrease in quality of life at six months, however, suggests that monitoring must be continued to manage complications like stent obstruction or recurrence of disease. By implementing systematic follow-up evaluations, clinicians are not only able to maximize the patient-centered care model but also allow for prompt resolution of any unfavorable effects that arise, thereby significantly affecting long-term management of biliary illnesses (Roy et al., 2024). Moreover, inclusion of adjuvant therapy, such as S-1 in biliary tract cancer, has a significant effect on long-term survival and relapse-free survival outcomes. A five-year follow-up trial emphasized the survival benefit of S-1, which maximized patient outcome far better than observation alone. This type of evidence encourages the implementation of these adjunct therapies as part of standard care for patients with resected biliary tract malignancies. This extended management and follow-up strategy moves beyond acute symptom control to the maintenance of treatment efficacy and extended survival. The application of these practices improves not only the clinical pathway but also the quality of holistic care of the patient with gallbladder and biliary tract diseases (Nakachi et al., 2024) (Figure 10.21).

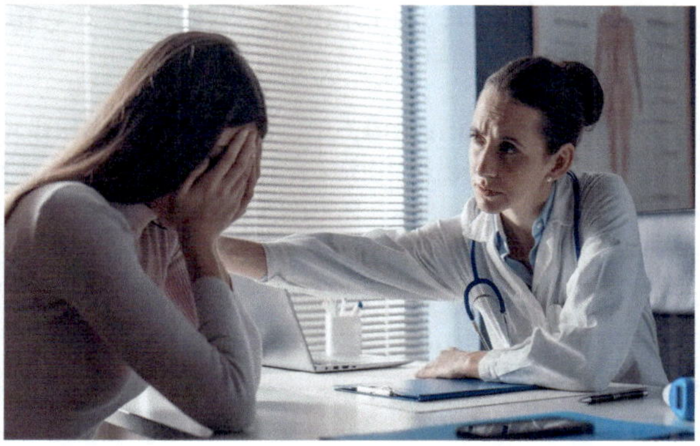

Figure 10.21. Long-term management and follow-up care.

Source: https://hlthd-prod.b-cdn.net/wp-content/uploads/2025/05/shutterstock_1926698816.jpg.

CLOSER LOOK

GALLBLADDER ATTACK:

A gallbladder attack, often referred to as biliary colic, is a painful episode caused by a temporary obstruction of the cystic duct—typically by gallstones. A closer look at gallbladder attacks reveals how subtle disruptions in bile flow can trigger intense, sudden pain and associated gastrointestinal symptoms. These attacks frequently occur after meals, especially those high in fat, because the gallbladder contracts to release bile, increasing the likelihood that a stone will block the bile duct. The hallmark symptom is sharp, steady pain in the right upper abdomen or epigastric region, sometimes radiating to the back or right shoulder blade. Unlike cramping or colicky pain, biliary colic tends to remain constant and can last from 30 minutes to several hours. Nausea, vomiting, bloating, and a sense of abdominal fullness may accompany the pain. Once the obstructing stone falls back into the gallbladder, symptoms typically resolve, leaving the patient feeling fatigued but otherwise normal.

Although the pain may subside, a gallbladder attack is a warning sign of underlying gallstone disease. Repeated episodes are common, and more serious complications may arise if the blockage persists or worsens. Prolonged obstruction can lead to acute cholecystitis, an inflammatory condition marked by fever, persistent pain, and marked tenderness of the abdomen. In more severe cases, stones may migrate into the common bile duct, causing choledocholithiasis, pancreatitis, or life-threatening infections such as cholangitis. Risk factors for gallbladder attacks include female sex, obesity, rapid weight loss, pregnancy, certain medications, and a family history of gallstones. Conditions that increase cholesterol saturation in bile—such as metabolic syndrome or high-fat diets—also contribute. Though gallstones are common, not all individuals develop symptoms; many stones remain silent throughout life.

Diagnosis often involves ultrasound imaging, which can detect gallstones and signs of inflammation. Blood tests may show elevated liver enzymes or markers of infection during complicated attacks. Management depends on symptom severity and recurrence. For uncomplicated biliary colic, pain control, dietary adjustments, and observation may be recommended. However, surgical removal of the gallbladder (cholecystectomy) is the definitive treatment for recurrent gallbladder attacks and is highly effective at preventing future episodes.

A closer examination shows that gallbladder attacks are more than temporary episodes of abdominal pain—they signal functional disruptions and potential complications within the biliary system. Early recognition, appropriate evaluation, and timely treatment are essential to preventing serious outcomes and restoring quality of life.

SUMMARY

In short, gallbladder and biliary tract disease complexities require a multi-dimensional approach and management (Starzl et al., 1979). The endemic nature of diseases , such as cholelithiasis renders it very important to detect them early and manage them accordingly. Pharmacological developments utilizing ursodeoxycholic acid (UDCA) have been very promising in managing gallstone dissolution and biliary sludge, as exhibited in comparative analysis showing the strength of Ursofalk over other UDCA drugs. The results affirm gradual regression of biliary sludge in patients given Ursofalk, giving insight into the potential of certain pharmacotherapy in managing biliary disease (Буторова et al., 2020). These findings indicate the critical need for ongoing research and development in the specialty to enhance patient outcomes. Furthermore, the public health significance of gallbladder disease extends beyond the individual to affect broader public health settings. Understanding the epidemiology of gallbladder disease enables healthcare professionals to allocate resources effectively and tailor prevention strategies. For instance, the linkage between gallbladder disease and noncommunicable diseases is an indicator of the significance of environmental factors and lifestyle in the disease burden. The Global Burden of Disease study highlights the disparity in the diagnosis, treatment, and outcomes of cancer by socio-demographic characteristics as a clarion call for equitable healthcare interventions (Fitzmaurice et al., 2019). An equitable approach to gallbladder and biliary tract disease can strengthen health systems and develop resilience to health crises. Ultimately, the combined management of gallbladder and biliary tract disease is an interdisciplinary approach with preventive, curative, and patient-centered interventions. Education and awareness activities can empower patients to make informed choices regarding their health and recognize early warning signs of biliary malfunction. The integration of clinical guidelines and patient education into clinical practice is essential in improving treatment adherence and global health literacy. Through the evolving research environment, the collaboration of policymakers, researchers, and healthcare providers will be instrumental in managing the complexities of biliary tract and gallbladder disease and ensuring quality care to the suffering population.

The gallbladder and biliary tract disease debate also underscores the interactive nature of various kinds of gastrointestinal disease and the general state of health conditions. Obesity, for instance, has been emphasized as an epidemic globally with the World Health Organization estimating that over 1.5 billion adults are overweight and about 500 million clinically obese. This condition directly increases the rate of gallbladder pathology, including gallstones and cholecystitis, due to disturbed lipid metabolism and a change in bile composition. Therefore, the rising cases of obesity are directly linked with a high prevalence of gallbladder complications, reflecting the need for public health intervention aimed at weight control and education to avoid such risks. The recognition of obesity as a causative agent for gallbladder disease emphasizes the interconnectedness of the ailments and requires treatment and prevention with interdisciplinary measures (Kyrou et al., 2010). In conjunction with obesity, cholestatic liver disease offers basic knowledge of the pathophysiology associated with gallbladder dysfunctions. Cholestasis, as expressed through bile flow dysfunction and intracellular liver bile acid accumulation, can significantly influence the biliary apparatus, such as gallbladder trauma. Symptomatology may arise due to acute or chronic inflammation, cholelithiasis, and even neoplasia. Recent studies support the need for an understanding of how gallbladder health relates to diseases affecting the intrahepatic biliary apparatus, e.g., cholangiopathies and fatty liver diseases. Notably, the gallbladder also shares developmental and functional ties with the biliary epithelium and consequently requires complete clinical evaluations that appreciate such ties.

The fine appreciation of how liver illness leads to gallbladder illness adds power to the holistic approach in diagnosis and treatment interventions (Alpini et al., 2023). The clinical importance of the appreciation of gallbladder and biliary tract disease overflows into environments of diagnosis and treatment. It is possible through advanced diagnostic techniques, including imaging and serology, to make a diagnosis of gallbladder disease in the setting of liver disease. Therapeutic interventions must also be able to address problems created by concurrent conditions, for instance, managing gallstones in cholestatic liver disease. This emphasizes the importance of integrated care pathways that balance gallbladder and hepatic health. By encouraging collaboration among specialists in gastroenterology, hepatology, and nutrition, medical professionals are able to tailor interventions for better patient outcomes. As comprehension of these interconnections is becoming ever deeper, so is the possibility of developing policy to meet the prevention and treatment of gallbladder and biliary tract disease as part of an international framework of metabolic disease (Alpini et al., 2023).

References

1. Starzl, T. E., Koep, L. J., Halgrimson, C. G., Hood, J., Schroter, G. P., Porter, K. A., & Weil, R., 3rd (1979). Fifteen years of clinical liver transplantation. Gastroenterology, 77(2), 375–388. (accessed on 16th July 2025).
2. Di Carlo, P., Serra, N., D'Arpa, F., Agrusa, A., Gulotta, G., Fasciana, T., Rodolico, V., Giammanco, A., & Sergi, C. (2019). The microbiota of the bilio-pancreatic system: a cohort, STROBE-compliant study. Infection and drug resistance, 12, 1513–1527. https://doi.org/10.2147/IDR.S200378(accessed on 16th July 2025).
3. Alebouyeh, M., Alizadeh, A. H. M., Majidi, M. R. S., Sherafat, et al. (2016). Association of diverse bacterial communities in human bile samples with biliary tract disorders: A survey using culture and polymerase chain reaction-denaturing gradient gel electrophoresis methods. https://core.ac.uk/download/52205553.pdf (accessed on 16th July 2025).
4. Aleksandrova, K., Boeing, H., Nöthlings, U., Jenab, M., Fedirko, V., Kaaks, R., Lukanova, A., et al. (2014). Inflammatory and metabolic biomarkers and risk of liver and biliary tract cancer. Hepatology (Baltimore, Md.), 60, 858–871. https://www.semanticscholar.org/paper/02520a457519c365edc3ee85e69c55c0bcbf18e6 (accessed on 16th July 2025).
5. Tamborini, A., Jahns, H., McAllister, H., Kent, A., Harris, B., Procoli, F., Allenspach, K., Hall, E. J., Day, M. J., Watson, P. J., & O'Neill, E. J. (2016). Bacterial Cholangitis, Cholecystitis, or both in Dogs. Journal of veterinary internal medicine, 30(4), 1046–1055. https://doi.org/10.1111/jvim.13974 (accessed on 16th July 2025).
6. Alpini, G., Baiocchi, L., Ceci, L., Francis, H., Gaudio, E., Han, Y., Kennedy, L., et al. (2023). Gallstone and gallbladder disease: Biliary tract and cholangiopathies. https://core.ac.uk/download/599513205.pdf (accessed on 16th July 2025).
7. Beeson, M. S., Ankel, F., Bhat, R., Broder, J., Paradise, S., Gorgas, D. L., Jones, J. S., et al. (2020). The 2019 model of the clinical practice of emergency medicine. Journal of Emergency Medicine, 59, 96–120. https://doi.org/10.1016/j.jemermed.2020.03.018 (accessed on 16th July 2025).
8. Brindley, P. J., Bachini, M., Ilyas, S. I., Khan, S. A., Loukas, A., Sirica, A. E., Teh, B. T., et al. (2021). Cholangiocarcinoma. Nature Reviews Disease Primers, 7. https://doi.org/10.1038/s41572-021-00300-2 (accessed on 16th July 2025).
9. Butorova, L. I., Ardatskaya, M. D., Osadchuk, M. A., Drobysheva, A. E., Zagrebina, E. A., Kadnikova, N. G., et al., (2020). Comparative effectiveness of ursodeoxycholic acid preparations in the treatment of biliary sludge. Terapevticheskii Arkhiv, 92, 60–65. https://doi.org/10.26442/00403660.2020.08.000700 (accessed on 16th July 2025).
10. Dai, F., Cai, Y., Yang, S., Zhang, J., & Dai, Y. (2025). Global burden of gallbladder and biliary diseases (1990–2021) with healthcare workforce analysis and projections to 2035. BMC Gastroenterology, 25. https://www.semanticscholar.org/paper/b7aa107a63fda0e6e0a43bf07038609f9b6a107f (accessed on 16th July 2025).
11. Davies, M. J., D'Alessio, D. A., Fradkin, J., Kernan, W. N., Mathieu, C., Mingrone, G., Rossing, P., et al. (2018). Management of hyperglycemia in type 2 diabetes, 2018: A consensus report by the American Diabetes Association (ADA) and the European Association for the Study of Diabetes (EASD). Diabetes Care, 41, 2669–2701. https://doi.org/10.2337/dci18-0033 (accessed on 16th July 2025).

12. Ferfetska, K., Hontsaryuk, D., Pits, L. O., & Pits, V. A. (2024). Biliary pancreatitis: Modern approaches to treatment (literature review). Herald of Pancreatic Club. https://www.semanticscholar.org/paper/85c6f128c3e88508ed77a325811b436a85f9f371 (accessed on 16th July 2025).

13. Fitzmaurice, C., Abate, D., Abbasi, N., Abbastabar, H., Abd-Allah, F., Abdel-Rahman, O., Abdelalim, A., et al. (2019). Global, regional, and national cancer incidence, mortality, years of life lost, years lived with disability, and disability-adjusted life-years for 29 cancer groups, 1990 to 2017. JAMA Oncology, 5, 1749. https://doi.org/10.1001/jamaoncol.2019.2996 (accessed on 16th July 2025).

14. Gochanour, E., Jayasekera, C. R., & Kowdley, K. V. (2020). Primary sclerosing cholangitis: Epidemiology, genetics, diagnosis, and current management. Clinical Liver Disease, 15, 125–128. https://doi.org/10.1002/cld.902 (accessed on 16th July 2025).

15. Lerut, J., Gordon, R. D., Iwatsuki, S., & Starzl, T. E. (1987). Surgical complications in human orthotopic liver transplantation. Acta chirurgica Belgica, 87(3), 193–204.(accessed on 16th July 2025).

16. He, L., Li, J., Cheng, X., Luo, L., & Huang, Y. (2025). Association between GLP-1 RAs and DPP-4 inhibitors with biliary disorders: Pharmacovigilance analysis. Frontiers in Pharmacology, 16. https://www.semanticscholar.org/paper/191565ae9a8b8f184b82d7aff9b7a0cc90ad3fb5 (accessed on 16th July 2025).

17. Khan, S. A., Tavolari, S., & Brandi, G. (2019). Cholangiocarcinoma: Epidemiology and risk factors. Liver International, 39, 19–31. https://doi.org/10.1111/liv.14095 (accessed on 16th July 2025).

18. Khomenko, V. S., Perepelitsia, V. P., Strotskyi, K. P., Dykyi, O., Prokopchuk, O., Kuchynskyi, I. O., Andruschenko, S., et al. (2021). Bouveret Syndrome (Clinical Case). https://www.semanticscholar.org/paper/fe0fae13f3225738d11e6a613690fa47eb226ec3 (accessed on 16th July 2025).

19. Konorev, M. R. (2008). Lecture Notes by Internal Diseases. https://core.ac.uk/download/80150474.pdf (accessed on 16th July 2025).

20. Kyo-Sang, Y, Woo, T. L., & Ho Soon, C. (2016). Biology of Cholangiocytes: From Bench to Bedside. https://core.ac.uk/download/185644754.pdf (accessed on 16th July 2025).

21. Kyrou I, Randeva HS, Tsigos C, et al. Clinical Problems Caused by Obesity. [Updated 2018 Jan 11]. In: Feingold KR, Ahmed SF, Anawalt B, et al., editors. Endotext [Internet]. South Dartmouth (MA): MDText.com, Inc.; 2000-. Available from: https://www.ncbi.nlm.nih.gov/books/NBK278973/

22. (accessed on 16th July 2025).

23. Lee, S. H., & Song, S. Y. (2024). Recent advancement in diagnosis of biliary tract cancer through pathological and molecular classifications. Cancers, 16. https://www.semanticscholar.org/paper/cba28b8d3a0b74a923d7daf98520b6d058bfe04b (accessed on 16th July 2025).

24. Liu, Q., Zhang, P., & Li, Q. (2024). Exploring molecular mechanisms in the second-line treatment of biliary tract malignant tumors. Discovery Medicine, 36(180), 48–60. https://www.semanticscholar.org/paper/6fae359ad21523620d2cdb2ecd63dd462a5a533a (accessed on 16th July 2025).

25. Minushkin, O., Maslovsky, L. V., Lvova, N., Legkova, K. S., Gordienko, E. S., Protsenko, O. A., Magomedrasulova, A. V., et al. (2020). Biliary dysfunction (according to recommendations of Rome IV): Diagnosis, treatment. https://www.semanticscholar.org/paper/4a899c7c30b9f4c49a88070e82316b0724e29e8f (accessed on 16th July 2025).

26. Molinero, N., Ruíz, L., Milani, C., Gutiérrez-Díaz, I., Sánchez, B., Mangifesta, M., Segura, J., et al. (2019). The human gallbladder microbiome is related to the physiological state and the biliary metabolic profile. Microbiome, 7. https://doi.org/10.1186/s40168-019-0712-8 (accessed on 16th July 2025).

27. Murray, C. J. L., Ikuta, K. S., Sharara, F., Swetschinski, L. R., Robles Aguilar, G., Gray, A. P., Han, C., et al. (2022). Global burden of bacterial antimicrobial resistance in 2019: A systematic analysis. The Lancet, 399, 629–655. https://doi.org/10.1016/s0140-6736(21)02724-0 (accessed on 16th July 2025).

28. Nakachi, K., Ikeda, M., Konishi, M., Mizusawa, J., Katayama, H., Sano, Y., Uesaka, K., et al. (2024). Adjuvant S-1 vs. observation for resected biliary tract cancer: 5-year follow-up of the JCOG1202/ASCOT. Journal of Clinical Oncology. https://www.semanticscholar.org/paper/5120389c2c5774ee0bd803b539e6a864254e7a39 (accessed on 16th July 2025).

29. Perino, A., Demagny, H., Velázquez-Villegas, L. A., & Schoonjans, K. (2020). Molecular physiology of bile acid signaling in health, disease, and aging. Physiological Reviews, 101, 683–731. https://doi.org/10.1152/physrev.00049.2019 (accessed on 16th July 2025).

30. Pivsaeva, V. M., Agafonov, A. O., Shatokhina, M. G., & Prosalova, N. V. (2025). CT and MRI imaging features as illustrated by a clinical case of biliary tract cancer. Diagnostic Radiology and Radiotherapy. https://www.semanticscholar.org/paper/d25322b6f8479dc67b669a0c6dd4b41d499a55f2 (accessed on 16th July 2025).

31. Rose, T. C., Pennington, A., Kypridemos, C., Chen, T., Subhani, M. M., Hanefeld, J., Ricciardiello, L., et al. (2022). Analysis of the burden and economic impact of digestive diseases and investigation of research gaps and priorities in the field of digestive health in the European Region—White Book 2: Executive summary. United European Gastroenterology Journal, 10, 657–662. https://doi.org/10.1002/ueg2.12298 (accessed on 16th July 2025).

32. Roth, G. A., Abate, D., Abate, K. H., Abay, S. M., Abbafati, C., Abbasi, N., Abbastabar, H., et al. (2018). Global, regional, and national age-sex-specific mortality for 282 causes of death in 195 countries and territories, 1980–2017: A systematic analysis for the Global Burden of Disease Study 2017. The Lancet, 392, 1736–1788. https://doi.org/10.1016/s0140-6736(18)32203-7 (accessed on 16th July 2025).

33. Roy, A., Chakraborty, S., & Thakur, A. (2024). Improvement in quality of life following percutaneous transhepatic biliary drainage for malignant obstructive jaundice: An institution-based observational study. International Journal of Advanced Research. https://www.semanticscholar.org/paper/45f6143014f0cf0d534dd45ecaf1b41b80f16ac7 (accessed on 16th July 2025).

34. Sharipov, A. M., Shamszoda, K. A., Mazabshoev, S. A., & Umarov, U. L. (2022). The diagnostic challenges presented by patient with duplication of gallbladder with the distal common bile duct stricture. Avicenna Bulletin. https://www.semanticscholar.org/paper/770044b227d6b05bf4a9ba27dae1c650def50366 (accessed on 16th July 2025).

35. Shaw, A. T., Ou, S. H. I., Bang, Y. J., Camidge, D. R., Solomon, B., Salgia, R., Riely, G. J., et al. (2014). Crizotinib in ROS1-rearranged non–small-cell lung cancer. New England Journal of

Medicine, 371, 1963–1971. https://doi.org/10.1056/nejmoa1406766 (accessed on 16th July 2025).

36. Shcherbynina, M. (2024). Clinical experience of application Holoplant®-Tau for biliary lesions. Modern Gastroenterology. https://www.semanticscholar.org/paper/517718332a3a4c4664f1d75cbbf4a593d418f8e2 (accessed on 16th July 2025).

37. Shulpekova, Y., Popova, I. R., & Nechaev, V. M. (2024). Functional disorders of the biliary tract and cholelithiasis: Analysis of a possible relationship. Russian Journal of Gastroenterology, Hepatology, Coloproctology. https://www.semanticscholar.org/paper/06ddbe2dde36c4a6e913281cc4d64861af39bb96 (accessed on 16th July 2025).

38. Sukhija, G., Baldwin, C., Elfar, E., Thoroughgood, J., Rutherford, A., Wincup, C., & Mahto, A. (2024). P08 Vanishing bile duct syndrome in hemophagocytic lymphohistiocytosis precipitated by Stevens-Johnson syndrome: A rare case report. Rheumatology Advances in Practice, 8. https://www.semanticscholar.org/paper/5104de139cae57625c31e9f85a66384d233f4714 (accessed on 16th July 2025).

39. Tenner, S., Baillie, J., DeWitt, J. M., & Vege, S. S. (2013). American College of Gastroenterology guideline: Management of acute pancreatitis. The American Journal of Gastroenterology, 108, 1400–1415. https://doi.org/10.1038/ajg.2013.218 (accessed on 16th July 2025).

40. Van der Merwe, R., van Wanrooij, L. J., Bronswijk, M., Everett, S., Lakhtakia, S., Rimbaş, M., Hucl, T., et al. (2021). Therapeutic endoscopic ultrasound: European Society of Gastrointestinal Endoscopy (ESGE) guideline. Endoscopy, 54, 185–205. https://doi.org/10.1055/a-1717-1391 (accessed on 16th July 2025).

41. Vannucchi, A. M., Kiladjian, J. J., Grießhammer, M., Masszi, T., Durrant, S., Passamonti, F., Harrison, C., et al. (2015). Ruxolitinib versus standard therapy for the treatment of polycythemia vera. New England Journal of Medicine, 372, 426–435. https://doi.org/10.1056/nejmoa1409002 (accessed on 16th July 2025).

42. Williamson, C., & Geenes, V. (2014). Intrahepatic cholestasis of pregnancy. Obstetrics and Gynecology, 124, 120–133. https://doi.org/10.1097/aog.0000000000000346 (accessed on 16th July 2025).

43. Yakub, Z. A., Aebisher, D., Woźnicki, P., Łabądź, J. M., Myśliwiec, A., Dynarowicz, K., & Bartusik-Aebisher, D. (2025). Different diagnostic methods for biliary tract cancer: A review. Advances in Radiotherapy & Nuclear Medicine. https://www.semanticscholar.org/paper/301703aba79bfe5338b189c28660b6c571e8d625 (accessed on 16th July 2025).

44. Yarchoan, M., Cope, L., Anders, R. A., Noonan, A., Goff, L., Goyal, L., Lacy, J., et al. (2020). Abstract CT043: A multicenter randomized phase 2 trial of atezolizumab as monotherapy or in combination with cobimetinib in biliary tract cancers (BTCs): A NCI Experimental Therapeutics Clinical Trials Network (ETCTN) study. Tumor Biology. https://www.semanticscholar.org/paper/93b7a740be9c085c8cb3de66b2f64604949a9035 (accessed on 16th July 2025).

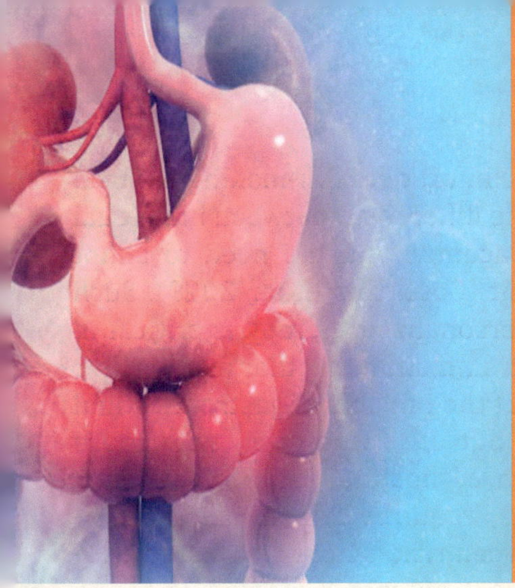

Chapter 11

GASTROINTESTINAL BLEEDING

Contents

Introduction

Gastrointestinal bleeding (GIB) is a significant clinical condition, encompassing a broad spectrum of pathological processes that may have a detrimental effect upon both morbidity and mortality. Bleeding can be classified into upper and lower gastrointestinal sources, the latter being generally generated by the esophagus, stomach, and duodenum, while the former is the colon and rectum. Awareness of the underlying mechanism and potential etiologies of GIB is crucial to initiate appropriate diagnostic and therapeutic interventions. These may vary from peptic ulcer disease, diverticulosis, malignancies, and inflammatory bowel disease to other causes. Prompt recognition of hematemesis or melena is important in the management of clinicians towards the appropriate interventions and avoiding life-threatening effects of uncontrolled blood loss. Evaluation of gastrointestinal bleeding involves an integrated process that includes patient history, physical examination, and focused diagnostic workup. It is in this sense that health authority recommendations play a pivotal role since they summarize current scientific evidence and provide a template for clinical decision-making. Clinical professionals must apply these guidelines while being sensitive to the differences between individual patient cases. Specifically, the ESC Guidelines point out clinical acumen and the need to adapt broad recommendations to individual medical needs of the patient (Cosentino et al., 2019). Such back-and-forth interplay between predetermined protocols and personalized therapy is critical in managing GIB well and can guide the development of customized treatment plans that may involve pharmacotherapy, endoscopy, or surgery. Additionally, awareness of the impacts of gastrointestinal bleeding is not only confined to practical clinical management but also associated with more general public health issues. The economic burden of GIB, such as hospitalization, diagnostic procedures, and extended care for long-term chronic conditions, requires effective preventive strategies. Public health initiatives that increase awareness and screen risk factors associated with GIB can significantly reduce the incidence rates and improve patient outcomes. According to the ESC Guidelines, health care providers should implement these preventive interventions without diminishing their ethical obligations to provide care that is specific to individual patients' needs (Kirchhof et al., 2016). Appreciation of the heterogeneity of gastrointestinal bleeding as both a clinical and public health problem is also important for maximizing the effectiveness of health systems as well as patient care quality (Figure 11.1).

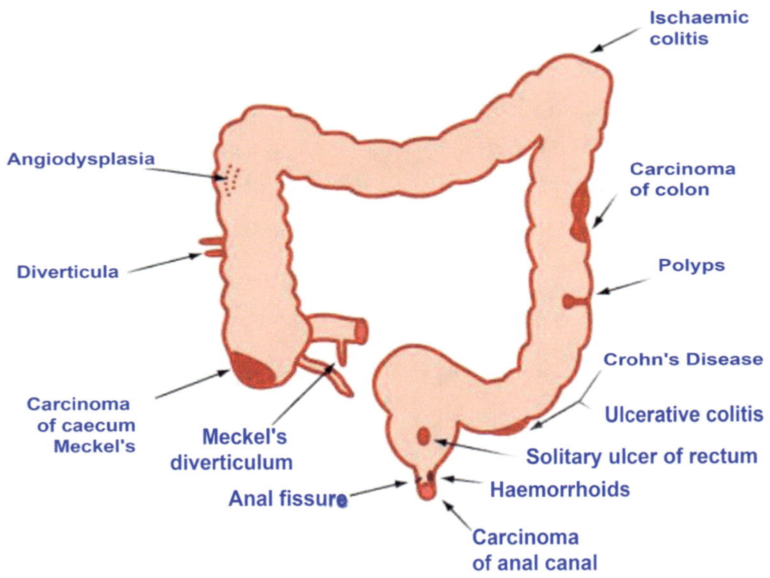

Figure 11.1. Gastrointestinal bleeding.

Source: https://www.mechealth.com/wp-content/uploads/2014/03/gastrointestinal-GI-bleeding.gif.

Definition of Gastrointestinal Bleeding

Gastrointestinal bleeding, a life-threatening medical condition, refers to any bleeding occurring within the gastrointestinal tract, which extends from the mouth to the anus. It is usually classified as upper or lower gastrointestinal bleeding depending on where it occurs. Urgent upper GI bleeding typically encompasses sources , such as peptic ulcers, esophageal varices, and gastritis, whereas lower GI bleeding is typically caused by diverticulosis, inflammatory bowel disease, or colorectal carcinoma. Presentation can be hematemesis, melena, or hematochezia, each of which occurs with varying degrees of severity and potential underlying pathology. Identification of these differences is crucial for diagnosis and subsequent management, as the etiology and implications of gastrointestinal bleeding can be quite diverse based on the site and nature of bleeding. Accurate classification of gastrointestinal bleeding is crucial for the guidance of appropriate treatment modalities. Patients presenting with gastrointestinal bleeding need to be urgently assessed, frequently highlighted by the need to stabilize the circulation and to measure the bleeding. The initial assessment generally encompasses a thorough history and physical examination, as well as diagnostic procedures , such as endoscopy or imaging studies. Such techniques allow clinicians to localize the source of bleeding and initiate focused therapies. For example, treatments range from medical therapy, e.g., proton pump inhibitors in the case of upper GI bleeding, to surgery in the case of malignancy or severe hemorrhage. In addition to this, understanding the complications arising from gastrointestinal bleeding is also essential because high-risk patients, like comorbid individuals, may require more intense management methods to avoid considerable morbidity due to the condition, as emphasized by recent studies (Shaw et al., 1985). Existing studies further emphasize the complicated interaction between gastrointestinal bleeding and various management strategies, like the use of non-steroidal anti-inflammatory drugs (NSAIDs). Though NSAIDs are popular among the analgesics used for pain control in postoperative scenarios, their link with gastrointestinal complications like anastomotic leaks after colorectal resection is an area of ongoing research (Bhangu et al., 2014). This emphasizes the importance of careful preoperative risk assessment and exercising caution in patients with a history of gastrointestinal bleeding. In short, the definition and significance of gastrointestinal bleeding are far-reaching in their areas of consideration, including their classification, etiology, and risks of treatment, all of which are significant factors to patient outcomes and management regimens.

Importance of Understanding Gastrointestinal Bleeding

In-depth knowledge of gastrointestinal bleeding is important in the early diagnosis and management of various pathologies. Gastrointestinal bleeding can manifest itself in a wide range of ways, ranging from acute presentation to chronic complications, which typically require immediate medical attention to prevent dire outcomes on the health of the patient. Pathogenesis of gastrointestinal bleeding is complex and includes conditions like peptic ulcers, cancers, and vascular malformations, each with unique diagnostic and therapeutic challenges. Recognition of these diverse causative factors enables personalized care to be provided by health professionals, significantly improving patient outcomes. Early treatment and diagnosis are able to prevent further development of diseases related to gastrointestinal bleeding, most notably those with long-term sequelae like gastric cancer and mucosa-associated lymphoid tissue disorders, as recent research has emphasized clinician identification and the efficacy of treatment (Obleaga et al., 2016). In addition, understanding the outcomes of gastrointestinal bleeding extends beyond short-term clinical benefits to encompass greater issues involving public health. Disorders like Cronkhite-Canada syndrome (CCS) that may lead to gastrointestinal bleeding are the need of greater awareness and research on uncommon disorders that have life-threatening complications (Hibi et al., 2016). The clinical prognosis for CCS has also been improved with the deployment of effective treatments , such as corticosteroids and dietary management, which underscore the importance of ongoing clinical education and observation of patients. The association of CCS with malignancies underscores the importance of monitoring systems that will ensure maximum patient safety and quality of life. Thus, comprehensive education on gastrointestinal bleeding not only equips clinicians to combat common diseases but also allows them to handle rare, complex disorders that may arise and need specialized care. Lastly, knowledge of gastrointestinal bleeding is important in its relevance to patient education and involvement.

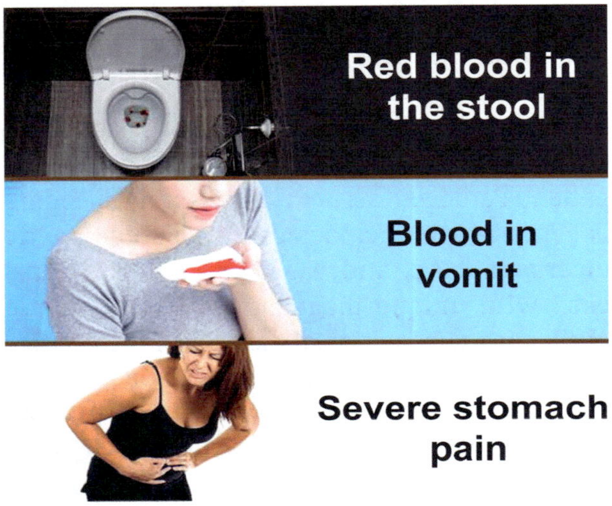

Figure 11.2. Importance of understanding gastrointestinal bleeding.

Source: https://images.medindia.net/patientinfo/950_400/symptoms-and-signs-of-gastrointestinal-bleeding.jpg.

Educated patients who are knowledgeable about the signs and symptoms of gastrointestinal bleeding can participate in their care, leading to earlier and better outcomes. Informational programs on risk factors and treatment regimes for diseases like helminthic infection or conditions arising out of *Helicobacter pylori* infection can make it possible for individuals to adopt a proactive approach to health by seeking medical advice early when they develop issues. Involving patients in their care plans, either through routine screenings or lifestyle modifications, empowers them to play an active part in managing their GI health. Educating oneself about the nuances of GI bleeding, then, meets not only the pragmatic clinical requirements but also adheres to a model of well-educated, engaged patients responding to enhanced overall health outcomes (Figure 11.2).

11.1. Types of Gastrointestinal Bleeding

The classification of gastrointestinal bleeding is largely dichotomized into two groups: upper gastrointestinal (UGI) bleeding and lower gastrointestinal (LGI) bleeding. UGI bleeding originates its location in the esophagus, stomach, or duodenum. Gastritis, peptic ulcers, and esophageal varices are the usual etiologies. The patient can be clinically manifested by hematemesis, e.g., vomiting blood or coffee ground material, and melena, manifesting as black, tarry stools due to the breakdown of blood. Considering the fact that UGI bleeding is usually associated with severe illnesses, e.g., *Helicobacter pylori* infection, which can exacerbate mucosal barrier damage and predispose to peptic ulcers, prompt diagnosis and therapy are warranted. Effective treatment not only eradicates the bleeding cause but also prevents future complications, e.g., chronic anemia or the development of a more dangerous disease, highlighting the importance of early clinical intervention in these cases (Obleaga et al., 2016). Conversely, lower gastrointestinal bleeding is more commonly from colonic or rectal sites and frequently is associated with per rectal bright red blood (hematochezia). Diverticular disease, IBD, colorectal cancer, or hemorrhoids are the usual causes of such bleeding. LGI bleeding diagnosis needs an attentive evaluation because the variety of etiologies necessitates a personalized therapeutic approach. For instance, diverticulosis may result in acute bleeding; even though spontaneous regression is feasible, however, severe attacks must be treated by surgery or endoscopy. In addition, surveillance for cancer must be done, especially in the elderly, since early detection can significantly help in enhancing the patient's status. Lastly, understanding these varying kinds of gastrointestinal bleeding has central significance in treatment as well as preventive medical care strategies (Mirambo et al., 2010). In the majority of cases, gastrointestinal bleeding is managed in a multi-system fashion that could include endoscopy, angiography, and surgery based on where and how severe the bleeding is. For upper GI bleeding, endoscopic therapies are able to address varices or ulcers by cauterizing the areas or applying clips directly.

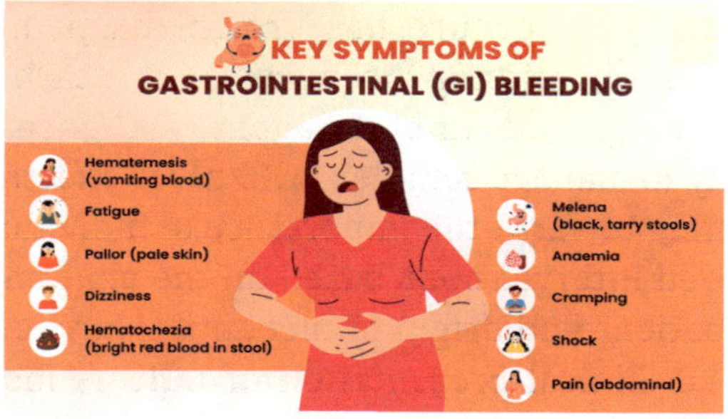

Figure 11.3 Types of gastrointestinal bleeding.

Source: https://www.manipalhospitals.com/uploads/image_gallery/key-symptoms-of-gastrointestinal-gi-bleeding.png.

On the other hand, minimal gastrointestinal bleeding may need more complex evaluations like colonoscopy to accurately identify the site of bleeding and provide space for therapeutic intervention. Also, understanding the pathophysiologic mechanisms involved, such as the consequences of chronic inflammatory conditions or malignancies, can assist in the development of tailored treatment capable of avoiding potential hazards in the future. Greater awareness and education among healthcare professionals on these forms of bleeding are essential to enable early and effective intervention, ultimately enhancing the outcomes of patients and lowering life-threatening complications of gastrointestinal bleeding (Mirambo et al., 2010; Obleaga et al., 2016) (Figure 11.3).

11.1.1. Upper Gastrointestinal Bleeding

Upper gastrointestinal bleeding (UGB) is a significant clinical issue due to its severity and many potential causes. UGB is any bleeding from the esophagus to the duodenum, and the most frequent cause is peptic ulcer disease. UGB may be secondary to esophageal varices, gastritis, or malignancy, all of which need emergent diagnosis and management. Notably, clinically, presentation is often hematemesis or melena, and there is a requirement for emergent medical evaluation. For effective UGB management, clinical professionals must utilize a complete history and physical examination, supplemented by diagnostic endoscopy, for site determination of the bleeding. Through the use of timely intervention, including intravenous fluid resuscitation, transfusion of blood products, or endoscopic therapy, patient outcomes can also be significantly improved in this critical setting. Current evidence highlights the complexity introduced by the coexistence of co-existing health conditions, particularly in patients with SARS-CoV-2 infection. Evidence indicates that these subjects have heightened risks related to UGB, as the virus can directly impair gastrointestinal tissues, and this may subsequently cause hemorrhagic complications. For example, a study reveals that ulcers in the duodenum have become the most prevalent reason for GI bleeding in SARS-CoV-2-positive patients. This group had more hospitalizations, anemia, and blood transfusions than non-virus-carrying individuals. This relationship underscores the necessity of heightened awareness and personalized management strategies to address the unique needs of

COVID-19 patients presenting with UGB. It also raises questions about the adequacy of current treatment protocols during a pandemic, which warrants continuous evaluation of therapeutic approaches. The effect of various treatment modalities on outcomes from UGB cannot be overlooked. Duodenal ulcer patients also often present with associated complications in the form of high Blood Urea Nitrogen (BUN) levels and anemia, further complicating their clinical management. Mainstream treatments predominate, but complementary therapies in the form of homeopathic individualized treatment should be investigated as adjuvants to mainstream therapy. Excellent results have been demonstrated with homeopathic therapy in a case report regarding duodenal ulcers, providing relief from crippling symptoms along with addressing the fundamental condition. These findings justify further research into ascertaining the efficacy of such treatments in larger groups. Ultimately, awareness of the integrative character of UGB, particularly within the context of evolving patient comorbidities and treatment strategies, is required for maximizing clinical results in the context of gastrointestinal bleeding.

11.1.2. Lower Gastrointestinal Bleeding

Lower gastrointestinal bleeding (LGIB) is a significant medical disorder that is defined as bleeding from the distal to the ligament of Treitz. The pathophysiology of LGIB is heterogeneous, ranging from nonmalignant conditions , such as hemorrhoids and diverticulosis to serious pathologies , such as inflammatory bowel disease and malignancy. Clinical presentation may be very variable; an acute hemorrhage in massive quantity in some patients and in others, chronic low-grade blood loss leading to anemia. Identification of the causes and presentation of LGIB is crucial to successful diagnosis and therapy because the method employed will vary with the particular condition and presentation of the patient. As elaborated in various studies, including among patients who were attended at Hospital Regional do Mato Grosso do Sul, sex and age are demographic variables that play a critical role in the occurrence and outcome of such gastrointestinal bleeding (Nantes et al., 2024). The management of LGIB involves multidisciplinary care that includes the skill of gastroenterologists, surgeons, and interventional radiologists. Initial management is stabilization of the patient, such as establishing hemodynamic status and blood transfusion if needed. Diagnostic evaluation by colonoscopy is then critical in localizing the source of bleeding. Not only can interpretation be done with direct visualization, but also therapeutic intervention, such as clipping or cauterization of bleeding lesions, is feasible. With improvements in medical technology, the interventional radiology procedure has grown, particularly for embolization procedures. Microcatheter technology and embolic agents enhance the ability to manage complex LGIB cases effectively, pointing towards the importance of individually tailored interventions based on the anatomy of the patient and origin of bleeding (Marri et al., 2024). Clinical presentation of LGIB is mostly dictated by the nature of the bleed and the intervention modalities applied. Previous studies have established that the nature of bleeding, enterorrhagia, melena, or hematochezia, bears certain relationships with clinical outcomes like mortality. It has been observed, for instance, that patients who present with melena have lower hemoglobin levels and a higher likelihood of poor outcomes compared to other bleeding presentations. Colonoscopy results not only aid in localizing the source of bleeding but can also be related to long-term mortality, in that certain pathologies, such as colitis, have increased mortality. Thus, a good appreciation of the risk of different types of LGIB is important in developing efficient management strategies so that patient care and outcome are improved overall within this rich clinical spectrum (Nantes et al., 2024) (Figure 11.4).

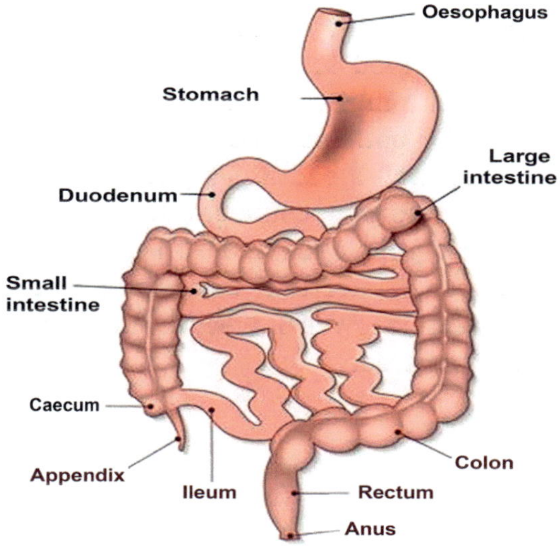

Figure 11.4. Lower gastrointestinal bleeding.

Source: https://deccanclinic.com/wp-content/uploads/2021/06/images_medium_bjha.2018.12.3.110_f04.jpg.

11.1.3. Occult Gastrointestinal Bleeding

Occult gastrointestinal bleeding is a clinical syndrome in which blood loss in the gastrointestinal tract is not clearly apparent in terms of outward symptoms , such as hematemesis or melena. The bleeding in most instances is insidious and becomes apparent through more subtle markers , such as iron deficiency anemia or unusual laboratory findings. The problem with occult bleeding is that it tends not to be discovered until later, which then makes it challenging to treat timely. Such a complication can result from numerous etiologies like gastric ulcers, malignancies, and vascular malformations. The need for aggressive investigation and diagnostic modalities like endoscopy and imaging studies becomes critical in identifying the etiology of gastrointestinal bleeding and preventing its progression to more complicated outcomes. The occurrence of occult gastrointestinal bleeding warrants high suspicion, particularly in at-risk populations. Chronic gastrointestinal disease patients, for instance, inflammatory bowel disease, are particularly vulnerable, since the underlying inflammation can lead to intermittent bleeding that is not necessarily detectable. Furthermore, patients who are at risk for , such as older age, anticoagulant therapy, and comorbid disease can have occult bleeding. In postoperative patients, as well highlighted by a recent survey, the risk of complications like marginal ulcers and anastomotic leaks can cause delayed diagnosis of gastrointestinal bleeding (Liu et al., 2025).

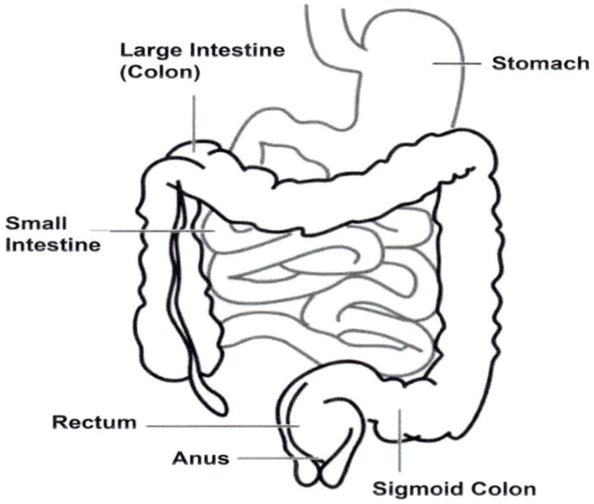

Figure 11.5. Occult gastrointestinal bleeding.

Source: https://i.ytimg.com/vi/-ZwiXSmev1Y/maxresdefault.jpg.

These observations emphasize the need for routine follow-up and the implementation of preventive measures to diagnose and manage occult bleeding in a proper manner. Most notably, occult gastrointestinal bleeding's relation to infectious conditions cannot be overlooked. Specifically, a parasitic infection of strongyloidiasis can lead to acute gastrointestinal manifestations, such as occult bleeding, particularly in immunocompromised individuals. As demonstrated from recent clinical findings, HIV patients who previously had a history of strongyloidiasis can develop gastrointestinal bleeding due to hyperinfection, thus complicating their clinical management (Badar et al., 2024). This highlights the need for a wide differential diagnosis while evaluating patients with suspected occult gastrointestinal bleeding, with the entire spectrum of potential aetiologies in mind. Familiarity with these diverse etiologies can assist clinicians in developing proper treatment strategies and improving patient outcomes within the context of gastrointestinal health (Figure 11.5).

11.2. Causes of Gastrointestinal Bleeding

The causes of gastrointestinal (GI) bleeding are multicausal and can be broadly categorized as upper and lower GI sources. Upper GI bleeding is frequently due to causes , such as peptic ulcer disease, esophageal varices, and gastric erosions. Peptic ulcers, which are due to *Helicobacter pylori* infection or chronic NSAID use, account for a high proportion of upper GI hemorrhage. Esophageal varices, which are a frequent complication in patients with chronic liver disease, can rupture and lead to catastrophic bleeding. In research, a top reason for upper GI bleeding has been recognized as esophageal varices, which occurs in about 57% of patients undergoing endoscopy for the condition. This renders it vital for clinicians to carefully assess liver function and variceal status in patients with such symptoms since early intervention can be lifesaving. Lower gastrointestinal bleeding is more frequently caused by diverticular disease, colorectal cancer, and inflammatory bowel disease. Diverticulosis, an outpouching of tiny pouches on the colon, can lead to diverticulitis and subsequent bleeding. Colorectal cancer, which is on the rise in varying populations, is a significant risk factor for bleeding in older people. Inflammatory bowel diseases like Crohn's disease and ulcerative colitis also cause inflammation and ulceration of the mucosa, resulting in blood loss. Notably, a study has shown that chronic liver disease occurs in about 30.6% of the patients who experience upper gastrointestinal bleeding, highlighting how systemic illness may connect and heighten GI bleeding (Northup et al., 2020). Therefore, it is important to be aware of the risk of systemic disease affecting lower GI bleeding to effectively diagnose and treat.

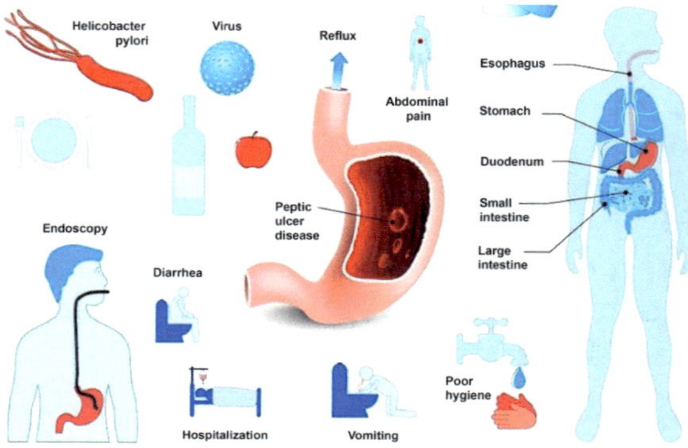

Figure 11.6. Causes of gastrointestinal bleeding.

Source: https://www.news-medical.net/image.axd?picture=2016%2F11%2FStomach_disease_infrographic_-_Designua_1000x_.jpg.

The contributions of comorbidities and systemic conditions to GI bleeding cannot be underestimated. Conditions , such as chronic liver disease, chronic and acute kidney disease, and cardiovascular disease contribute significantly to the risk of bleeding. Chronic liver disease patients have abnormal hemostasis that not only predisposes them to bleeding but also makes intervention difficult. Portal hypertension and associated variceal bleeding, for instance, pose enormous challenges that need careful follow-up and management to prevent serious outcomes. In addition, metabolic conditions, such as coagulation disorders, may also contribute to the presentation. Health care practitioners should recognize the interdependence of these systemic illnesses in assessing patients and formulating individualized treatment options for GI bleeding (Northup et al., 2020). This holistic approach facilitates enhanced risk stratification and offers evidence in decision-making for urgent therapy and potential endoscopic interventions (Figure 11.6).

11.2.1. Peptic Ulcers

Peptic ulcers, or open sores on the gastric or duodenal mucosa, are a significant gastrointestinal health issue and are particularly concerning due to their potential to bleed. These ulcers often arise due to an imbalance between injurious factors, such as gastric acid and pepsin, and protective factors, such as mucosal integrity and bicarbonate secretion. One of the more significant etiologic factors responsible for causing peptic ulcers is *Helicobacter pylori* infection, a pathogen that compromises the mucosal barrier. *H. pylori* not only leads to ulcer development but has also been determined to induce mucosal erosion that can cause gastrointestinal bleeding, and thus why its contribution to peptic ulcer pathology must be elucidated (Obleaga et al., 2016). This multi-factorial pathogenesis of ulcer formation needs to be treated so as to correct both the ulcerative lesions and the etiology. Management of peptic ulcers is both pharmacologic and non-pharmacologic, with healing and prevention of recurrence, particularly of bleeding, as goals. Patients were often previously treated with antisecretory drugs or surgery to reduce gastric acid secretion. However, with the advent of eradication regimens for *H. pylori*, treatment processes have been revolutionized. Studies have proven that eradication of the organism not only cures symptoms but also reduces recurrence of ulcers and occurrence of bleeding to a significant level (Lai et al., 1999). Bleeding remains a major complication with serious morbidity and mortality implications for its victims. Early peptic ulcer bleeding detection and control are required to prevent complications and thus serve as a reason for health practitioners to come up with guidelines on monitoring and intervention. Overall, the connection between peptic ulcers and gastrointestinal bleeding highlights the need for an all-around understanding of their pathophysiology, treatment, and long-term management. The present practice underlines the significant role of *Helicobacter pylori* eradication in the prevention of ulcer complications like bleeding, thereby enhancing patient outcomes. As the prevalence of *H. pylori* is maintained, sustained surveillance needs to be carried out to ensure effective treatment regimens and patient education regarding compliance with treatment regimens. Research in the future must pursue new forms of overcoming resistance to *H. pylori* treatments and improve overall treatment success, hence prospectively reducing peptic ulcer bleeding rates and their accompanying health outcomes. Understanding the association between these diseases is significant for both patients and clinicians alike for the best and complete care.

11.2.2. Inflammatory Bowel Disease

Inflammatory bowel disease (IBD), which encompasses disorders , such as Crohn's disease and ulcerative colitis, severely impacts gastrointestinal health and can lead to severe complications, including gastrointestinal bleeding. The pathophysiology of IBD is a dysregulated immune response to intestinal microbiota with resultant chronic inflammation. The inflammation can weaken the mucous layer that covers the intestines and cause blood vessels susceptible to damage. Consequently, the patient may complain of hematochezia or melena based on the severity and site of the lesion. Furthermore, the severity of the inflammation is related to the risk of bleeding; widespread ulceration of the intestinal mucosa, as in late stages, may result in significant loss of blood, prompting urgent medical attention to prevent potentially fatal consequences. Management of gastrointestinal bleeding in IBD is extremely challenging and is likely to require a multidisciplinary approach to target the multifaceted character of the illness. Acute haemorrhage needs cautious diagnostic investigation, e.g., endoscopy, to determine the source of the bleeding and direct therapy. Treatment may vary from conservative management, i.e., fluid resuscitation and transfusions, to aggressive interventions like surgery resection in complicated disease or failure to establish hemostasis.

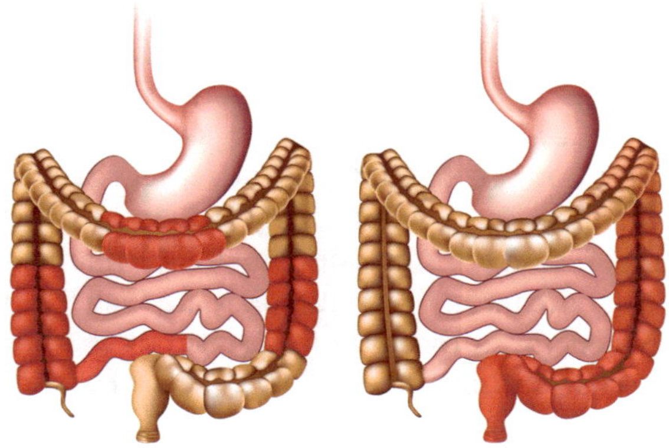

Figure 11.7. Inflammatory bowel disease.

Source: https://privategastrolondon.com/wp-content/uploads/2018/10/Picture14.png.

Gastroenterologists, surgeons, and radiologists all need to be involved since timely interventions can significantly alter clinical courses and improve patient quality of life. Because of the chronic and relapsing nature of IBD, frequent follow-up and tailored therapeutic strategies are indicated to prevent rebleeding and manage the underlying inflammatory process optimally. Recent advances in imaging and treatment technologies have led to better prognosis of gastrointestinal bleeding in IBD. Techniques , such as capsule endoscopy and device-assisted enteroscopy allow for total small intestine examination, facilitating the early recognition and treatment of bleeding sources, particularly in obscure gastrointestinal bleeding. Additionally, continuous research on the genetic and inflammatory mechanisms of IBD has the potential to improve the understanding of disease mechanisms and therapeutic outcomes. This information can result in more personalized treatment approaches, such as biologic therapies that target particular pathways to mitigate inflammation and, by extension, the threat of bleeding. As our insight increases, clinicians are in an even better position to navigate the intricacies of IBD, ultimately with a view to optimizing outcomes and reducing the burden of gastrointestinal bleeding (Siddiqui et al., 2024; Gonçalves et al., 2025) (Figure 11.7).

11.2.3. Gastrointestinal Tumors

The presence of gastrointestinal tumors is a high risk for gastrointestinal bleeding, with colorectal cancer ranking among the most common types. The number of incidents and mortality rates of colorectal cancer are still on the increase, placing a high load on healthcare systems globally. Genetic predispositions, lifestyle, and food intake are the key factors in establishing whether one will get colorectal tumors, as revealed by research. Additionally, the identification of such tumors at later stages is associated with more cases of complications, including bleeding. With the growth of the tumor, it invades neighboring tissues and disrupts vascular structures, which can cause hematochezia or melena. Early diagnosis is necessary because it can possibly allow preventive interventions or procedures to be used that are able to lower the risk of gastrointestinal bleeding as well as improve overall patient outcomes (Rawla et al., 2019). Besides colorectal tumors, there are some other forms of gastrointestinal cancers that also have serious complications of bleeding. Gastric cancers, for instance, are notorious for gastric mucosal erosion and ulceration, typically causing massive hemorrhagic manifestations. Cancers in the upper GI tract, including esophageal and pancreatic cancers, can likewise cause disastrous complications , such as hemorrhage through invasion or occlusion of major blood vessels. These bleeding attacks not only contribute to morbidity but also complicate surgery as they carry an increased risk of hemorrhage during and after surgery. This necessitates a multidisciplinary approach in managing gastrointestinal tumors when oncologists collaborate with gastroenterologists and surgeons to deliver comprehensive care to patients that minimizes complications like gastrointestinal bleeding (Sigrist et al., 2017). Research has been instrumental in the development of advanced diagnostic methods for identifying gastrointestinal tumors, thus broadening the chances of intervention at the early stage. Endoscopy, imaging, and the least invasive treatments are among the most significant methods in tumor identification before they progress to stages requiring bleeding complications. Besides, emerging imaging methods , such as elastography, hold promise for non-invasive diagnosis of tumor characteristics and associated tissue changes and thus can be used to facilitate improved diagnosis and treatment plans for patients. Along with improving detection, these techniques also help identify invasiveness and potential bleeding risks of tumors. By coordinating diagnostic development with treatment possibilities, healthcare providers can effectively reduce the frequency of tumor-associated gastrointestinal bleeding, improving survival and quality of life in affected patients (Rawla et al., 2019).

11.3. Symptoms and Diagnosis

Identification of the symptoms related to gastrointestinal bleeding is crucial for early treatment and diagnosis. Variable manifestations can be presented by patients, and the most common are hematemesis, melena, and hematochezia. Hematemesis, or vomiting blood, is typically suggestive of upper gastrointestinal sources , such as esophageal varices or peptic ulcer, while melena is indicative of blood that has been digested in the stool, indicative of bleeding occurring higher in the gastrointestinal tract. Conversely, hematochezia, or the passing per rectum of obviously red blood, typically describes lower GI bleeding, typically arising from such causes as diverticulosis or colon carcinoma. Identification of these symptoms aids clinicians in establishing a differential diagnosis, finally culminating in the ensuing investigation and treatment protocols to efficiently counteract the root cause of the bleeding effectively. True diagnosis of gastrointestinal bleeding necessitates a multi-factorial process. Health care professionals would begin with a detailed patient history and physical examination, which are cardinal factors in determining the etiology of the bleeding. Other tests, including laboratory examination and imaging studies, are also vital in demystifying the illness. For instance, a full blood count would illustrate anemia as a result of blood loss, while endoscopic examinations would visualize the site of hemorrhage. Methods , such as upper endoscopy and colonoscopy prove useful in diagnosing conditions such as ulcers or tumors, and may even facilitate therapeutic maneuvers, such as cauterization of the causative vessel. Utilization of imaging modalities , such as CT scans further helps in fine-tuning diagnosis by identifying vascular lesions, such as pseudoaneurysms, causative of such atypical presentations of gastrointestinal bleeding , such as hemosuccus pancreaticus (Lee et al., 2007). A thorough understanding of the potential complications of gastrointestinal bleeding is required for enhancing patient management. For instance, the relationship between *Helicobacter pylori* infection and the formation of bleeding lesions, such as peptic ulcers, is well-documented. The bacteria compromise the gastric mucosal barrier, leading to tissue erosion and subsequent hemorrhage (Obleaga et al., 2016). Clinicians must be cognizant of treatment efficacy monitoring because successful elimination of *H. pylori* may forestall the onset of severe complications , such as gastric cancer and mucosa-associated lymphoid tissue lymphoma. Patient education and follow-ups about the chronicity of the infections are essential in controlling expectations and outcomes. Thus, comprehension of symptomatology along with meticulous diagnostic techniques is essential not just for the detection of gastrointestinal bleeding but also in the prevention of its potentially fatal outcome (Figure 11.8).

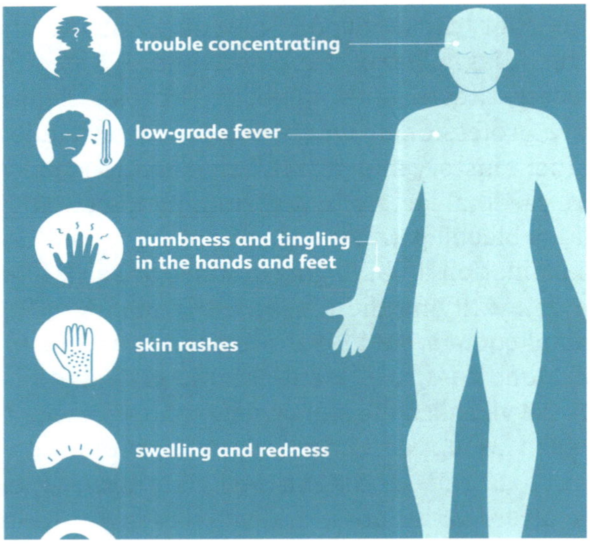

Figure 11.8. Symptoms and diagnosis.

Source: https://www.verywellhealth.com/thmb/kP5SwDnwHMYInmYKeNe1ZRLFz-g=/6251x4168/filters:no_upscale():max_bytes(150000):strip_icc()/3232847_color1-5c0191cec9e77c00013b3053.png.

11.3.1. Common Symptoms of Gastrointestinal Bleeding

The clinical presentation of gastrointestinal bleeding is very diverse but certain symptoms are most commonly seen with this disorder. Hematemesis, vomiting of blood of varying colors between bright red to coffee grounds because of the commingling of gastric secretions with blood, is the most frequently seen symptom by patients. Also, melena or black, tarry stools, is usually the most important sign of upper gastrointestinal bleeding due to the breakdown and transformation of blood when it travels through the intestines. These signs immediately bring a patient to see a doctor because these may be the manifestation of serious underlying conditions like peptic ulcers or esophageal varices. Recognition of these symptoms is critical to the timely diagnosis and treatment of gastrointestinal bleeding because untreated bleeding will have high morbidity and mortality. Other common presentation of gastrointestinal bleeding, in addition to hematemesis and melena, is hematochezia, which is the discharge of fresh blood with stools. Hematochezia typically indicates lower gastrointestinal bleeding and can be associated with conditions , such as diverticulitis, colorectal carcinoma, or hemorrhoids. Depending upon the volume of blood lost, patients may also present with anemic symptoms like fatigue, pallor, and dyspnea secondary to reduced cardiac output based on low hemoglobin. Clinicians typically employ laboratory results, such as complete blood count, to assess the severity and guide further management. Presentation of hematochezia emphasizes the need to differentiate between bleeding from the upper and lower parts of the gastrointestinal tract, a consideration that can significantly impact the treatment plan and prognosis. Another fascinating aspect of gastrointestinal bleeding is its relationship to hemodynamic instability, particularly in the most critical cases. Lightheadedness, syncope, or confusion can be presentations of severe blood loss, causing hypovolemic shock. For instance, an effectiveness study of intravenous ferric carboxymaltose in acute gastrointestinal bleeding patients highlights the imperative need to manage hemoglobin levels upon admission (Ballester-Clau et al., 2019). Hemodynamically unstable patients require instant resuscitation and often need interventions like blood transfusion or iron supplementation to restore blood volume and improve oxygen delivery. Detection of such complex manifestations of gastrointestinal bleeding is essential in order to deliver appropriate treatment and prevent complications of this fatal disease (Figure 11.9).

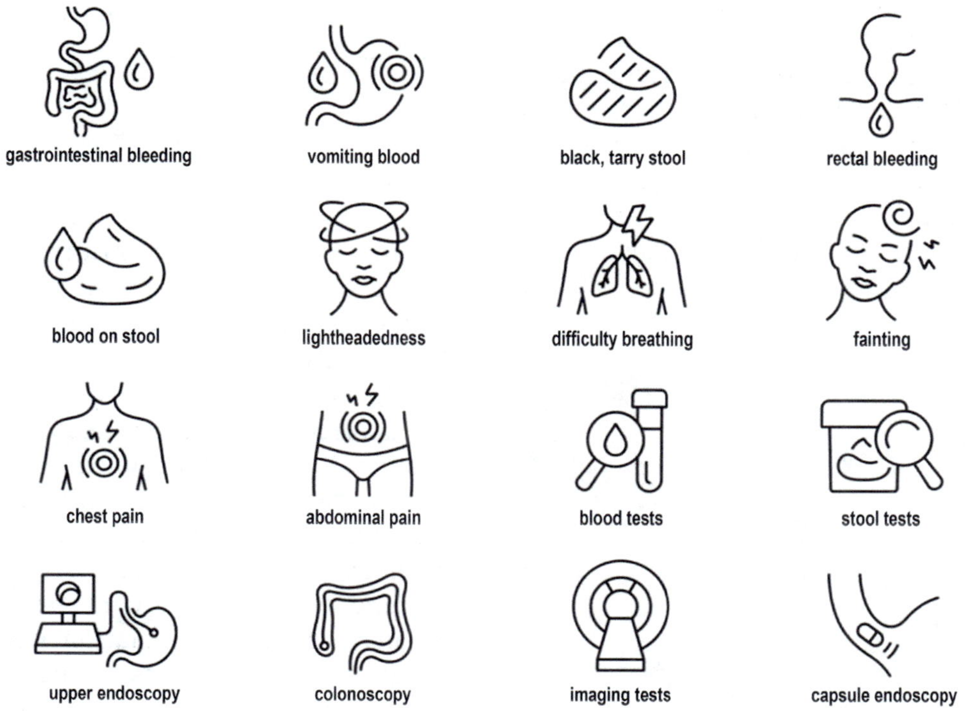

Figure 11.9. Common symptoms of gastrointestinal bleeding.

Source: https://www.manipalhospitals.com/uploads/image_gallery/gastrointestinal-bleeding-symptoms-manipal-hospitals.jpg.

11.3.2. Diagnostic Procedures (e.g., Endoscopy, Colonoscopy)

Endoscopy and colonoscopy are very valuable diagnostic tests in the management and evaluation of gastrointestinal bleeding. They are less invasive techniques through which practitioners are able to look at the interior of the gastrointestinal tract for diagnosis and treatment. Endoscopy, typically applied for upper gastrointestinal disease, employs a flexible scope with a camera system to inspect ulcers or variceal bleeding. Meanwhile, colonoscopy focuses on the lower GI tract, making it possible to explore the colon for bleeding causes like polyps or tumors. Both are essential to diagnose the cause of bleeding and thus guide follow-up therapeutic interventions. Direct visualization provided by these diagnostic approaches makes possible discrimination between the various causes of gastrointestinal bleeding with precision and is essential for enhancing patient outcomes. The diagnostic value of tests does not end in visualization; they also aid in therapeutic management. In certain cases, the conditions causing gastrointestinal bleeding can be treated therapeutically during the same procedure. For instance, if a Dieulafoy lesion is identified by colonoscopy, as mentioned in remarks on the management of gastrointestinal bleeding, the physician can employ techniques , such as clipping or injection to arrest the bleeding instantaneously (Farag et al., 2025). Early treatment is most crucial in preventing complications due to massive blood loss. Moreover, the fact that therapeutic and diagnostic procedures can be carried out in parallel reduces the need for further surgical intervention, as it underscores the efficacy and efficiency of gastroenterological endoscopy in dealing with patients suffering from acute bleeding. Despite their benefits, diagnostic tests like endoscopy and colonoscopy are not without danger.

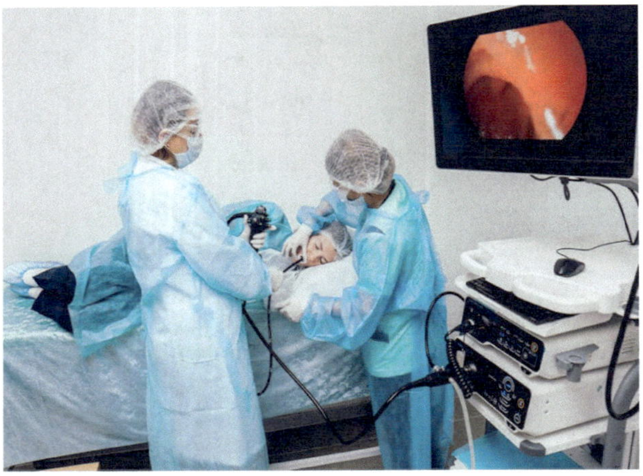

Figure 11.10. Diagnostic procedures (e.g., endoscopy, colonoscopy).

Source: https://www.srikotamedical.com/wp-content/uploads/2021/01/endoscopy-1.jpg.

Several studies have yielded variable complication rates, e.g., perforation or hemorrhage, after these procedures with vast variability related to facility volume and experience (Jung et al., 2022). For instance, the risk of perforation during therapeutic colonoscopy can be as high as 0.731% in high-volume centers, highlighting the need for procedure expertise and appropriate patient selection (Jung et al., 2022). Consequently, while endoscopic studies are of prime importance to diagnose and treat gastrointestinal hemorrhage, physicians have to weigh the advantages against the dangers of such interventions. Through this process, not only is the safety of the patient enhanced, but the therapeutic utility of these life-saving diagnostic imaging modalities is also optimized (Figure 11.10).

11.3.3. Laboratory Tests and Imaging Studies

In the evaluation of gastrointestinal bleeding, imaging studies and laboratory testing play a significant role in the diagnosis of the underlying etiology and guiding therapeutic management. The routine laboratory tests, including prothrombin time (PT) and international normalized ratio (INR), are frequently employed to determine hemostatic function but are of little utility in cirrhotic patients. Patients with chronic liver disease exhibit composite alterations of their hemostatic systems, which cannot be captured by these conventional indices. For instance, in a population with cirrhosis, global tests for hemostasis , such as thrombin generation tests and viscoelastic tests, including thromboelastography (TEG), provide improved information on the status of coagulation and risk of bleeding than can be obtained using conventional tests individually (Northup et al., 2020). Therefore, more importance is placed on the application of these newer assays in accurately assessing the risk of bleeding in those patients who present with both pro- and antithrombotic changes. Imaging studies are similarly essential in the diagnosis of the cause of gastrointestinal hemorrhage, particularly for diseases that include vascular disorders or neoplasms. Imaging methods , such as ultrasound, computed tomography (CT), and magnetic resonance imaging (MRI) help to provide gross anatomical data that can be utilized for guiding management strategies. Examples of the same include Doppler ultrasound for assessing portal vein patency and the diagnosis of conditions like portal vein thrombosis, which may cause bleeding attacks (Northup et al., 2020). Furthermore, CT scans can identify ongoing bleeding via contrast extravasation or elucidate the presence of tumors , such as hepatocellular carcinoma, which mimics bleeding signs. Of specific mention, the atezolizumab and bevacizumab combination has been promising in unresectable hepatocellular carcinoma patients, a trend evolving in therapeutic approaches for bleeding-defined liver pathologies. In combination, however, both laboratory exams and imaging studies enhance the clinician's diagnostic and therapeutic power in the case of gastrointestinal bleeding.

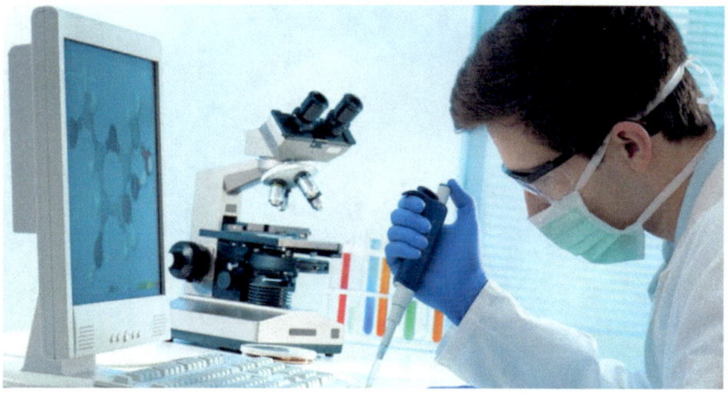

Figure 11.11. Laboratory tests and imaging studies.

Source: https://www.828urgentcare.com/Sites/B35EE094-1733-4F45-AE3A-184C3FAB532F/images/wp-content/uploads/2018/03/Onsite-Laboratory-Investigations-and-Screening-Services.jpg.

Not only does this multidisciplinary approach enable a more accurate definition of hemostatic equilibrium in cirrhotic patients, but it also enables early detection of potential sites of bleeding through the use of high-resolution imaging. Owing to the complexity of bleeding disorders in this patient population, it is necessary that an advanced analysis of laboratory and imaging findings takes place in order to develop appropriate management plans. Implementation of these newer diagnostic technologies can lead to improved patient outcomes, especially in addressing the dynamic course of gastrointestinal bleeding in patients with preexisting liver disease (Figure 11.11).

11.4. Treatment Options

In the management of gastrointestinal bleeding, early identification and appropriate treatment modalities are essential, particularly since this condition can have potentially fatal consequences. Initial treatment modalities may involve resuscitation to stabilize the patient, such as intravenous replacement and blood transfusions to manage severe blood loss. The latter focuses on determining the source of bleeding can have an impact on specific therapeutic interventions. For the situation of upper gastrointestinal bleeding, endoscopy is now the leading underlying modality of treatment, allowing for the intervention directly through cauterization, band ligation, or clipping to address lesions , such as ulcers or varices. Pharmacotherapy has its role in such interventions as being routinely recommended by proton pump inhibitors owing to their efficacy in inhibiting gastric acid secretion and causing healing of ulcers, pointing to their pivotal role in treatment regimens (Menichelli et al., 2024). The management of lower gastrointestinal hemorrhage is very variable according to the etiology and severity of the bleeding, and therefore triggers certain treatment options. The initial approach can include an extensive examination through colonoscopy, which not only allows for diagnosis but also for therapeutic intervention , such as polypectomy or cauterization of lesions diagnosed. In more complex instances, imaging studies like angiography are employed to localize the bleeding and enable transcatheter arterial embolization, a less invasive procedure with the aim of occluding the blood vessels supplying the hemorrhage. Interventional decision is also largely determined by the general well-being of the patients, comorbidities, and specific characteristics of the lesions identified, providing evidence for the necessity of personalized treatment approaches in managing lower GI bleeding (Menichelli et al., 2024). Treatment modalities presently on the horizon also encompass newer techniques that address specific etiologies of gastrointestinal hemorrhage, such as hemobilia. Given that the disease presents complex diagnostic and therapeutic cases, interventions like ERCP, alongside angiographic techniques, can be started in an effort to cure bile duct injury or anomalous vascular communication adequately. Such intervention techniques will significantly enhance outcomes in patients by sealing off bleeding sites in a minimally invasive approach. Furthermore, novel pharmacologic interventions and optimized management in high-risk populations, such as elderly patients with bleeding complications secondary to drug therapy, indicate further evolution in gastrointestinal management. With novel treatment on the horizon and with increasing options, it is increasingly necessary that a multidisciplinary approach to management is employed from diagnosis through recovery.

11.4.1. Medical Management (e.g., Medications)

Effective medical treatment of gastrointestinal bleeding (GIB) depends on a multi-disciplinary strategy mainly founded on drug administration, considering the etiology of the bleeding. Anticoagulants , such as direct oral anticoagulants (DOACs) and vitamin K antagonists (VKAs) are prevalent in patients with diseases requiring thromboprophylaxis. With the growing popularity of DOACs because of their ease of use and predictable pharmacokinetics, the risk of GIB has an intricate relationship with them. Recent studies indicate DOAC users may be at a higher rate of GIB than VKA users, as evidenced by the Turkish Ministry of Health's e-Nabız system retrospective study. These results emphasize the requirement for close tracking and control of anticoagulation in high-risk populations, and suggest that clinicians must balance the benefits of anticoagulation with the potential for significant adverse effects , such as GIB (Racharla et al., 2024). GIB management is further complicated by the need for immediate action and medication adjustment for bleeding. After a bleed is identified, it is then imperative to examine the patient's current medications and deal with the risk of an interaction or an increase in the bleeding episode.

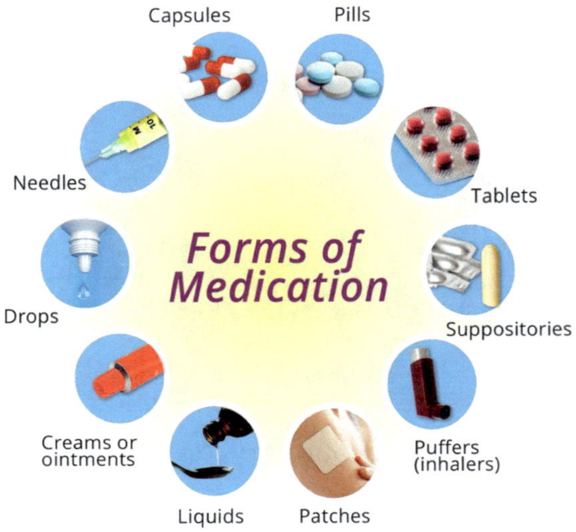

Figure 11.12. Medical management (e.g., medications).

Source: https://www.mygrief.ca/pluginfile.php/2868/mod_lesson/page_contents/2647/M5%20-%20medications%20image.jpg.

For instance, continuing or altering anticoagulant therapy must be approached very carefully, taking into consideration the involved risk factors, including comorbidities and the global anticoagulation level of the patient. Anticoagulation in patients with left ventricular assist devices (LVADs) is particularly problematic. Studies show that aspirin exclusion in LVAD recipients does not correlate with pump thrombosis or stroke risks, thus showing that titration of the drug regimen can be cautiously pursued while avoiding GIB risks (Racharla et al., 2024). Under the current management of GIB, health practitioners are supposed to consider patient compliance with medication regimens, particularly following bleeding. Half of all patients, in a great majority, lose anticoagulation after GIB occurs, posing a challenge in terms of prevention of thromboembolic events and long-term risk management. Continuation rates of some anticoagulants differ, with rivaroxaban exhibiting a higher continuation rate compared to comparators like apixaban. Such practices highlight the importance of intensifying education and counseling coupled with rigorous follow-up treatment to ensure patient safety. Lastly, medication control of GIB demands an inclusive approach that involves drug management as well as measures to prevent recurrence, along with the management of the lifestyles of the patients after the episode (Çakmak et al., 2024) (Figure 11.12).

11.4.2. Surgical Interventions

Surgery is at the heart of the management of gastrointestinal hemorrhage if conservative measures are unable to achieve hemostasis. Endoscopic therapy is commonly employed as a first treatment modality due to its less invasive nature and control of hemorrhage in circumscribed lesions. However, when endoscopy fails, surgery becomes necessary. The goals of surgical control are not only to control bleeding but also to diagnose and, when needed, resect the underlying pathologies that led to the bleed, such as tumors, ulcers, or vascular malformations. Because bleeding complications may lead to life-threatening medical emergencies, urgent surgical treatment is indicated to avoid complications and improve patient outcomes. Severity and location of gastrointestinal bleeding dictate the type of surgical procedure carried out. For instance, patients presenting with lower gastrointestinal bleeding may have varying strategies compared to those presenting with upper gastrointestinal sources. Based on a study evaluating complications following percutaneous coronary intervention, it has been established that non-access site bleeding, like gastrointestinal bleeds, had significant mortality risks due to its intricate anatomical basis and associated conditions (Buchan et al., 2015). So, when a patient exhibits signs of gastrointestinal instability, the surgical teams must assess the cause of bleeding carefully, possibly involving exploratory laparotomy or localized resections in case of bleeding caused by some anatomical anomalies.

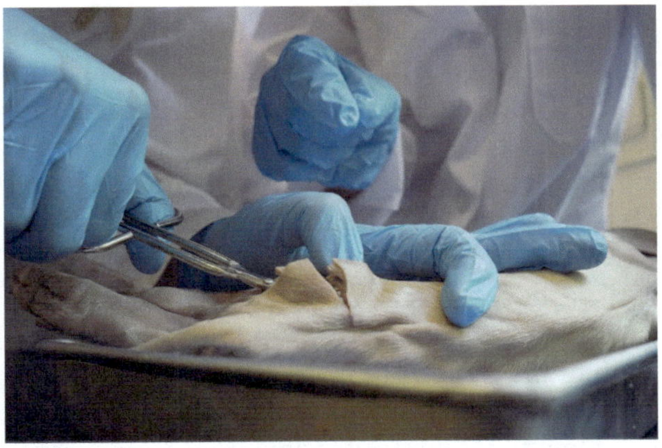

Figure 11.13. Surgical interventions.

Source: https://blog.explo.org/hubfs/yale/academics/slideshows/20170629_103615/6-29_Surgical_Interventions_-_12_of_20.jpg.

These specialized surgical treatments guarantee complete control of the bleeding episode, along with dealing with the patient's overall clinical condition. In addition to the early challenges of controlling bleeding, postoperative care has an important function in ensuring the patient's recovery and preventing recurring bleeding episodes. A recent study highlighted the importance of identifying risk factors that can predict severe complications following lower gastrointestinal bleed events, which might include the requirement for surgery (Leafloor et al., 2020). Age, hemoglobin, and INR were variables related to greater adverse outcomes, illustrating the importance of risk estimation in surgical planning. With appropriate postoperative management and monitoring schemes, recovery may be enhanced and complications prevented. Surgical procedures are a critical component of the surgical armamentarium to treat gastrointestinal bleeding, eventually aiming towards healing of the patient's condition and prevention from recurrence of such life-threatening activity (Figure 11.13).

11.4.3. Endoscopic Treatments

Endoscopic procedures are now the turning point technique in gastrointestinal bleeding control, especially in acute non-variceal upper gastrointestinal bleeding (ANVUGIB). Endoscopic techniques not only achieve hemostasis but also provide visualization of the bleeding. Through technological advancement, endoscopic techniques , such as the use of thermal coagulation, band ligation, and hemoclips, have been found beneficial in control and prevention of re-bleeding. The potential for reducing the need for surgical intervention makes endoscopic therapy an invaluable component of the therapeutic armamentarium of gastrointestinal bleeding. Refinement in training and facilities has improved clinical outcomes, particularly with the added advantage of early patient assessment and appropriate risk stratification techniques. Thus, the evolution of endoscopic treatment is a pivotal shift in the management of gastrointestinal bleeding by doctors to improve patient prognosis and minimize complications (Lee et al., 2025). Early management of gastrointestinal bleeding cannot be overstressed since endoscopic treatment in a timely fashion has a profound effect on patient outcomes. Growing evidence proves that standardized peri-endoscopy care will significantly enhance the handling of UGIB cases. With the application of a systematic approach to risk assessment, physicians can possibly ensure high-risk patients receive definitive interventions that are crucial in preventing morbidity and mortality associated with gastrointestinal bleeding. Moreover, integration of more sophisticated scoring systems—, such as the ABC score, is a valuable aid to clinicians in estimating mortality and making clinical judgments and ensures effective resource allocation (Maity et al., 2024). Through effective communication between gastroenterologists and emergency health professionals, early recognition and management of gastrointestinal bleeding can lead to improved patient care and results, thus eventually enhancing the overall management paradigm.

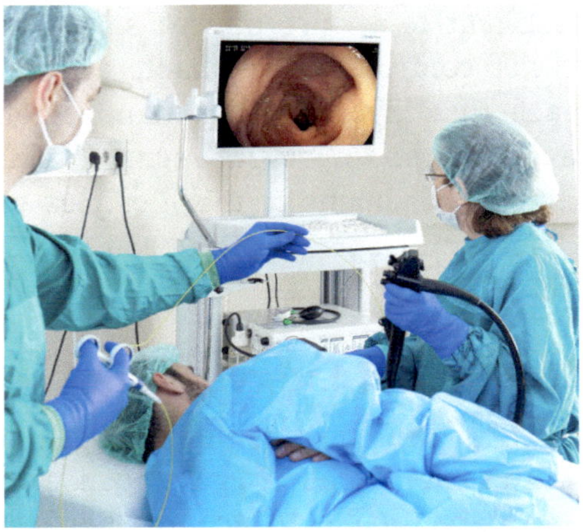

Figure 11.14. Endoscopic treatments.

Source: https://gastro-md.com/wp-content/uploads/2020/01/UGIE-Graphics3-min-2048x2048.jpg.

New endoscopic interventions continue to evolve, and they present promising avenues for the control of refractory cases of gastrointestinal bleeding where conventional interventions have failed. The advancement of hemostatic powders and the use of over-the-scope clips have recently been established, providing alternative options to clinicians faced with the challenge of achieving hemostasis. These advancements have the potential to be very beneficial in high-risk situations or in anatomical contraindications that prevent conventional interventions. The emphasis placed on the validation and construction of these emerging techniques is in alignment with the trend toward personalized medicine, allowing for patient-specific treatment modalities to be designed to fit each patient's profile and comorbidities. With additional studies to further elucidate the safety and effectiveness of these treatments, the overall picture of endoscopic treatment of gastrointestinal bleeding is soon to improve significantly, hence reducing the medical burden imposed by this common though severe disease (Maity et al., 2024; Lee et al., 2025) (Figure 11.14).

11.5. Complications of Gastrointestinal Bleeding

Complications of gastrointestinal bleeding can cause massive morbidity and mortality among patients. NVUGIB patients are at greater risk when they also have a condition , such as NAFLD. According to existing research, admission following NVUGIB reveals a shocking trend: patients who have NAFLD have noticeably high mortality rates when compared with those who do not have this condition. For instance, the adjusted odds ratio of mortality in this cohort is 1.018, which demonstrates a statistically significantly higher risk. This enhanced mortality is attributed to various factors, such as the impaired liver function in NAFLD, which has the tendency to aggravate the complications arising from bleeding per se from the gastrointestinal tract, i.e., shock and acute respiratory failure, and thus makes patient outcomes gravely complicated (Soni et al., 2023). The impacts of gastrointestinal bleeding also extend beyond the acute clinical sequelae, influencing the economic burden placed on healthcare systems. Patients hospitalized with NVUGIB and NAFLD tended to have higher total charges, averaging around $2,148, which highlights the economic burden involved in managing these complications. These patients usually need intensive treatment and prolonged hospitalization because their conditions tend to be complex in nature, particularly for advanced complications like acute liver failure. Most significantly, even though such patients tend to have extended hospitalizations, they are not necessarily encumbered with an increased occurrence of sepsis or acute kidney injury.

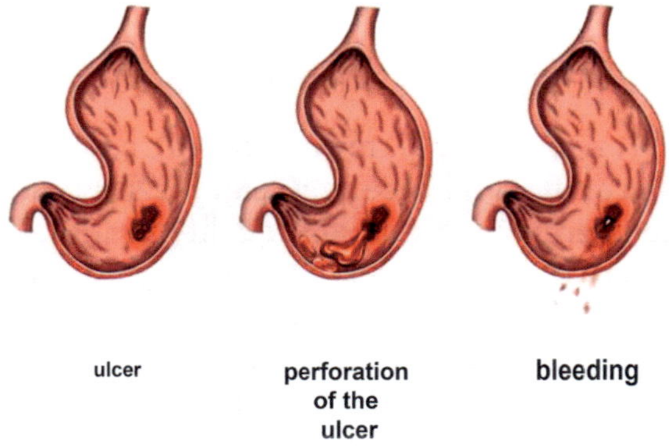

Figure 11.15. Complications of gastrointestinal bleeding.

Source: https://c8.alamy.com/zooms/9/1049932063bd43fea1c44c9578cd85fb/2a3ce5x.jpg.

This apparent paradox indicates that even while the economic cost is significant, some outcomes may not necessarily align with the expected rise in morbidity rates, presenting an intricate clinical situation needing further research (Soni et al., 2023). The interaction between surgical interventions and gastrointestinal complications adds another layer of complexity to patient management of gastrointestinal bleeding. Surgical patients, especially those who have undergone cardiac surgery, have a much higher prevalence of gastrointestinal complications, with studies showing an approximate incidence of about 2.51% incidence. Risks are much more pronounced in elderly patients as well as in patients with comorbidities, since longer cardiopulmonary bypass times are associated with complications. In-hospital mortality rose to 25.8% in patients who developed such complications during their hospital stay, reflecting the gravity of the clinical scenario. The extremely heightened risk of mortality for this group indicates that gastrointestinal complications are not simple run-of-the-mill difficulties but decisive determinants that have significant effects on patient survival and recovery following surgery (Figure 11.15).

11.5.1. Anemia and Its Effects

Anemia, a common complication of gastrointestinal bleeding, significantly affects the overall condition and quality of life of the patient. Anemia is characterized by a decrease in the red blood cell count or hemoglobin, leading to decreased oxygenation of the body. Particularly in the case of chronic gastrointestinal bleeding, blood loss quickly exhausts iron stores, exacerbating anemia. Symptoms of such weakness, fatigue, and mental impairment are typically due to this condition and can render daily functioning impossible and reduce the functional capacity of patients to perform daily activities. Severity and frequency of such symptoms typically point to the need for early diagnosis and treatment of anemia and the causes of anemia, particularly gastrointestinal bleeding, as a leading cause of chronic blood loss. Among a variety of conditions, hereditary hemorrhagic telangiectasia (HHT) is a key disorder that is accompanied by chronic GI bleeding and resulting anemia. Vascular defects occurring in HHT patients lead to periodic bleeding, lowering their hemoglobin values quite significantly. Evidence from a multicenter clinical trial assessing the use of bevacizumab, a vascular endothelial growth factor antibody, indicates a favorable use in controlling bleeding from HHT. Following therapy, the patients demonstrated remarkable improvement with a rise in mean hemoglobin by 3.2 g/dL, reflecting therapeutic response to manage anemia due to gastrointestinal bleeding. This supports the complex association between gastrointestinal function and systemic diseases , such as anemia, emphasizing the extreme significance of specific therapies that address both control of bleeding and hemoglobin replenishment in patients under assault (H-Samkari et al., 2020).

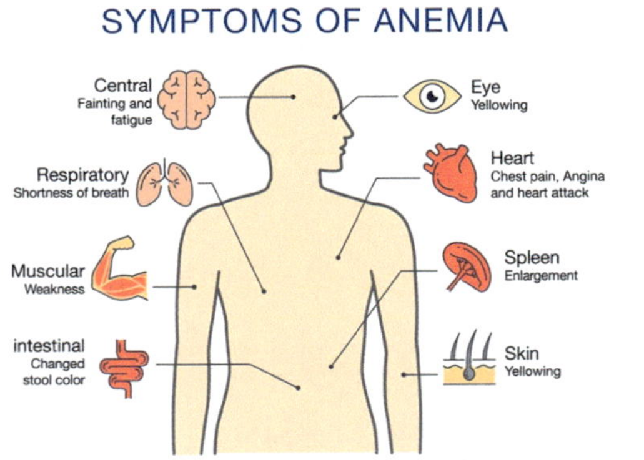

Figure 11.16. Anemia and its effects.

Source: https://biodesignwellness.com/wp-content/uploads/2018/10/Anemia_Symptoms.jpg.

Treating anemia does not only involve treating the immediate effects of blood loss but also implies there is a necessity for an effective understanding of its implications, particularly on cardiovascular health. Research has shown that individuals with high triglyceride levels are vulnerable to ischemic events, and hence metabolic health is linked with complications of anemia. The ethyl ester of eicosapentaenoic acid, which lowers triglycerides and is a function of Icosapent ethyl, illustrates the potential of pharmacologic treatment in altering cardiovascular risk from anemia. Thus, management of anemia and its effects should be properly controlled through a multidisciplinary approach that includes control of nutritional deficiencies, implementation of therapy for etiologies like gastrointestinal bleeding, and choice of preventive therapy for associated conditions. This comprehensive approach is necessary to enhance patient outcomes and deepen understanding of the widespread repercussions of anemia (Bhatt et al., 2018) (Figure 11.16).

11.5.2. Shock and Hemodynamic Instability

Development of shock and hemodynamic instability is an avid interest in the setting of gastrointestinal bleeding, particularly in the case of upper gastrointestinal bleeding (UGIB). This is typically due to significant loss of blood that compromises the body's compensatory mechanisms to maintain adequate perfusion of the vital organs. Because the gastrointestinal tract is highly vascular, gastrointestinal tract hemorrhage can lead to a very rapid development of worsening in a patient. Shock is also classified based on the mechanism underlying, such as hypovolemic shock due to fluid loss secondary to hemorrhage. The presentation clinical assessment can classify patients into hemodynamically unstable or stable, which is particularly important in defining the initial management strategy. Scores like the Glasgow Blatchford score enable clinicians to predict outcomes based on patient-specific circumstances and laboratory results and permit deferred interventions in those at higher risk of instability (Khayyat, 2024). Hemodynamic instability is also closely associated with greater morbidity and mortality in UGIB patients. The mortality rate can be increased from approximately 10% to 15% in hemodynamically unstable patients. If patients exhibit signs of shock, such as tachycardia or hypotension, prompt recognition is essential. These initial signs do not just indicate the extent of the bleeding but also guide the urgency and type of intervention to be undertaken. Early detection of shock has been established through evidence to enhance survival rates, with immediate interventions like fluid resuscitation and blood transfusion being the primary methods. It is imperative to understand the relationship between bleeding and shock to effectively manage them because early management has the potential to decrease the cascading effect of hemodynamic instability (Sarıbaş et al., 2024). In the acute setting, the possible use of predictive factors like the Shock Index (SI) and its variants is helpful for risk stratification in UGIB patients. These scoring systems can be used to quantify the extent of hemodynamic compromise, enabling clinicians to adjust their management plan accordingly. In the research on the effectiveness of these scoring systems, modifications like the AMSI have been shown to have better predictive value for in-hospital mortality rates. These evaluations are particularly important in determining patients at high risk who would require immediate diagnostic or surgical interventions. In general, a focus on the monitoring of hemodynamic parameters in assessing gastrointestinal bleeding adds value to the importance of prompt and accurate management towards improved patient outcomes (Khayyat, 2024; Sarıbaş et al., 2024).

11.5.3. Long-Term Gastrointestinal Issues

Chronic gastrointestinal diseases typically present significant hazards following acute events like gastrointestinal bleeding, which can be induced by diverse etiologies , such as peptic ulcers, diverticulosis, and malignancies. Such bleeding can lead to long-term anemia, iron deficiency, and chronic intestinal inflammation complications and significantly affect patients' quality of life. Chronic blood loss anemia may lead to fatigue, reduced physical function, and mental impairment, which necessitate ongoing management strategies. Additionally, the etiologies of bleeding per se may also contribute to late morbidities; e.g., conditions , such as diverticulitis may recur, leading to recurring treatments and further complications. Thus, accurate control of the acute bleeding episode as well as etiology is necessary to minimize long-term gastrointestinal complications and obtain optimal patient outcomes (Mack et al., 2019). Long-term gastrointestinal complications arising due to previous bleeding episodes also often require comprehensive, multidisciplinary treatment protocols. These may include pharmacologic therapy, dietary adjustments, and continued follow-up in an attempt to prevent recurrence and treat any complications. For instance, proton pump inhibitors can be prescribed to patients to suppress acid production, preventing further bleeding and ulceration. Dietary modification may involve the use of food and supplements rich in iron in an attempt to treat resulting anemia, and follow-up appointments are paramount for surveillance and timely intervention in recurrent gastrointestinal disease. Moreover, those patients who have received surgery as a result of gastrointestinal bleeding also present with impaired bowel habits or with malabsorption syndromes, thus showing the importance of customized healthcare interventions addressing each patient's individual needs (Cosentino et al., 2019). Finally, the psychological aspect of coping with long-standing gastrointestinal disorders due to episodes of bleeding are also secondary but no less important. Many patients are anxious and depressed regarding the threat of recurrence, need for repeated interventions, and lifestyle modifications. These mental burdens further aggravate physical symptoms, and emotional distress leads to deteriorating gastrointestinal health. Therefore, integrating psychological support into the management protocol is highly recommended to ensure a comprehensive approach to care. By addressing the physical and mental health effects of chronic gastrointestinal illness, medical practitioners can better empower patients to heal and improve their overall health. This holistic model of treatment is needed in order to avoid the long-term effects of gastrointestinal bleeding and to promote long-term health (Mack et al., 2019) (Figure 11.17).

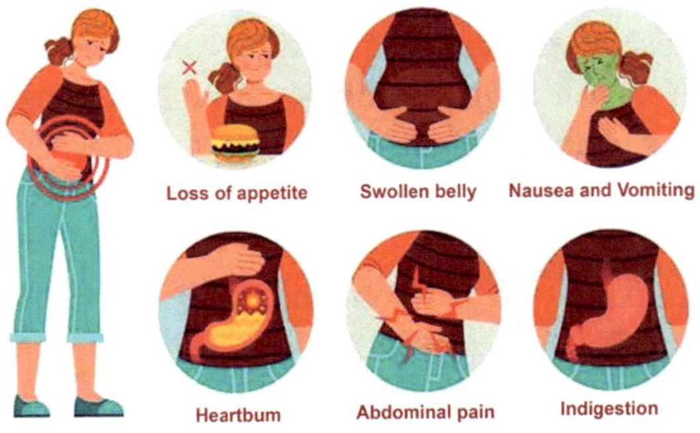

Figure 11.17. Long-term gastrointestinal issues.

Source: https://cdn.medizzy.com/Te2CsBwvuBSdh3CjNUM6URDrecs=/600x400/img/posts/91d4fbd2-3cac-41a7-94fb-d23caca1a789.

11.6. Prevention Strategies

Prevention of the situation of gastrointestinal bleeding (GIB) is important in an attempt to manage risk factors for possible underlying conditions. One common risk factor is the use of non-steroidal anti-inflammatory drugs (NSAIDs), which are commonly used because of their analgesic and anti-inflammatory properties. Although NSAIDs are useful, they also carry the risk of gastrointestinal harm, including dyspepsia and increased bleeding tendency. Research has indicated that while all NSAIDs are dangerous, the occurrence of enteropathy and resultant complications is possible even outside of the duodenum, making prevention strategies also consider the overall impact of such drugs on the gut (Rudichenko & Sokolenko, 2023). Therefore, practitioners must perform thorough patient assessments, encouraging alternative routes of analgesia or protective drugs like PPIs as a precaution when prescribing NSAIDs to avoid GIB risk. An additional preventive measure is modifying anticoagulant therapy in patients with a history of GIB, particularly if they are about to undergo procedures related to left ventricular assist devices (LVAD). The current research on LVAD patients showed that various secondary GIB prophylaxis strategies resulted in comparable recurrence rates, with the implication that optimizing anticoagulation could be a way to increase safety without taking away from patient outcomes. Initiatives like offering personalized INR target ranges or employing hemostatic agents like danazol may provide insight into the limitations of reducing GIB events (Gerrald et al., 2022). The findings emphasize the need to continuously monitor those patients who are under increased risk of bleeding and thus complement preventive interventions with patient-specific factors in consideration and individualized therapeutic strategies.

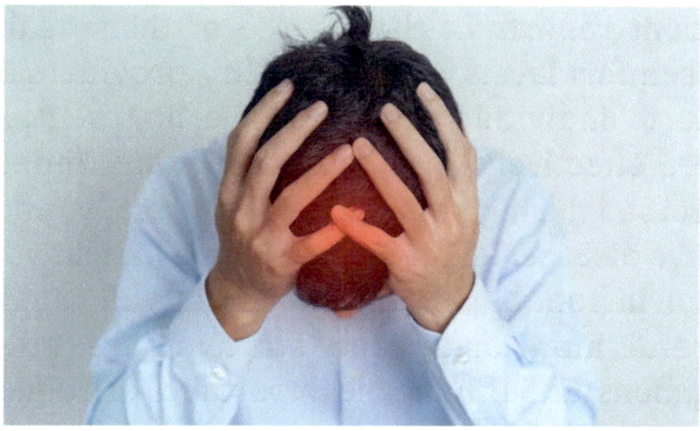

Figure 11.18. Prevention strategies.

Source: https://images.moneycontrol.com/static-mcnews/2024/06/20240618061847_Brain-stroke.jpg?impolicy=website&width=770&height=431.

Education also forms a primary part of the prevention programs against GIB, directed to healthcare providers as well as patients. By heightened awareness of GIB symptoms and signs, clinicians are able to ensure early diagnosis and intervention, eventually reducing the severity of hemorrhage episodes. Patient education programs are required to emphasize adherence to medication regimens, awareness of dietary effects, and frequent follow-up visits. Moreover, the integration of supportive resources , such as nutritional counseling to complement gastrointestinal care, enables patients to make the best lifestyle choices that minimize risk factors for GIB. These integrative approaches that integrate education, drug management, and patient activation are integral components within the comprehensive plan to efficiently prevent gastrointestinal bleeding (Figure 11.18).

11.6.1. Lifestyle Modifications

Lifestyle changes are important both in preventing and managing gastrointestinal bleeding. Among the most powerful tools is dietary change to support digestive health. The addition of fiber to one's diet is key since fiber ensures that bowel movements are regular and prevents constipation, one of the factors that causes straining and, possibly, bleeding. Secondly, a diet consisting of whole grains, vegetables, and fruits not only aids in digestion but also provides essential nutrients that add to the overall gastrointestinal well-being. Lifestyle changes must extend beyond basic dietary patterns; more hydration must be included, since adequate water intake makes the stool softer and more easy to pass, reducing the risk of damage to the lining of the intestine, which has been linked with most gastrointestinal disorders (Gupta et al., 2025). Physical exercise is another valuable lifestyle alteration that can go a long way in ensuring gastrointestinal health and reducing bleeding risk. Daily exercise has been shown to improve metabolic function and the ability of the body to manage stress, factors known directly to influence digestive health. Sedentary living has been associated with all sorts of gastrointestinal syndromes, from constipation to reduced circulation within the digestive tract. Including regular physical activity, such as walking, swimming, or yoga, not only trains muscular control of the abdomen but also promotes proper digestion and gut motility. Moreover, exercise will also aid in weight management, reducing the risk of gastrointestinal disorders of obesity, which are said to exacerbate bleeding symptoms (Shen et al., 2025). Through intense engagement in physical activity, a person can create a more consistent internal setting conducive to the prevention of gastrointestinal complications. In addition to exercise and food changes, avoidance of some toxic chemicals is also essential for gastrointestinal health maintenance and the prevention of bleeding. Lifestyle changes should initially aim at the prevention or reduction of tobacco consumption and alcohol use, both of which have been implicated in the exacerbation of gastrointestinal disease. Smoking has also been identified as a causative factor in the development of such diseases as gastroesophageal reflux disease (GERD), which can result in inflammation and bleeding in the esophagus. Similarly, binge drinking will cause inflammation of the gastrointestinal tract lining and the formation of ulcers. By implementing these lifestyle changes, individuals can effectively lower their risks of serious complications of gastrointestinal bleeding, ensuring a healthier digestive system. In the long term, a balanced lifestyle change enhances not only the quality of life but also long-term gastrointestinal health (Gupta et al., 2025; Shen et al., 2025).

11.6.2. Regular Screenings and Check-Ups

Regular screenings and check-ups are of the utmost significance for the early detection and management of gastrointestinal bleeding, a very often overlooked but lethal illness. This should be treated in the early stages because early detection renders successful intervention for causative agents , such as peptic ulcers, hemorrhoids, or malignancies. For individuals over a certain age or those with risk factors , such as a history of gastrointestinal disease in their family, regular check-ups with medical professionals are especially vital. Routine checks typically involve a combination of examination of the patient's history, physical examination, and diagnostic tests , such as endoscopies, which can visualize and diagnose the gastrointestinal tract, enhancing the accuracy of diagnoses. As a preventive health practice, routine screening not only promotes consciousness of gastrointestinal health but also allows patients to alert their providers to symptoms and risk factors. Beyond individual consciousness, periodic check-ups are important because they allow systematic management of gastrointestinal bleeding and illnesses associated with it. During these tests, clinicians need to assess clinical symptoms , such as abdominal pain, change of bowel habits, or signs of anemia, which can be suggestive of underlying gastrointestinal pathology. Moreover, patient-reported outcomes, or the self-perceived experience of symptoms spontaneously reported by patients, are becoming more commonly employed as part of these evaluations. By adding patient reports of their sense of their health, discomfort levels, and life quality, providers are able to individualize preventive interventions more effectively. Also, remember that findings observed during a visit do not necessarily reflect active disease. Instead, they will be indicative of prior infections or conditions that will require careful monitoring and strategic treatment regimens, underlining the importance of frequent check-ups in maintaining gastrointestinal health under control (Salvi et al., 2023). Adding to the importance of screenings, public health also underlines the importance of wide-based education in relation to gastrointestinal health and the value of periodic monitoring. Many patients are not even cognizant of the possible warning signs that can develop into more serious complications , such as gastrointestinal bleeding or cancer. Educational programs, especially among target populations, can permit earlier treatment and diagnosis, thereby reducing mortality and morbidity from such diseases. Greater knowledge regarding gastrointestinal health can empower patients to become responsible for incorporating routine check-ups in their lives. In addition, the healthcare systems should prioritize accessibility to preventive services such that these screenings become an integral part of extensive care. By adopting a preventive culture of health management, we can aim to minimize the potential impacts of gastrointestinal bleeding and enhance the overall quality of life for those involved (Chakraborty et al., 2021) (Figure 11.19).

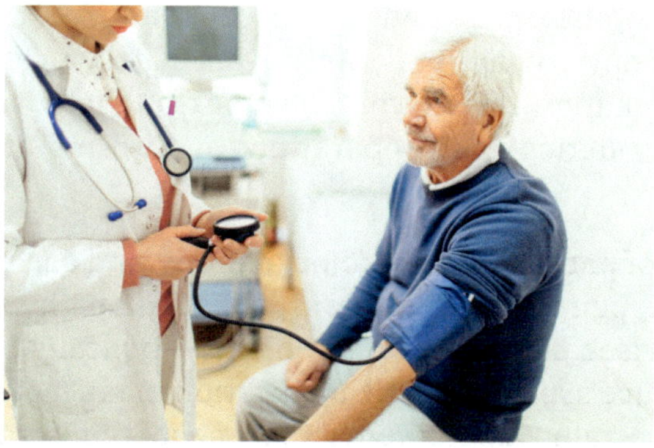

Figure 11.19. Regular screenings and check-ups.

Source: https://www.nurseregistry.com/wp-content/uploads/2017/01/iStock-500457696-1024x683@2x.jpg.

11.6.3. Management of Underlying Conditions

Effective control of the underlying disease is essential in the control of gastrointestinal bleeding, as these diseases will generally serve as contributing factors. Processes , such as chronic liver disease, inflammatory bowel disease, and malignancy can significantly increase the risk of bleeding events. Identification and treatment of these underlying pathologies through the delivery of healthcare can not only mitigate the acute risks of gastrointestinal hemorrhage but also enhance overall health outcomes in patients. For instance, pharmacologic control of portal hypertension in cirrhotic patients can reduce the risk of variceal bleeding, an common complication. Similarly, adjustable therapy of inflammatory bowel diseases can have the ability to reduce mucosal inflammation, eventually minimizing the risk of bleeding. These interventions demonstrate that integrated treatment of affiliated diseases plays a pivotal role in preventing cases of gastrointestinal bleeding. Moreover, medical communities' standards underscore the need to integrate best practice recommendations within the management of underlying conditions. Health professionals must handle complex clinical cases, balancing evidence-based therapy with the distinct needs of the patient. For this reason, the ESC Guidelines prioritize individualized care, advising clinicians to use these guidelines while adjusting them according to the patient's individualized health context. This tailored approach ensures that practices utilized to manage bleeding underlying conditions are aligned with current scientific evidence and public health recommendations, particularly when considering the disparities in causes of bleeding within the gastrointestinal tract. Through a systematic process, clinicians are able to analyze and prioritize interventions for both bleeding and the underlying causes of the bleeding, thereby advancing better therapeutic results. The fusion of clinical acumen with adherence to formal protocols is equally important in forging successful treatment regimens. Ultimately, ongoing monitoring and education of the patient are fundamental components of the management of comorbidities related to gastrointestinal bleeding. Follow-up appointments allow clinicians to gauge the success of treatment and make the required adjustments in order to ensure that any complications arising are addressed promptly. Furthermore, patient education on their disease and the importance of treatment regimen compliance plays a central role. Patient information is essential to better engage patients in the tracking of their disease, and they will recognize early warning signals for likely bleeding to enable early action by the healthcare team. In addition, enhancing an open communication channel between patients and healthcare teams may enhance treatment compliance and, hence, management of chronic disease.

CLOSER LOOK

PERI-ENDOSCOPY CARE:

Peri-endoscopy care encompasses the comprehensive management of patients before, during, and after endoscopic procedures to ensure safety, optimize outcomes, and enhance patient comfort. Endoscopy, including upper gastrointestinal (GI) endoscopy, colonoscopy, and advanced therapeutic procedures, carries risks such as bleeding, perforation, sedation-related complications, and infection. A closer look at peri-endoscopy care highlights how meticulous preparation, monitoring, and follow-up are critical components of quality care.

Pre-procedure care begins with a thorough assessment of patient history, comorbidities, and current medications. Risk factors such as cardiovascular disease, pulmonary conditions, or coagulopathy are identified to guide procedural planning. Patients are advised on fasting requirements—typically 6–8 hours for solids and 2–4 hours for clear liquids—to reduce aspiration risk. Medication management is crucial; anticoagulants, antiplatelet agents, and certain supplements may need temporary adjustment, while chronic medications such as antihypertensives are generally continued. Patient education forms a cornerstone of pre-procedure care, ensuring informed consent and addressing anxieties about sedation, procedural sensations, and potential complications.

Intra-procedure care focuses on continuous monitoring and support. Vital signs, oxygen saturation, and level of consciousness are observed throughout the procedure, particularly if sedation or anesthesia is administered. Proper positioning and equipment setup reduce injury risk, while trained personnel remain ready to respond to adverse events. Infection control practices—including hand hygiene, sterilization of endoscopes, and use of personal protective equipment—minimize cross-contamination and protect both patients and staff. Communication between the endoscopist, nurses, and anesthetists ensures smooth coordination and rapid intervention if needed.

Post-procedure care emphasizes recovery, complication surveillance, and patient education. Patients are monitored until sedation effects diminish, with attention to airway safety, hemodynamic stability, and pain control. Potential complications, such as bleeding, perforation, or post-polypectomy syndrome, are recognized early through observation and appropriate laboratory or imaging tests if indicated. Discharge instructions include activity restrictions, diet progression, signs of complications, and follow-up plans. Clear communication improves adherence and reduces preventable readmissions.

In addition to patient-centered care, peri-endoscopy practices support quality outcomes through standardized protocols, checklists, and documentation. This structured approach minimizes variability, enhances safety, and ensures regulatory compliance.

Peri- endoscopy care underscores that successful endoscopic procedures extend beyond technical skill. Comprehensive pre-, intra-, and post-procedure management is essential for minimizing risks, optimizing patient experiences, and improving overall clinical outcomes.

SUMMARY

In summary of this essay on gastrointestinal bleeding, there is a fine balance to be noted between the benefits and risks of treatments aimed at lessening bleeding episodes in vulnerable populations. The increased prevalence of gastrointestinal bleeding with chronic use of aspirin is a major clinical concern. Even though prophylactic aspirin therapy is universally known for its cardiovascular protective effects, particularly in secondary prevention, up-to-date evidence indicates that the complications of such usage, such as gastrointestinal hemorrhage, necessitate a cautious evaluation of patient profiles. The question of whether the potential benefit, like reduced mortality from cardiovascular disease and certain cancers, justifies the risk of increased gastrointestinal bleeding remains central to clinical practice and patient safety (Battistoni et al., 2017). In acknowledging that the effects of aspirin therapy can profoundly impact quality of life, health care providers must be careful in determining whether or not to prescribe aspirin for primary prevention. Recent studies have reported impressive increases in the relative risks of severe bleeding and gastrointestinal adverse effects, ranging from 37% to more than 60%, depending on bleeding severity (Clarke et al., 2013). In consideration of such evidence, the practitioner is spurred to critically evaluate the patient's individual risk factors, including age, active comorbid illnesses, and other medications, before undertaking aspirin therapy. An informed approach not only enhances patient outcomes but also fosters a collaborative process of decision-making, thereby allowing healthcare professionals and patients to weigh the potential risks against the potential therapeutic benefits maximally. Finally, aspirin remains a cornerstone of cardiovascular disease prevention on the first level and offers potential anti-cancer benefits, but at the expense of which the consequences of gastrointestinal bleeding cannot be overlooked. With the new evidence that is emerging, particularly ongoing clinical trials examining the efficacy of aspirin in cancer prevention, future suggestions for its use should still be based on an overall risk assessment of the harms involved (Battistoni et al., 2017). The weighing of benefits versus harms highlights the importance of individualized treatment protocols so that clinical practice is rooted in evidence-based practice. Lastly, focus on patient safety, informed consent, and ongoing research will be essential to maximizing outcomes in high-risk patients for gastrointestinal bleeding.

Gastrointestinal bleeding (GI bleeding) is a severe medical illness that has a wide differential diagnosis of causes, from potentially life-threatening illness to benign disease. The investigation for GI bleeding is usually begun with a complete clinical assessment, such as history, physical examination, and targeted diagnostic studies like endoscopy or imaging. Key presentations of GI hemorrhage may be divided into upper or lower, with symptomatology being different based on the location and severity of bleeding. Hematemesis or melena might present with upper GI hemorrhage, while lower GI hemorrhage is typically associated with hematochezia. Recognition of these clinical presentations should be achieved to ensure timely diagnosis and treatment with increased patient recovery. Moreover, prompt recognition of the severity of bleeding, along with associated risk factors like hemodynamic instability and coagulopathy, is crucial to effective management and treatment planning, pointing towards the need for an individualized treatment strategy for every patient. The cause of gastrointestinal bleeding is multifactorial and includes a variety of conditions like malignancy, diverticular disease, and peptic ulcers, necessitating an extensive workup to identify the individual etiology. Peptic ulcer disease remains one of the most common causes for upper GI bleeding, often complicated by the chronic use of non-steroidal anti-inflammatory drugs (NSAIDs) and alcohol abuse. Diverticulosis is also a common cause of significant lower GI bleeding, particularly in older adults. More complex disease processes, such as colorectal cancer, must also be considered, particularly in the patient with chronic, occult gastrointestinal bleeding. Surveillance of these conditions is critical, especially in risk groups, and recommendations favor the implementation of screening programs. Effective control of the underlying conditions may prevent recurrent bleeding and thus enhance the quality of life of the individuals involved. Management of gastrointestinal bleeding varies with the severity of the event and the etiology. Early stabilization involves the stabilization of hemodynamic instability with fluid resuscitation and blood transfusion when needed. Endoscopic management often plays a central role in the treatment of upper GI and lower GI hemorrhages and allows for direct manipulation of the site of bleeding. Pharmacotherapy can also be applied, particularly for conditions like peptic ulcer disease, where proton pump inhibitors are widely utilized. Apart from this, multidisciplinary team collaboration among healthcare professionals is also required to optimize the treatment outcome and address potential complications like the risk of re-bleeding. With growing knowledge of gastrointestinal bleeding, novel treatments and technologies are emerging, highlighting ongoing research and education within this vital area of health care (Crabb et al., 2019; Rychik et al., 2019).

References

1. Al-Samkari, H., Kasthuri, R. S., Parambil, J. G., Albitar, H. A. H., Almodallal, Y., Vázquez, C., Serra, M., et al. (2020). An international, multicenter study of intravenous bevacizumab for bleeding in hereditary hemorrhagic telangiectasia: The InHIBIT-Bleed study. *Hematologica, 106*, 2161–2169. https://doi.org/10.3324/haematol.2020.261859 (accessed on 16th July 2025).
2. Badaró, P. F. M., Machado, C. A. C., de Freitas, L. A. R., Branco, R. D. A., & da Silva, B. C. (2024). Gastrointestinal bleeding as a clinical manifestation of *Strongyloides stercoralis* hyperinfection in a patient with HIV: A case report. *Journal of Gastrointestinal Infections.* https://www.semanticscholar.org/paper/2f7129913e6dbfc0d81c737e54834297ae15df69 (accessed on 16th July 2025).
3. Ballester-Clau, R., Cucala-Ramos, M., López-Barroso, L., Planella de Rubinat, et al. (2019). *Clinical experience with ferric carboxymaltose in the management of anemia in acute gastrointestinal bleeding.* https://core.ac.uk/download/187430167.pdf (accessed on 16th July 2025).
4. Battistoni, A., Coluccia, R., De Caterina, R., Gallo, et al. (2017). *Aspirin and the primary prevention of cardiovascular diseases: An approach based on individualized, integrated estimation of risk.* https://core.ac.uk/download/127586997.pdf (accessed on 16th July 2025).
5. Bhangu, A., Chapman, S. J., Fitzgerald, J. E., Glasbey, et al. (2014). *Multicenter observational cohort study of NSAIDs as risk factors for postoperative adverse events in gastrointestinal surgery.* https://core.ac.uk/download/29411424.pdf (accessed on 16th July 2025).
6. Bhatt, D. L., Steg, P. G., Miller, M., Brinton, E. A., Jacobson, T. A., Ketchum, S., Doyle, R. T., et al. (2018). Cardiovascular risk reduction with icosapent ethyl for hypertriglyceridemia. *New England Journal of Medicine, 380*, 11–22. https://doi.org/10.1056/nejmoa1812792 (accessed on 16th July 2025).
7. Bhattacharya, S., Pal, G., Manoharan, R., Mondal, M., Sahoo, S., Srivastava, T., Mondal, B. K., et al. (2022). Homoeopathic management of duodenal ulcer: A case report. *International Journal of Homoeopathic Sciences.* https://www.semanticscholar.org/paper/5a9c4c23f75119b7440302eb8cdb7ecbfbf07bf0 (accessed on 16th July 2025).
8. Buchan, I., de Belder, M. A., Khan, M. A., Kinnaird, et al. (2015). *Access and non–access site bleeding after percutaneous coronary intervention and risk of subsequent mortality and major adverse cardiovascular events: Systematic review and meta-analysis.* https://core.ac.uk/download/41991341.pdf (accessed on 16th July 2025).
9. Carmona, T. C., Hooper, C. T., Abbagoni, V., Al Shakkakee, H., Devani, A., Illan, J. D. M., Valencia, M., et al. (2024). Hemobilia: A narrative review of current diagnostic techniques and emerging management strategies. *Cureus, 16.* https://www.semanticscholar.org/paper/5143a41381c497946a8363c57b4763c4766211ef (accessed on 16th July 2025).
10. Chakraborty, T., Jamal, R. F., Battineni, G., Teja, K. V., Marto, C. M., & Spagnuolo, G. (2021). A review of prolonged post-COVID-19 symptoms and their implications on dental management. *International Journal of Environmental Research and Public Health, 18*, 5131–5131. https://doi.org/10.3390/ijerph18105131 (accessed on 16th July 2025).
11. Obleaga CV, Vere CC, Valcea ID, Ciorbagiu MC, Moraru E, Mirea CS. Helicobacter pylori: Types of Diseases, Diagnosis, Treatment and Causes of Therapeutic Failure. *Journal of Mind and Medical Sciences.* 2016; 3(2):150-161. https://doi.org/10.22543/2392-7674.1048(accessed on 16th July 2025).

12. Clarke, A., Connock, M., Freeman, K., Grove, et al. (2013). *Aspirin for prophylactic use in the primary prevention of cardiovascular disease and cancer: A systematic review and overview of reviews.* https://core.ac.uk/download/17180813.pdf (accessed on 16th July 2025).

13. Cosentino, F., Grant, P. J., Aboyans, V., Bailey, C. J., Ceriello, A., Delgado, V., Federici, M., et al. (2019). 2019 ESC Guidelines on diabetes, pre-diabetes, and cardiovascular diseases developed in collaboration with the EASD. *European Heart Journal, 41*, 255–323. https://doi.org/10.1093/eurheartj/ehz486 (accessed on 16th July 2025).

14. Crabb, D. W., Im, G. Y., Szabó, G., Mellinger, J. L., & Lucey, M. R. (2019). Diagnosis and treatment of alcohol-associated liver diseases: 2019 practice guidance from the American Association for the Study of Liver Diseases. *Hepatology, 71*, 306–333. https://doi.org/10.1002/hep.30866 (accessed on 16th July 2025).

15. Duman, Z., Bayram, M., Timur, B., Kaplan, M. C., & Aksu, T. (2023). Predictors and outcomes of gastrointestinal complications after cardiac surgery: A systematic review and meta-analysis. *Turkish Journal of Thoracic and Cardiovascular Surgery, 31*, 45–55. https://www.semanticscholar.org/paper/e674ca5fe8998787bd990bbf3623e8594cda28e4 (accessed on 16th July 2025).

16. Farag, M., Diaz, Y., & Patel, H. (2025). Colonic Dieulafoy lesion as a rare cause of lower gastrointestinal bleeding. *Case Reports in Gastroenterology, 19*, 52–56. https://www.semanticscholar.org/paper/c0b2ecca554de4d8c8768d44b395f2db0a5ab9f4 (accessed on 16th July 2025).

17. MARIAM M. MIRAMBO,1 HUMPHREY D. MAZIGO,2 HYASINTA M. JAKA,3 RODRICK KABANGILA,3 HAMIS KOMBO,4 STEPHEN E. MSHANA,1 LUCAS FAUSTINE,5 JEREMIAH SENI,1 and MARIA M. ZINGA (2010). *Case report: Unsuspected uterine choriocarcinoma with lung metastasis.* JRuralTropPublicHealth 2010, VOL 9, p. 121 - 123 https://core.ac.uk/download/pdf/18410769.pdf (accessed on 16th July 2025).

18. Finn, R. S., Qin, S., Ikeda, M., Galle, P. R., Ducreux, M., Kim, T.-Y., Kudo, M., et al. (2020). Atezolizumab plus bevacizumab in unresectable hepatocellular carcinoma. *New England Journal of Medicine, 382*, 1894–1905. https://doi.org/10.1056/nejmoa1915745 (accessed on 16th July 2025).

19. Gerrald, J. E., Ather, A., Schadler, A. D., Birks, E., Kolodziej, A., & Kuan, W. (2022). Retrospective review of secondary prevention strategies for gastrointestinal bleeding and associated clinical outcomes in left ventricular assist device patients. *Artificial Organs.* https://www.semanticscholar.org/paper/ccf6d25b75ca4a010cd77630d1c8ca1349ec3f31 (accessed on 16th July 2025).

20. Gonçalves, J., Rosa, B., & Cotter, J. (2025). Small bowel vasculitis? What a gastroenterologist should know—From diagnosis to management. *Current Opinion in Gastroenterology, 41*, 132–138. https://www.semanticscholar.org/paper/96ebf12137f83122eeee72fdaaca06125af360a0 (accessed on 16th July 2025).

21. Gupta, T., Gupta, R., Mishra, S., & Garg, S. (2025). Exploration of herbs to overcome the constipation. *African Journal of Biomedical Research.* https://www.semanticscholar.org/paper/ce5f1753d81817c4754caec749ea3ff02ee0b8ef (accessed on 16th July 2025).

22. Hibi, T., Hirata, I., Hokari, R., Kaunitz, et al. (2016). *Endoscopic and clinical evaluation of treatment and prognosis of Cronkhite-Canada syndrome: A Japanese nationwide survey.* https://core.ac.uk/download/323078062.pdf (accessed on 16th July 2025).

23. Jung, Y., Kim, J. W., Im, J., Cho, Y., Lee, T., & Jang, J. (2022). Safety of gastrointestinal endoscopy in Korea: A nationwide survey and population-based study. *Journal of Korean Medical Science, 37.* https://www.semanticscholar.org/paper/17a54e9663cce33f6fb01513dbe85b0536ee0185 (accessed on 16th July 2025).

24. Khayyat, Y. (2024). Trends in upper gastrointestinal bleeding management. *World Journal of Clinical Cases, 12*, 6007–6010. https://www.semanticscholar.org/paper/7c77fa9c553445fbd9d2d2f7962452467af4ba15 (accessed on 16th July 2025).

25. Kirchhof, P., Benussi, S., Kotecha, D., Ahlsson, A., Atar, D., Casadei, B., Castellá, M., et al. (2016). 2016 ESC Guidelines for the management of atrial fibrillation developed in collaboration with EACTS. *European Heart Journal, 37*, 2893–2962. https://doi.org/10.1093/eurheartj/ehw210 (accessed on 16th July 2025).

26. Lai, K. C., & Lam, S. K. (1999). The need for *Helicobacter pylori* eradication therapy in patients with peptic ulcer bleeding. https://core.ac.uk/download/37883930.pdf (accessed on 16th July 2025).

27. Leafloor, C., Perry, J., Ramaekers, R., Thiruganasambandamoorthy, et al. (2020). *Prediction model for 30-day outcomes among emergency department patients with lower gastrointestinal bleeding.* https://core.ac.uk/download/287622003.pdf (accessed on 16th July 2025).

28. Lee, E. W., Wilson, M. W., & Yang, L. (2007). *Hemosuccus Pancreaticus as a Rare Complication of Bariatric Surgery.* https://core.ac.uk/download/323078002.pdf (accessed on 16th July 2025).

29. Lee, H. S., & Lee, D. K. (2025). Emerging diagnostic techniques and therapies for upper gastrointestinal bleeding. *The Korean Journal of Gastroenterology = Taehan Sohwagi Hakhoe Chi, 85*(2), 153–159. https://www.semanticscholar.org/paper/3df91bd7f2a88ef6b6dcc70f386845f7ef4bd6ea (accessed on 16th July 2025).

30. Liu, Z.-J., Hong, J.-Y., Zhang, C., She, J., & Zhai, H.-H. (2025). Gastrointestinal bleeding after pancreatoduodenectomy: Report of four cases. *World Journal of Gastrointestinal Surgery, 17.* https://www.semanticscholar.org/paper/ff8cce7b3ca2f1bf33e2231a6e9cd3c426f20ed2 (accessed on 16th July 2025).

31. Mack, C. L., Adams, D. H., Assis, D. N., Kerkar, N., Manns, M. P., Mayo, M. J., Ling, S. C., et al. (2019). Diagnosis and management of autoimmune hepatitis in adults and children: 2019 practice guidance and guidelines from the American Association for the Study of Liver Diseases. *Hepatology, 72*, 671–722. https://doi.org/10.1002/hep.31065 (accessed on 16th July 2025).

32. Maity, R., Dhali, A., & Biswas, J. (2024). Importance of risk assessment, endoscopic hemostasis, and recent advancements in the management of acute non-variceal upper gastrointestinal bleeding. *World Journal of Clinical Cases, 12*, 5462–5467. https://www.semanticscholar.org/paper/a927937266c5364c274f8fa007032afea47a71c3 (accessed on 16th July 2025).

33. Marri, U., Singh, J. R., Pal, P., & Modak, S. (2024). Lower gastrointestinal bleeding (nonvariceal): Concepts and technique. *Digestive Disease Interventions.* https://www.semanticscholar.org/paper/d55a42f32a3eb18ae8b012e87d992c9fd71f1961 (accessed on 16th July 2025).

34. Menichelli, D., Gazzaniga, G., Del Sole, F., Pani, A., Pignatelli, P., & Pastori, D. (2024). Acute upper and lower gastrointestinal bleeding management in older people taking or not taking anticoagulants: A literature review. *Frontiers in Medicine, 11.* https://www.semanticscholar.org/paper/20cd04b04542dce644e8fa85c7a71d35f792924b (accessed on 16th July 2025).

35. Moledina, S. M., & Komba, E. (2017). Risk factors for mortality among patients admitted with upper gastrointestinal bleeding at a tertiary hospital: A prospective cohort study. *BMC Gastroenterology, 17.* https://doi.org/10.1186/s12876-017-0712-8 (accessed on 16th July 2025).

36. Nantes, A. G., Abreu, G. M., Borges, G. H. P. de Á., Momm, I. C., Mazzini, K. de A., Lani, L. G., de Araujo, R. L., et al. (2024). Main characteristics of lower gastrointestinal bleeding in patients treated at a reference hospital. *Journal of Coloproctology, 45*, e1–e7. https://www.semanticscholar.org/paper/18a3a69f509d35af8b37b2669a26bc2cf5dae8e8 (accessed on 16th July 2025).

37. Northup, P. G., García-Pagán, J. C., García–Tsao, G., Intagliata, N. M., Superina, R., Roberts, L. N., Lisman, T., et al. (2020). Vascular liver disorders, portal vein thrombosis, and procedural bleeding in patients with liver disease: 2020 practice guidance by the American Association for the Study of Liver Diseases. *Hepatology, 73*, 366–413. https://doi.org/10.1002/hep.31646 (accessed on 16th July 2025).

38. Racharla, L., Sidhu, K., & Vidula, H. (2024). New advances in medical management of left ventricular assist devices recipients. *Current Treatment Options in Cardiovascular Medicine.* https://www.semanticscholar.org/paper/09ba94a013cb17a3e48fcf10774be160fe71bf22 (accessed on 16th July 2025).

39. Rawla, P., Sunkara, T., & Barsouk, A. (2019). Epidemiology of colorectal cancer: Incidence, mortality, survival, and risk factors. *Gastroenterology Review, 14*, 89–103. https://doi.org/10.5114/pg.2018.81072 (accessed on 16th July 2025).

40. Rudichenko, V., & Sokolenko, A. (2023). Importance of prophylactic strategies in prevention of gastrointestinal injuries by nonsteroidal anti-inflammatory drugs (clinical case). *Family Medicine. European Practices.* https://www.semanticscholar.org/paper/5ac26b9fc88a81bde559137cd31480fafa66f176 (accessed on 16th July 2025).

41. Rychik, J., Atz, A. M., Celermajer, D. S., Deal, B. J., Gatzoulis, M. A., Gewillig, M., Hsia, T.-Y., et al. (2019). Evaluation and management of the child and adult with Fontan circulation: A scientific statement from the American Heart Association. *Circulation, 140.* https://doi.org/10.1161/cir.0000000000000696 (accessed on 16th July 2025).

42. Salvi, G. E., Roccuzzo, A., Imber, J.-C., Stähli, A., Klinge, B., & Lang, N. P. (2023). Clinical periodontal diagnosis. *Periodontology 2000.* https://doi.org/10.1111/prd.12487 (accessed on 16th July 2025).

43. Sanzone, E., Gheysens, K., Hunter, K., Chaaya, A., & Phadtare, S. (2025). Incidence and outcomes of upper GI bleeding in hospitalized SARS-CoV-2 patients. *Gastroenterology Research and Practice, 2025.* https://www.semanticscholar.org/paper/df4125076b3f3b574a5f220d3f6ba659b2eaae3c (accessed on 16th July 2025).

44. Sarıbaş, M., Aygun, A., Kara, F., Koksal, A., & Çaltekin, İ. (2024). The role of shock index and its derivatives in predicting mortality in patients with upper gastrointestinal bleeding. *Medicine Science | International Medical Journal.* https://www.semanticscholar.org/paper/06f192cc8ecb5ff2b7fa40294cba1dc724cd3ae4 (accessed on 16th July 2025).

45. Shaw, B. W., Starzl, T. E., & Wood, R. P. (1985). *Extrahepatic Complications of Liver Transplantation.* https://core.ac.uk/download/12204047.pdf (accessed on 16th July 2025).

46. Shen, J., Guo, Y., & Cao, R. (2025). The relationship between amino acids and gastroesophageal reflux disease: Evidence from a Mendelian randomization analysis combined with a

meta-analysis. *Frontiers in Immunology, 16.* https://www.semanticscholar.org/paper/bd84ad722facce704b48c735d4bca47ef9927541 (accessed on 16th July 2025).

47. Siddiqui, A., Zafar, N., Hakiminezhad, M., Jamal, Z., Alam, I., & Khawaja, Z. (2024). Beyond the usual suspects: Appendiceal bleeding as the surprising cause of lower gastrointestinal (GI) bleeding. *Cureus, 16.* https://www.semanticscholar.org/paper/3d789a2f83c4c8ea20df677cdb3b597ab8df158c (accessed on 16th July 2025).

48. Sigrist, R., Liau, J., El Kaffas, A., Chammas, M. C., & Willmann, J. K. (2017). Ultrasound elastography: Review of techniques and clinical applications. *Theranostics, 7,* 1303–1329. https://doi.org/10.7150/thno.18650 (accessed on 16th July 2025).

49. Soni, A., Yekula, A., Singh, Y., Sood, N., Dahiya, D., Bansal, K., & Abraham, G. M. (2023). Influence of non-alcoholic fatty liver disease on non-variceal upper gastrointestinal bleeding: A nationwide analysis. *World Journal of Hepatology, 15,* 79–88. https://www.semanticscholar.org/paper/8bc86c95fd721fe5529c3b2594f405bd14fe0653 (accessed on 16th July 2025).

50. Visseren, F. L. J., Mach, F., Smulders, Y. M., Carballo, D., Koskinas, K. C., Bäck, M., Bénétos, A., et al. (2021). 2021 ESC Guidelines on cardiovascular disease prevention in clinical practice. *European Heart Journal, 42,* 3227–3337. https://doi.org/10.1093/eurheartj/ehab484 (accessed on 16th July 2025).

51. Yılmaz Çakmak, N., Ata, N., Güven, S., Gemcioğlu, E., Çağlayan, M., Ülgü, M., & Birinci, Ş. (2024). Gastrointestinal bleeding among oral anticoagulant users: A comprehensive 7-year retrospective review using Türkiye's national health data system. *Turkish Journal of Medical Sciences, 54,* 1005–1012. https://www.semanticscholar.org/paper/f85f1c8360673bf2e7eba455c670fb617d6708ab (accessed on 16th July 2025).

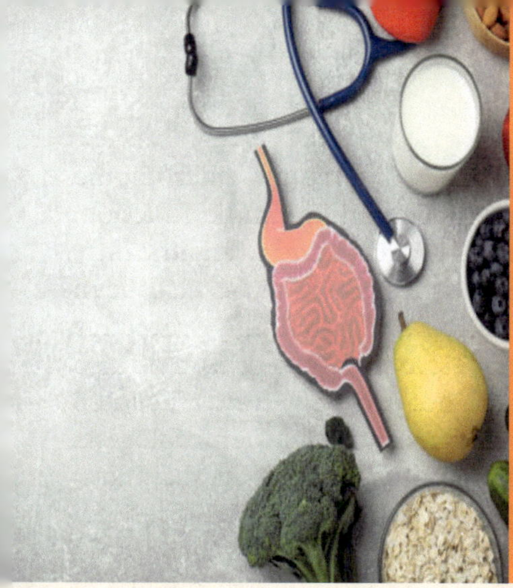

Chapter 12

NUTRITIONAL ASPECTS IN GASTROENTEROLOGY

Contents

Introduction

Gastroenterology is a critical branch of medicine that is concerned with the research and management of the gut and its ailments. It is the intensive study of various anatomical organs like the esophagus, stomach, intestines, liver, pancreas, and gallbladder. Knowing the functioning of the GI tract is crucial as it is responsible for nutrient absorption and waste excretion. The interactive dynamics between food intake and GI health are what highlight the necessity for attentive dieting within gastroenterology. Nutrition not only plays a role in initiating and progressing gastrointestinal disease but is also absolutely necessary for controlling it. Thus, physicians must gain a grasp of how nutrients impact the health of the entire gut and, thus, the health of the patient. By treating nutritional constituents, gastroenterologists can enhance the outcomes of treatment and enable higher levels of well-being among patients with digestive ailments. The gut microbiota-gastrointestinal health connection has been an extremely emphasized area of study in recent decades, leading to greater investigation of the role on the microbiome composition. Evidence indicates that a healthy, diverse gut microbiome is required to ensure gastrointestinal health and influence both metabolic and immune function. Antibiotic usage, the method of delivery during birth, infection, and even diet can tend to significantly affect people's microbiota. Specific nutrients, including prebiotics and probiotics, have also been discovered to increase beneficial flora in the gut, thus aiding digestion and providing protective barriers against infection and disease. The progressive science in the microbiota-gut-brain axis also highlights the mechanisms by which diet and nutrition could influence not just body health but also mental well-being. These factors are central to advancing the continuing need for gastroenterologists to include dietary recommendations in their practice, hence optimal patient management plans. Nutrition becomes central in prevention and therapy interventions in the situation of gastrointestinal disease. For patients who have diseases like inflammatory bowel disease (IBD), celiac disease, or even liver disease, certain dietary modifications can prevent symptoms and enhance quality of life. Dietary recommendations in these disorders are generally focused on individualized dietary modification that serves to reduce inflammation, restore gut flora, and decrease the symptoms of malabsorption. The AASLD/EASL Practice Guideline Subcommittee points out the importance of evidence-based treatment of liver complications, underlining the contribution of nutrition to effective care plans. As gastroenterologists continue to respond to evolving research and clinical data, the incorporation of nutritional factors into care plans will be included. Lastly, an interdisciplinary treatment protocol that entails gastroenterological and nutrition protocols can significantly improve patient outcomes in terms of controlling difficult digestive diseases (Vilstrup et al., 2014; Cryan et al., 2019) (Figure 12.1).

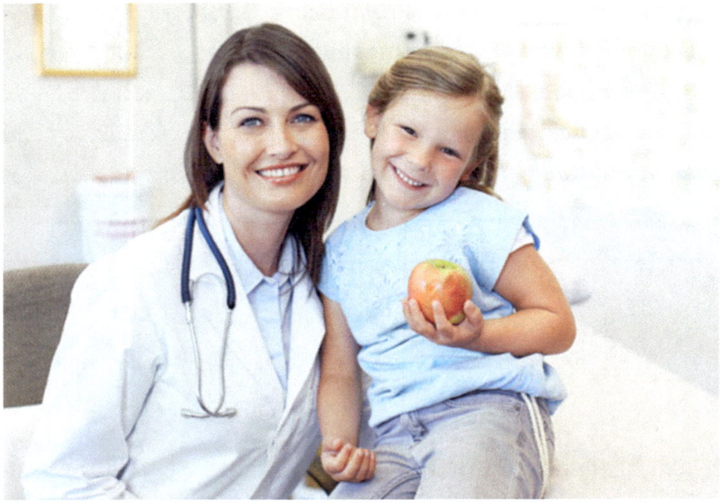

Figure 12.1. Nutritional aspects in gastroenterology.

Source: https://my.clevelandclinic.org/-/scassets/images/org/pediatrics/departments/gastroenterology.jpg.

Definition and Scope of Gastroenterology

Gastroenterology is the medical science that is responsible for the study, diagnosis, and treatment of the gastrointestinal (GI) diseases, which run from the esophagus to the rectum. Gastroenterology involves clinical practice and research to understand various disorders of digestion, including inflammatory bowel disease (IBD), gastrointestinal cancers, gastrointestinal bleeding, and functional gastrointestinal disorders like irritable bowel syndrome (IBS). The specialty of gastroenterology is wide, and its application necessitates integration from several specializations, like nutrition, pathology, and surgery. For example, nutrition is vital in the scenario of chronic diseases like ulcerative colitis, where therapeutic diets are a crucial factor in disease severity and patient outcome. The foundation of gastroenterology, thus, is not only pathology but also focuses on the therapeutic process, and nutrition, therefore, becomes a component of integral care in this discipline. Nutritional factors are the central theme in the practice of gastroenterology and have relevance to both preventive and therapeutic interventions in GI diseases. Individualized dietary focus can improve symptomatology and quality of life in patients with several gastrointestinal disorders. The integration of nutritional science into gastroenterology clinical practice is founded upon the understanding that a large number of digestive disorders are indelibly linked to diet and dietary insufficiency. Processes by which nutrition affects GI health involve modulation of gut microbiota, nutrient absorption, and immunity. Research findings indicate that some eating patterns can avoid inflammation and promote mucosal healing, particularly in disorders , such as Crohn's disease and ulcerative colitis. As more is known on these matters, gastroenterologists are now more and more adopting a patient-oriented approach, leading to tailor-made nutrition therapy to enhance the health outcome in individuals suffering from such afflictions. The definition and boundaries of gastroenterology continue to evolve, particularly with new research developments in medicine, highlighting the imperative for a multidisciplinary approach. New evidence concerning what is known about postbiotics, a term in part defined as inactive microorganisms and their components that are health-promoting, mirrors the growing overlap between nutrition and gastroenterology (Salminen et al., 2021). With more research into the interactive relationship between diet and the gut, clinicians are now encouraged to integrate emerging treatments into clinical practice. Moreover, organizations like the American Society of Colon and Rectal Surgeons emphasize the guidelines for high-quality treatment in gastrointestinal disorders that include the role of nutritional therapy in the treatment of specific conditions (Holubar et al., 2021). The ongoing development of gastroenterology as a field demonstrates the potential for the progress of patient treatment by evidence-based dietary management and multidisciplinary treatment (Figure 12.2).

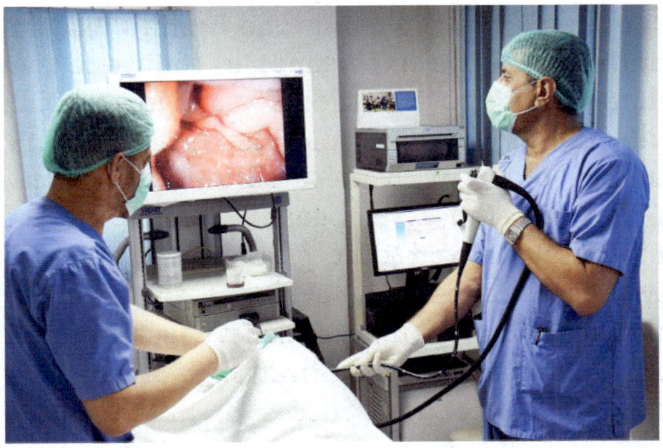

Figure 12.2. Scope of gastroenterology.

Source: https://www.fmic.org.af/OurServices/Clinics/PublishingImages/Dr-Atiqullah-Halimi-Gastronterology--Adult-Clinic-(2).jpg.

Importance of Nutrition in Gastrointestinal Health

Nutrition is of critical value in the maintenance of gastrointestinal health, with diet determining function and structure within the gut. An adequate diet can promote diverse and wholesome gut microbiota, which are critical in digestion, nutrient uptake, and protection against pathogens. Synbiotics, a combination of probiotics and prebiotics, have recently been found to confer synergistic health benefits. These food products are capable of enhancing gut barrier function and immune function modulation, thus reducing inflammation and overall gastrointestinal well-being. The International Scientific Association for Probiotics and Prebiotics brings to light a diet that promotes these prebiotics and probiotics, citing the impact on host health through the balance of microbiome and moderation of digestive function (Swanson et al., 2020). Lastly, nutrition knowledge and implementation of measures in nutrition can evidently enhance gastrointestinal function and prevent various gastrointestinal disorders. The interrelationship between nutrition and gastrointestinal illnesses, particularly inflammatory bowel diseases (IBD) , such as ulcerative colitis and Crohn's disease, underscores the importance of individualized diet treatment. Nutritional management can alleviate symptoms and improve patients' quality of life with these chronic conditions. Clinicians tend to emphasize the importance of individualized diet plans in compliance with guideline-based evidence to meet the nutritional needs of the patients. Macronutrient and micronutrient modifications, for instance, may influence the process of inflammation and healing of mucosal linings. Comprehensive guidelines, developed by a coalition of health care practitioners, advance the application of nutritional interventions as a key component of treatment modalities in IBD, enhancing the efficacy of therapies and outcomes of the patients (Lamb et al., 2019). These integrative approaches can very effectively improve the overall well-being and gastrointestinal health of these patients. Also, the prevention and control of gastrointestinal disease can be significantly determined by an active intervention in nutrition. Physicians are increasingly realizing that nutrition is not a supplement to therapy but part of disease prevention. For example, some dietary fibers have prebiotic action to nourish beneficial bacteria in the gut, which play a role in the health of the gut. Plant foods and vegetable antioxidants might also reduce oxidative stress, one of the factors in the development of gastrointestinal disease. As recognition of these relationships becomes increasingly common, nutrition education must be part of disease-preventive and therapeutic strategies for gastroenterology. By promoting good eating habits, patients can be empowered by health practitioners to take an active role in their gastrointestinal health and consequently better control their present ailments in addition to preventing future gastrointestinal ailments (Figure 12.3).

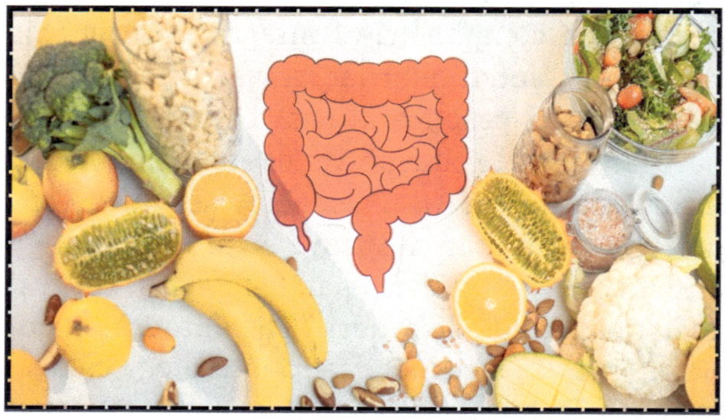

Figure 12.3. Importance of nutrition in gastrointestinal health.

Source: https://www.healixhospitals.com/tinyimages/Nutrition%20in%20Gastrointestinal%20Health%20-%20Healix%20Hospitals.jpg.

Overview of Common Gastrointestinal Disorders

Gastrointestinal (GI) illnesses are a wide range of digestive system diseases that have significant nutritional and overall health implications. The most prevalent disorders include gastroesophageal reflux disease (GERD), inflammatory bowel disease (IBD), and celiac disease, each with its own specific symptoms and physiologic effects. GERD is defined by recurring acid reflux, which may lead to pain and esophageal damage, whereas IBD, such as Crohn's disease and ulcerative colitis, is defined by inflammatory manifestations that disrupt nutrient absorption. Celiac disease is caused by a toxic reaction to gluten, causing villous atrophy of the small bowel and malabsorption of nutrients. These conditions are treated with focused dietary regimens to reduce symptoms and promote healing, highlighting the dynamic interaction between diet and gastrointestinal health, as numerous alterations in diet can alter the course and severity of these conditions. Obesity is a leading factor influencing the course of GI disorders. Not only does obesity increase the severity of such conditions as GERD and NAFLD, but it also renders them more difficult to treat. For instance, obesity complications are associated with a higher risk of developing chronic diseases that threaten digestive health, including metabolic syndrome and gallbladder disease. The etiology of obesity being multifactorial necessitates a multifaceted treatment strategy that frequently includes nutritional counseling and lifestyle modifications. Evidence indicates that obesity management in specific interventions is imperative to improved outcomes for individuals afflicted with GI disorders, according to the European Guideline on Obesity management in patients with gastrointestinal and liver diseases, joint ESPEN/UEG guideline, which gives more significance to the utilization of precise nutritional interventions to control weight as imperative to effective treatment and symptom reduction (Krznarić, 2022). New gastrointestinal disorders, such as food allergies and intolerances, also demonstrate the intricacy of dietary management of GI disorders. These conditions can result in severe nutritional deficiency if not managed appropriately due to the avoidance of offending foods, which limits the intake of critical nutrients. Food-allergic children, for instance, can suffer from stunted growth and developmental impairment from restricted diets, necessitating critical assessment and counseling. Also, the process of curing such allergies is often multidisciplinary, involving allergists and nutritionists to prepare a balanced diet that would include the requirements necessary for the patient but not the allergens. Research offers a comprehensive overview of such conditions, offering perspectives on the intersectionality of gastrointestinal health and nutritional surveillance, leading to the imperative for tailor-made dietary regimens that consider both the clinical presentation and nutritional needs of the affected (Sibal et al., 2015) (Figure 12.4).

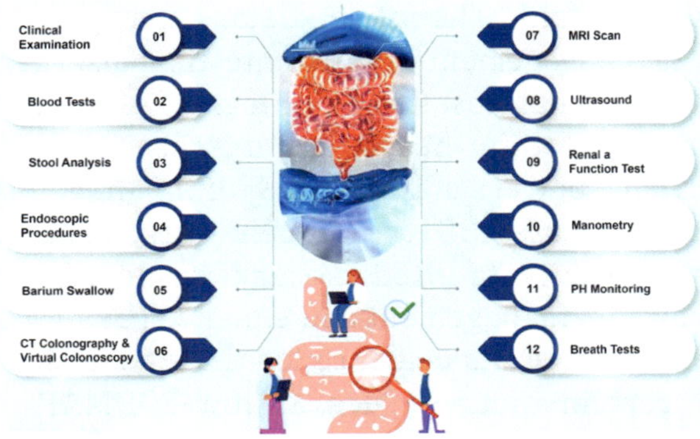

Figure 12.4. Overview of common gastrointestinal disorders.

Source: https://www.reddit.com/media?url=https%3A%2F%2Fi.redd.it%2Fa-cool-guide-diagnostic-tests-for-gastrointestinal-v0-jt43ibgi167b1.jpg%3Fs%3D451416c51b09052d929cf606644f10279a0a7918.

12.1. Role of Nutrition in Digestive Health

Nutrition is also essential to maintaining digestive health as a factor determining gastrointestinal (GI) tract efficiency. The composition of one's diet significantly influences the gut's microbial content and, in turn, creates an environment conducive to supporting or protecting against digestive function. Dietary fiber, for instance, serves as an important substrate for gut microbes that facilitates the development of a symbiotic relationship promoting digestive and nutrient absorption functions. These interactions illustrate the intricate relationship between our dietary patterns and gut microbiome health. Furthermore, some nutrients, vitamins A and E, for instance, with antioxidant functions, are crucial in protecting the gut wall from oxidative stress, thereby reducing inflammation. This relationship highlights not only the importance of a balanced diet but also the importance of concentration on specific nutritional components that are good for the digestive system and overall health. The role of dietary management in the management of gastrointestinal disorders also emphasizes the significance of diet to gastrointestinal health. Conditions , such as irritable bowel syndrome (IBS) or inflammatory bowel disease (IBD) are frequently best managed by specially tailored dietary strategies for symptom management and enhanced quality of life. There exists evidence for the effectiveness of certain diets—, such as low-FODMAP or Mediterranean diet—in the prevention of these disorders' symptoms. By targeting specific foods that improve inflammation and promote gut health, such interventions demonstrate the strong role that nutrition can play in clinical gastroenterology. In addition, there is some new evidence to suggest that nutrition influences the efficacy of drug therapy, demonstrating the need for a multisided strategy combining dietary modification with conventional treatment. This multiaspect approach reasserts the central role of nutrition in the prevention and treatment of gastrointestinal diseases. In addition to direct dietary impact on digestive health, the sharing of quality health information through social media channels has never been more crucial. Since many are turning to such avenues for health information, gastroenterologists need to come forward to provide evidence-based nutrition practices that help foster digestive health. Misinformation spreads so rapidly, and the benefits of sound dietary decisions get obscured. Both patients and members of the public can be reached via education to create a realization of ideal feeding habits needed for gastrointestinal health. Professional associations are also urged to support training in how to use social media effectively so that clinicians and scientists may be able to present crucial nutritional information effectively. This effort not only combats misinformation but also enables patients to make well-informed food selections that enhance their digestive health, showcasing the evolving relationship between nutrition, technology, and patient education (Figure 12.5).

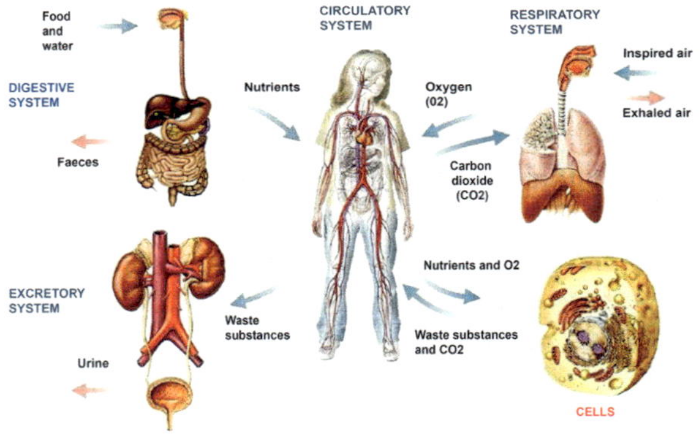

Figure 12.5. Role of nutrition in digestive health.

Source: https://image.jimcdn.com/app/cms/image/transf/dimension=origxorig:format=jpg/path/s37af0fcd02709117/image/ica73bf103ef3ba75/version/1474310319/image.jpg.

12.1.1. Impact of Diet on Gut Microbiota

The intricate relationship between diet and gut microbiota has garnered widespread attention in the last decade, particularly as research has unveiled how specific dietary habits can influence microbial composition and function. Diet is one of the most modifiable influences on the gut microbiome, with various foods acting as prebiotics or probiotics that can stimulate beneficial bacteria. For instance, fiber-rich foods , such as fruits, vegetables, and whole grains serve as substrates for the gut bacteria to ferment and form SCFAs that promote gut health and are anti-inflammatory. A high intake of processed foods and sugars, on the other hand, has been linked with reduced microbial diversity and overgrowth of potentially pathogenic microorganisms and exacerbation of gastrointestinal diseases. Hence, dietary choices not only have direct consequences for health but also affect the microbial populations residing within the gut. Recent research has suggested that specific dietary interventions could be vital in alleviating conditions related to an imbalanced gut microbiota. For example, the diet of the Mediterranean region, which is rich in plant foods, healthy fats, and fish and dairy foods in moderation, has been discovered to support the high presence of health-supporting bacteria like most Lactobacillus and Bifidobacterium species. High-sugar and high-fat diets, however, have been discovered to lead to dysbiosis, excessive growth of pathogen microbiota, which leads to diseases like inflammatory bowel disease (IBD). Evidence also indicates that dysbiosis may be involved in an impaired mucosal barrier, where opportunistic pathogens break the integrity and trigger an immune reaction, thereby indicating the critical role of dietary elements in the management of gastrointestinal health. These findings confirm that dietary interventions can be significant in reversing the risk factors associated with disease conditions like IBD and, potentially restore microbial homeostasis. Understanding dynamic relationships between gut microbiota and eating habits directs the development of customized nutrition strategies to support optimal gut health. The use of adjunctive probiotics and prebiotics in nutritional regimens can enhance the functionality and diversity of gut microbiota, with suggested therapeutic benefits. Clinical trials increasingly demonstrate that dietary modification to encourage a healthy microbiome can lead to increased digestive wellness, immune capacity, and even mood. With further research, more studies of the specific mechanisms through which food constituents regulate the gut microbiome will be essential. By providing a greater understanding of such correlations, healthcare professionals can prescribe more personalized dietary recommendations to individuals that promote healthy long-term consequences and safeguard against gastrointestinal disorders. More systematic incorporation of these dietary components into gastroenterological treatment is also necessary to successfully optimize patient outcomes (Figure 12.6).

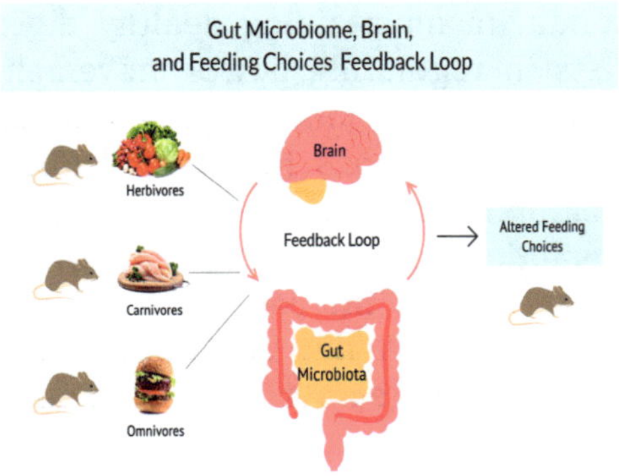

Figure 12.6. Impact of diet on gut microbiota.

Source: https://www.nutritional-psychology.org/wp-content/uploads/2022/05/unnamed-1-1.jpg.

12.1.2. Nutritional Deficiencies and Their Effects on Digestion

Nutrient deficiencies come in a wide variety of forms and can have a significant impact on digestion. Vitamins and minerals , such as B vitamins, magnesium, and zinc are among the most crucial to the digestive system's health. For instance, vitamin B12 is essential for optimal gastrointestinal function and facilitates the absorption of nutrients. Deficiency of this vitamin can cause malabsorption syndromes and play a role in gastrointestinal pathology , such as anemia, a reflection of defective digestion. Magnesium also plays an important role in muscular activity, including the muscles of the gut tract. Constipation and other gastrointestinal symptoms can result from a lack of magnesium, a demonstration of nutritional and gastrointestinal interdependence. The rectification of these deficiencies through appropriate dietary interventions is essential in the prevention of digestive disorders and attaining the highest level of digestive health. The role of fiber intake towards digestive health cannot be overstated, particularly in the prevention of nutritional deficiencies. Dietary fiber, which is supplied mainly in the form of fruits, vegetables, and whole grains, is essential in maintaining healthy digestion. It assists in regulating bowel movements by bulkifying the stool and plays a critical role in avoiding conditions like diverticulitis and constipation. In addition to that, fiber also serves as a prebiotic, nourishing gut microbiota, which consequently can increase nutrient uptake, including vital vitamins and minerals. In the absence of adequate fiber, one can be subjected to digestive disturbances that can aggravate or lead to nutritional deficiencies. This is aimed at emphasizing the importance of fiber diets not only in efficient digestion but as a main strategy in preventing nutrient deficiencies, emphasizing diet diversity and balance as needed. Further, recent research describes the potential of future food sources, such as Azanza garckeana, in nutritional inadequacy management. Azanza garckeana fruit has a high protein and crude fiber content, which can aid in digestion by promoting gut health. Non-nutritional constituents , such as oxalates, are, however, their limiting factors since they question their influence on nutrient bioavailability and gut health. Therefore, even though this plant is a potential functional food candidate in preventing nutrient deficiency, caution should be taken on potential anti-nutritional factors. Strategic preparation and cooking methods can minimize such undesirable consequences and enhance the nutritional aspect. Further research on emerging food sources will increase our understanding of dietary sources in gastroenterology, providing more opportunities for combating nutritional inadequacies through diet (Sabo et al., 2024) and employing new ingredients to enhance overall digestive well-being and health (Figure 12.7).

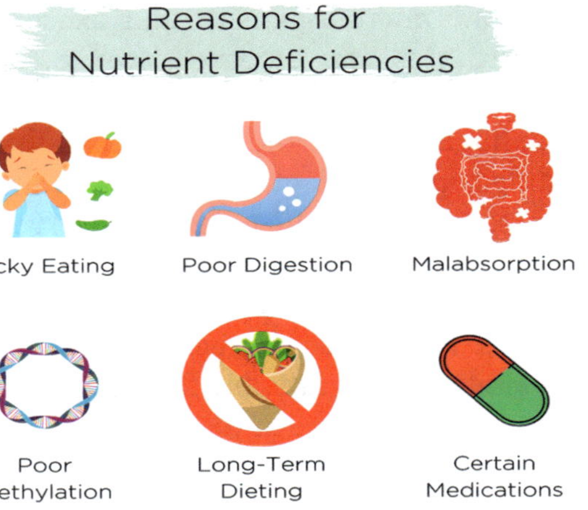

Figure 12.7. Nutritional deficiencies and their effects on digestion.

Source: https://images.squarespace-cdn.com/content/v1/64f2616ca380351b0c174792/1693706961335-SUJ6ZVFB85MTTZ4EVI2B/image-asset.png.

12.1.3. Importance of Hydration in Gastrointestinal Function

Hydration is an integral component of maintaining adequate gastrointestinal (GI) function, influencing both the digestive processes and general health. The GI system relies on adequate water intake for the digestion and absorption of nutrients. Hydration impacts saliva production, which is essential to facilitate the breakdown of food and initiate the digestion process. Water is also integral to the production of gastric juices employed to digest food in the stomach. Without proper hydration, people can suffer from digestive issues, including constipation, which can further result in more serious ailments like fecal impaction or bowel blockage. Hence, maintaining proper fluid levels is critical not just for proper digestion but also to avoid painful and possibly life-threatening gastrointestinal ailments. In addition, hydration is crucial for mucosal function and integrity in the GI tract. The intestinal mucosa requires adequate moisture to be able to function and preserve its structural and functional capacities, which are of critical importance for the absorption of nutrients as well as the preservation against pathogen invasion. Research has established that dehydration heightens intestinal permeability, also referred to as leaky gut.

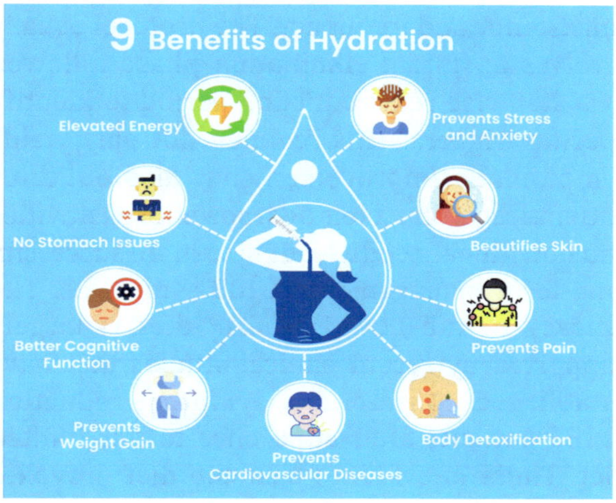

Figure 12.8. Importance of hydration in gastrointestinal function.

Source: https://lumispareview.com/wp-content/uploads/2023/03/benefits-of-hydration-for-the-body.png.

This enhances the penetration of toxins and bacteria into the bloodstream, thus inducing systemic inflammation. Additionally, an adequately hydrated intestinal environment favors good gut microbiota, which improves digestive function and boosts immune status. Proper hydration thus, is not only ancillary but is actually mandatory to preserve the integrity of the GI tract and avoid disease associated with impaired mucosal function. In critically ill patients, hydration is even more important since alterations in fluid status will exacerbate gastrointestinal impairment. Fluid resuscitation is generally needed to support hydration status, especially in sepsis or significant fluid loss. This dehydration has the added effect of worsening gastrointestinal dysmotility in terms of delayed gastric emptying and risk for feeding intolerance. As per organizational guidelines from A.S.P.E.N. and SCCM, hydration status plays a key role in the management of critically ill patients in order to enhance recovery and avoid complications during nutrition therapy (McClave et al., 2016; Chaudhury et al., 2017). Therefore, hydration should be given due emphasis by healthcare professionals in combination with nutritional support to optimize gut function and overall patient outcomes in the critical care environment (Figure 12.8).

12.2. Dietary Recommendations for Gastrointestinal Disorders

The intricate relationship between diet and gastrointestinal disease necessitates customized dietary counseling that can significantly affect patient outcomes. In individuals with conditions , such as irritable bowel syndrome (IBS), inflammatory bowel disease (IBD), and gastroesophageal reflux disease (GERD), identifying foods that may exacerbate or ease symptoms becomes crucial. Fiber-rich diets, and particularly soluble fiber diets, can benefit most patients since they stabilize the bowel movements and contribute to gut health. Steer clear of usual irritants , such as caffeine, alcohol, and very processed foods to minimize the symptoms and promote healing. These individualized strategies highlight the importance of nutritional therapy in the management of gastrointestinal disorders and suggest that healthcare practitioners need to work with patients to identify their specific precipitating factors and nutritional needs. The use of probiotics and prebiotics is also a critical consideration for individuals with gastrointestinal disorders. Probiotics, in the form of live microbes, can restore balance to the gut microbiome, while prebiotics act as substrates that provide nutrition to beneficial bacteria in the gut. To gain maximal health benefits, experts recommend that patients use synbiotics, foods that contain both probiotics and prebiotics, yet again enhancing their digestive system. This approach aligns with emerging research evidence revealing gut microbiomes' key role in maintaining overall health, particularly in gastrointestinal health and immune function. Additionally, eating a diet rich in fruits, vegetables, whole grains, and fermented foods can improve gut flora diversity and immune function so that a holistic approach to managing gastrointestinal disorders is possible (Swanson et al., 2020). Another crucial element of dietary therapy for gastrointestinal disorders is individualized nutrition therapy. As highlighted by recent guidelines, one-size-fits-all is insufficient due to the variation in people's needs according to their health status, food choices, and cultures. Continued collaboration between patients and healthcare professionals is required to create effective dietary plans, considering the individual situation of each patient. A personalized strategy will best help maintain glycemic targets, achieve weight loss goals, and manage cardiovascular risk factors. Thus, nutrition counseling is a critical component of the management of gastrointestinal disorders to facilitate symptom relief and improved quality of life (Evert et al., 2019). Such a demand for individualization of diet therapy highlights the complex interlink between nutrition and gastrointestinal health, reiterating the necessity of individualized interventions in clinical practice.

12.2.1. Low FODMAP Diet for Irritable Bowel Syndrome

The Low FODMAP diet has been a vital tool for dietary management of Irritable Bowel Syndrome (IBS), a disorder characterized by chronic gastrointestinal discomfort and irregular bowel function. The diet centers on restriction of certain fermentable carbohydrate substrates known as FODMAPs, highly fermentable oligosaccharides, disaccharides, monosaccharides, and polyols, which are implicated in increased symptoms for patients with IBS. With a gradual reduction in FODMAP intake, patients typically experience marked symptom relief, including decreased abdominal pain, bloating, and alterations in stool consistency and frequency. The protocol usually involves an initial elimination phase followed by a stepwise reintroduction period to identify specific triggers. This regimen not only yields symptomatic improvement but also educates patients regarding their own specific sensitivities and nutritional needs, leading to more successful long-term management of IBS symptoms. The efficacy of the Low FODMAP diet is largely supported by recent clinical studies that have established considerable symptom reduction in IBS patients after adherence to this limited diet. There is evidence that the diet provokes changes in the metabolome and gastrointestinal microbiome, the variables that are positively associated with symptom reduction. Notably, there is evidence appearing that indicates that adhering to the Low FODMAP diet may lead to increased diversity of actinobacteria in stool samples, responsible for maintaining gut health. This alteration of the gut flora is indicative of a healthier absorption and digestion environment. However, despite its worth, the low FODMAP diet is generally recommended as a short-term treatment against acute exacerbations with regard to nutrient intake in mind as the diet limits most nutrients that are otherwise high in vitamins and minerals (Jo et al., 2024). It is difficult to maintain long-term adherence to the Low FODMAP diet, particularly because it may lead to nutritional imbalance and lower nutrient variety. Thus, healthcare practitioners would favor the inclusion of aspects of this diet within other sensible dietary paradigms , such as the Mediterranean diet, which may be a longer term sustainable answer to the management of IBS symptoms. The Mediterranean diet, as it consists of whole foods, healthy fats, and fiber, proves to successfully replace symptoms with its anti-inflammatory properties and density of nutrients and is still able to incorporate the concepts of the Low FODMAP diet. This dual approach offers patients flexibility and variety in the foods they can have, ultimately making the long-term food selection choices appealing and obtainable. Therefore, an extensive understanding of the Low FODMAP and the Mediterranean diets offers a robust strategy in the dietary treatment of IBS that is adequate to address both long-term and short-term health complications (Staudacher et al., 2017) (Figure 12.9).

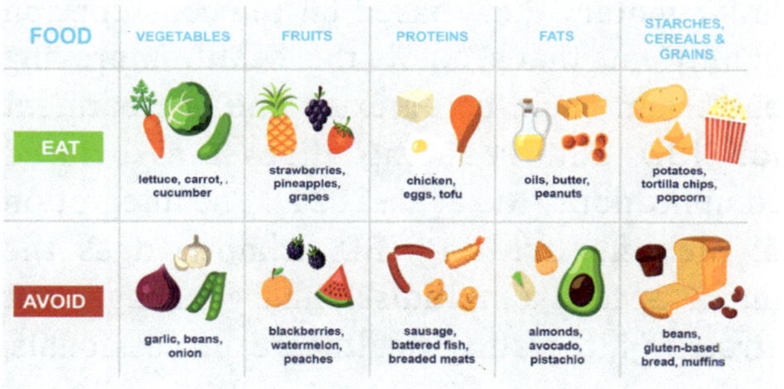

Figure 12.9. Low FODMAP diet for irritable bowel syndrome.

Source: https://charlestongi.com/wp-content/uploads/2021/03/21-CGI-0862-FB-09.png.

12.2.2. Gluten-Free Diet for Celiac Disease

The gluten-free diet is the cornerstone of the treatment of celiac disease, an autoimmune disorder that encompasses an abnormal reaction to gluten, a protein found in wheat, barley, and rye. Compliance with this dietary restriction is necessary to minimize the deleterious effects of gluten on the gastrointestinal tract and prevent long-term sequelae, such as malabsorption of nutrients and increased predisposition to other autoimmune diseases. Since celiac disease affects approximately 1% of the global population, this dietary therapy is very important as it contributes to the recovery of health in patients who show a wide array of symptoms, from gastrointestinal to nonspecific symptoms of fatigue and iron deficiency anemia (Chandrakar, 2024). Effective management through a gluten-free diet not only manages to eradicate physical symptoms but also induces normalcy and well-being in patients, thereby enhancing the overall quality of life. Studies show the significant role played by health-related quality of life (HRQoL) in the case of patients on a gluten-free diet. Factors that promote improved HRQoL include perceived self-efficacy and illness perception, which involve the manner in which individuals perceive the consequences of celiac disease and how they can manage the condition (Chandrakar, 2024). The adult presentation of celiac disease revealed that those who maintained a positive outlook and showed positivity about following their diet regimen had better psychological adjustment and quality of life. Alternatively, negative attitudes towards celiac disease or low belief levels concerning its severity were associated with more adverse outcomes. Hence, the psychological dimensions of adjusting to celiac disease become important when considering multifaceted treatment and support systems that can ultimately lead to increased dietary compliance and health outcomes. Although the gluten-free diet is effective in treating celiac disease, its use is fraught with challenges of dietary restriction and social difficulty, which can influence adherence. The patient may experience challenges with food selection, particularly in social situations where foods containing gluten are more common. Additionally, the gluten-free diet is costly and can restrict the range of suitable food availability, with resultant potential nutritional insufficiency. Health care providers have an important part to play in instructing patients with the information and resources they require to successfully maintain a gluten-free diet, and in identifying alternative sources of food that offer comprehensive nutrition (Ford et al., 2012). By including nutritional counseling and diet education in the treatment plan, health care providers can enhance rates of adherence and decrease psychological distress associated with celiac disease, resulting in better health outcomes for this population (Figure 12.10).

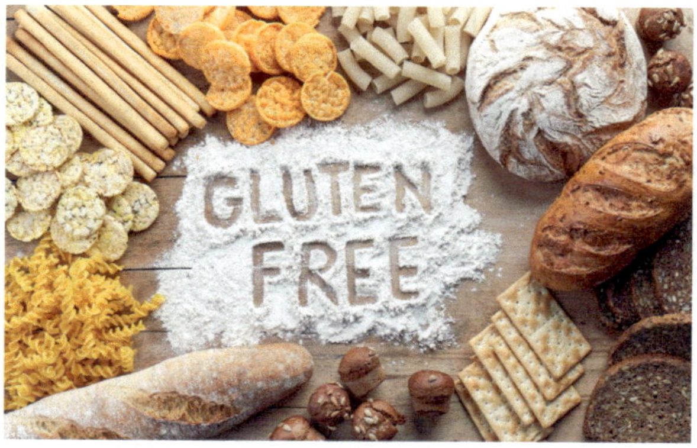

Figure 12.10. Gluten-free diet for celiac disease.

Source: https://content.presspage.com/uploads/1483/1920_glutenfree-362847.jpg?10000.

12.2.3. Anti-Inflammatory Diets for Inflammatory Bowel Disease

The multifaceted interaction between diet and inflammatory bowel disease (IBD) indicates the potential therapeutic benefit of anti-inflammatory diets in ulcerative colitis and Crohn's disease. Profound gastrointestinal inflammation is characteristic in IBD patients, and dietary influence could be a method for symptom relief and remission induction. Recent studies have found that specific diets, with their anti-inflammatory constituents, can heavily impact the gut microbiome, which is crucial to balancing an equilibrated intestinal environment. Notably, diets rich in omega-3 fatty acids, fiber, and fermented foods have the potential to increase the concentration of healthy bacteria capable of maintaining a healthy gut and reducing inflammation. By adhering to a carefully planned anti-inflammatory diet, individuals with IBD might be able to reduce their symptoms, leading to improved overall well-being. Research has indicated that specific gut microbiota, such as *Roseburia intestinalis*, could impart therapeutic benefit to IBD patients. The species is defined by its ability to produce the short-chain fatty acid butyrate, which is an effective anti-inflammatory agent and preserves the mucosal health. Scientific findings indicate a disrupted abundance of R. intestinalis among IBD patients, which translates into a dietary target. Adding food with prebiotic and probiotic content, favoring the growth of beneficial bacteria, can boost the number of R. intestinalis in the gut, which may have implications in lowering inflammation and improving energy homeostasis.

Thus, interest in the adoption of anti-inflammatory diets based on the consumption of nutrients that promote this health-improving bacterium could be an extra line of treatment for IBD and reducing disease-associated complications (Nie et al., 2021). The integration of diet into treating IBD acknowledges the importance of a multidisciplinary management strategy integrating healthcare professionals, patients, and nutritionists. Multidisciplinary plans can optimize treatment strategies tailored based on individual dietary patterns in considering the complexity of IBD. Evidence-based dietary recommendations, coupled with medication therapies, can enhance treatment outcomes and adherence. The guidelines of the UK in managing inflammatory bowel disease emphasize multidisciplinary care, which should incorporate dietary counseling as an essential component of overall management (Lamb et al., 2019). Through the combination of nutrition interventions with clinical best practice and patient-centered care, health practitioners can better address the unique needs of those who live with IBD, resulting in improved health outcomes and better long-term management of this chronic condition (Figure 12.11).

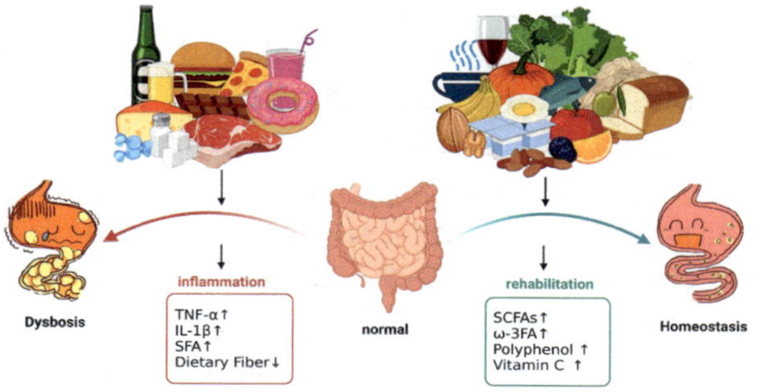

Figure 12.11. Anti-inflammatory diets for inflammatory bowel disease.

Source: Hou Y, Wang S-F, Zhou K and Dai S-X (2023) Comparison and recommendation of dietary patterns based on nutrients for Eastern and Western patients with inflammatory bowel disease. Front. Nutr. 9:1066252. doi: 10.3389/fnut.2022.1066252

12.3. Nutritional Interventions in Gastrointestinal Diseases

The relationship between diet and gastrointestinal (GI) disease is multifaceted and pivotal to the understanding of illness prevention and control. Recent evidence suggests that dietary factors have a major role in inflammatory bowel disease (IBD) etiology and pathogenesis, with alterations in gut microbiota and environmental factors interacting within genetically predisposed subjects. The D-ECCO working group has collated evidence that underscores the significance of dietary interventions and grouped them into three broad areas: etiological role of diet in disease, induction and maintenance treatment using diet, and nutritional status evaluation. The systematic review identifies areas of research that need to be bridged to develop a strong therapeutic profile for IBD, emphasizing the necessity of an individualized nutrition plan for patients. Besides IBD, acute pancreatitis is also a context where nutritional interventions are of the greatest importance. The position of dietary fiber in the management of pancreatic disease is currently a debated topic. There is evidence to suggest that a diet rich in prebiotics can provide positive outcomes, such as reduced infection rates of pancreatic necrosis and shorter hospital stays. This protective effect can be explained by the fiber's capacity for stabilizing the intestinal barrier and suppressing systemic inflammatory reactions. The picture, however, becomes complicated in the case of exocrine pancreatic insufficiency, where a high-fiber diet has the potential for promoting fecal fat excretion, involving fibers inhibitory influence on pancreatic enzymes. Thus, the optimal dietary strategy should weigh carefully the putative benefits and risks of fiber intake in this patient population (Ribichini et al., 2019). The usefulness of tailored nutritional therapy is not unique to the entire spectrum of gastrointestinal diseases. The diet is not merely preventive but also therapeutic, and it impacts the management of conditions , such as celiac disease, irritable bowel syndrome (IBS), and diverticular disease. For example, for someone with celiac disease, a gluten-free diet is required, but implementing such a dietary restriction requires strict attention to micronutrient intake and dietary balance as a whole. Likewise, with IBS, patients can be helped with certain dietary patterns, like low-FODMAP diets, which have been shown to improve symptoms for the majority of patients. Furthermore, nutritional assessment and supportive nutritional therapy remain integral parts of a comprehensive management strategy for gastrointestinal diseases. With evolving technology, the need for tailored dietary methods considering the unique pathophysiology of each disease remains critical to optimizing patient outcomes (Sigall-Boneh et al., 2017).

12.3.1. Role of Probiotics and Prebiotics

Increasing awareness of nutritional components of gastroenterology has placed on center stage the crucial roles of probiotics and prebiotics in gut health. Probiotics, being live bacteria or yeast, have gained prominence for their ability to restore gut microbial equilibrium. Probiotics are known through research to have the capacity to influence the gut-brain axis, linking gastrointestinal well-being with mental well-being. Some probiotic strains have also become promising therapy for symptom diminishment in depression, hence specifying their usefulness for more than gut functioning. Moreover, heterogeneity in the composition of the gut microbiota plays a major role in providing many physiological functions, and hence probiotics are beneficial for treating diseases , such as IBS and inflammatory bowel disease (IBD) that are prevalent in the field of gastroenterology (Clerici et al., 2025). Aiding probiotics, prebiotics are dietary fibers that are fermented in the colon to selectively stimulate the growth of good gut bacteria. These undigestible fibers are vital in facilitating the metabolic functions of probiotics, which result in a healthier gut in the long term. By elevating the concentration of short-chain fatty acids (SCFAs) generated during fermentation, prebiotics can potentially alleviate inflammation and increase gut barrier function. New studies have underlined the curative potential of some prebiotic fibers to reduce the incidence and severity of gastrointestinal disease, further solidifying their position in nutritional therapy (Sionek et al., 2025). As consumers continue to pay attention to functional food, the inclusion of prebiotics in diets is a new strategy to maximize overall gut health and disease prevention. Both the pairing of probiotics and prebiotics supports the trend in the dieting guidance in gastroenterology, and functional foods. The market trend has shifted to one of embracing foods that offer additional health benefits rather than just nutrition. Probiotic and prebiotic foods, especially those derived from vegetable sources, are now being considered for their potential to have a healthy microbiome and well-being (Sionek et al., 2025). This movement is mirroring growing consumer demands for health-positive and sustainable products, not just to feed but also to foster long-term health results. As ongoing research continues to associate the wide range of health effects with these substances, gastroenterologists and nutritionists are forced to encourage eating habits full of prebiotics and probiotics as key elements of gastrointestinal health strategy in clinical practice (Clerici et al., 2025) (Figure 12.12).

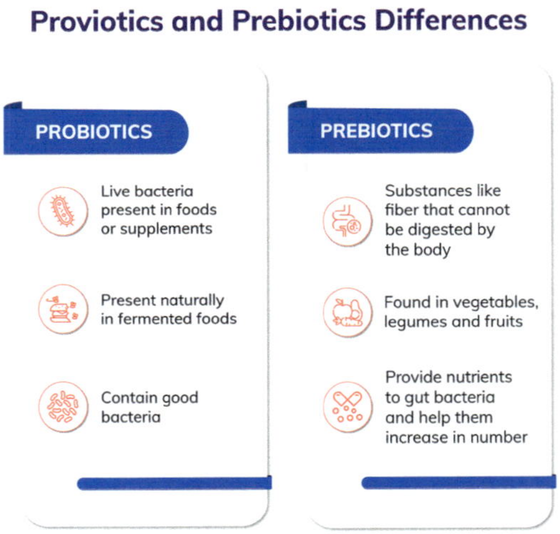

Figure 12.12. Role of probiotics and prebiotics.

Source: https://wordpresscmsprodstor.blob.core.windows.net/wp-cms/2022/02/16-633190e41f0c7.jpg.

12.3.2. Use of Enteral Nutrition in Malnutrition

The management of malnutrition, particularly gastroenterology, often involves the employment of enteral nutrition (EN). Enteral nutrition, or the delivery of nutrients directly into the GI tract, is a significant intervention for patients who cannot meet their nutritional requirements through oral intake. This policy is not merely linked with improved patient outcomes for patients with malnutrition but also ensures gut integrity and function. Early enteral nutrition has been shown to substantially reduce the risk of complications of malnutrition, resulting in improved recovery and general health among diverse categories of patients. Considering the multifactorial nature of conditions leading to malnutrition , such as inflammatory bowel disease and alcoholic liver disease, personalized enteral nutrition plans can effectively meet individual nutritional needs and manage the disease as a whole. The use of enteral nutrition in gastroenterological disorders highlights the importance of its role in clinical medicine. For instance, in IBD patients, enteral nutrition is utilized both for induction and maintenance therapy with the potential for suppressing inflammation as well as providing required nutrients. One systematic review highlighted dietary intervention in IBD management, concluding that specific nutrient profiles have been shown to influence the activity of the disease as well as the quality of the patient's life (Sigall-Boneh et al., 2017). Furthermore, enteral nutrition can reduce the need for corticosteroid therapy in such patients, restricting potential side effects observed with prolonged use. Consequently, the inclusion of enteral nutrition as part of therapeutic treatment not only normalizes malnutrition but also provides an opportunity to counteract the pharmacological loads so far experienced by such patients. In alcoholic liver disease (ALD), enteral nutrition also plays a pivotal role in the treatment of malnutrition and convalescence. The relationship between nutrition and ALD has received more scrutiny in recent years, particularly with the adverse effects of malnutrition on liver function and overall health. Presentations at a recent symposium documented how some nutritional components, such as fats and carbohydrates, could influence the progression of ALD and the potential role of nutritional support within patient management overall (Feldstein et al., 2018). Enteral nutrition can normalize disturbed metabolic processes caused by alcohol intake and support the restoration of nutritional status, crucial for liver rehabilitation and regeneration. Before enteral nutrition in the management of malnourished gastroenterological patients, health professionals can offer complete care encompassing both nutritional needs and the underlying medical illnesses.

12.3.3. Dietary Modifications for Liver Disease Management

Nutritional management is significantly improved by dietetic alterations, which can optimize liver function and delay disease progression. A high-nutrient diet comprising unrefined foods is essential in patients with liver conditions , such as nonalcoholic fatty liver disease (NAFLD) and cirrhosis. Specifically, the supplementation with fruits, vegetables, whole grains, and lean proteins optimizes metabolic activities and promotes the regeneration of liver cells. This dietary alteration not only helps with weight regulation but also enhances insulin sensitivity, particularly important for individuals who suffer from metabolic syndrome that typically accompanies liver disease. Pivotal nutrient elements, such as omega-3 fatty acids found in fish, can lower fat in the liver and have anti-inflammatory properties, further underscoring the role of nutrition towards the regulation of the liver (Caio et al., 2019). Thus, dietary modification has to be taken into account as a central element in total liver disease treatment regimens. Moreover, limiting processed food intake and avoiding saturated fats, sugar, and refined carbohydrates can contribute to the control of liver disease. Literature emphasizes that overconsumption of alcohol, fructose, and trans fatty acids triggers inflammation of the liver and steatosis, which speeds up diseases like NAFLD and alcoholic liver disease. It is critical that individuals suffering from liver disease are aware of these nutritional traps. Instead, adoption of a Mediterranean-type diet, with rich unsaturated fat, fiber, and antioxidants content, has shown to have promise in promoting liver health and minimizing the risk of fibrosis (Chalasani et al., 2017). Care through diet is also required, as rigorous adherence to the same can lead to significant declines in liver enzymes and overall metabolic function, finally leading to the betterment of the health and quality of life of the patients. Apart from overall dietary interventions, case-specific nutritional therapy is also essential.

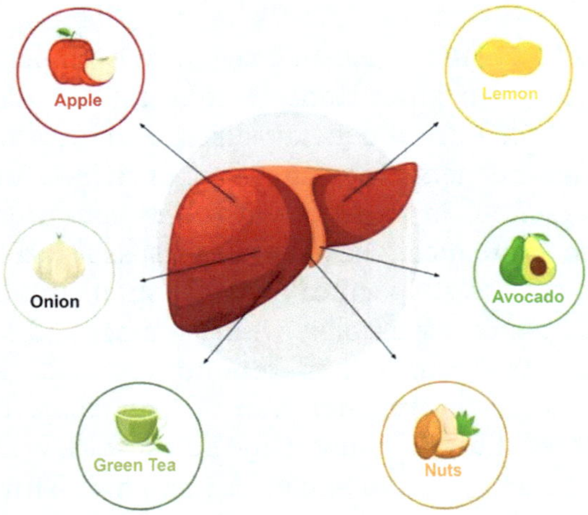

Figure 12.13. Dietary modifications for liver disease management.

Source: https://www.kaizengastrocare.com/wp-content/uploads/2023/04/Diet-for-Liver-Disease.jpg.

For example, patients with end-stage liver disease will develop protein intolerance, and therefore, a careful balance of protein intake needs to be maintained to prevent complications , such as hepatic encephalopathy without sacrificing muscle mass preservation. Nutritional assessment is necessary for tailoring these diets, and practitioners should consider caloric needs, food preferences, and comorbid conditions. Vitamin and mineral supplementation, particularly B vitamins, vitamin D, and selenium, may also prove to be useful in alleviating deficiency, which is prevalent in patients with liver disease (Caio et al., 2019). Integrating personalized nutritional advice into the treatment strategy can significantly influence patient outcomes and reiterates the importance of nutrition as an integral component of the management of liver disease (Figure 12.13).

12.4. The Gut-Brain Axis and Nutrition

Gut-brain axis refers to two-way communication between the gastrointestinal tract and the central nervous system, highlighting the intricate interaction between diet and psychological health. The axis is supported by several mechanisms, including neuroendocrine signaling, immune system function, and the effect of gut microbiota on intestinal and neuronal functions. Breaking research points to how food choice affects gut microbiota structure and consequently neurochemical signaling pathways that modulate mood and cognition. For instance, consumption of a high-fiber diet can nourish beneficial gut bacteria that produce short-chain fatty acids, which have been linked to improved mood and cognitive processes. These findings underscore the importance of including nutritional interventions as part of mental health treatment and thereby the promise that modifications in diet can affect both gut and brain health. Dysbiosis, or the impairment of the balance between gut microbial communities, has been linked to many neurological and psychiatric diseases, reinforcing the influence of the gut-brain axis in nutrition. The metabolic products of the gut microbiota can modulate the permeability of the intestinal epithelial barrier, which is crucial to homeostasis maintenance. Its derangement can induce high intestinal permeability, whereby potentially toxic antigens penetrate into the circulation and trigger systemic inflammation and contribute to psychological stress and other brain-associated issues. Single microbial populations, such as Roseburia intestinalis, demonstrate the capacity for restoring balance to gut microbiota and lowering inflammation by releasing health-boosting metabolites like butyrate, which have been shown to support barrier function and modulate immunity. Gut microbial populations can hence be addressed through dietary interventions, which may offer a novel approach to the treatment of mental illness and fortifying the gut-brain axis. Nutrition's role in maintaining the intestinal epithelial barrier (IEB) is also at the core of uncovering the gut-brain axis.

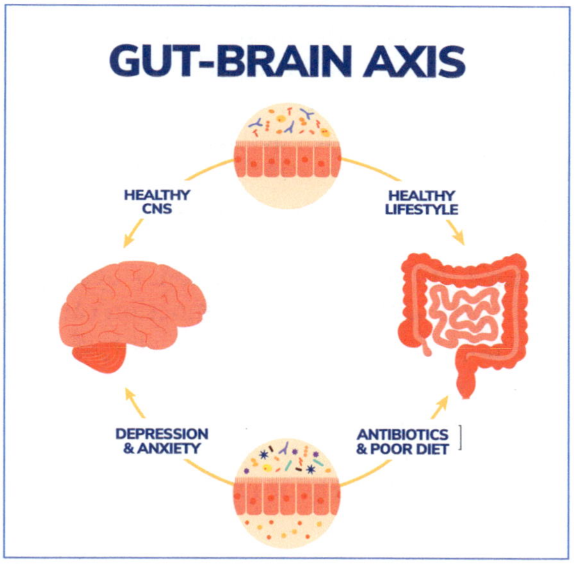

Figure 12.14. The gut-brain axis and nutrition.

Source: https://greaterorlandogi.com/wp-content/uploads/2023/06/GBA4-min.jpg.

The IEB is a significant interface, dictating what enters the bloodstream while permitting nutrient absorption. All of these elements, including diet, gut microbiota, and cytokine function, act in concert to control IEB integrity and permeability. When the IEB is disturbed by dysbiosis or poor diet, it has the potential to initiate inflammatory responses that affect gut and neurological well-being. More specifically, the regulation of tight junctions is important for maintaining barrier function and preventing the translocation of inappropriate antigens, which can exacerbate diseases like IBS and IBD. Recent research stresses the relationship between the IEB, gut microbiota, and immune system in such diseases and also further describes the rationale for nutritional therapy in gastroenterology (Figure 12.14).

12.4.1. Connection Between Gut Health and Mental Well-Being

The relationship between intestinal health and psychological well-being has attracted increasing attention from the scientific community, and it is here that the gut microbiome is cited as an important factor in this relationship. The gut, or the second brain, contains approximately 100 million neurons and talks to the central nervous system via several avenues. These are the neural, immune, and endocrine systems. This complex communication substantiates the importance of maintaining a healthy gut microbiome in enhancing mental well-being. Changes in the gut microbiota have been linked to mood disorders, anxiety, and cognitive impairment, suggesting that a deficiency might be the cause of adverse psychological consequences. As researchers continue to investigate such relationships in greater depth, they hypothesize that nutritional interventions and gut health upkeep can be effective methods towards the prevention of mental illnesses and general well-being, opening the door to future research in nutritional psychiatry and gastroenterology (Mishra & Mewani, 2025). In addition, nutritional psychiatry is an innovative field of study that highlights the intricate overlap between food choices and mental health consequences. Payers to nutrient-rich, anti-inflammatory diets, including the Mediterranean diet, have been promising in improving mood and symptom reduction in depression and anxiety. Principal nutrients , such as omega-3 fatty acids, B vitamins, and magnesium have been shown to be essential in brain function and emotional regulation. These nutritional factors support the health of the gut microbiome, which in turn exerts influence on mood and behavior through the gut-brain axis. With nutritional interventions becoming more common as part of mental health care, collaboration between healthcare professionals and dietitians is crucial in order to provide the specific nutritional requirements of an individual. Recognition of this connection not only underscores the significance of digestive health to mental well-being but also drives the necessity for interdisciplinary approaches in optimizing the outcome of the patient (Julius, 2025). In summary, the connection between digestive health and mental well-being is a critical research area under nutritional dimensions within gastroenterology.

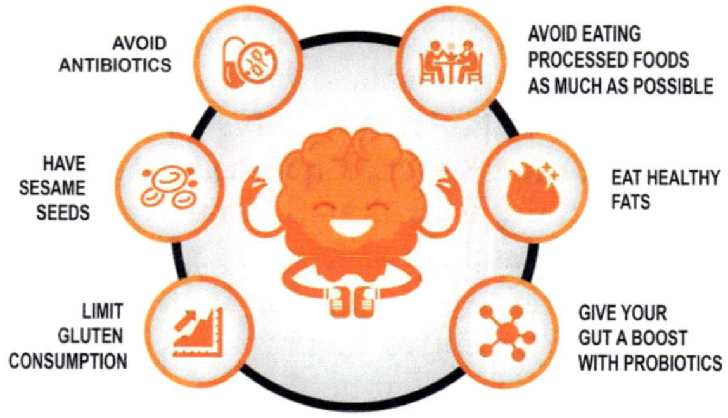

Figure 12.15. Connection between gut health and mental well-being.

Source: https://thefitvision.com/wp-content/uploads/2019/04/Gut-brain-768x566.jpg.

As increasingly more evidence mounts for bidirectional interaction between the gut and the brain, it is more apparent that gut health is crucial to promoting psychological resilience. The harmonics of this association extend beyond individual health and raise significant public health issues around the prevention and management of chronic disease as well as mental illness. More research must continue to investigate interventions like dietary modifications and probiotic consumption to gain more insights into how gut microbiota can be optimized for the upkeep of mental health. By combining research from both gastroenterology and nutritional psychiatry, healthcare professionals can formulate strong plans that completely address the demands of their patients, and this eventually leads to a healthier society (Julius, 2025; Mishra & Mewani, 2025) (Figure 12.15).

12.4.2. Influence of Stress on Digestive Health

The relationship between gastrointestinal wellness and stress is a multifaceted issue that also underscores the significance of the gut-brain axis in gastroenterology. Stress may cause numerous physiological alterations, including changes in gut motility, augmented secretion of gastric acid, and changes in the composition of the gut microbiota. Stress-induced changes may also cause a wide range of gastrointestinal disorders, including IBS, IBD, and functional dyspepsia. Interference with normal gut function can have severe implications for nutrient absorption and overall well-being. Indeed, there is evidence to suggest that chronic stress may lead to dysbiosis, and the pathogenic and beneficial gut flora are disturbed, leading to enhanced inflammation and gut disturbance. Given this, understanding the mechanisms whereby stress impacts digestive health is fundamental to the development of nutritional and therapeutic strategies to oppose these effects. In addressing the nutritional aspects of gastrointestinal health, it's worth mentioning that food can either exacerbate or reduce the effect of stress on digestion. Nutrient-rich foods that promote gut health, such as those rich in fiber, prebiotics, and probiotics, play an important role in maintaining a healthy gut microbiome. Probiotics, or live microorganisms conferring benefit on the host, have gained much attention for their potential to enhance gastrointestinal symptoms related to stress. Certain strains of probiotics have been shown to enhance a better gut environment and may potentially alter neurochemical signaling, therefore possibly mitigating the physiological symptoms of stress. The ingestion of these probiotics into the diet could be of immense benefit to the stressed individuals with gastrointestinal disturbances, thereby proving the contribution of diet in the overall management of the gastrointestinal wellness. Further research on some of the gut microbiota , such as *Roseburia intestinalis* sheds more light on how stress, diet, and gastrointestinal well-being are connected. This probiotic anaerobic bacterium is butyrate-producing, a short-chain fatty acid linked with gut health and anti-inflammatory responses. Research suggests that the amount of R. intestinalis is usually lower in patients with stress-driven ailments like inflammatory bowel disease. The improvement of gastrointestinal diseases caused by stress via the promotion of beneficial microbes like R. intestinalis could be a novel therapeutic avenue. As the latest research goes deeper and deeper into these interactions, and especially into the development of advanced methodologies for gut microbiota analysis, it becomes ever clearer that encouraging a well-functioning microbiome in addition to healthy stress management can bring a very tangible benefit to digestive health. Such observations underscore the interconnected nature of nutrition, gut microbiota, and psychological wellbeing in gastroenterology (Figure 12.16).

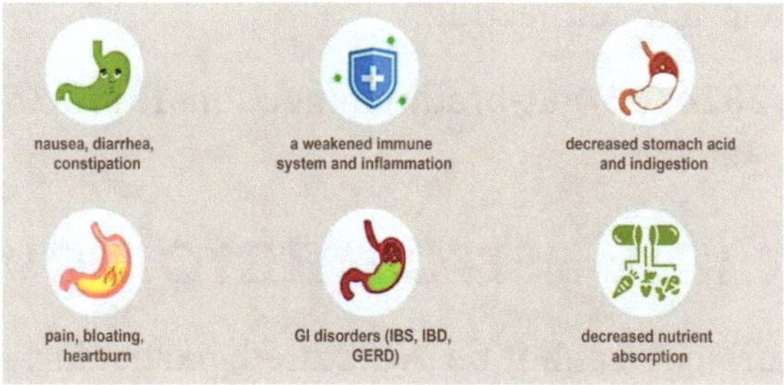

Figure 12.16. Influence of stress on digestive health.

Source: https://www.planetnaturopath.com/wp-content/uploads/2021/05/How-Stress-Affects-Your-Digestive-System1-1024x558.jpg.

12.4.3. Nutritional Strategies to Support the Gut-Brain Connection

The intricate relationship between diet and the gut-brain axis has been a subject of increasing interest in gastroenterology. An excellent diet containing high levels of some nutrients can profoundly influence gut microbiota, impacting brain function. It has been proven that the presence of the good bacteria , such as *Roseburia intestinalis*, is crucial for maintaining healthy guts and preventing disorders of inflammation and metabolic disorders. This butyrate-producing microbe plays a pivotal function in energy homeostasis and intestinal barrier function. As the dietary pattern shifts towards processed food with high sugar and fat content, this resultant dysbiosis can induce gastrointestinal and neurological symptoms, making it important to have targeted nutritional interventions aimed at improving microbial richness and optimizing the gut-brain axis (Nie et al., 2021). Dietary strategies targeting the consumption of prebiotics and probiotics must be employed in order to stimulate the gut-brain interface. Prebiotics, such as are found in fiber-rich fruits, vegetables, and whole grains, are substrates for beneficial gut bacteria, which may stimulate their growth and activity. Through the promotion of microbial diversity, these food substances can lead to beneficial effects in conditions , such as irritable bowel syndrome and inflammatory bowel disease, where gut-brain communication is impaired. Probiotics, on the other hand, introduce live healthy bacteria into the diet that can restore balance. Taken together, these approaches not only preserve the integrity of the intestinal epithelial barrier but also influence the release of neurotransmitters , such as serotonin. This close interaction underscores the importance of a diet intervention that includes functional foods in order to promote overall well-being (Barbara et al., 2021). Supplementation with omega-3 fatty acids, found in fatty fish and walnuts, is another potent dietary intervention for enhancing the gut-brain connection. Essential fatty acids, omega-3s, are anti-inflammatory and neuroprotective. Evidence suggests that omega-3s can control gene expression associated with gut and brain health and, in response, influence mood and cognition. Since most gastrointestinal and neurological diseases have inflammation as a central causative factor, the supplement of omega-3 fatty acids can decrease intestinal inflammation and result in a healthier gut microbiota. Also, the fatty acids may heal the intestinal epithelial barrier function, improving its defense against pathogenic antigens and reducing the risk of dysbiosis. This exchange yet again highlights how dietary choices are utilized for therapeutic intents in managing neurological dysfunction of the gut (Nie et al., 2021) (Figure 12.17).

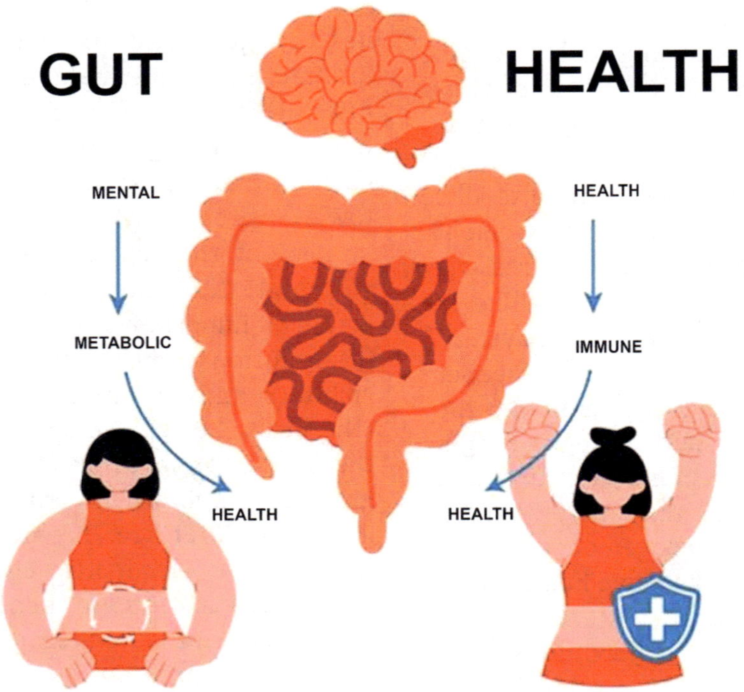

Figure 12.17. Nutritional strategies to support the gut-brain connection.

Source: https://incontact.com.sg/wp-content/uploads/2024/06/gut-brain-connection-1.webp.

12.5. Nutritional Assessment in Gastroenterology

The contribution of nutritional assessment to gastroenterology cannot be overstated, particularly of gastrointestinal illnesses , such as inflammatory bowel disease (IBD). Emerging evidence suggests that diet is integral to the pathogenesis and management of IBD. Researchers have begun examining how environmental factors, including diet, interact with gut microbiota in susceptible subjects. The D-ECCO working group emphasizes the importance of exploring the role of diet, not just as an environmental factor in IBD, but also as a therapeutic intervention. Establishing the specific nutritional deficiencies and implementing dietary intervention would create an avenue for improving patient outcomes and quality of life (Sigall-Boneh et al., 2017). Thus, nutritional status estimation plays a primary role in the treatment regimen of the patient with gastrointestinal disease, so that individual therapeutic measures can be applied according to individual nutritional needs. The development of new nutritional treatments, such as blenderized food for tube-feeding (BFTF), has sparked interest in recent years, especially within pediatric gastroenterology. A big survey among pediatric dietitians revealed heterogeneity regarding the efficacy and safety of BFTF. Although there were concerns from some dietitians around nutritional inadequacy and complications , such as tube blockage and increased infection rates, most saw the potential advantages of decreased reflux and increased caregiver involvement in food care (Armstrong et al., 2016). Such ambivalence in opinion responds to the necessity for a comprehensive nutritional assessment in pediatric patients, particularly those under tube feeding. By identifying unique needs and wants, clinicians can tailor nutrition interventions that not only meet metabolic needs but also family and personal circumstances, thus enhancing compliance and overall outcomes. Aside from basic caloric intake, nutritional evaluation includes the identification of macronutrient and micronutrient deficiencies that may arise due to gastrointestinal malabsorptive disorders. For instance, patients with chronic pancreatitis or celiac disease typically present with significant impairment of nutrient absorption. In such patients, a comprehensive nutritional assessment allows the clinician to formulate elaborate dietary plans that may include supplementation to compensate for some shortages. Physiology of the gut requires the evaluation to be longitudinal and multi-dimensional and to account for changing dynamics of a patient's condition over time. In the end, effective nutrition assessment is a cornerstone in gastric and digestive disease management, connecting diet intervention and improved clinical results and decreasing the risk of further complications.

12.5.1. Methods for Evaluating Nutritional Status

Proper nutritional assessment plays a critical role in the treatment of patients with gastrointestinal disease, as such a diagnosis can have a direct impact on treatment outcome. The correct assessment of nutritional status is typically achieved by clinical examination, anthropometry, laboratory tests, and dietary study. Clinical examination typically begins with a thorough medical history and physical examination that identifies symptoms indicative of malnutrition, such as weight loss, wasting of muscles, and also symptoms of micronutrient deficiencies. Furthermore, anthropometric measurements, such as body mass index (BMI) and waist-to-hip ratio, provide data on fat distribution and body composition, which are of relevance in understanding the repercussions of obesity or undernutrition in gastroenterology patients. A multimodal strategy , such as this, allows health practitioners to devise tailored measures to address the complex interface between nutrition and gastrointestinal health. Biochemical markers play an essential part in the evaluation of nutritional status among patients with gastrointestinal disease. Biochemical tests are able to measure some parameters, like serum albumin, prealbumin, and transferrin levels, that are indicative of protein status and adequacy of nutrition. Reduced levels of serum albumin, for example, may indicate the development of malnutrition or inflammation such that clinicians must place these results in the clinical context. In addition, the measurement of micronutrient concentrations, such as vitamin D, folate, and iron, reveals more about the diet of patients and potential deficiencies that may complicate gastrointestinal illness. All these biochemical markers are combined with the clinical and anthropometric measurements with the purpose of creating a complete picture of a patient's nutritional status and inform proper intervention actions based on specific needs and circumstances, as it is extremely important in gastroenterology. Dietary assessment, including 24-hour dietary recalls and food frequency questionnaires, supplements other instruments by assisting in the identification of patients' consumption patterns and nutrient intake. This information is particularly valuable in gastroenterology, where diet will play a role in disease advancement and treatment. Full dietary evaluation not only identifies areas of deficit or excess but also evaluates suspected food intolerance or allergy contributing to gastrointestinal symptoms. Furthermore, telemedicine technology in the form of food logging software and web-based dietary consultation optimizes access to diet assessment so that patients can actively participate in treatment. Awareness of the patient's diet and food likes/dislikes not only allows them to make better informed choices but also fosters a patient-provider collaborative partnership. Multidisciplinary assessment methods need to be integrated in order to develop balanced nutritional treatment plans in gastroenterology, as food choice and nutrition status are intimately linked with patient outcomes.

12.5.2. Importance of Individualized Nutrition Plans

In gastroenterology, the requirement for individualized nutrition regimens is identified by the unique physiological responses of patients to specific dietary therapy. Gastrointestinal disorders preferentially manifest in dissimilar ways in different individuals based on genetic, environmental, and lifestyle factors. This dissimilarity necessitates individualized nutrition respecting each patient's inherent health conditions, requirements, and preferences. For example, a celiac patient needs a totally gluten-free diet, while a patient with irritable bowel syndrome would need to adhere to a low-FODMAP diet to prevent symptoms. Such an appreciation of the delicate interactions between them enables clinicians to create nutrition recommendations that enhance digestive function and general health efficiently. It is obvious that there is no single-fits-all diet in this multifaceted field, pointing to the paramount importance of personalized nutrition in the therapy of gastrointestinal disease. Taking into account the unique nutritional needs of elderly patients again underlines the necessity of individualized nutritional programs in gastroenterology. As highlighted by more recent research, nutrient requirements also differ according to age, based on comorbidities, medications, and mobility status (Oliveira & Lima, 2025). Personalized nutrition not only addresses the nutritional inadequacies that lead to frailty and deteriorating health status but also preserves cognitive function and quality of life in older people. Personalized nutrition education for this population must be supported by comprehensive knowledge of their health history and daily lifestyle, which can translate into habitual food consumption in health-focused interventions. Moreover, by providing a facilitating environment that includes social and cultural factors, physicians can empower older patients to make food-related decisions in an informed way, thus promoting autonomy and engagement in health care. Technological advancements have also contributed significantly to the development of customized diet plans, making it possible to provide more precise recommendations based on patient choice and nutritional needs. Machine learning and big datasets on diets have enabled nutritionists and medical practitioners to design meal plans in a whole new manner (Ashmitha et al., 2025). One can use these technologies to provide personalized meal recommendations based on individual tastes, nutritional requirements, and even ethnicity. Enhanced recipe recommendation and meal planning features motivate individuals to adhere to dietary guidelines, yet also optimize the cooking satisfaction of healthy food. This technological integration could revolutionize how patients engage with food, making it simpler to adhere to tailored nutrition programs that are good for their gut microbials and lifestyles. Thus, with the continued advancement of personalized nutrition, there are promising paths for addressing the diverse issues posed in gastroenterology (Figure 12.18).

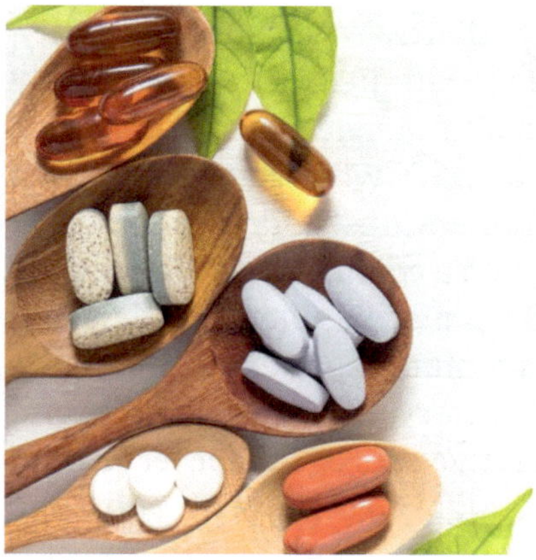

Figure 12.18. Importance of individualized nutrition plans.

Source: https://harborhealth.net/wp-content/uploads/2021/12/importance-of-planning-individual-nutrition-1080x675.jpg.

12.5.3. Role of Dietitians in Gastroenterology

Dietitians play a vital role in the management and treatment of many gastrointestinal illnesses in gastroenterology. Dietitians assess patients' nutritional status and develop individualized dietary treatments addressing specific conditions , such as inflammatory bowel disease (IBD), celiac disease, and nonalcoholic fatty liver disease (NAFLD). These specialists are equipped with the knowledge to identify nutritional deficiencies that may arise as a consequence of compromised absorption or digestion that characterizes these disorders. With medical nutrition therapy (MNT), dietitians guide patients to optimal dietary habits that not only alleviate symptoms but also optimize overall well-being. Their clinical expertise in diet planning facilitates the application of customized approaches considering patients' cultural backgrounds, personal food habits, and comorbidities, ensuring a holistic and effective gastroenterological nutritional program. Furthermore, collaboration between gastroenterologists and dietitians guarantees improved patient outcomes by way of interprofessional practice. Dietitians often work with physicians to develop inclusive care plans that integrate both clinical care and nutritional care. Patient education to educate them on food choices and their implications on gastrointestinal health is paramount in this context. Current studies indicate that proper nutrition counseling will maintain patients on their treatment regimen, thereby leading to enhanced control of disease and quality of life. As a member of the healthcare team, the dietitian's input not only helps improve clinical results but also empowers patients to take an active role in their own nutritional health, which is essential to long-term management of gastrointestinal disease.

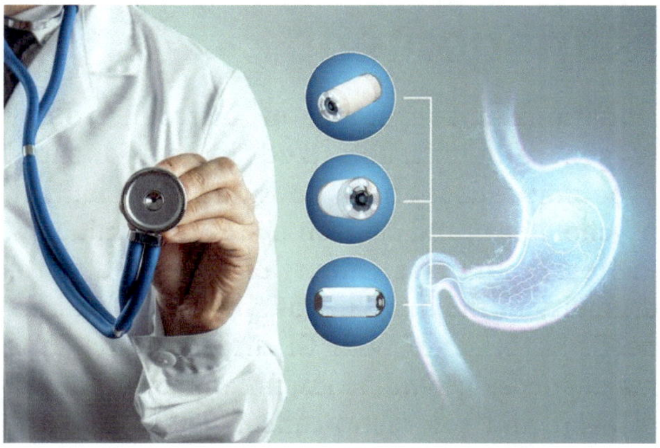

Figure 12.19. Role of dietitians in gastroenterology.

Source: https://www.medicalindependent.ie/wp-content/uploads/2021/05/Page-28-Clinical-Gastroenterology.jpg.

Research and the development of evidence-based dietary advice are also part of the gastroenterologist's role as a dietitian. Because gastrointestinal disease is increasingly the domain of complex understanding of disease and diet interaction, dietitians are contributors to continuous research to determine effective dietetic interventions. Dietary guidance, food behavior, and nutritional skills are all shed light on by their input into clinical recommendations, which reflect current best evidence. This includes identification of particular dietary patterns that may prevent gastrointestinal disease or improve the management of established disease. By keeping current with the most recent scientific evidence, dietitians are able to make recommendations that are not only realistic but also built on solid evidence, setting the stage for improved nutritional futures for patients struggling with difficult gastrointestinal issues (Figure 12.19).

12.6. Challenges in Nutritional Management

Nutritional management in gastroenterology is generally characterized by complicated problems susceptible to multiple medical, psychological, and environmental determinants. Professionals are most often faced with difficulty in the handling of specific nutritional needs of patients with GI diseases, including malabsorption syndromes, inflammatory bowel disease, and colorectal cancer. These diseases are likely to be associated with a variety of complications, from malnutrition and electrolyte imbalance to more critical outcomes, including the necessity for special dietary management. For instance, inflammatory bowel disease patients may require special anti-inflammatory, nutrient-dense diets to heal and bring about inflammation suppression. However, adhering to these diets can be hindered by ignorance or caregiver failure, making the process of nutrition even more difficult. Overcoming these challenges is important to improve the outcomes of patients as well as the overall quality of life for individuals suffering from GI disorders. Another problematic condition is the management of neurodevelopmental disorders , such as autism spectrum disorder (ASD). Nutritional issues are present in such patients, with food selectivity, refusal, and other mealtime issues that greatly complicate adequate nutrient absorption. With the correlation of ASD with gastrointestinal symptoms, practitioners must address nutritional management through a comprehensive approach with modifications in diet, supplementation, and behavioral management. Evidence highlights that while dietary intervention can yield useful outcomes, the effectiveness of such intervention is uncertain and highly contingent upon the individual child's needs and circumstances. Furthermore, the construction of a successful mealtime environment focused on the sensory comfort of ASD children plays an important role in promoting better eating behavior. Thus, addressing the nutritional needs of such patients requires an all-encompassing strategy that is responsive to the interplay of behavioral, nutritional, and psychological factors. Lastly, the onus of the health professionals in bridging the gap between knowledge and practice in nutrition cannot be overstressed. Registered dietitians often encounter key obstacles that hinder effective management, such as caregiver nonadherence and inadequate training in specialized care in nutrition. For instance, a study of South African registered dietitians reported that while the majority had learned some aspect of the management of conditions like cerebral palsy, the training was poor and not in line with policy. Issues mentioned were a lack of adequate communication and inter-professional working among practitioners, undermining the support network for effective nutrition management. These obstacles are recognized and solved by numerous studies as being crucial to enhancing the nutritional literacy of healthcare professionals and outcomes of patients in gastroenterology. Prioritizing professional cooperation and ongoing education in nutrition can help eliminate these challenges significantly and ultimately contribute to better health outcomes for patients in need of it (Figure 12.10).

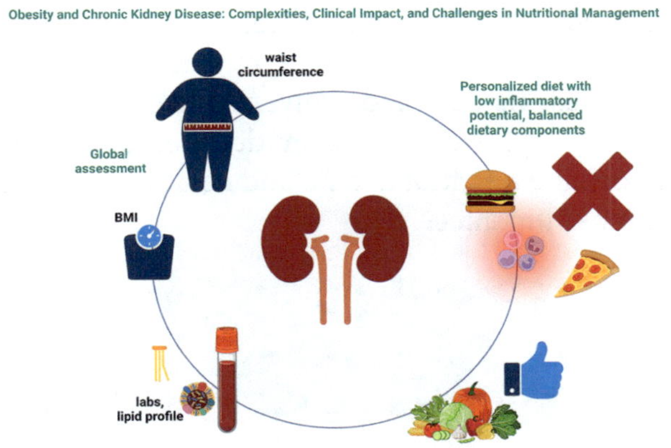

Figure 12.20. Challenges in nutritional management.

Source: https://www.frontiersin.org/files/Articles/1212700/fnut-10-1212700-HTML-r1/image_m/fnut-10-1212700-g001.jpg.

12.6.1. Barriers to Dietary Adherence in Patients

Adherence to prescribed dietetic regimens is inevitable in the treatment of the majority of gastrointestinal disorders. However, patients typically experience overwhelming obstacles that make them unable to adhere to the dietary advice. The primary challenges are that they lack sufficient information regarding the dietetic changes they must adopt and will be advantageous to their conditions, and the diets are complex. They become upset at having to alter well-established eating habits, and non-compliance may follow. In addition, sociocultural factors, including family preference, economic cost, and working environments, also complicate compliance with suggested alterations in diet. Those patients who report that their diets are too limiting may be unable to make these alterations a part of their daily routines, resulting in a cycle of non-compliance that has negative effects on their overall health outcomes (Sharaiha et al., 2023). Psychological considerations are also central to dietary compliance in gastroenterology patients. The majority of individuals suffer from emotional or psychological challenges , such as anxiety and depression, that undermine their capacity to be motivated towards compliance with dietary recommendations. Psychological burdens prevent patients from caring about their health and could lead to consumption depending on psychological comfort rather than nutritional necessity. In addition, the embarrassment associated with certain health ailments can exacerbate guilt or shame and hence induce avoidance behavior related to diet adherence. Those patients judged by medical experts or family members are more likely to shun active participation with dietary advice, creating further distance from efficient control over their health situations. Thus, psychological support for mental well-being is essential for helping patients overcome such challenges and improving diet adherence (Kanth & Inadomi, 2021). Lastly, the patient-physician relationship is also vital in determining diet adherence. Patients frequently report barriers in terms of not having sufficient time to communicate with healthcare workers, lowering the chance of receiving personalized dietary advice and encouragement. When patients are not given the impression that their concerns are being handled appropriately, they will be demotivated and less inclined towards making the necessary adjustments. Effective communication is key to overcoming such barriers, as it develops confidence and commitment in the treatment process. Furthermore, practitioners must adopt a multidisciplinary approach by integrating nutritionists, psychologists, and healthcare experts to ascertain that an integrated support system is developed for patients. An emphasis on establishing definite, doable dietary goals is likely to empower individuals and aid them in surmounting such obstacles to a higher level of compliance with dietary recommendations (Sharaiha et al., 2023).

12.6.2. Cultural and Socioeconomic Factors Affecting Nutrition

Today, cultural and socioeconomic factors profoundly affect dietary habits with a critical impact on health outcomes, particularly in the field of gastroenterology. Globalization has led to a shift where a number of populations have abandoned traditional diets that were characterized by high intake of fruits and vegetables and replaced them with energy-dense foods but nutrient-poor foods , such as fast food and processed food. Consequently, people now more often experience chronic conditions due to food intake, setting the stage for such conditions as obesity, diabetes, and gastrointestinal disease. This dietary change highlights the importance of investigating the interdependence between culture and nutrition since food habits tend to be an indicator of what a community values and how it performs on health. Failure to maintain such practices has the potential of eliciting negative consequences not just for the individuals but also for public health systems that are dealing with diet-related diseases, emphasizing the need for policies that facilitate healthier dieting amid different cultural settings (Bhatoolaul et al., 2024). Socioeconomic status plays a significant role in determining nutritional patterns since it dictates individuals' ability to access food and their capability to make healthy choices. Those who have lower socioeconomic status frequently encounter barriers like reduced access to supermarkets with fresh produce, as well as financial limitations that make it less affordable to buy healthier foods. This, coupled with the availability of fast food and processed foods, exacerbates dietary issues among the poor. Evidence indicates that such socioeconomic disparities not only lead to poorer diets but also have an immense impact on health outcomes, with the underprivileged groups having greater rates of gastrointestinal illnesses. All efforts to reverse such disparities should be directed towards making food more affordable and accessible, improving nutrition knowledge, and establishing an environment that promotes healthy food choices, thus responding to both individual and community health needs (Kabata, 2021). Also, cultural identity determines dietary patterns and practices, often dictating what is healthy and acceptable to eat in various societies. Established conventional foods and feeding styles shaped over decades or longer determine nutritional data and health behaviors in most instances.

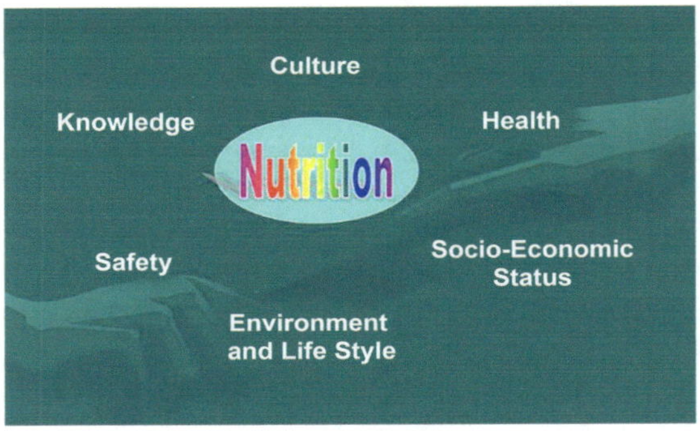

Figure 12.21. Cultural and socioeconomic factors affecting nutrition.

Source: https://image.slideserve.com/1296738/factors-affecting-nutrition-l.jpg.

However, food system changes resulting from globalization have broken these domestic food cultures, pushing individuals towards dietary practices that may be discordant with their culture of origin. The resulting loss of identity not only affects physical health, in terms of a decrease in typical healthy food intake, but also potentially produces psychological distress, which is itself likely to affect eating behaviors. Identification and promotion of culturally sensitive nutritional interventions that honor traditional practices are able to give a sense of belonging, ultimately promoting nutritional health and reducing gastrointestinal symptoms prevalent among various populations, as they navigate the subtleties of food contexts in the modern world (Bhatoolaul et al., 2024) (Figure 12.21).

12.6.3. Addressing Misinformation About Diets and Supplements

Misinformation about diets and supplements is one of the biggest problems in the specialty of gastroenterology, particularly in treating conditions , such as irritable bowel syndrome (IBS). They typically derive themselves from anecdotal experience or from news transmitted via social media and not evidence-based scientific facts. Such an approach can lead to inappropriate dietary habits that exacerbate gastrointestinal symptoms. To face this challenge, one needs to have a holistic view of nutritional science that combines different disciplines , such as biology and psychology. The Academy of Nutrition Sciences strongly argues that providing effective dietary advice must consider the intricate interaction between personal health requirements and accessible scientific evidence. Effective communication among patients and health practitioners is critical in dispelling myths and facilitating adherence to evidence-based nutritional protocols, thereby enhancing patient outcomes in gastrointestinal disorders (Hickson et al., 2024). Further, the rapid dissemination of information, particularly through the internet, has contributed to the marketing of unsubstantiated information regarding dietary supplements. The majority of patients with gastrointestinal illness, in a last attempt to attain quick relief, are still susceptible to the allure of products marketed as "miracle cures." Scrutiny of those claims, though, reveals that most supplements are unproven or lack more than limited supporting evidence, as explained through various paradigms of nutrition (Pasta et al., 2024). The lack of regulation in the supplement sector only adds to the complexity; most will carry unstated ingredients or not live up to stated benefits. Therefore, there is a part for healthcare professionals to play in counseling patients on reading critically dietary supplement labels and making informed decisions based on evidence and not hype-laden marketing. To win the battle against misinformation about diets and supplements effectively, one needs a multi-level approach. Clinical education of healthcare professionals and patients can develop awareness of reliable dietary habits. This includes learning how to assess the validity of diet-related information and distinguish between evidence-based advice and unsubstantiated assertions. Individualized management of conditions like IBS through diet, which is sensitive to the patient's specific symptoms and eating history, holds the key to success (Pasta et al., 2024). Facilitating media literacy and critical examination of nutrition can allow medical professionals to empower patients to make informed choices. Joint efforts among nutrition experts, healthcare practitioners, and reputable groups can raise additional public awareness and facilitate the utilization of evidence-based eating habits, significantly improving overall gastrointestinal health care (Hickson et al., 2024).

CLOSER LOOK

PERSONAL FOOD HABITS:

Personal food habits encompass the choices, patterns, and routines that shape an individual's daily diet. A closer look at these habits reveals how they influence overall health, energy balance, and risk for chronic diseases. Food habits are shaped by a complex interplay of cultural norms, socioeconomic factors, personal preferences, lifestyle, and psychological influences, making them highly individual and variable over time. One key aspect of personal food habits is meal frequency and timing. Some people follow traditional three-meal patterns, while others prefer smaller, more frequent meals or intermittent fasting. Timing can affect metabolism, energy levels, and even digestive health. For instance, late-night eating has been associated with impaired glucose regulation and weight gain, whereas consistent meal schedules support better appetite control and nutrient utilization.

Food choices and preferences are central to dietary habits. These choices are influenced by taste preferences, cultural traditions, beliefs about health, and convenience. Diets rich in fruits, vegetables, whole grains, lean proteins, and healthy fats are linked to lower risk of obesity, cardiovascular disease, and diabetes. Conversely, frequent consumption of ultra-processed foods, sugary drinks, and high-fat snacks can contribute to nutrient deficiencies, inflammation, and metabolic disorders. Understanding one's own tendencies—such as reliance on fast food during busy periods or emotional eating in response to stress—helps identify areas for improvement.

Portion control and eating environment also shape habits. Mindful eating, which emphasizes paying attention to hunger and fullness cues, can prevent overeating. Eating while distracted, such as in front of screens, often leads to larger portions and reduced awareness of satiety signals. Social factors—family meals, peer influence, and workplace culture—further impact what, when, and how much people eat.

Psychological and emotional aspects of food habits are increasingly recognized. Stress, mood, and mental health can drive food choices, often promoting comfort foods high in sugar or fat. Conversely, individuals who cultivate positive relationships with food and prioritize balanced meals tend to experience better mental and physical outcomes. Monitoring and reflecting on personal food habits can be transformative. Keeping food diaries, planning meals, and gradually incorporating healthier options can improve nutrient intake, support sustainable weight management, and enhance overall well-being. Personalized nutrition approaches, which consider individual preferences, health status, and lifestyle, are particularly effective.

A closer examination of personal food habits highlights that diet is more than mere sustenance—it is a dynamic interplay of behavior, culture, psychology, and physiology. By understanding and adjusting these habits thoughtfully, individuals can promote long-term health and foster a positive relationship with food.

SUMMARY

Overall, the relationship between nutrition and gastrointestinal health is paramount, particularly in patients with inflammatory bowel diseases (IBD) , such as Crohn's disease and ulcerative colitis. Several studies have demonstrated that such disorders are linked to severe nutritional deficits, which can compromise patient health. For example, evidence indicates that even those patients with a normal Body Mass Index (BMI) can have their muscle mass reduced as a result of malabsorption syndromes, which are frequently seen in IBD. This highlights the need for detailed nutritional evaluations, incorporating the use of bioimpedance analysis to find and correct underlying nutritional deficits effectively. Without these observations, patients will remain undiagnosed and untreated, leading to further complications and deteriorating health conditions, highlighting the imperative for ongoing nutritional evaluation in clinical practice (Makharia et al., 2024). Furthermore, the need for education on nutritional issues in gastroenterology cannot be overstated. The global response to the COVID-19 pandemic has demonstrated the relevance of virtual education programs in disseminating information on important topics in the area of applicability to nutritional support. WGO survey results reflect an overwhelming consensus for ongoing education programs on nutrition as a priority topic, followed by clinical gastroenterology and endoscopy. By providing primary emphasis on educational outreach through the spheres of virtual platforms, gastroenterology professionals not only improve the knowledge and application of nutritional principles but also enhance patient care at the global level. This shift towards distant forms of learning is a hopeful opportunity to improve the clinical knowledge base across different geographic areas (Makharia et al., 2024). In summary, the nutritional aspect of gastroenterology presents both challenges and opportunities in clinical practice. Incorporation of nutrition in the disease management of gastrointestinal conditions is essential and can significantly enhance patient outcomes. As increased knowledge of the interaction between nutrition and gastrointestinal health is made available, our approach to treating patients should also evolve. Future discussion and research must be focused on simplifying educational curricula that incorporate these nutritional standards, promoting interdisciplinary practice that incorporates dietitians alongside gastroenterology specialists. Ultimately, creating an environment where nutritional well-being is recognized as an integrated part of gastrointestinal care will not only benefit specific patients but also the development of gastroenterological practice and education in general. Through this integrated approach, the practice can shift toward greater patient well-being and overall health results.

Understanding the nutritional aspect of gastroenterology is crucial in managing most gastrointestinal diseases effectively. Nutrition plays a crucial role in the prevention as well as management of diseases , such as inflammatory bowel disease, celiac disease, and peptic ulcers. An individually tailored diet significantly mitigates symptoms and improves the quality of life for patients with these conditions. For instance, prebiotic and probiotic dietary interventions have been shown to enhance gut health by modulating the microbiome and thus sustaining gastrointestinal function. Moreover, adequate intake of micronutrients, particularly vitamins and minerals, is required because gastrointestinal diseases lead to malabsorption and subsequently deficiencies. The healthcare professionals should thus prioritize nutritional evaluation to enable holistic care. Individualization of diet to address the requirements of a subject improves clinical outcomes and management of chronic gastrointestinal disease. In gastroenterology, some nutrients and dietary habits have been particularly helpful. For example, inclusion of soluble fiber materials , such as oats and legumes, contributes to the mitigation of gastrointestinal disease symptoms through improvement in regularity of bowel movements and maintenance of gut barrier function. Fatty acids, particularly omega-3s in fish and flaxseeds, also have anti-inflammatory properties that would benefit inflammatory bowel disease patients. Moreover, do not take hydration lightly; the right fluid intake is crucial in ensuring healthy digestion and avoiding problems , such as dehydration, particularly for patients who experience diarrhea or vomiting. These high-nutrient-dense foods and a well-balanced hydration regimen form a basis for a therapeutic dietary regimen that can be used to complement conventional medical therapies and improve the overall health of patients suffering from gastrointestinal ailments. Finally, there is a need to pay attention to the wider implications of food interventions in gastroenterology by recognizing the effect of social, economic, and cultural influences on food intake. For instance, there is limited access to healthy food in certain populations, which contributes to a higher incidence of gastrointestinal disease. This necessitates a response to diet education from an inter-professional perspective involving the scientific rationale behind nutrition as well as socio-economic factors for patients. Tailored interventions should then focus on responding to provision, education, and support to facilitate patients in making beneficial dietary choices. Integration of environmental factors, such as sustainable food consumption, can further enhance the efficacy of nutritional support in gastroenterology clinics. Therefore, advocacy of a holistic understanding of nutritional elements, grounded in both private and public health issues and social processes, is critical to effective management in this regard.

References

1. Ford, S., Howard, R., & Oyebode, J. (2012). Psychosocial aspects of coeliac disease: a cross-sectional survey of a UK population. *British journal of health psychology*, *17*(4), 743–757. https://doi.org/10.1111/j.2044-8287.2012.02069.x (accessed on 16th July 2025).
2. Al-Beltagi, M. (2024). Nutritional management and autism spectrum disorder: A systematic review. *World Journal of Clinical Pediatrics, 13.* https://www.semanticscholar.org/paper/da40f0f83cb419bbda59a4060b723d0cc5e312d9 (accessed on 16th July 2025).
3. Sigall-Boneh, R., Levine, A., Lomer, M., Wierdsma, N., Allan, P., Fiorino, G., Gatti, S., Jonkers, D., Kierkus, J., Katsanos, K. H., Melgar, S., Yuksel, E. S., Whelan, K., Wine, E., & Gerasimidis, K. (2017). Research Gaps in Diet and Nutrition in Inflammatory Bowel Disease. A Topical Review by D-ECCO Working Group [Dietitians of ECCO]. *Journal of Crohn's & colitis, 11*(12), 1407–1419. https://doi.org/10.1093/ecco-jcc/jjx109(accessed on 16th July 2025).
4. Armstrong, J., Buchanan, E., Duncan, H., Gerasimidis, K., et al. (2016). *Dietitians' perceptions and experience of blenderized feeds for pediatric tube-feeding.* https://core.ac.uk/download/46559249.pdf (accessed on 16th July 2025).
5. Ashmitha, B. M., Tom, A., Paul, A. M., Abhiroop, M. P., & Aswathy, T. S. (2025). Recipe recommendation system using NLP, deep learning. *International Journal of Scientific Research in Engineering and Management.* https://www.semanticscholar.org/paper/41a6e3d6716d86cddfc88965985dce3f575958d8 (accessed on 16th July 2025).
6. Ribichini, E., Stigliano, S., Rossi, S., Zaccari, P., Sacchi, M. C., Bruno, G., Badiali, D., & Severi, C. (2019). Role of Fibre in Nutritional Management of Pancreatic Diseases. *Nutrients, 11*(9), 2219. https://doi.org/10.3390/nu11092219(accessed on 16th July 2025).
7. Barbara, G., Barbaro, M. R., Fuschi, D., Palombo, M., Falangone, F., Cremon, C., Marasco, G., et al. (2021). Inflammatory and microbiota-related regulation of the intestinal epithelial barrier. *Frontiers in Nutrition, 8.* https://doi.org/10.3389/fnut.2021.718356 (accessed on 16th July 2025).
8. Bhatoolaul, Y., Alrefaei, A., & Jeewon, R. (2024). Narrative review on the factors affecting fast food consumption among adults. *Current Research in Nutrition and Food Science Journal.* https://www.semanticscholar.org/paper/3a786a90ff499ff242e4a96995a36ad94b179e53 (accessed on 16th July 2025).
9. Caio, G., Volta, U., Sapone, A., Leffler, D. A., De Giorgio, R., Catassi, C., & Fasano, A. (2019). Celiac disease: A comprehensive current review. *BMC Medicine, 17.* https://doi.org/10.1186/s12916-019-1380-z (accessed on 16th July 2025).
10. Chalasani, N., Younossi, Z. M., Lavine, J. E., Charlton, M., Cusi, K., Rinella, M. E., Harrison, S. A., et al. (2017). The diagnosis and management of nonalcoholic fatty liver disease: Practice guidance from the American Association for the Study of Liver Diseases. *Hepatology, 67,* 328–357. https://doi.org/10.1002/hep.29367 (accessed on 16th July 2025).
11. Chandrakar, A. (2024). *Exploring Diverse Aspects of Celiac Disease – A Review.* https://core.ac.uk/download/617706676.pdf (accessed on 16th July 2025).
12. Chaudhury, A., Duvoor, C., Dendi, V. S., Kraleti, S., Chada, A., Ravilla, R., Marco, A., et al. (2017). Clinical review of antidiabetic drugs: Implications for type 2 diabetes mellitus management. *Frontiers in Endocrinology, 8.* https://doi.org/10.3389/fendo.2017.00006 (accessed on 16th July 2025).

13. Clerici, L., Bottari, D., & Bottari, B. (2025). Gut microbiome, diet and depression: Literature review of microbiological, nutritional and neuroscientific aspects. *Current Nutrition Reports, 14.* https://www.semanticscholar.org/paper/b7b3a7403b0fc0d6821b5d30849bb67f12e27439 (accessed on 16th July 2025).

14. Cryan, J. F., O'Riordan, K. J., Cowan, C. S. M., Sandhu, K. V., Bastiaanssen, T. F. S., Boehme, M., Codagnone, M. G., et al. (2019). The microbiota-gut-brain axis. *Physiological Reviews, 99*, 1877–2013. https://doi.org/10.1152/physrev.00018.2018 (accessed on 16th July 2025).

15. Evert, A. B., Dennison, M., Gardner, C. D., Garvey, W. T., Lau, K. H. K., MacLeod, J., Mitri, J., et al. (2019). Nutrition therapy for adults with diabetes or prediabetes: A consensus report. *Diabetes Care, 42*, 731–754. https://doi.org/10.2337/dci19-0014 (accessed on 16th July 2025).

16. Feldstein, A. E., Kharbanda, K. K., Kirpich, I. A., McClain, C., et al. (2018). *Role of nutrition in alcoholic liver disease: Summary of the symposium at the ESBRA 2017 Congress.* https://core.ac.uk/download/323064796.pdf (accessed on 16th July 2025).

17. Gainutdin, A. E., Nersesov, A. V., Raisova, A. M., Suleimenova, D. S., Ashimova, N. A., Madenova, S. S., Shamshidinova, M. A., et al. (2024). *Determination of nutritional status in patients with inflammatory bowel diseases using bioimpedance research: Analysis of clinical cases.* Наука и здравоохранение. https://www.semanticscholar.org/paper/154abf68f7136c272bda0eba6f2cba5b7b322da1 (accessed on 16th July 2025).

18. Guarner, F., Sanders, M. E., Szajewska, H., Cohen, H., Eliakim, R., Herrera-deGuise, C., Karakan, T., et al. (2024). World Gastroenterology Organisation global guidelines: Probiotics and prebiotics. *Journal of Clinical Gastroenterology, 58*, 533–553. https://doi.org/10.1097/mcg.0000000000002002 (accessed on 16th July 2025).

19. Hickson, M., Papoutsakis, C., Madden, A., Smith, M. A., & Whelan, K. (2024). Nature of the evidence base and approaches to guide nutrition interventions for individuals: A position paper from the Academy of Nutrition Sciences. *British Journal of Nutrition.* https://doi.org/10.1017/s0007114524000291 (accessed on 16th July 2025).

20. Holubar, S. D., Lightner, A. L., Poylin, V., Vogel, J. D., Gaertner, W. B., Davis, B. R., Davis, K. G., et al. (2021). The American Society of Colon and Rectal Surgeons clinical practice guidelines for the surgical management of ulcerative colitis. *Diseases of the Colon & Rectum, 64*, 783–804. https://doi.org/10.1097/dcr.0000000000002037 (accessed on 16th July 2025).

21. Staudacher, H. M., Irving, P. M., Lomer, M. C. E., & Whelan, K. (2017). The challenges of control groups, placebos and blinding in clinical trials of dietary interventions. *The Proceedings of the Nutrition Society, 76*(3), 203–212. https://doi.org/10.1017/S0029665117000350(accessed on 16th July 2025).

22. Jacobson, D., van Niekerk, E., & Marais, M. (2024). Current practices and challenges of registered dietitians in the nutritional management of children with cerebral palsy in South Africa. *South African Journal of Clinical Nutrition, 37*, 84–91. https://www.semanticscholar.org/paper/f1294a86bed34a3d50f9f77751631a0f7d7b4a35 (accessed on 16th July 2025).

23. Jo, N. J., & Ortega-Santos, C. (2024). *The impacts of the low-FODMAP diet on the management of irritable bowel syndrome symptoms: Possibilities, feasibility, and alternatives.* https://core.ac.uk/download/604655390.pdf (accessed on 16th July 2025).

24. Julius, S. (2025). Nutritional psychiatry: The impact of diet on mental health. *Newport International Journal of Research in Medical Sciences.* https://www.semanticscholar.org/paper/114c76239915c51148b054874d59404c14300675 (accessed on 16th July 2025).

25. Kanth, P., & Inadomi, J. M. (2021). Screening and prevention of colorectal cancer. *BMJ.* https://doi.org/10.1136/bmj.n1855 (accessed on 16th July 2025).

26. Kapoor, T., Kansal, A., Jaffar, M., Venkatesan, D., Sarmah, R. G., Jyothi, R., & Verma, S. (2025). Nutritional innovations in aquafeed for sustainable and eco-friendly fish farming. *International Journal of Aquatic Research and Environmental Studies.* https://www.semanticscholar.org/paper/fadeb293d35ba8c0da21940902b4254e1a256521 (accessed on 16th July 2025).

27. Khan, H. T., Siddiqui, S., Tahir, S., Siddiqui, S., Akhlaq, M., & Alum, M. K. (2025). *Cichorium intybus* (Beekhe Kasni): A comprehensive analysis of traditional, pharmacological, and nutritional aspects. *Insights – Journal of Health and Rehabilitation.* https://www.semanticscholar.org/paper/5116007455faa9f6fdfb4ee9262fce55a227c914 (accessed on 16th July 2025).

28. Krznarić, Ž. (2022). Burden of obesity in gastrointestinal and liver diseases. *United European Gastroenterology Journal, 10*, 629–630. https://www.semanticscholar.org/paper/faa5e4329fc0ede5001218e3f86e462f76781968 (accessed on 16th July 2025).

29. Lamb, C. A., Kennedy, N. A., Raine, T., Hendy, P., Smith, P. J., Limdi, J. K., Hayee, B., et al. (2019). British Society of Gastroenterology consensus guidelines on the management of inflammatory bowel disease in adults. *Gut, 68*, s1–s106. https://doi.org/10.1136/gutjnl-2019-318484 (accessed on 16th July 2025).

30. Makharia, G., Agrawal, S., Hansen-Barkun, C., Sadgehi, A., Moreira, L., Lee, Y. Y., Leung, W., et al. (2024). Virtual education is the need of the hour for the global gastroenterology community: A survey of leaders of professional gastroenterology organizations. *Journal of Gastrointestinal and Liver Diseases, 33*(3), 418–423. https://www.semanticscholar.org/paper/c0b914c3b341820ab23fd8e321b819ac6b7f8659 (accessed on 16th July 2025).

31. McClave, S. A., Taylor, B., Martindale, R. G., Warren, M., Johnson, D. R., Braunschweig, C., McCarthy, M. S., et al. (2016). Guidelines for the provision and assessment of nutrition support therapy in the adult critically ill patient. *Journal of Parenteral and Enteral Nutrition, 40*, 159–211. https://doi.org/10.1177/0148607115621863 (accessed on 16th July 2025).

32. Mishra, C., & Mewani, A. (2025). Exploring gut microbiome, gut-brain axis and relationship with exercise; exploring the impact of exercise on metabolic and mental well-being. *International Journal of Horticulture, Agriculture and Food Science.* https://www.semanticscholar.org/paper/09cab30d0452f05e029540078398067a836aefb9 (accessed on 16th July 2025).

33. Nie, K., Ma, K., Luo, W., Shen, Z., Yang, Z., Xiao, M., Tong, T., et al. (2021). *Roseburia intestinalis*: A beneficial gut organism from the discoveries in genus and species. *Frontiers in Cellular and Infection Microbiology, 11.* https://doi.org/10.3389/fcimb.2021.757718 (accessed on 16th July 2025).

34. Oliveira, R., & Lima, J. (2025). Desafios e oportunidades na nutrição geriátrica: Rumo a um envelhecimento saudável. *RIAGE – Revista Ibero-Americana de Gerontologia.* https://www.semanticscholar.org/paper/2f35a5f37ff90ed2bc9d596fd1aece6f3f92b8b8 (accessed on 16th July 2025).

35. Pasta, A., Formisano, E., Calabrese, F., Plaz Torres, M., Bodini, G., Marabotto, E., Pisciotta, L., et al. (2024). Food intolerances, food allergies and IBS: Lights and shadows. *Nutrients, 16*, 265–265. https://doi.org/10.3390/nu16020265 (accessed on 16th July 2025).

36. Qiu, P., Ishimoto, T., Fu, L., Zhang, J., Zhang, Z., & Liu, Y. (2022). The gut microbiota in inflammatory bowel disease. *Frontiers in Cellular and Infection Microbiology, 12.* https://doi.org/10.3389/fcimb.2022.733992 (accessed on 16th July 2025).

37. Sabo, U., Jamilu, M., & Ali, M. (2024). Assessment of nutritional value of *Azanza garckenia* (Goron Tula/Apple Snot) in Maiduguri metropolis. *International Journal of Convergent and Informatics Science Research.* https://www.semanticscholar.org/paper/6138e7aed1c9a17b8aa9e5893e7cb7c069fa56ac (accessed on 16th July 2025).

38. Salminen, S., Collado, M. C., Endo, A., Hill, C., Lebeer, S., Quigley, E. M. M., Sanders, M. E., et al. (2021). The International Scientific Association of Probiotics and Prebiotics (ISAPP) consensus statement on the definition and scope of postbiotics. *Nature Reviews Gastroenterology & Hepatology, 18*, 649–667. https://doi.org/10.1038/s41575-021-00440-6 (accessed on 16th July 2025).

39. Sharaiha, R. Z., Shikora, S. A., White, K. P., Macedo, G., Toouli, J., & Kow, L. (2023). Summarizing consensus guidelines on obesity management. *Journal of Clinical Gastroenterology, 57*, 967–976. https://doi.org/10.1097/mcg.0000000000001916 (accessed on 16th July 2025).

40. Sibal, A., Gopalan, S., Kapoor, A., & Bhatia, V. (2015). *Textbook of pediatric gastroenterology, hepatology and nutrition.* https://www.semanticscholar.org/paper/71cc2844a3eded1cd1377d4be6156a4a88570851 (accessed on 16th July 2025).

41. Silverman, J. A., Chugh, A., Hollier, J., Martin, N., Raghu, V., Rosas-Blum, E., van Tilburg, M. A. L., et al. (2024). Using social media for patient care, research, and professional development: A North American Society of Pediatric Gastroenterology, Hepatology, and Nutrition position paper. *Journal of Pediatric Gastroenterology and Nutrition.* https://www.semanticscholar.org/paper/0fa7b08841a6de06d503f0a136f9a061d3550260 (accessed on 16th July 2025).

42. Sionek, B., & Szydłowska, A. (2025). Probiotics and prebiotics in the aspect of health benefits and the development of novel plant-based functional food. *Applied Sciences.* https://www.semanticscholar.org/paper/539d10aaf5d0d203e8fbc0f8ddc420ad1b097cf3 (accessed on 16th July 2025).

43. Swanson, K. S., Gibson, G. R., Hutkins, R., Reimer, R. A., Reid, G., Verbeke, K., Scott, K. P., et al. (2020). The International Scientific Association for Probiotics and Prebiotics (ISAPP) consensus statement on the definition and scope of synbiotics. *Nature Reviews Gastroenterology & Hepatology, 17*, 687–701. https://doi.org/10.1038/s41575-020-0344-2 (accessed on 16th July 2025).

44. Triana, A. J., Gusdorf, R. E., Shah, K. P., & Horst, S. (2020). Technology literacy as a barrier to telehealth during COVID-19. *Telemedicine Journal and e-Health, 26*, 1118, 1119. https://doi.org/10.1089/tmj.2020.0155 (accessed on 16th July 2025).

45. Vašková, J., Stupák, M., Vidová Ugurbaş, M., Židzik, J., & Mičková, H. (2025). Therapeutic uses of retinol and retinoid-related antioxidants. *Molecules, 30.* https://www.semanticscholar.org/paper/553a5b45a117189c1d4692f3d228ee720c14dcd3 (accessed on 16th July 2025).

46. Vilstrup, H., Amodio, P., Bajaj, J. S., Córdoba, J., Ferenci, P., Mullen, K. D., Weißenborn, K., et al. (2014). Hepatic encephalopathy in chronic liver disease: 2014 practice guideline by the American Association for the Study of Liver Diseases and the European Association for the Study of the Liver. *Hepatology, 60*, 715–735. https://doi.org/10.1002/hep.27210 (accessed on 16th July 2025).

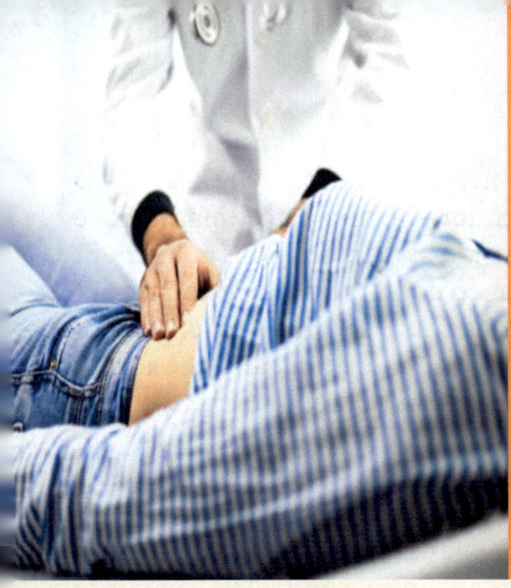

Chapter 13

PEDIATRIC GASTROENTEROLOGY

Contents

Introduction

Pediatric gastroenterology is a specialist field that is committed to the diagnosis and management of gastrointestinal diseases in infants, children, and adolescents. The field encompasses a wide range of diseases, from common ailments like gastroesophageal reflux and constipation to severe illnesses , such as inflammatory bowel disease and cow milk protein allergy (CMPA). Understanding the unique physiological and developmental characteristics of a child's gastrointestinal system is essential to its proper care and treatment. Advances in pediatric gastroenterology have been achieved through an increasing body of evidence, leading to stricter diagnostic criteria and treatment plans tailored to younger patients. As highlighted in current bibliometric studies, the growth in research on CMPA is a sign of a growing concern with tackling gastrointestinal complications in children, thus informing clinical practice and enhancing patient outcomes (Zhou et al., 2025). Nutrition in the treatment of child patients is also a critical component of pediatric gastroenterology. Food at the appropriate time not only supports development and growth in young patients but also helps considerably in treating a number of gastrointestinal system disorders. For instance, preterm low-birth-weight infants have been of particular interest in clinical guidelines for their feeding. The latest advancement in nutrient intake and care of these vulnerable groups accentuates the importance of great research to present solid evidence to support sound feeding strategies (Konchakovska & Shunko, 2024). Additionally, their care includes making tough choices regarding breastfeeding, formula-feeding, and the use of fortified milk, all of which require knowing about the pathophysiology behind their gastrointestinal issues. Multidisciplinary treatment approaches in pediatric gastroenterology are necessary to ensure comprehensive care for patients. The collaboration of pediatricians, gastroenterologists, nutritionists, and dietitians ensures that all aspects of a child's well-being are taken care of. Such integration is important in aspects of chronic disease management, where intervention can significantly alter the trajectory of a child's well-being. Emerging trends in research also bring into focus the significance of the gut microbiome and the development of therapeutic interventions, for example, immunotherapy for diseases like CMPA (Zhou et al., 2025). Over time, the area is likely to progress even more, with continued exploration of new treatments and prevention regimens being a major driving force in shaping future practice and quality of care provided to children with gastrointestinal disorders (Figure 13.1).

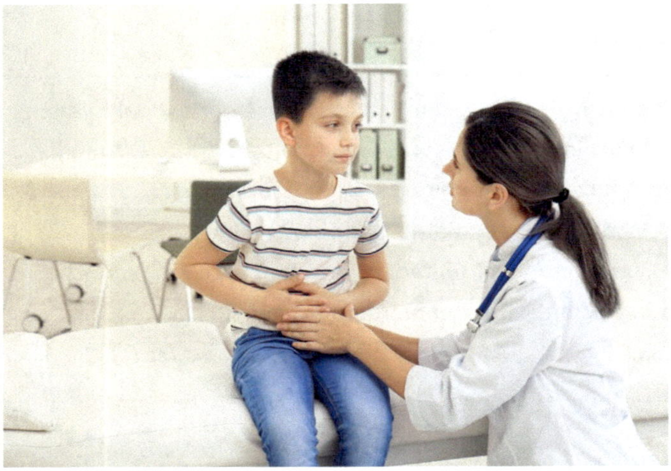

Figure 13.1. Pediatric gastroenterology is diagnosing and treating.

Source: https://productimages.withfloats.com/serviceimages/tile/6503ea7a6c38a85a3eec7042pediatric-gastroenterology-1024x705.

Definition and Scope of Pediatric Gastroenterology

The subspecialty of pediatric gastroenterology is a very specialized branch of medicine dedicated to the diagnosis, management, and treatment of gastrointestinal diseases in children from infancy through adolescence. The subspecialty focuses on a wide range of conditions, including but not limited to gastroesophageal reflux disease, inflammatory bowel disease, celiac disease, and many liver disorders. Pediatric gastroenterologists are not only capable of handling the complexity of such diseases in a developing body but are also attuned to the psychological and emotional aspects of childhood illnesses. The way children develop and grow necessitates a special handling in treatment, distinguishing pediatric gastroenterology from its adult counterpart. Furthermore, educational approaches to family and caregivers are a common denominator in this specialty, acknowledging the importance of support systems in being able to handle these chronic diseases effectively. Prevention and early detection of gastrointestinal diseases are also part of the pediatric gastroenterology field. Pediatric gastroenterologists also perform various preventive measures, like nutritional counseling and lifestyle modifications, to curb the increasing trend of obesity, a growing public health problem in America, spreading to approximately 17% of children and adolescents. The gravity of this problem is underscored by the associated health complications, like type 2 diabetes and coronary heart disease (Ameer & Weintraub, 2018). Thus, combating obesity through effective communication and intervention is essential. Pediatric clinicians emphasize the need for comprehensive management plans with dietary intervention, physical activity, and behavioral treatment to reverse obesity as well as its related gastrointestinal complications. Assessment of these interventions highlights the importance of early pediatric developmental health, eventually translating to better outcomes. In addition, technology and methodological progress have significantly broadened the diagnostic capability in pediatric gastroenterology. Techniques , such as endoscopy, ultrasound, and advanced imaging allow proper estimation of gastrointestinal function and structure. Of special interest are innovations , such as the Endocuff Vision, which have been shown to improve lesion identification during colonoscopies while reducing examination time (Garcia et al., 2019). Such technology is particularly valuable because it supports the identification of precursors to more severe conditions that can affect children's health in the long run. Further, the emphasis on the use of state-of-the-art technology underscores the need for continuing professional development in pediatric gastroenterologists so that clinicians apply optimal practices both in diagnostics and therapeutics. The call for new approaches indicates the commitment of the profession to advance patient care, ultimately benefiting children with gastrointestinal ailments in terms of improved quality of life (Figure 13.2).

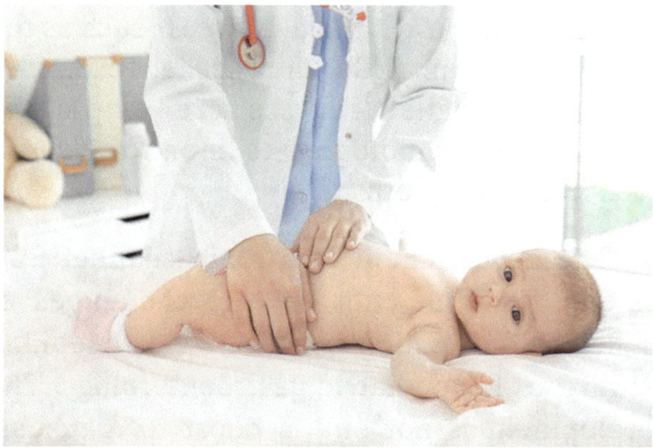

Figure 13.2. Pediatric gastroenterology is a specialized.

Source: https://gastrohealth.com/-/media/decorative-images/specialty-services/baby-gets-an-examination.ashx.

Importance of Specialized Care for Children

In pediatric gastroenterology, there should be specialized treatment for accommodating the children's individual physiological and psychological needs. The gastrointestinal diseases in children are very different compared to adults and thus need certain diagnostic and therapeutic approaches. For instance, conditions , such as NAFLD need developmental factors and special intervention strategies to be taken into account. Literature indicates that a large majority of children with NAFLD require dyslipidemia interventions as per guidelines, which reinforces the necessity for pediatric professionals with expertise in the complexity of lipid management in children (Harlow et al., 2018). Advanced practitioners' ability to deconstruct complex clinical cases enhances the effectiveness of treatment protocols with better child health outcomes. One of the important areas of specialized pediatric treatment involves the application of the newer diagnostic technology that can potentially provide more accurate diagnoses in gastrointestinal conditions. The majority of the functional and motility disorders in children are typically underdiagnosed, as the traditional tests are limited. Devices , such as the electrogastrogram (EGG) are excellent examples of how specialist centers are employing noninvasive technologies to monitor gastric electrical activity effectively.

The development of a multi-channel EGG system, one that cuts out the challenges of single-channel testing, is a future worth looking forward to for pediatric gastroenterology. The development is not only a boost to diagnosis but also allows specialists to be better able to observe patients and customize treatment schemes based on real-time data (Coleman et al., 2018). Due to this reason, the presence of such advanced diagnostic equipment in expert facilities is paramount to optimizing patient care. The psychological aspects of gastrointestinal illnesses in children also illustrate the necessity of specialty treatment.

Children with chronic gastrointestinal illness can suffer deeply from emotional and psychological distress, which exacerbates the physical symptomology. Specialty pediatric gastroenterologists are more likely to work in conjunction with mental health professionals in an effort to adopt an integrated treatment approach that involves both the medical and psychosocial aspects of treatment. This integrated practice ensures that children and their families receive comprehensive care throughout diagnosis and treatment, fostering an environment of healing. Also, by addressing the physiological symptoms and the emotional condition of children, specialized care significantly enhances the quality of life of children, affirming the need for specialist intervention in pediatric gastroenterology.

Overview of Common Gastrointestinal Disorders in Children

Gastrointestinal illness in children consists of a range of diseases that can have far-reaching effects on their growth, development, and overall well-being. Functional gastrointestinal diseases , such as irritable bowel syndrome (IBS) and functional abdominal pain, are some of the most prevalent disorders. The illnesses consist of recurrent digestive symptoms with no apparent organic etiology. The outcomes of these illnesses can be formidable, leading to a poor quality of life in children. Intensive management and assessment protocols are needed to manage these conditions properly, with a focus on relief from symptoms and enhancement of coping strategies. Cognizant of the likelihood of misdiagnosis, pediatric gastroenterologists must employ guarded clinical practice in discriminating these functional disorders from more serious underlying pathologies, in a timely and appropriate way, in a way to avoid their long-term consequences. Inflammatory bowel disease (IBD), consisting of Crohn's disease and ulcerative colitis, is a major issue in pediatric gastroenterology. IBD prevalence has considerably risen, indicating changes in environmental and dietary forces could be altering its cause. Symptoms of IBD in children can vary from pain in the abdomen to excessive weight loss, impacting their growth patterns. Recent publications focus on the importance of nutrition as a potential environmental factor in the induction and sustenance of IBD in genetically predisposed patients. The evidence reveals the need for diet control as a therapeutic intervention to manage IBD, emphasizing nutrition in both treatment and prevention protocols (Sigall-Boneh et al., 2017). Continued research into the complex interaction between diet, microbiota, and genetic predisposition is critical in seeking effective treatments for this disabling illness in children. Another critical issue in pediatric gastroenterology is the growing trend of childhood and adolescent obesity. Recent statistics reveal that approximately 17% of American kids are obese comes as a shocking revelation, and severe obesity is the fastest-growing subgroup (Ameer & Weintraub, 2018). Aside from its marker by weight, there are various comorbidities of obesity , such as type 2 diabetes and cardiovascular disease. Pediatric obesity needs to be addressed with multimodal treatment alternatives, including behavioral management, nutritional guidance, and increased physical exercise. However, the effectiveness of such treatments may be limited, particularly in cases of extreme obesity. With evolving scientific knowledge in this area, there is an increasing demand for new therapeutic approaches, including pharmacologic treatments tailored to adolescents, to adequately treat the obesity epidemic and promote successful long-term health outcomes in adolescent patients (Figure 13.3).

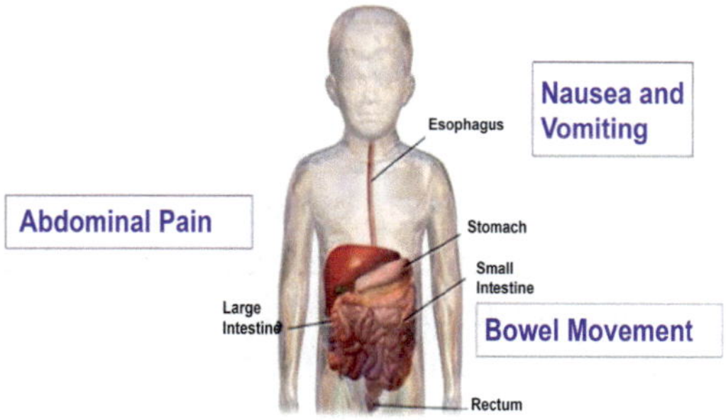

Figure 13.3. Overview of common gastrointestinal disorders in children.

Source: https://i.ytimg.com/vi/i3YoviYtPts/hq720.jpg?sqp=-oaymwEhCK4FEIIDSFryq4qpAxMIARUAAAAAGAElAADIQj0AgKJD&rs=AOn4CLBENSuFryPzFaj4_20w51DlOG72_Q.

13.1. Anatomy and Physiology of the Pediatric Gastrointestinal System

The pediatric GI system anatomy is specifically adapted to the growth and developmental needs of children. Unlike adults, the structure of the pediatric GI tract changes radically as the child progresses from infancy to adulthood. The esophagus, for instance, is shorter in infants and thereby predisposes them to gastroesophageal reflux disease (GERD). The stomach is larger in proportion because it has a capacity to hold more food, but also has different motility characteristics and pH that affect digestion. There are anatomical variations in the intestines as well, for example, the small intestine which is longer in proportion and the colon which is shorter, and these play a critical role in nutrient absorption and an important part of lactose and other macromolecule digestion. Understanding these anatomical components illuminates the prevalent gastrointestinal disorder in children, which enhances clinical evaluation and management. Physiologically, the GI system of children is marked by stages of development that influence its function in childhood. The digestive enzymes amylase and lipase are secreted in minimal amounts in neonates, influencing the digestion of carbohydrates and fats. As the gastrointestinal tract develops, so does its enzymatic function, allowing for better digestion and absorption of nutrients. In addition, the gut microbiota, which is accountable for immune system maturation, begins forming in infancy, and this process is significantly affected by mode of delivery and diet. The efforts of recent research have increasingly underscored the interlinkage between the well-being of the gastrointestinal system and general health in children, since a good microbiome promotes homeostasis and allows for better functioning of the gastrointestinal system. These physiological findings are fundamental to the understanding of disorders , such as Pediatric Feeding Disorders (PFD), in which impaired oral intake can lead to nutrition impairment and psychosocial issues, highlighting the significance of integrated assessment and intervention measures (Browne et al., 2019). The pediatric gastrointestinal tract is not spared from a plethora of pathophysiological conditions, most of which significantly impact the quality of life and overall health. Conditions like gastroesophageal reflux, constipation, and inflammatory bowel disease are all consequence of multifactorial interactions between genetics, environment, and diet. Clinical presentation can be highly heterogeneous and may vary from feeding intolerance, malnutrition, or growth failure.

For instance, pediatric feeding disorders (PFDs) could be characterized by oral intake dysfunction as well as associated medical, nutritional, and psychosocial dysfunctions. Professionals have to overcome these escalated disorders through an interdisciplinary diagnosis and treatment approach that combines various healthcare specialties to best address the needs of unique patients. Through knowledge of the relationship between the anatomy, physiology, and pathology of the pediatric GI system, clinicians and investigators can develop greater knowledge about these conditions and improve therapeutic interventions (Kinney, 2007) (Figure 13.4).

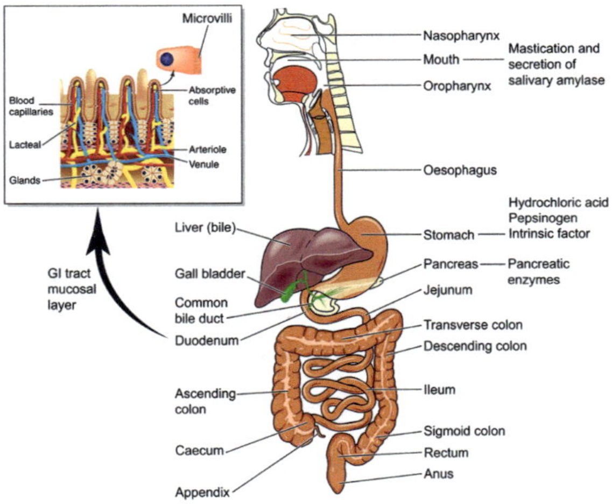

Figure 13.4. Anatomy and physiology of the pediatric gastrointestinal system.

Source: https://www.liveoaksurgery.com/wp-content/uploads/2020/05/GI-Tract-copy.jpg.

13.1.1. Differences Between Pediatric and Adult Gastrointestinal Anatomy

Analysis of the differences between pediatric and adult gastrointestinal (GI) anatomy reveals significant differences that have a major impact on pediatric gastroenterology practice. The GI tract in infants and children is narrower and shorter proportionally compared with adults. For example, the esophagus is smaller and more susceptible to motility alteration, predisposing children to conditions like gastroesophageal reflux disease (GERD). Moreover, the capacity of infants' stomachs is much lower and needs frequent high-frequency feeding. The anatomical positioning of organs is also different; the stomach in infants is more horizontally oriented and affects the mechanisms of digestion and absorption of nutrients. All these physiological differences require higher-level knowledge and skills in pediatric gastroenterology for a correct diagnosis and treatment of GI pathology in this age group, and therefore, health professionals must be aware of pediatric differences in anatomy. The difference in digestive organ development between children and adults only contributes to pediatric gastrointestinal health. To illustrate, the liver of the infant is significantly larger in proportion to size than that of an adult and develops throughout childhood. The child possesses a special microbiome that develops significantly during infancy, depending on mode of birth, early nutrition, and environment. This unique microbial material can influence not just digestion, but also immunity and metabolic processes. Furthermore, the infant pancreas has different enzymatic activities that mature over time and influence nutrient digestion and absorption and thus modulate the manner in which health conditions , such as malnutrition or metabolic disease, present differently across pediatrics. It is essential to admire these developmental differences when developing effective treatment regimens and interventions designed to maximize pediatric GI well-being.

Moreover, the differential presentation of disease in children versus adults is underscored by the anatomical differences outlined. Diseases , such as inflammatory bowel disease (IBD) and celiac disease present differently due to anatomical and physiological variations in the GI tract.

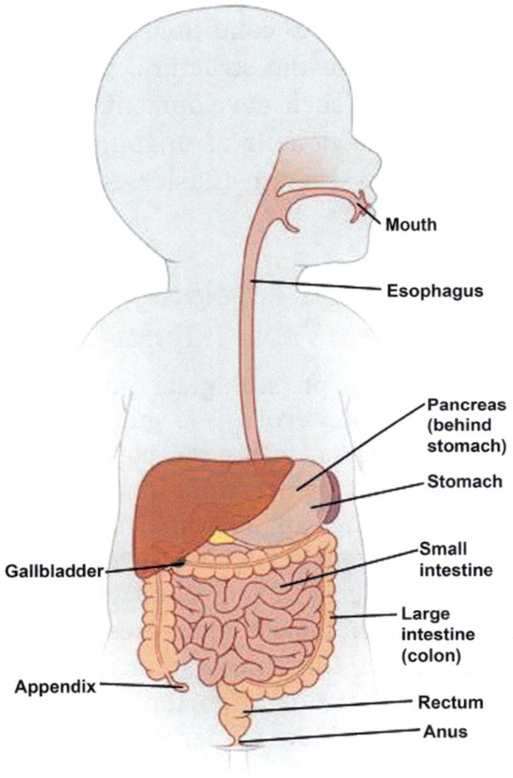

Figure 13.5. Differences between pediatric and adult gastrointestinal anatomy.

Source: https://api.kramesstaywell.com/Content/6066ca30-310a-4170-b001-a4ab013d61fd/ucr-images-v1/Images/outline-of-baby-with-head-turned-to-side-showing-mouth-esophagus-pancreas-behind-stomach-stomach-small-intestine-large-in.

Children can have growth retardation or delayed development as a direct consequence of their GI diseases, which again complicates therapy. Diagnostic modalities are likely to have to be modified in pediatric patients since the common techniques piloted on adults will not yield acceptable results in younger patients due to their anatomical variations. A case is the endoscopic process that might significantly vary, and pediatric specialists will have to adapt methods for effectiveness as well as safety. For this purpose, understanding the anatomical differences between pediatric and adult GI is essential to provide comprehensive care, as seen in guidelines from professional societies (Pennazio et al., 2022) and general guidelines acknowledging unique pediatric challenges (Barker et al., 2020) (Figure 13.5).

13.1.2. Developmental Changes in the Gastrointestinal System

Throughout early development, the GI system also makes dramatic morphological and functional changes that are key to responding to the nutritional demands of the expanding pediatric populace. At first, an infant's GI tract is immature and incompetent to digest intricate nutrients. Upon birth, the stomach is proportionally small, and the acidic environment of the stomach is less mature compared to adults and prevents the enzymatic activity necessary for effective digestion. Once babies transition to a diet of breast milk and formula, their GI tract begins to adapt, a process that parallels development, including alterations , such as gastric acid production maturation and pancreatic enzymatic function. These alterations, such as increased intestinal villi and microvilli development, facilitate nutrient absorption required for development and growth. An understanding of these developmental changes is critical in the management of pediatric GI disorders and in the administration of adequate nutrition during infancy. With increasing age, the gastrointestinal tract continues to mature, defined by alterations in motility, secretory function, and microbial colonization. In early childhood, GI motility undergoes significant alteration, with infants demonstrating more sluggish intestinal transit times compared with older children. This diminished gut transit time is typically associated with physiological conditions like constipation that are fairly prevalent in pediatric patients. Moreover, the trillions of microbes comprising the gut microbiome, which begins to develop during infancy, play a pivotal role in immune regulation and metabolic activities. Dysbiosis of microbial composition can lead to any of the GI complications, ranging from inflammatory bowel disease to obesity, so nutritional well-being becomes imperative. The interaction of eating habits and microbial diversity highlights the need for particular nutritional intervention to promote gastrointestinal well-being. The pattern of growth of the gastrointestinal tract is also influenced by the differences in eating habits and lifestyle factors as children develop into adolescents.

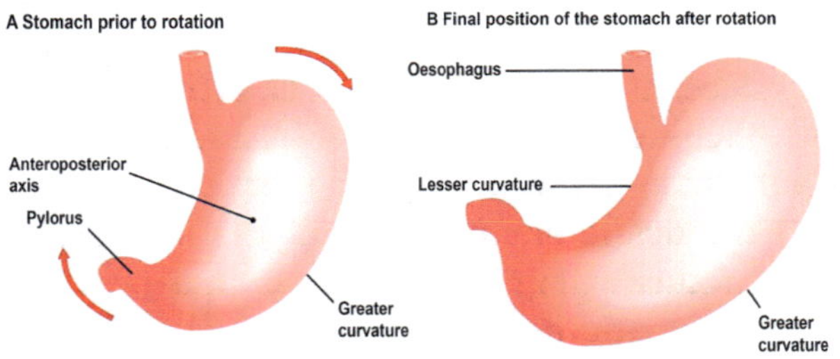

Figure 13.6. Developmental changes in the gastrointestinal system.

Source: https://static.cambridge.org/binary/version/id/urn:cambridge.org:id:binary:20161116082711659-0544:9781107587519:66713fig13_2.png?pub-status=live.

As more complex diets, including solid food and rising levels of processed foods, are introduced, the GI system is required to be able to harbor a range of nutrients without compromising its structure. This level of dietary innovation is evidenced by the recent surge in diseases like obesity among children and young adolescents to highlight the consequences of such dietary reforms on the GI system, as evidenced by the rising comorbidities that accompany obesity at this age. Chronic obesity is often accompanied by shifts in metabolic and gastrointestinal function, requiring an advanced understanding of the interplay between development, nutrition, and disease in pediatric gastroenterology (Ameer & Weintraub, 2018). Furthermore, conditions like annular pancreas illustrate the structural defects that may accompany such developmental changes, highlighting the benefit of ongoing research and clinical observation (Easler et al., 2019) (Figure 13.6).

13.1.3. Common Physiological Functions and Their Implications

One of the key physiological processes in pediatric gastroenterology is gut microbiota homeostasis, which forms the core of overall health. The gastrointestinal tract is home to a diverse range of microbial species in a symbiotic relationship with the human host. This complex ecosystem plays a vital role in numerous physiological processes, including nutrient uptake, immune system modulation, and the synthesis of important vitamins. A healthy gut microbiota is marked by a state of eubiosis where microbial communities function in a harmonious arrangement to sustain body functions. Imbalances of this sort, referred to as dysbiosis, can have serious consequences for pediatric health and may result in gastrointestinal disease, as well as impacting the outcome of systemic health. The intricate interplay between gut microbiota and physiological processes highlights the importance of understanding how such microbes affect children's growth and development, and hence exploration of treatments for re-establishing normal microbiota equilibrium in children is a priority area (Iebba et al., 2016). When inflammatory bowel diseases (IBD) occur, dietary factors and interactions with gut microbiota are particularly relevant for children. Recent research points to the possible role of individual nutritional exposures in the pathogenesis of IBD, especially in response to rising incidence and prevalence in children. There is an intricate balance between environmental stimuli, such as diet, and genetic susceptibility that lies behind the development and maintenance of IBD. For example, some nutrients and eating habits can continue or dampen inflammatory activity in the bowel. The Dietary Exposure and Crohn's Disease Cooperation Consortium (D-ECCO) highlights the potential contribution that nutrition can make not only as an environmental stressor but also as a therapeutic pathway. Clinicians are required to grasp the dietary significance for the administration of IBD because they must support families in informed nutritional choices that will lead to better health outcomes in children (Sigall-Boneh et al., 2017).

The influence of gut microbiota and diet extends beyond local gastrointestinal symptoms and impacts other systemic physiological processes. For instance, gut health has been implicated in immune system function, brain development, and control of metabolism in children. Well-natured microbiota aids in the maturation of the immune system and the suppression of uncontrolled inflammatory reactions, which are particularly relevant in food-allergic and autoimmune-disease-prone children. Additionally, early introduction to a diverse range of nutrient-rich foods can potentially fortify the microbiome, with far-reaching health consequences. Dysbiosis, in contrast, has potential correlations with negative outcomes , such as obesity and metabolic syndromes. Such factors further establish the need for a holistic approach in pediatric gastroenterology, encompassing nutritional counseling and management focused on the preservation of intestinal health as well as comprehending its extensive impact on the range of physiological processes in children.

13.2. Common Gastrointestinal Disorders in Children

Gastrointestinal diseases in children are particularly challenging, and this is due to the anatomical and physiological differences between pediatric and adult subjects. Inflammatory bowel disease (IBD) is one of the most common gastrointestinal disorders in children and encompasses Crohn's disease and ulcerative colitis. These conditions are characterized by chronic inflammation of the gastrointestinal tract and can cause extreme morbidity if not properly controlled. Evidence indicates that diet can be closely correlated with the pathogenesis and treatment of IBD in children. The D-ECCO working group has highlighted that diet must be conceived as an environmental stimulus in the pathogenesis of IBD as well as a potential therapeutic strategy for managing symptoms. This increasing understanding of the role of diet can aid in tailoring treatment regimens responsive to the child's general well-being and quality of life, underlining the need for more research in this direction (Sigall-Boneh et al., 2017). Another frequent disorder in the pediatric population is eosinophilic gastrointestinal disorders (EGIDs), a group of conditions with eosinophilic infiltration of the gastrointestinal tract. They typically have a variety of symptoms , such as abdominal cramps, vomiting, and difficulty feeding and are notoriously difficult to diagnose. EGIDs are thought to be caused by an abnormal immune reaction to allergens that provokes inflammation that, unless the causative allergen is identified and removed, will lead to chronic disease. Treatment today ranges from elimination dietary strategies to medications, but is marked by a vital deficiency of randomized, controlled trials to properly address treatment efficacy. The ongoing need for extensive research to explain the pathogenesis and optimal management strategies for EGIDs cannot be overestimated, especially since the treatments currently available can adversely impact a child's quality of life alongside their physiological health (Naramore & Gupta, 2018). In pediatric gastroenterology, the overlap between various gastrointestinal diseases demands a multidisciplinary approach to management. In addition to the more prevalent diseases of IBD and EGIDs, children can have a wide range of gastrointestinal diseases, including functional gastrointestinal disorders , such as irritable bowel syndrome (IBS) and gastroesophageal reflux disease (GERD). The variable nature of these diseases often makes them challenging to diagnose and treat and demands scrupulous evaluation and coordination between pediatricians, gastroenterologists, dietitians, and mental health professionals. In addition, understanding the psychological impact of gastrointestinal conditions in children is essential, since anxiety and stress can exacerbate symptoms. With a comprehensive strategy to treat both the physiological and psychological bases of gastrointestinal conditions, healthcare providers can treat these conditions more efficiently and improve health outcomes in children with them.

13.2.1. Gastroesophageal Reflux Disease (GERD)

Gastroesophageal reflux disease (GERD) is a frequent illness in children that is characterized by the pathological regurgitation of gastric contents into the esophagus. Its presentation is not uniform in all infants and children, ranging from benign diseases , such as simple regurgitation to complicated diseases that lead to serious health consequences. Unlike the classical symptoms of GERD in adults, for instance, heartburn, children present with unusual presentations that complicate diagnosis and management. The elevated risk factors among children include gastrointestinal immaturity and environmental stimuli, and the significance of learning GERD thoroughly in the context of children cannot be overstated. As expounded by Borrelli et al. (2017), the recognition of the distinct patterns of GERD among pediatric patients is the cornerstone of successful therapy, separating it from normal reflux that may not need treatment. Diagnosis of GERD in children is typically a combination of clinical evaluation and testing. Pediatric gastroenterologists employ a range of tools, including pH testing and endoscopy, to quantify the degree of esophagitis and the severity of reflux. Clinical presentation typically dictates the test modality of choice, with children presenting with respiratory symptoms in one category and with failure to thrive or irritability in another. Therefore, an all-encompassing strategy is required for the correct diagnosis of GERD and its potential complications. Moreover, differentiation of GERD from other pathologies, such as allergies or respiratory illnesses, can be particularly challenging. As demonstrated through the evidence provided in Lorenzo et al. (2017), esophageal acid clearance pathophysiological differences among patients with such diseases as cystic fibrosis compared to control children emphasize the complexity in GERD diagnosis in pediatric gastroenterology. Treatment of GERD in children is a multifaceted approach consisting of lifestyle modification, pharmacotherapy, and, in rare cases, surgery. Primary treatment involves diet modification, positioning, and education of caregivers in the management of reflux. If symptoms are unresponsive or worsen, pharmacotherapy in the form of proton pump inhibitors might be tried to reduce acid exposure in the esophagus. Surgery, such as fundoplication, is reserved for those cases that do not respond to medical management. Ongoing research must be done to more effectively individualize these treatment modalities, especially in the context of the variable response rates found among children. Lastly, understanding the nuances of GERD management in children, as identified in (Borrelli et al., 2017), is required in order to maximize patient outcomes and adapt to their developmental needs (Figure 13.7).

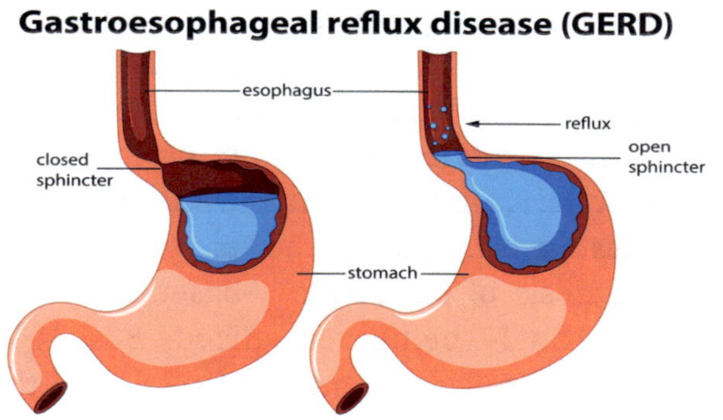

Figure 13.7. Gastroesophageal reflux disease (GERD).

Source: https://sonosif.com/wp-content/uploads/2020/10/Gastroesophageal-Reflux-Disease-GERD.jpg.

13.2.2. Inflammatory Bowel Disease (IBD)

The growing incidence of inflammatory bowel disease (IBD) among children is of concern and reflects a complex interaction between environmental factors, such as diets, and genetic susceptibility. New evidence highlights the contribution of diet to IBD pathogenesis, and that recent changes in diet are possibly responsible for the increased prevalence of the disease. The D-ECCO work group highlighted crucial thematic issues on the role of diet in IBD, including its impact on disease onset, maintenance treatment, and nutritional monitoring. These are critical factors for pediatric gastroenterologists as they strive to re-engineer interventions that can prevent the occurrence of IBD in children, who may be more susceptible than adults to the negative impacts of poor diet. As research into diet's influence on IBD expands, caution must be exercised with regard to responding to a child's nutrition status as part of their overall clinical evaluation and management (Sigall-Boneh et al., 2017). Inflammatory bowel disease treatment in children often involves multi-faceted treatment interventions, including pharmacologic interventions and lifestyle modifications. One of the more prominent therapies for the management of Crohn's disease is biologic therapy with agents , such as Adalimumab (Ada). Current research observations highlight Ada's efficacy, particularly as an alternative in the treatment of children who have shown resistance to previous infliximab therapy. In the cohort evaluation, important clinical improvement in disease activity, measured using the Pediatric CD Activity Index (PCDAI), was observed after six months of therapy, revealing that nearly half of the patients were in clinical remission.

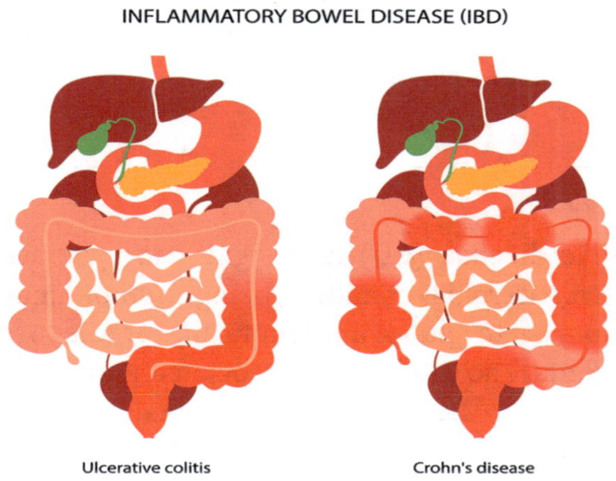

Figure 13.8. The rising incidence of inflammatory bowel disease (IBD) among pediatric.

Source: https://www.hopkinsmedicine.org/-/media/images/health/1_-conditions/stomach-and-gut/inflammatory-bowel-disease-graphic-large.ashx.

These findings add strength to the existing body of knowledge on the efficacy of biologic agents in early intervention regimens, hope for the afflicted families with the chronicity of IBD (Alvisi et al., 2019). The multifactorial etiology of inflammatory bowel disease cannot be covered by pharmacologic management alone and needs a comprehensive approach to patient management. Impartial attention to dietetic therapy and dietary interventions is important in maximizing overall health outcomes in pediatric patients in situations of critical growth periods. Pediatric gastroenterologists must assess not only clinical IBD symptoms but also the patient's nutritional status since malnutrition can be caused by disease as well as by treatment side effects. Individualized dietary care strategies, as part of appropriate supplementation where necessary, are part of a complete management of IBD. This emphasis on a model of care in its entirety will not only manage disease more effectively but also provide for the psychosocial well-being of children in terms of quality of life and developmental milestones, responding to the multifactorial impact of IBD (Sigall-Boneh et al., 2017) (Figure 13.8).

13.2.3. Celiac Disease and Gluten Sensitivity

Celiac disease (CD) is a significant pediatric gastroenterology condition, being an autoimmune response to gluten in genetically predisposed patients. The condition is associated with villous atrophy of the small intestine, malabsorption of nutrients, and numerous gastrointestinal as well as extraintestinal symptoms.

The presentation may be very variable in the clinical setting, with some of the children presenting classical symptoms of failure to thrive and diarrhea, while others present with atypical presentations , such as anemia or neurological presentation. Early and proper diagnosis is critical to avoid long-term complications , such as osteoporosis, infertility, and malignancy susceptibility. It requires a multidisciplinary approach involving healthcare professionals, including pediatric gastroenterologists, dietitians, and family doctors, in screening and treating CD for better care of the pediatric population and for raising awareness of the disease among parents and teachers. Determination of the prevalence of celiac disease in the pediatric population necessitates reviewing current practice in its diagnosis and management. Published literature documents a high degree of variability among the clinical practices of pediatric gastroenterologists in North America. For instance, while biopsy of the intestine is frequently the gold standard for the diagnosis of CD, serology-based diagnosis is increasingly being recognized. Based on the recent surveys, as many as 47.5% of the practitioners have embraced serology as an acceptable diagnostic criterion (Singh et al., 2024). These messages could be due to variation in training and the capacity of clinicians to identify celiac disease and reflect the need for ongoing education in this area. Problems of optimum management, such as restricted access to dietetic management and variability in the level of clinicians' experience, emphasize the need for formal celiac disease training within pediatric gastroenterology fellowship programs. Gluten sensitivity, while distinct but connected with celiac disease, poses other challenges in the management of children. Unlike celiac disease, gluten sensitivity lacks the autoimmune response and intestinal damage of CD but can still have a significant effect on a child's quality of life. Gluten-sensitive children have non-specific presentations , such as abdominal pain, fatigue, or behavior problems and are not easy to diagnose. Pediatric gastroenterologists need to be able to accurately differentiate between the two entities as awareness regarding gluten sensitivity grows. Synthesis of symptomatology, patient history, and appropriate testing modalities is then essential to arrive at the proper diagnosis and intervention. Ongoing research into the pathophysiology of gluten sensitivity will be necessary to develop inclusive guidelines that include celiac disease as well as gluten sensitivity and ultimately move pediatric gastroenterological practice forward and enhance outcomes for these children.

13.3. Diagnostic Approaches in Pediatric Gastroenterology

Diagnosis of pediatric gastrointestinal illness typically involves unique problems based upon symptom heterogeneity and variation in developmental levels. A thorough understanding of pediatric anatomy and physiology is required to differentiate between normal and pathological states. Physical examination and detailed patient history must be relied upon to a great extent by practitioners, with special emphasis on dietary habits, growth patterns, and accompanying symptoms. As most gastrointestinal disorders are asymptomatic in the initial stages, high clinical suspicion is required to avoid late diagnoses. This is particularly important in chronic liver illnesses, in which early presentations may be subtle or uncharacteristic. Delayed diagnosis in children of such conditions has devastating impacts; therefore, the upgrading of diagnostic methods is central to optimizing outcomes in children (Della Corte et al., 2016). Advancements in diagnostic imaging technology have increased the ability to evaluate gastrointestinal diseases in children. Imaging techniques , such as ultrasound, magnetic resonance imaging (MRI), and computed tomography (CT) scans are beneficial in providing useful information in terms of structural defects and functional tests. Of these, ultrasound is particularly advantageous in that it is a radiation-free procedure and therefore safer for children. In addition, it can be performed at the bedside with minimal sedation needed and for rapid evaluation. For additional benefit, the utilization of endoscopic techniques provides visualization of the gastrointestinal system directly, and it can both diagnose and treat. However, interpretation of these imaging investigations necessitates specific training, hence expertise in pediatric gastroenterology is necessary to make appropriate judgments and effective management plans in children (Coleman et al., 2018). Functional gastrointestinal disorders, i.e., motility disorder, are another point of focus in pediatric gastroenterology. Diagnosis of these disorders is typically dependent on meticulous clinical assessment since conventional types of imaging do not help. In the recent past, new noninvasive technologies like the electrogastrogram (EGG) have become accessible, offering novel methods of continuous measurement of gastric electrical activity. The technology has the potential to enhance the accuracy of diagnosis and increase the number of patients who can be effectively screened and managed. By targeting the underlying physiological mechanisms, such diagnostic approaches have the capability of fine-tuning treatment modalities, eventually maximizing the quality of life in affected children. However, there are still practical concerns , such as a need for improved signal interpretation methods and more access to advanced facilities, which itself creates a need for ongoing innovations in this field (Coleman et al., 2018) (Figure 13.9).

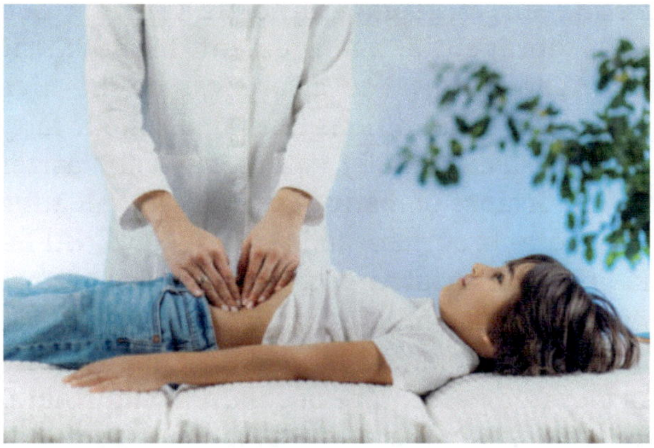

Figure 13.9. Diagnostic approaches in pediatric gastroenterology.

Source: https://media.istockphoto.com/id/1474101958/photo/pediatric-gastroenterology-abdominal-examination.jpg?s=612x612&w=0&k=20&c=fDgRYypPFndDhCGRsvxw1KzBgbjPXZyMVGUCMjDVybE=.

13.3.1. Clinical Evaluation and History Taking

Thorough clinical evaluation and meticulous history taking are pillars of pediatric gastroenterology, enabling practitioners to diagnose and manage gastrointestinal disorders to the best possible extent. Initial contact with patients and families is also most revealing about medical history, chief complaints, and psychosocial factors that may impact the health of the child. In children, history-taking extends beyond mere symptom collection; it is about an understanding of milestones in development, dietary habits, and the family history of disease. The participation of parents in this process is also critical, as they are able to provide meanings of symptoms that would otherwise be foreign to the child. A comprehensive approach provides clinicians with the opportunity not to overlook important information that may guide diagnosis and management, hence enhancing the quality of care provided. Finally, accurate clinical examination lays the ground for targeted diagnostic work-up and best therapeutic management in pediatric gastroenterology. The awareness of the high prevalence of conditions like nonalcoholic fatty liver disease (NAFLD) in children emphasizes the importance of meticulous clinical evaluation and the appropriate taking of history. NAFLD has been associated with various risk factors like obesity and metabolic syndrome, which are increasingly common in pediatric populations. An elevated percentage of children with NAFLD are at risk for increased blood pressure due to the interaction of these factors, underlining the significance of regular cardiovascular assessment within this group (Behling et al., 2014). Physicians must inquire about diet, exercise, and cardiovascular disease family history in their patients in order to identify individuals with a higher risk. This prospective clinical evaluation not only facilitates early detection of complications but also promotes preventive interventions to reduce these risks, thereby maximizing worldwide patient outcomes in pediatric gastroenterology. The integration of clinical evaluations with novel diagnostic technologies further elevates the importance of early and comprehensive history taking. Non-invasive diagnostic methods , such as ultrasound and liver wellness biomarkers complement routine evaluation regimens and can be directed by history drawn from interviews of the patient. Furthermore, as increasing understanding of gut wellness and microbiota comes to light, clinicians must be careful in questioning that helps elucidate underlying gastrointestinal illness. These would include inquiries about bowel habits, food intolerance, and past gastrointestinal symptoms. Through the combination of scrupulous history taking and clinical examination, medical professionals can create a detailed profile for each patient that guides future interventions and enhances their approach to managing complex pediatric gastroenterological illness (Kinney, 2007). Consequently, the incorporation of cautious history taking and clinical evaluation generates a more subtle awareness of individual patient needs, leading to better care management and outcomes.

13.3.2. Laboratory Tests and Imaging Studies

In pediatric gastroenterology, the diagnosis of liver disease often necessitates the combination of laboratory examination and imaging studies to establish etiology. A vital component of this evaluation is the evaluation of hepatobiliary disease, which may have nonspecific manifestations like abdominal pain, jaundice, or failure to thrive. Laboratory investigations that measure liver function, including serum aspartate aminotransferase (AST) and serum alanine aminotransferase (ALT), play a crucial role in evaluating hepatocellular injury and liver health. In cases where nonalcoholic fatty liver disease (NAFLD) is being suspected, additional markers like insulin are also considered, as liver dysfunction due to obesity may lead to systemic insulin resistance, further obscuring clinical presentation and necessitating more investigation (Batens et al., 2019). Imaging modalities are an essential aspect of pediatric gastroenterology by complementing laboratory findings and providing visual confirmation of suspected diagnoses. The most frequently used first-line imaging study is ultrasonography due to its non-invasive nature and ability to identify hepatic steatosis, biliary tract disease, or gallstones. Elastography is a helpful tool, particularly for the assessment of liver stiffness that correlates with fibrosis, with the advancement of imaging technology. While liver biopsy remains the gold standard for liver disease staging and diagnosis, non-invasive diagnostics are increasingly employed, especially among children, in an effort to decrease pain and procedure-related complication risks associated with biopsies. Non-invasive biomarkers accompanied by imaging studies might facilitate closer assessment while minimizing the number of invasive repeat procedures (von Eckardstein, 2017). The simultaneous application of laboratory testing and imaging tests not only aids the diagnosis of diseases like NAFLD but also directs the treatment process and prognosis. For instance, lobular inflammation in liver biopsy has been correlated powerfully with metabolic derangements like insulin resistance (Batens et al., 2019). Thus, correlating with biochemical markers, the histological evidence can enhance our understanding of a child's liver condition, with specialists then being able to use directed therapy. Through further research, constant verification of non-invasive biomarkers and imaging techniques continues to be a prime focus, as such advances are sure to deliver greater diagnostic accuracy and better patient outcomes in pediatric gastroenterology. Integration of information from laboratory and imaging tests encourages a multidisciplinary plan, optimizing the care for children with liver conditions and ensuring a more individualized health approach.

13.3.3. Endoscopic Procedures and Their Role

The landscape of pediatric gastroenterology has seen an increased reliance on endoscopic procedures, which are both of primary diagnostic and therapeutic significance. Endoscopic techniques are minimally invasive and offer significant benefits over traditional open surgery, enabling faster recovery and shorter hospitalization. Children who lack tolerance for invasive treatment have endoscopy as a solution that minimizes discomfort while providing the best clinical outcomes. The methods have a wide range of indications, ranging from the investigation of unexplained gastrointestinal symptoms to therapeutic interventions , such as polypectomy or dilatation of strictures. The application of the methods is evidence of their contribution not only to the diagnosis of gastrointestinal disorders but also to the management of conditions that would otherwise necessitate additional surgery, thus maximally advancing general pediatric gastroenterology patient care. Additionally, clinical guidelines and criteria development, such as the Rome II criteria for pediatric functional gastrointestinal disorders, have been instrumental in optimizing the appropriateness of endoscopic procedures in children. Research shows that 26% of pediatric gastrointestinal endoscopies performed prior to the implementation of these criteria were inappropriate. Since the introduction of the Rome II guidelines, there has been a significant decrease in unwarranted procedures, leading to increased diagnostic yield and better management of gastrointestinal disease. Specifically, studies showed that correct endoscopies following implementation had higher rates of significant findings, illustrating the positive effect of governed guidelines on the decision-making process in pediatric endoscopy. This trend accentuates the significant interface between evidence-based treatment and clinical practice in pediatric gastroenterology. In addition to increased diagnostic sensitivity, endoscopic interventions also speak to an escalating shift toward tailoring interventions in the pediatric population. The evolution of advanced endoscopic techniques, such as endoscopic mucosal resection and balloon enteroscopy, not only provides direct treatment of gastrointestinal diseases but also helps create a long-term treatment plan for chronic diseases. The versatility of endoscopy allows real-time intervention, where the therapeutic intervention is possible based on the outcome during the procedure, reducing the need for multiple interventions. As technology becomes more advanced, one can anticipate the scope and effectiveness of pediatric endoscopic techniques to further broaden, resulting in even improved outcomes in children with a wide array of gastrointestinal conditions. It is therefore paramount that these methods are incorporated into pediatric gastroenterology to enhance the overall quality of care provided to this vulnerable group of patients (Figure 13.10).

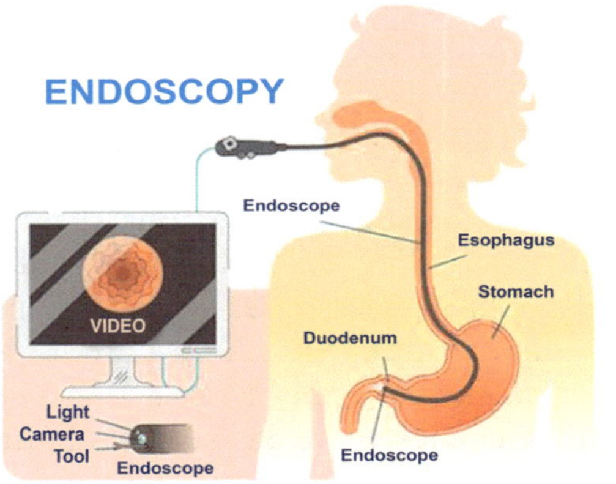

Figure 13.10. Endoscopic procedures and their role.

Source: https://www.hopkinsmedicine.org/-/media/images/health/2_-treatment/gastroenterology/endoscopic-procedure-illustration.ashx?h=400&iar=0&mh=400&mw=670&w=582&hash=8B3D71297CEAB6E90AF42E816D6865C6.

13.4. Treatment Modalities in Pediatric Gastroenterology

Clinical practice of pediatric gastroenterology encompasses the vast array of therapeutic modalities applied in the management of gastrointestinal diseases in children. One of the areas of clinical interest is eosinophilic gastrointestinal disorders, with the latter representing a complex clinical situation with the mechanism of uncharacteristic inflammatory responses to allergens. Treatment of disorders includes the application of corticosteroids and elimination diets, which, however, carry significant side effects. Corticosteroids pose long-term side effects concerns for usage, while the elimination diets may severely compromise the quality of a child's life. Current literature emphasizes that more research should be done on other treatment modalities that can yield effective outcomes without compromising the health of child patients (Naramore & Gupta, 2018). Therefore, utmost consideration of these treatment modalities is warranted to continue promoting the care of children with eosinophilic disorders and enhancing overall treatment efficacy. Another major focus area of pediatric gastroenterology is inflammatory bowel disease (IBD), which has been on the rise globally. The difficulty in treating IBD is since it is etiologically multifactorial and likely to be genetic and environmental in origin. More recent studies have revealed that epigenetic changes, such as DNA methylation, in the colonic mucosa can be a critical mechanism of pediatric IBD pathogenesis. Characterization of these epigenetic markers in treatment-naive individuals offers a fantastic opportunity for improving diagnostic and therapeutic strategies. For example, widespread gene expression alterations associated with differentially methylated regions indicate specific pathways engaged in immune and inflammatory responses.

The potential impact of such research could result in developing novel interventions based on the specific requirements of IBD children (Bronsky et al., 2014). In addition, a synergistic strategy that combines pharmacologic therapy with lifestyle modification is crucial in providing holistic treatment to pediatric patients with gastrointestinal illness. The multidimensionality of these conditions requires that healthcare providers not only attend to pharmacotherapy but also to the psychosocial dimensions of treatment. Tailoring interventions that are sensitive to a child's eating habits, psychological state, and general lifestyle can have a profound effect on their health outcomes. Education of families and patients can encourage adherence to treatment regimens and education about early symptoms of illness, which can result in earlier medical intervention. Finally, coordination between specialists, families, and patients themselves is key to optimizing treatment modalities and improving the course of pediatric gastrointestinal illness.

13.4.1. Dietary Management and Nutritional Support

Good nutritional care and dietary control are crucial components in the treatment of disorders that are commonly encountered in pediatric gastroenterology. Malnutrition and growth retardation are common among children with gastrointestinal diseases, such as Crohn's disease, often due to disrupted nutrient absorption and increased nutrient requirements. Individualized nutritional therapy can play an important role in both clinical response and quality of life. For instance, as therapy agents, focused nutritional formulas have become the preferred treatment for pediatric Crohn's disease, with studies indicating that the formulas can heal the mucosa and sustain remission in the long run. More patients on specialized formula have significant therapeutic landmarks when compared to patients receiving standard nutrition, even though direct comparison between both interventions is needed to further develop clinical recommendations for clinicians (Russell et al., 2025). At the other end of the disease spectrum, with more serious gastrointestinal disease , such as biliary atresia, nutritional management comes to the forefront even more. These patients also suffer from severe nutritional issues due to compromised bile secretion, and digestion and absorption of fats and fat-soluble vitamins are an issue. A tailored dietary regimen using the use of medium-chain triglyceride (MCT) oil as an energy source that can bypass bile salt dependence corrects malabsorption issues of fats. In addition, specialty nutritional formulations that contain primary fat-soluble vitamins are also important in counteracting the deficiencies that may arise in such patients. Implementing these dietary interventions not only assists in managing the symptoms but also is significant in the children's overall development and growth needs during their waiting period for liver transplantation (Choe, 2025). The role of caregivers and medical personnel in implementing dietary management interventions cannot be overemphasized. The transition of children with gastrointestinal disease to proper nutritional regimens involves cooperation between pediatric gastroenterologists, dietitians, and families. Ongoing monitoring and adaptation according to growth rates, clinical course, and individual dietary limitations are necessary to maximize care. Furthermore, when oral feeding is insufficient or insufficient for the sustainment of nutritional status, alternative feeding strategies, including nasogastric or gastrostomy tube feeding, may be utilized. These methods provide a means of observing proper caloric and nutritional intake, especially among children who are faced with significant growth problems. Through comprehensive planning of dietary management, children who are faced with gastrointestinal complications are capable of achieving better health status, thereby promoting their potential toward a healthy growth process.

13.4.2. Pharmacological Interventions

Pharmacological therapy plays a very critical role in the management of a variety of gastrointestinal ailments in pediatric gastroenterology. Cyclic Vomiting Syndrome (CVS) is one such ailment that severely affects the quality of life of children due to recurring vomiting spells. Recent guidelines clearly indicate the utility of pharmacological therapy, particularly with anti-migraine medication, for aborting an acute CVS attack. These are evidence-based treatments that allow for targeted treatment plans based on individual patient presentations. For instance, intravenous 5-hydroxytryptamine 3 (5-HT3) receptor antagonists have been reported as a conditional recommendation in order to effectively treat acute symptoms, particularly in situations where prompt action is required.

This multidimensional approach facilitates ongoing clinical evaluation and realignment of treatment plans based on the development of new evidence (Karrento et al., 2025). In addition to acute treatment, drug therapy also assists in the preventive role of pediatric gastroenterology. Functional constipation in children generally requires a combination of dietary modifications and medication for guaranteed relief of symptoms and normal bowel habits. In this case, laxatives, like osmotic agents, play a central role in treatment. These elevate stool consistency and ease defecation, which is both physical relief and treats psychological issues in regularity of the bowel. Pharmacological interventions have to be complemented with educational interventions among children and parents to cement behavior changes that support long-term gastrointestinal health. As pharmacologic agents are realized in greater detail, medication can be integrated with non-pharmacological care in improved, optimized care plans for the effective management of pediatric constipation (Burgos et al., 2025).

Pharmacologic intervention is also used for the management of more complex conditions , such as inflammatory bowel disease (IBD) in children. Aminosalicylates and corticosteroids are selected according to disease severity and specific patient needs. These drug therapies not only induce and maintain remission but also significantly enhance the overall quality of life for the children concerned. One of the matters for consideration in the management of these drugs is the assessment of likely side effects and vigilance for untoward reactions, requiring a comprehensive clinical evaluation on treatment. With ongoing elucidation of the IBD pathophysiology by investigators, improvement in targeted therapy use and biologic drugs further empowers clinicians with the capability for personalized care. Therefore, the strategic use of pharmacological management in pediatric gastroenterology practice continues to be a fundamental component of effective treatment regimens for chronic gastrointestinal disease (Karrento et al., 2025) (Figure 13.11).

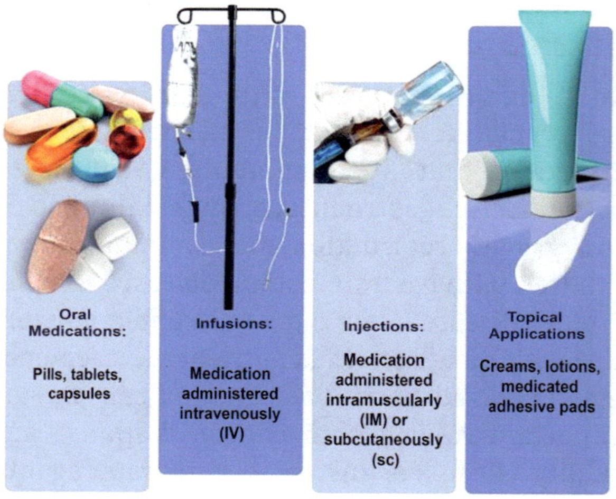

Figure 13.11. In the pharmacological interventions.

Source: https://www.neuroinjuryspecialists.com/wp-content/uploads/2024/09/types-of-pharmacological-intervention.jpg.

13.4.3. Surgical Options and When They Are Indicated

In pediatric gastroenterology, operative treatment is a key option when nonoperative treatment fails to achieve desired outcomes. Some conditions , such as biliary atresia, need surgical treatment for the correction of bile flow anatomical defects. Biliary atresia, in infants, can lead to severe liver damage if treated outside the surgical approach. The Kasai procedure is one of the more common operations and attempts to restore bile flow by directly attaching the small intestine to the liver. Timing is important for this surgery; an early operation greatly improves long-term survival, illustrating the importance of early diagnosis and referral to specialty care. Therefore, symptomatic presentations resulting from such conditions necessitate early surgical evaluation as a key element in the management of diseases that commonly involve the pediatric age group, frequently determining the prognosis of different gastrointestinal pathologies. Pediatric patients presenting with obesity-related complications that defy traditional therapy also have an important surgical option. Childhood severe obesity, as measured by a body mass index of at or above 120% of the 95th percentile, is increasing and results in major health consequences like type 2 diabetes and cardiovascular disease (Ameer & Weintraub, 2018). If lifestyle treatment and pharmacotherapy are unsuccessful, bariatric surgery can be used to ensure weight reduction as well as improve metabolic performance. Surgical procedures , such as gastric bypass or sleeve gastrectomy can significantly reduce obesity-associated comorbidities, but extensive pre-operative workups should be done. Surgical treatment typically involves a multidisciplinary assessment, considering the child's age, growth patterns, and psychological maturity to ensure surgical treatment concurs with long-term health goals. Surgical intervention in pediatric gastroenterology also comprises the repair of congenital abnormalities of the gastrointestinal tract, such as Hirschsprung's disease. The disease, caused by a lack of ganglion cells within a segment of the colon, leads to severe constipation and bowel obstruction in affected infants. Surgical correction, typically by a pull-through procedure, is indicated for the resection of the aganglionic segment in order to allow normal bowel function. The timing of this procedure is significant, with early intervention preventing complications , such as enterocolitis or perforation of the bowel. Multidisciplinary management of such children, nutrition and psychosocial issues, is crucial after surgery in order to maximize optimal recovery and development. By considering the specific needs of each patient, pediatric gastroenterologists can optimize surgical results and overall quality of life in children with gastrointestinal disease.

13.5. Impact of Gastrointestinal Disorders on Child Development

The influence of gastrointestinal disease on development in children is staggering, crossing beyond the physical into cognitive and emotional development. Diseases , such as celiac disease, inflammatory bowel disease, and chronic constipation can impair absorption, with deficiencies that are absolutely critical to cognitive development. Iron, zinc, and certain vitamins are necessary nutrients with critical roles in neurological and body development during early development. They tend to exhibit delays in developmental milestones, and the conditions present themselves as challenges not just to their education but to their overall well-being. Detection of such impact has come to center stage for pediatricians as well as healthcare providers, hence presenting the need for complete treatment approaches, combining the treatment of the gastrointestinal condition and its far-reaching developmental impacts (Caffarelli et al., 2019). Moreover, the social-emotional aspects of childhood development can be significantly altered by gastrointestinal illness. These children can experience social rejection, peer rejection, and worry. Decreased engagement in activities characteristic of a child follows. When food avoidance or abdominal pain excludes participation in usual childhood activities, the psychological effect is profound. The chronic cycle of somatic pain and social exclusion can have dire mental health implications, which may even continue into adolescence and adulthood. Hence, medical practitioners must incorporate psychological support into treatment plans so that interventions are not only adequate for dietary and medical needs but also for emotional resilience and social integration (Ameer & Weintraub, 2018). This integrative approach is critical in facilitating healthy growth among impacted children and families. Besides, the management of gastrointestinal pathologies is a significant challenge in the field of pediatric medicine. Treatment can be successful through a multidisciplinary team comprising pediatric gastroenterologists, nutritionists, and mental health professionals. Such groups must work together to design overall treatment plans that address not just the physiological but also the psychosocial aspects of the child. Progress in pediatric gastroenterology has added to treatment modalities , such as pharmacologic therapy and dietary interventions, yet the nature of such diseases necessitates future studies and innovation. For instance, the understanding of the pathophysiology of obesity among children has broader implications, given that the disease is intimately linked with various gastrointestinal-related complications, thereby complicating treatment regimens further (Ameer & Weintraub, 2018). Therefore, constant improvements and integrated care methods are paramount in preventing long-term impacts of gastrointestinal illness on the development of children (Figure 13.12).

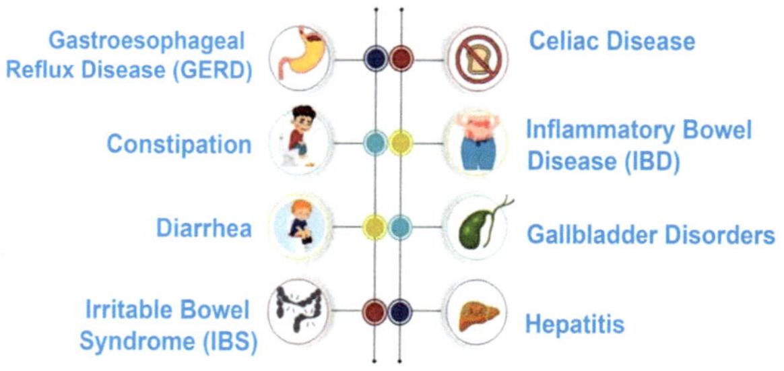

Figure 13.12. Impact of gastrointestinal disorders on child development.

Source: https://drmagnusjayaraj.b-cdn.net/wp-content/uploads/2023/10/Digestive-Disorders-in-Children-1024x671.webp.

13.5.1. Physical Growth and nutritional Status

Physical growth and nutritional status are central to pediatric gastroenterology, especially in the context of conditions , such as inflammatory bowel disease (IBD). IBD can produce abnormal intestinal function and hence, malabsorption and deficiencies of nutrients, severely detrimental to children's growth and development. Pediatric patients thus most frequently present with growth impairment, most frequently resulting from nutritional deficiency and impaired absorption. The increasing prevalence of IBD calls for a better understanding of the role of diet in the pathogenesis of the disease and how nutrition becomes an integral part of therapeutic interventions. Current evaluations by the D-ECCO working group highlight the contribution of food exposure to explaining the increased incidence of IBD, thus the need for thorough nutritional assessment and management to facilitate the best growth outcome in affected children (Sigall-Boneh et al., 2017). The impact of medication on physical growth and nutrition in children with gastrointestinal illness is of particular concern to practitioners. A cross-sectional analysis among children with Crohn's disease indicated that the nature of medication significantly influenced anthropometric findings, where some therapies were linked with levels of growth outcomes. For instance, adalimumab and methotrexate treatment were linked with positive trends of skinfold measurements and body mass index (BMI) scores reflecting better nutritional status, whereas thiopurines exhibited negative correlations with various growth markers (Gupta et al., 2018). These findings emphasize the requirement for the employment of appropriate treatment regimens not only for the management of the initial gastrointestinal condition but also for the maintenance of nutritional status and physical growth of the pediatric group. Thus, pediatric gastroenterology requires integrative care through combined pharmacologic and nutritional therapy to ensure optimal growth patterns. Total physical growth control and nutritional status regulation in children demand continuous monitoring and individualized therapeutic regimens. Regular measurement of anthropometric parameters, including weight, height, and BMI, is mandatory to identify early growth failures and intervene early. Furthermore, every healthcare professional should have a high priority for the inclusion of nutritional education for patients and families, with emphasis on the importance of a well-balanced diet that includes essential nutrients. It entails emphasizing the importance of diet variety and supplementation when this is necessary in order to control specific deficiency that results secondary to underlying gut pathology. In addition, collaboration among pediatric gastroenterologists, dietitians, and other medical practitioners is key in the development of personalized treatment plans that not only take into account compliance and efficacy of medication but also the overall development and nutritional requirements of pediatric patients (Sigall-Boneh et al., 2017; Gupta et al., 2018). These multi-dimensional approaches are significant in the improvement of the quality of life and health conditions of children with growth and nutritional issues owing to gastrointestinal disorders.

13.5.2. Psychological Effects and Quality of Life

The psychological effect of pediatric gastrointestinal disorders is substantial and multifaceted, imposing a significant burden on the quality of life of the affected children and their families. Those that are chronic in nature, such as inflammatory bowel disease (IBD) and liver disease, can induce increased stress, anxiety, and depression in pediatric patients. The daily battle to manage symptoms can create an increased sense of vulnerability and isolation that can contribute to psychological suffering. Such children usually struggle with insecurity about their state of health, which translates into low self-esteem and social isolation. That inner turmoil must be thoughtfully addressed because the psychological condition of child patients is irrevocably linked with their general well-being and treatment compliance, making it crucial to use combined strategies that prioritize both physical and psychological well-being. Besides, the impact of these gastrointestinal disorders is not only on the patient but also on the social life of the family and their interactions. Parents and siblings may experience their own emotional response, including anxiety about the child's condition and changes in daily routines, which might be brought about by incessant hospitalization and diet restrictions. Research has shown that strong family support systems can reverse some of these effects and build resilience in ill children who have been exposed to chronic illness. However, when a child's illness is neglected or not treated, as is normally the case in pediatric liver diseases, according to Della Corte et al. (2016), family stressors may become compounded, and this can set off a chain reaction of increasing emotional burden on all. This underlines the importance of an integrated treatment plan considering the psychosocial factors of illness. Lastly, treatment of pediatric gastrointestinal disease can be extremely heterogeneous based on patient tolerance to therapy and dietary control. There is some new evidence that nutritional therapy plays a central role in not only the physical management of diseases like IBD but also psychological well-being. It is on (Sigall-Boneh et al., 2017) that dietary selection has the potential to influence the course of such diseases and, by proxy, the well-being of children. Through the incorporation of methods aiming to enhance nutritional status, the medical professional can help develop physical health as well as psychological resilience. As these patients reveal the numerous challenges that confront them, an encouraging environment that caters to both their gastrointestinal and psychological demands is the linchpin in establishing overall quality of life and maximizing optimal outcomes in pediatric gastroenterology.

13.5.3. Social Implications and Family Dynamics

The intricate interplay of pediatric gastroenterology and social impacts reflects an immediate need among families coping with chronic gastrointestinal conditions. Disorders , such as inflammatory bowel disease (IBD) affect not only the physical health of the affected child but also exert tremendous psychosocial pressures on the family. IBD are likely to have limitations in their daily lives, e.g., attending school, engaging in sports, or merely being socially active. These may lead to isolation and anxiety on the part of the child, as well as on the part of parents who are unable to provide emotional support, along with the weight of providing their child's medical care. Truancy from school will further lead to underachievement and poor self-esteem, further serving to complicate the psychosocial scenario for both children and their families. For effective treatment as well as overall family functioning, these social consequences must therefore be addressed. Moreover, nutritional care in pediatric gastroenterology also has important social consequences that have a negative impact on family relationships. As exemplified by the latest research, the interplay between diet and gastrointestinal illness demonstrates that nutritional treatment is a key element in the prevention as well as care for diseases like IBD. Parents often are put in the stressful situation of controlling diets, and this can result in conflict over meals and place extra pressure on the routine. A change in diet may require a tremendous amount of teaching materials and general family involvement, which is not always feasible. Financial limitations can also contribute to these problems because therapeutic diets may increase the family's overall food expenses. Understanding these implications helps clinicians develop protocols that do not just treat medicine but also support familial functioning and cohesion, with social context playing an important part in dietary control and outcomes (Sigall-Boneh et al., 2017). Transition from child to adult care for children with chronic gastrointestinal illnesses is another area where family dynamics come into the picture.

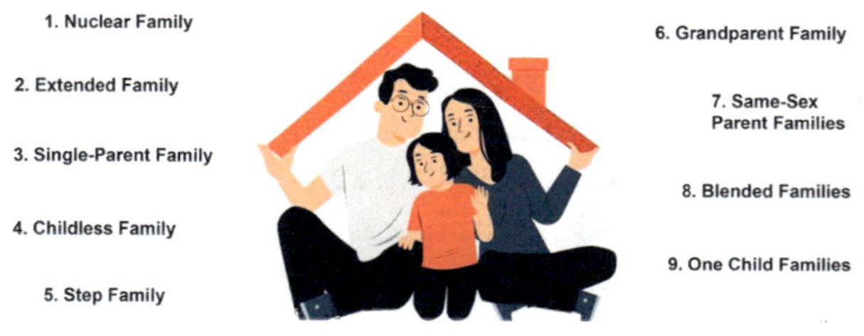

Figure 13.13. Social implications and family dynamics.

Source: https://www.parentingforbrain.com/wp-content/uploads/family-dynamics-types-1024x524.jpg.

This period of transition, particularly for those with long-term conditions like Type 1 diabetes, has a tendency to lead to breakdown in care and deteriorating health outcomes. A systematic review elucidates that effective transition involves various elements like family involvement and coordination between pediatrics and adult services. Disengagement by parents and increasing autonomy of youth can lead to unmanaged health behaviors that affect glycemic control and overall wellness. Therefore, close family support and structured transition processes are essential to empower youth to successfully navigate their healthcare journey. Through the placement of emphasis on family inclusion within this critical transition, healthcare providers are facilitated to reduce potential declines in health and foster an easier transition, encouraging an integrated, multidisciplinary system in pediatric gastroenterology (Bagnall et al., 2013) (Figure 13.13).

13.6. Advances in Pediatric Gastroenterology

The recent advances in pediatric gastroenterology have drastically improved the knowledge and management of inflammatory bowel diseases (IBD), i.e., ulcerative colitis (UC) and Crohn's disease (CD). IBD tends to present a unique challenge in children, hence requiring specific therapeutic protocols. Recent research emphasizes the relevance of a systems biology approach, involving genetic, epigenetic, and microbiomic factors in unraveling the complex pathogenesis of IBD in children. These strategies allow clinicians to identify the central regulatory hubs in the IBD interactome, which could guide the design of targeted therapies in these critical pathways. This worldwide view not only allows new drug targets to be discovered but also enhances predictive modeling of the onset of disease in kids with these debilitating diseases (Polytarchou et al., 2014). Apart from molecular data, identification of novel biomarkers is transforming the clinical management of IBD in children. Traditional assessment methods are largely reliant on clinical symptoms, which often do not reflect disease activity. Recent findings have delineated circulating microRNAs as new diagnostic and predictive markers for ulcerative colitis. Studies have shown that specific microRNA profiles are highly correlated with disease severity, offering greater sensitivity and specificity compared to conventional biomarkers like C-reactive protein (CRP). Implementing these microRNAs in routine clinical work could potentially enhance monitoring of patients and therapeutic decision-making, therefore fulfilling a specific clinical requirement for useful screening devices in pediatric gastroenterology (Touroutoglou et al., 2015). Besides, pediatric gastroenterology research is still striving towards maximizing therapeutic paradigms with personalized medicine approaches. With the convergence of omics technologies and clinical data, clinicians are now able to treat patients based on individual patient profiles, achieving maximum outcomes with minimal side effects. Utilization of molecular data to inform therapeutic strategy is especially significant in the pediatric setting, where concerns for growth and development take precedence. As a more available database of information on individual genetic history and response to therapy becomes available, the field of pediatric gastroenterology will be richly rewarded. Enhanced therapeutic specificity maximizes therapy while promoting a more anticipatory care of chronic gastrointestinal disease in children and eventually promising improved quality of life (Polytarchou et al., 2014; Touroutoglou et al., 2015).

13.6.1. Emerging Research and Clinical Trials

Fresh evidence in pediatric gastroenterology is significant, particularly in inflammatory bowel disease (IBD), where understanding the role of diet is expanding. Fresh evidence has indicated the interplay of genes, environmental exposure, and gut microbiota as etiologies of the rising incidence of IBD in children. A comprehensive review by the D-ECCO working group identifies diet as one important environmental determinant of IBD etiology, and an essential dialogue about nutritional interventions is invited. By investigating the potential of dietary change to evoke and maintain therapeutic remission, new studies might complement current treatment protocols. These studies are likely to fuel new strategies for meeting the nutritional needs of pediatric patients, thereby driving evidence-based pediatric gastroenterology practice guidelines recommending comprehensive disease management like that of IBD (Sigall-Boneh et al., 2017). With the increasing rise in obesity among children and adolescents, understanding the complex pathophysiology of its causation is also at the forefront of developing research. This disorder currently impacts approximately 17% of US adolescents, with extreme obesity, the most quickly expanding category, accounting for a crisis of pressing health. Recent studies show that the medical consequences of obesity, such as type 2 diabetes and cardiovascular disease, are dose-dependently linked to the degree of obesity. Treatment programs, as diverse as they are, often prove to be of limited value, particularly for the treatment of extreme obesity. This points towards the urgent need for clinical trials to establish multi-modal treatment programs including behavioral therapy, nutrition, and pharmacologic interventions, considering the unique developmental issues of children (Ameer & Weintraub, 2018). This is a challenge in progressing from holistic awareness to functional therapeutic interventions, and there is a need for more to be explored through emerging research. Against this background of emerging trends in pediatric gastroenterology, the ongoing work on effective clinical trials is a watershed for further studies that could impact clinical practice to a great extent. The studies of the role of dietary intervention in IBD and obesity management are an example of the call for interdisciplinarity. Securing the bridge between emerging research and clinical trials can lead to more comprehensive treatment models that not only consider the effectiveness of medication but also the overall psychosocial and nutritional health of children as patients. As researchers move to fill gaps identified in current therapeutic practice, integrating research across the disciplines will be essential to the advancement of better health outcomes for children with gastrointestinal disease. Such dedication to clinical innovation and research is critical in setting a platform that provides for maximum care in pediatric gastroenterology (Sigall-Boneh et al., 2017; Ameer & Weintraub, 2018) (Figure 13.14).

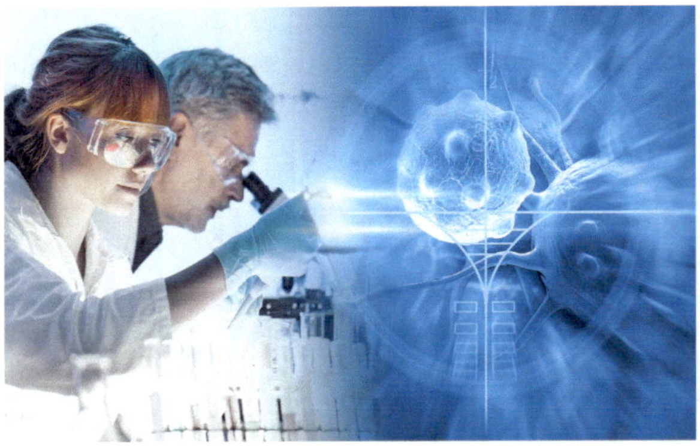

Figure 13.14. Emerging research and clinical trials.

Source: https://www.biospectrumasia.com/uploads/articles/sillajen-14477.jpg.

13.6.2. Innovations in Diagnostic Technology

Technological advancements in the field of diagnostics have transformed pediatric gastroenterology to a significant extent, leading to improved patient outcomes and a more accurate diagnosis. Among these developments, sophisticated imaging methods , such as ultrasound, magnetic resonance imaging (MRI), and computed tomography (CT) play a central role in evaluating gastrointestinal (GI) disease in children. For instance, real-time imaging has become possible with the aid of high-resolution ultrasound to diagnose abnormalities , such as congenital malformations or inflammatory disease. These non-invasive techniques, along with increasingly advanced image interpretation software, allow clinicians to make better decisions while minimizing the number of invasive tests required. Furthermore, advancements in gastrointestinal motility studies, with emphasis on the use of wireless motility capsules, have revolutionized the diagnostic approach to gastroparesis and constipation, providing full data on GI function in a less invasive manner. Machine learning algorithms and artificial intelligence (AI) are now beginning to influence diagnostic practice in pediatric gastroenterology, with the potential to revolutionize workflows and improve diagnostic precision. Such machines can integrate computerized amounts of information from various sources, including imaging studies and clinical notes, to discern patterns and predictive patterns for GI illness. Notably, endoscopic findings may be interpreted by AI, a move that would help reduce human error while also accelerating diagnosis. Pediatric gastroenterologists, in their turn, get the advantage of receiving more accurate and timely assessments, which allow for customized treatment protocols appropriate to the specific needs of each child. This capability maximizes patient care as well as reduces healthcare spending by optimizing interventions while limiting unnecessary procedures through enhanced diagnostic discrimination. Furthermore, the integration of new biomarkers and genetic testing into the diagnostic algorithms is revolutionizing disease knowledge and treatment in the pediatric GI tract. Studies have begun to determine the place of specific biomarkers in the diagnosis of illnesses , such as inflammatory bowel disease, celiac disease, and other functional gastrointestinal diseases. The capacity to develop urine and blood tests that can detect the subclinical alterations that accompany such conditions offers a less invasive means of diagnosing than traditional biopsy operations. Genetic testing has also been shown to be a critical resource, particularly when heredity is integral. By identifying genetic predispositions to gastrological illness, clinicians can utilize anticipatory surveillance and therapeutic intervention. These diagnostic technologies, complemented by traditional imaging modalities, offer a firm foundation for advancing pediatric gastroenterology, allowing physicians to offer timely, accurate, and individualized therapy that has a significant positive impact on patient outcomes.

13.6.3. Future Directions in Treatment and Management

With the expansion of pediatric gastroenterology, treatment and management directions in the future become increasingly aimed at newer therapies that tap state-of-the-art biotechnological advancement. Stem cell therapy, particularly through the application of intestinal stem cells (ISCs), is one of the primary lines of research. New advances in the ability to culture adult human ISCs and pluripotent stem cells bring new promise for the cure of diseases like intestinal failure that greatly impede normal development and hydration in children. The possibility of organoid technology replicating the cellular heterogeneity of the gut is that such stem cells can be employed to treat specific monogenic and polygenic diseases. These developments promise more therapeutic and targeted interventions, a paradigm shift in gastroenterological treatment approaches (Dunn et al., 2016). Moreover, integration of genome-editing technologies, such as CRISPR/Cas9, into the treatment arsenal of children promises a new strategy for the management of inherited gastrointestinal disease. Through these technologies, researchers are capable of correcting disease-triggering variants in the patient's own stem cells, enabling autologous ISC transplantation. This innovation diminishes organ rejection issues of allogeneic transplants and places treatment near the genetic identification of the patients, offering more tailored healthcare responses. There still remain issues with optimizing strategies , such as ISC expansion, ablation, and engraftment procedures that are critical for clinical safety and efficacy

(Dunn et al., 2016). As we go on to develop these methods, future studies need to focus on overcoming these challenges to facilitate wider clinical use. In addition to therapies with stem cells, advancing our understanding of the role of the gut microbiome in children's gastrointestinal health is another potentially thrilling area for future treatments. The gut microbiome, whose intricate dance of microbial populations is as varied as it is complicated, has been linked to a broad spectrum of gastrointestinal disorders, including inflammatory bowel disease and food allergy. Directed modulation of the microbiome by prebiotics, probiotics, and diet offers therapeutic avenues that might not only cure manifestations but also alter disease progression in infected children. Efforts should be made to study the identification of specific microbial profiles related to pediatric gastrointestinal diseases so as to guide interventions favoring a healthy microbiome. Ultimately, a multi-disciplinary approach including stem cell therapy, genomic editing, and microbiome management would transform treatment paradigms in pediatric gastroenterology with the promise of improved patient outcomes in the future (Figure 13.15).

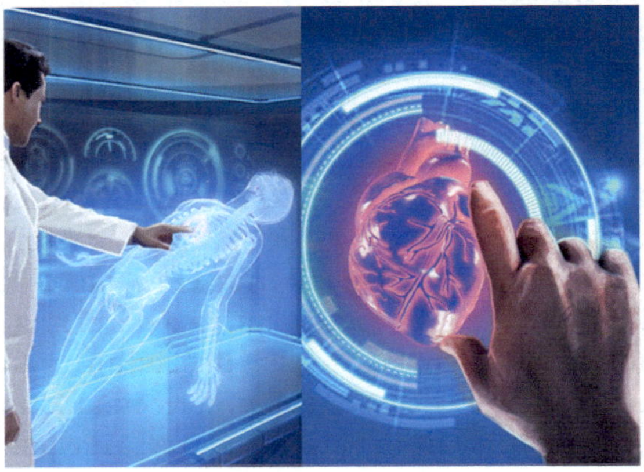

Figure 13.15. Future directions in treatment and management.

Source: https://www.appstudio.ca/blog/wp-content/uploads/2020/08/Major-AI-Trends-Revolutionizing-Healthcare-in-The-Future.jpg.

CLOSER LOOK

NON-INVASIVE BIOMARKERS:

Non-invasive biomarkers are measurable indicators of physiological, pathological, or therapeutic processes that can be detected without the need for invasive procedures such as biopsies or surgical sampling. A closer look at these biomarkers highlights their growing importance in diagnostics, disease monitoring, and personalized medicine. By providing critical information through easily accessible samples like blood, urine, saliva, breath, or imaging studies, non-invasive biomarkers reduce patient risk, improve compliance, and enable earlier detection of disease. One key advantage of non-invasive biomarkers is their ability to facilitate early diagnosis. For example, circulating tumor DNA in blood, specific microRNAs, or protein signatures can signal the presence of cancer before clinical symptoms appear. Similarly, biomarkers in urine, such as albumin or specific metabolites, allow early detection of kidney disease. These markers offer clinicians a window into disease processes at stages when intervention is most effective, improving prognosis and reducing the need for invasive testing.

Non-invasive biomarkers also play a crucial role in monitoring disease progression and treatment response. For chronic conditions like diabetes, heart disease, and liver disease, biomarkers such as glycated hemoglobin, natriuretic peptides, or liver enzyme ratios provide continuous, real-time insights into patient status. This allows physicians to adjust medications, dietary interventions, or other therapeutic strategies more precisely, supporting individualized care and minimizing complications.

Another area of advancement is the use of imaging-based biomarkers. Techniques such as MRI, CT scans, and PET imaging can quantify tissue changes, inflammation, or metabolic activity without requiring tissue extraction. When combined with artificial intelligence and machine learning, these imaging biomarkers can enhance disease prediction, track subtle changes over time, and guide clinical decision-making. Despite their promise, the application of non-invasive biomarkers presents challenges. Standardization is critical to ensure reproducibility across laboratories, while validation studies are necessary to confirm clinical relevance. Sensitivity and specificity vary among biomarkers, and false positives or negatives can impact diagnosis and management. Ethical and regulatory considerations—such as data privacy for genetic or metabolic markers—also require careful oversight.

Overall, a closer examination of non-invasive biomarkers reveals their transformative potential in modern healthcare. By minimizing patient risk, enabling early intervention, and supporting personalized treatment plans, these biomarkers are reshaping disease detection and management. Continued research, validation, and integration into clinical workflows are essential to fully harness their capabilities and translate scientific discovery into improved patient outcomes.

SUMMARY

In summarizing pediatric gastroenterology discussion, it is important to note the fine balance between inflammatory bowel disease (IBD) and autoimmune liver diseases in children. Research indicates that autoimmune liver disease has a predominant prevalence, affecting approximately 6.8% of children fighting IBD, particularly ulcerative colitis. The association with severe ulcerative colitis and autoimmune liver disease, or sclerosing cholangitis, is a significant association warranting further clinical attention. The identification of acute hepatobiliary complications, as uncommon as they are, necessitates close monitoring and evaluation of children to neutralize potential long-term consequences. Therefore, greater emphasis on the multifaceted character of these diseases is necessary to inform pediatric clinical practice, ultimately to promote improved results for affected children (Alexopoulou et al., 2016). Another fundamental perspective in pediatric gastroenterology concerns dietary problems as factors in the pathogenesis and management of IBD. Recent research has described the role of diet as a key environmental influence that may be involved in the rising incidence of IBD in genetically predisposed children. The D-ECCO working group describes how dietary exposures can affect both induction and maintenance of these diseases, with the understanding that nutrition therapy may double as induction and maintenance treatment for IBD. This new insight illuminates the requirement for clinicians to adopt a more integrated approach that includes nutritional assessment within treatment interventions. By integrating evidence-based nutrition interventions, medical practitioners are able to enhance the quality of the pediatric patient's life such that they can achieve improved symptom management and disease progression (Sigall-Boneh et al., 2017). Lastly, the application of science within pediatric gastroenterology induces an interdisciplinary system that intertwines care, nutritional therapy, and vigilant surveillance of accompanying conditions. As the scientific information regarding complex interdependencies between pediatric gastroenterological disorders, such as IBD and autoimmune liver diseases, is refined, future research must aim toward untapped territories, namely those related to diet and how it influences long-term health outcomes. Ongoing studies of nutritional components and their functions in the manifestation of disease will spur progressive avenues for maximizing patient care and practice guidelines. As clinicians aim to address the unique needs of children, devotion to integrative paradigms in gastroenterology will undoubtedly foster better health outcomes in this high-risk group.

In pediatric gastroenterology, the transition from pediatric to adult care is a critical milestone that poses serious implications for adolescents who have been diagnosed with diseases , such as eosinophilic esophagitis (EoE). Constant monitoring and interventions required are the priority as children with EoE mature into adulthood. A systematic critique examining the process of transition from pediatric gastroenterology (pGI) to adult gastroenterology (aGI) revealed significant issues like loss to follow-up and increased rates of non-adherence to medication, which were noted to rise from 7% in the pediatric setting to 26% after transfer to adult care. There was also a highly concerning increase in symptoms of heartburn that indicated that patients might have a decline in their overall management as they make this health transition. These findings highlight the importance of further optimizing the transitional care processes in pediatric gastroenterology clinics (Webber et al., 2025). The importance of having health services among young patients cannot be overemphasized, especially in cases of chronicity that require extended management over the long term. The study aimed at a cohort of 58 EoE patients converting to aGI, where researchers found that the median duration of time from the most recent pGI clinic visit and first visit with aGI was 299 days. This long duration not only corresponds to patient dropout but also suggests a potential fragmentation of continuity of care, which is detrimental to effective management of the disease. As quoted, endoscopic and histological outcomes were not altered, suggesting that delays in the care transition do not represent a reduction in the severity of the disease at the time but may reflect a future worsening in health outcomes if follow-up care is inadequately planned (Webber et al., 2025). Addressing these systemic problems necessitates the development of standard procedures that are meant to facilitate smoother transitions in teens entering adult healthcare environments. With pediatric gastroenterology, this means not only extending care continuity but also educating patients and families regarding the requirement for follow-up over time. Demand exists: an active process must be put into place, one that emphasizes clear communication and interprovider collaboration between pediatric and adult gastroenterology providers. With the growth of young patients, it is necessary to maintain them engaged in a manner that avoids gaps in care and adherence to care plans. Integration of pediatric and adult services in gastroenterology will eventually lead to better outcomes, a smooth care pathway, and enhanced quality of life for youth with chronic gastrointestinal disease (Webber et al., 2025).

References

1. Alvisi, P., Arrigo, S., Cucchiara, S., Lionetti, P., Miele, E., Romano, C., Ravelli, A., Knafelz, D., Martelossi, S., Guariso, G., Accomando, S., Zuin, G., De Giacomo, C., Balzani, L., Gennari, M., Aloi, M., & SIGENP IBD Working Group (2019). Efficacy of adalimumab as second-line therapy in a pediatric cohort of Crohn's disease patients who failed infliximab therapy: the Italian Society of Pediatric Gastroenterology, Hepatology, and Nutrition experience. *Biologics : targets & therapy*, *13*, 13–21. https://doi.org/10.2147/BTT.S183088(accessed on 16th July 2025).
2. Harlow, K. E., Africa, J. A., Wells, A., Belt, P. H., Behling, C. A., Jain, A. K., Molleston, J. P., Newton, K. P., Rosenthal, P., Vos, M. B., Xanthakos, S. A., Lavine, J. E., Schwimmer, J. B., & Nonalcoholic Steatohepatitis Clinical Research Network (NASH CRN) (2018). Clinically Actionable Hypercholesterolemia and Hypertriglyceridemia in Children with Nonalcoholic Fatty Liver Disease. *The Journal of pediatrics*, *198*, 76–83.e2. https://doi.org/10.1016/j.jpeds.2018.02.038 (accessed on 16th July 2025).
3. Alexopoulou, A., Alvarez, F., Block, G., Boonstra, K., Deneau, M., Dotson, J., Faubion, W., et al. (2016). *Clinical features and risk factors of autoimmune liver involvement in pediatric inflammatory bowel disease.* https://core.ac.uk/download/74318847.pdf (accessed on 16th July 2025).
4. Della Corte, C., Mosca, A., Vania, A., Alterio, A., Alisi, A., & Nobili, V. (2016). Pediatric liver diseases: current challenges and future perspectives. *Expert review of gastroenterology & hepatology*, *10*(2), 255–265. https://doi.org/10.1586/17474124.2016.1129274(accessed on 16th July 2025).
5. Sigall-Boneh, R., Levine, A., Lomer, M., Wierdsma, N., Allan, P., Fiorino, G., Gatti, S., Jonkers, D., Kierkus, J., Katsanos, K. H., Melgar, S., Yuksel, E. S., Whelan, K., Wine, E., & Gerasimidis, K. (2017). Research Gaps in Diet and Nutrition in Inflammatory Bowel Disease. A Topical Review by D-ECCO Working Group [Dietitians of ECCO]. *Journal of Crohn's & colitis*, *11*(12), 1407–1419. https://doi.org/10.1093/ecco-jcc/jjx109(accessed on 16th July 2025).
6. Ameer, B., & Weintraub, M. A. (2018). Pediatric Obesity: Influence on Drug Dosing and Therapeutics. *Journal of clinical pharmacology*, *58 Suppl 10*, S94–S107. https://doi.org/10.1002/jcph.1092(accessed on 16th July 2025).
7. Gupta, N., Lustig, R. H., Chao, C., Vittinghoff, E., Andrews, H., & Leu, C. S. (2018). Thiopurines are negatively associated with anthropometric parameters in pediatric Crohn's disease. *World journal of gastroenterology*, *24*(18), 2036–2046. https://doi.org/10.3748/wjg.v24.i18.2036(accessed on 16th July 2025).
8. Bagnall, A., Day, R., & Kime, N. H. (2013). *Systematic review of transition models for young people with long-term conditions: A report for NHS Diabetes.* https://core.ac.uk/download/29018738.pdf (accessed on 16th July 2025).
9. Barker, P., Lewin, M., Donofrio, M. T., Altman, C. A., Ensing, G. J., Arya, B., Swaminathan, M. (2020). Specific considerations for pediatric, fetal, and congenital heart disease patients and echocardiography service providers during the 2019 novel coronavirus outbreak: Council on Pediatric and Congenital Heart Disease supplement to the statement of the American Society of Echocardiography. *Journal of the American Society of Echocardiography, 33*, 658–665. https://doi.org/10.1016/j.echo.2020.04.005 (accessed on 16th July 2025).

10. Batens, A. H., Bekaert, M., Geerts, A., Hoorens, A., et al. (2019). *Insulin resistance associates with hepatic lobular inflammation in subjects with obesity.* https://core.ac.uk/download/237012237.pdf (accessed on 16th July 2025).

11. Behling, C., Donithan, M., Hallinan, E. K., Newton, K. P., et al. (2014). *Longitudinal assessment of high blood pressure in children with nonalcoholic fatty liver disease.* https://core.ac.uk/download/323064808.pdf (accessed on 16th July 2025).

12. Caffarelli, C., Santamaria, F., Mastrorilli, C., Santoro, A., Iovane, B., Petraroli, M., Gaeta, V., Di Pinto, R., Borrelli, M., Bernasconi, S., & Corsello, G. (2019). Report on advances for pediatricians in 2018: allergy, cardiology, critical care, endocrinology, hereditary metabolic diseases, gastroenterology, infectious diseases, neonatology, nutrition, respiratory tract disorders and surgery. *Italian journal of pediatrics*, *45*(1), 126. https://doi.org/10.1186/s13052-019-0727-6(accessed on 16th July 2025).

13. Blazeby, J., Blencowe, N., Chalmers, K., et al. (2017). *Methodological overview of systematic reviews to establish the evidence base for emergency general surgery.* https://core.ac.uk/download/79655849.pdf (accessed on 16th July 2025).

14. Borrelli, O., Pesce, M., Rybak, A., Thapar, N., et al. (2017). *Gastro-Esophageal Reflux in Children.* https://core.ac.uk/download/111029577.pdf (accessed on 16th July 2025).

15. Bronsky, J., Ferry, G. D., Frank, E., Harris, J., et al. (2014). *DNA methylation-associated colonic mucosal immune and defense responses in treatment-naïve pediatric ulcerative colitis.* https://core.ac.uk/download/29361673.pdf (accessed on 16th July 2025).

16. Browne, J., Cohen, S. S., de Camargo, O. K., Delaney, M. T., et al. (2019). *Pediatric Feeding Disorder: Consensus Definition and Conceptual Framework.* https://core.ac.uk/download/286544045.pdf (accessed on 16th July 2025).

17. Burgos, F., González, L., Leta, K., & Toca, M. C. (2025). Dyschezia or functional constipation: A frequent challenge in pediatric practice. *Archivos Argentinos de Pediatría.* https://www.semanticscholar.org/paper/1dd0c8291fcb2fe20f0b97ce4ef2923e4beecdd3 (accessed on 16th July 2025).

18. Iebba, V., Totino, V., Gagliardi, A., Santangelo, F., Cacciotti, F., Trancassini, M., Mancini, C., Cicerone, C., Corazziari, E., Pantanella, F., & Schippa, S. (2016). Eubiosis and dysbiosis: the two sides of the microbiota. *The new microbiologica*, *39*(1), 1–12. (accessed on 16th July 2025).

19. Choe, U. (2025). Nutritional management for pediatric biliary atresia patients preparing for liver transplantation. *Children, 12.* https://www.semanticscholar.org/paper/0abbabcf244f9254d80388207086bfd9e0cc76f2 (accessed on 16th July 2025).

20. Coleman, T. P., Gharibans, A. A., Kriegsfeld, L. J., Kunkel, D. C., et al. (2018). *Artifact rejection methodology enables continuous, noninvasive measurement of gastric myoelectric activity in ambulatory subjects.* https://core.ac.uk/download/323082131.pdf (accessed on 16th July 2025).

21. Di Lorenzo, C., Hayes, D., Jadcherla, S. R., Kaul, A., et al. (2017). *Not all children with cystic fibrosis have abnormal esophageal neutralization during chemical clearance of acid reflux.* https://core.ac.uk/download/323311033.pdf (accessed on 16th July 2025).

22. Dunn, J. C. Y., Hong, S. N., Martín, M. G., Stelzner, M., et al. (2016). *Concise review: The potential use of intestinal stem cells to treat patients with intestinal failure.* https://core.ac.uk/download/323078733.pdf (accessed on 16th July 2025).

23. Easler, J. J., El Hajj, I. I., Fogel, E. L., Gromski, M. A., et al. (2019). *Annular pancreas: Endoscopic and pancreatographic findings from a tertiary referral ERCP center.* https://core.ac.uk/download/227054194.pdf (accessed on 16th July 2025).

24. Garcia, J., Gross, S. A., Lahr, R., Rex, D. K., et al. (2019). *Endocuff Vision reduces inspection time without decreasing lesion detection in a randomized colonoscopy trial.* https://core.ac.uk/download/187423803.pdf (accessed on 16th July 2025).

25. Naramore, S., & Gupta, S. K. (2018). Nonesophageal Eosinophilic Gastrointestinal Disorders: Clinical Care and Future Directions. *Journal of pediatric gastroenterology and nutrition, 67*(3), 318–321. https://doi.org/10.1097/MPG.0000000000002040(accessed on 16th July 2025).

26. Polytarchou, C., Koukos, G., & Iliopoulos, D. (2014). Systems biology in inflammatory bowel diseases: ready for prime time. *Current opinion in gastroenterology, 30*(4), 339–346. https://doi.org/10.1097/MOG.0000000000000081(accessed on 16th July 2025).

27. Karrento, K., Rosen, J. M., Tarbell, S. E., Issenman, R. M., Gelfand, A. A., Gamboa, H., Parikh, S., et al. (2025). North American Society for Pediatric Gastroenterology, Hepatology, and Nutrition 2025 guidelines for management of cyclic vomiting syndrome in children. *Journal of Pediatric Gastroenterology and Nutrition.* https://www.semanticscholar.org/paper/d72ec6d07d177c17d7c83027a399a3a0efd4bf9f (accessed on 16th July 2025).

28. Khan, H. H., Kumar, S., & Lyons, H. (2025). Practices of North American pediatric gastroenterologists in the management of celiac disease—A survey study. *JPGN Reports, 6*, 137–145. https://www.semanticscholar.org/paper/114b777e329e6b36da7a563b919af752a1463e74 (accessed on 16th July 2025).

29. Kinney, A. L. (2007). *National Scientific Facilities and their Science Impact on Non-Biomedical Research.* https://arxiv.org/abs/0705.1797 (accessed on 16th July 2025).

30. Konchakovska, T., & Shunko, E. (2024). Enteral nutrition of preterm infants (2022): A position paper from the European Society for Pediatric Gastroenterology, Hepatology and Nutrition and invited experts. *Neonatology, Surgery and Perinatal Medicine.* https://www.semanticscholar.org/paper/66291ff4d774d77a0fb987fe2e585c8d3509f2b4 (accessed on 16th July 2025).

31. Kyryk, V. (2024). Stem cell therapy for cardiac regeneration: Key points. *Cell and Organ Transplantology.* https://www.semanticscholar.org/paper/6a1b536f3691ad0d162e4187a4a2e2ffd1507b5f (accessed on 16th July 2025).

32. Focal Spot, Fall/Winter 2010/2011. Bernard Becker Medical Library Archives. Washington University School of Medicine, Saint Louis, Missouri (accessed on 16th July 2025).

33. Pennazio, M., Rondonotti, E., Despott, E. J., Dray, X., Keuchel, M., Moreels, T. G., Sanders, D. S., et al. (2022). Small-bowel capsule endoscopy and device-assisted enteroscopy for diagnosis and treatment of small-bowel disorders: European Society of Gastrointestinal Endoscopy (ESGE) Guideline – Update 2022. *Endoscopy, 55*, 58–95. https://doi.org/10.1055/a-1973-3796 (accessed on 16th July 2025).

34. Russell, R. K., Fagbemi, A., Benyacoub, J., Capobianco, M. E., Wells, L. E., Shergill-Bonner, R., Sharma, P., et al. (2025). Specialized and standard nutritional formulas for the dietary management of pediatric patients with Crohn's disease: A systematic literature review. *Expert Review of Gastroenterology & Hepatology, 19*, 455–465. https://www.semanticscholar.org/paper/7e655269101068cc27bc47af3d38573448b9fa60 (accessed on 16th July 2025).

35. Singh, A., Silvester, J. A., Turner, J., Absah, I., Sparks, B. A., Walsh, C., Bracken, J. M., et al. (2024). Celiac disease in North America: What is the current practice of pediatric gastroenterology providers? *JPGN Reports, 5,* 276–283. https://www.semanticscholar.org/paper/eef2ed333b165701e8052301e3f16ade66cb3782 (accessed on 16th July 2025).

36. Touroutoglou, A., Oikonomopoulos, A., Baltimore, Baumgart, Cho, C., Polytarchou, C., CramaBohbouth, et al. (2015). *Assessment of circulating microRNAs for the diagnosis and disease activity evaluation in patients with ulcerative colitis by using the Nanostring technology.* https://core.ac.uk/download/30650084.pdf (accessed on 16th July 2025).

37. Tramontano, A., Giannetti, E., Greco, L., Martinelli, M., et al. (2010). *Impact of the Rome II pediatric criteria on the appropriateness of the upper and lower gastrointestinal endoscopy in children.* https://core.ac.uk/download/55044504.pdf (accessed on 16th July 2025).

38. von Eckardstein, A. (2017). *Laboratory Diagnostics of Non-Alcoholic Fatty Liver Disease.* https://core.ac.uk/download/85223615.pdf (accessed on 16th July 2025).

39. Webber, K. F., Slaughter, J. C., Patel, D., & Hiremath, G. (2025). Impact of transfer from pediatric gastroenterology to adult gastroenterology care in eosinophilic esophagitis. *Diseases of the Esophagus, 38.* https://www.semanticscholar.org/paper/80ce41d9b6f25d1f4d8de5bc6996739de03a96b4 (accessed on 16th July 2025).

40. Zhou, L., Li, T., Zheng, Q., Xu, J., Xu, C., Zhang, B., Wang, Z., et al. (2025). Research progress and future opportunities of pediatric cow milk protein allergy: A bibliometric overview and evidence mapping. *International Archives of Allergy and Immunology.* https://www.semanticscholar.org/paper/c57e04d92222d35fe54a9f5c7d7bc34a4d411caa (accessed on 16th July 2025).

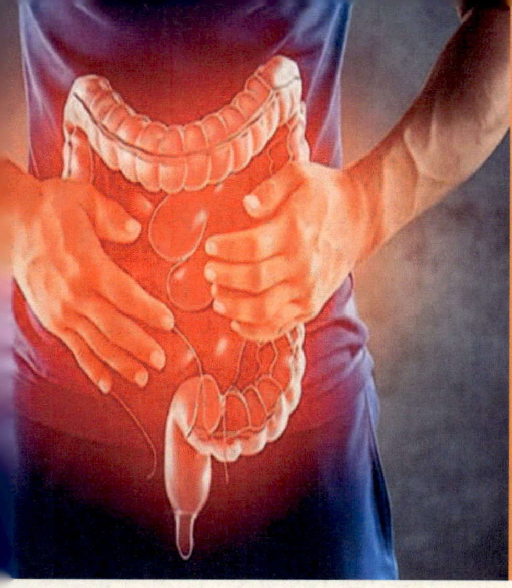

Chapter 14
GI ONCOLOGY

Contents

Introduction

The field of gastrointestinal (GI) oncology is an essential research and clinical field with the concern of cancers that develop in the digestive tract, including the esophagus, stomach, pancreas, liver, colon, and rectum. Understanding the complexities of such cancers is vital to moving along with patient care and improving outcomes. The research has highlighted significant survival rate variations and effectiveness of treatment among various GI cancers, necessitating the adopting a multi-faceted management technique involving precision medicine, surgery, and novel therapeutic agents. In addition, strategies , such as high-dose chemotherapy with autologous stem cell transplant demonstrate the advancement towards optimizing survival in extremely challenging scenarios like relapsed Wilms tumor, revealing an emerging need for continued investigation into therapy approaches that optimize outcomes in gastrointestinal cancers (Abdel-Azim et al., 2017). The use of extensive care in GI oncology applies beyond the immediate cancer treatments; it is used to address necessary support for lifestyle modifications and comorbid health conditions. Smoking is an established risk factor for a range of GI malignancies, ultimately impinging on patient outcome as well as therapeutic response. A prime model of intervention, as introduced by the Stanford Cancer Center, depicts a successful incorporation of tobacco cessation programs into the oncology clinics. This initiative led to a remarkable increase in patient referrals and screening rates for smoking abstinence, ultimately increasing treatment retention and encouraging better patient habits (Gali et al., 2020). These combined measures not only make the treatment more efficient but also address the larger goal of improving the overall quality of life for patients who are battling the intricacies of GI cancers. In addition, GI oncology development must incorporate the diverse spectrum of gastrointestinal cancers with unique biological and clinical behavior. Multidisciplinary intensive effort is required from oncologists, surgeons, radiologists, and palliative care physicians to create individualized therapeutic strategies toward fulfilling the patient's unique needs. Cutting-edge research continues to find novel molecular targets and biomarkers that have the promise of altering the treatment scenario of GI cancer, enhancing the specificity of the therapy and minimizing side effects. Along with developments in the department, new paradigms of therapy, including immunotherapy and targeted therapy, emerge, focusing on continuous education, clinical trials, and patient-centered care in GI oncology. It is the joint effort of patients, practitioners, and researchers that will ultimately decide the future course of this critical medical discipline (Figure 14.1).

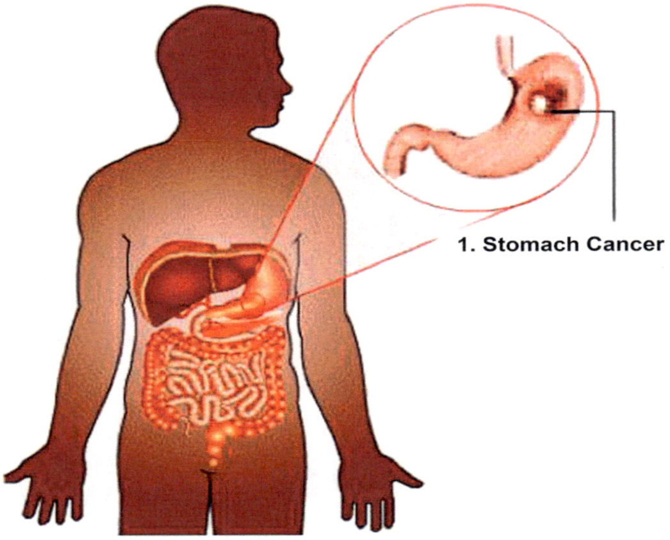

Figure 14.1. GI oncology.

Source: https://www.rainbowhospitalkolhapur.com/liver-specialist-kolhapur/gi-oncology/stomach-cancer-treatment-maharashtra.jpg.

Definition of GI Oncology

Gastrointestinal (GI) oncology is a specialty of oncology that deals with the diagnosis, management, and treatment of cancers that affect the gastrointestinal tract, such as organs like the esophagus, stomach, pancreas, liver, and intestines. GI oncology practice entails the entire spectrum of cancer care from early detection and diagnosis to therapy and palliation. Therefore, it requires a multidisciplinary insight that unifies the expertise of surgeons, medical oncologists, radiation oncologists, pathologists, and nutritionists. The multidisciplinary environment is crucial in optimizing the patient's outcome since it allows for the development of individualized treatment plans that are adjusted to the unique biological behavior of each category of cancer, as well as to the patient's unique requirements. With the variance and complexity of GI malignancies, the right definition of GI oncology is important to both patients and healthcare professionals as they consider their choice for treatment. In GI oncology, evidence-based care is becoming increasingly emphasized, particularly in assessing the quality of life and results of the treatment of cancer patients. More contemporary studies have highlighted the need for universally agreed outcome measures that are accurate representations of the complicated problems seen in patients following treatment for GI cancers. For instance, a systematic review of measures of female sexual dysfunction after cervical and endometrial cancer therapy has been conducted, and existing measures have been identified to have serious limitations with the necessity for distress at sexual change as defined by DSM-5 diagnostic criteria (White et al., 2016). Incorporation of such steps into clinical practice not only enhances the personalization of treatment plans but also raises the level of the patient experience overall to the point where quality of life is kept at the center of cancer treatment. In addition, GI oncology's interest is also focused on rare tumors like Pancreatic Neuroendocrine Neoplasms, which require a special diagnostic and treatment approach. Care of these tumors is a prototype of the necessity for specialized knowledge and expertise since these tumors are usually indolent but quite troublesome because of their peculiar biological characteristics (Almar et al., 2019). Treatment needs to be properly addressed through specialized biochemistry tests and a variety of medical treatments, based on the status of the individual patient, again with a demonstration of the absolute necessity of a multidisciplinary team in GI cancer care. This disciplined framework allows for the best care pathways that are attuned to the complexities of GI tumors, thereby cementing the definition of GI oncology not only as a medical specialty but also as a collaborative model dedicated to improving patient outcomes for a spectrum of gastrointestinal cancers.

Importance of GI Oncology in Cancer Treatment

GI oncology plays a very important role in cancer therapy because cancers of the digestive system present unique challenges. Esophageal, gastric, colorectal, pancreatic, and liver cancers, among others, have the potential to significantly influence nutrient absorption, digestion, and metabolic health. As such, these types of oncologists possess extremely valuable expertise in how to manage the multifaceted symptoms and complications of GI tumors. Effective management requires an interdisciplinarity that includes nutritional support, pain management, and symptom relief. Amidst the complexity of GI oncology is also the challenge to study special methods of therapy, like targeted therapies and novel immunotherapies that have shown significant efficacy in recent years. The continuous progress in knowing the biologic behavior of GI tumors thus positively influences patient outcomes and harmonizes therapeutic action with the patient's individual needs. In addition to the treatment complexity, side effects of standard cancer treatments are a significant concern in GI oncology. Systemic corticosteroids, to cite one example, which are commonly administered, can potentially induce undesirable events , such as hyperglycemia, dyspepsia, and oral candidiasis among cancer patients. A study at Boffa Hospital finds that such side effects were inadequately controlled in a large proportion of patients, only 36% having followed guidelines for managing hyperglycemia, though it was common among this patient population (Fsadni, 2015). Such findings indicate a wide gap in the implementation of best practice in cancer treatment, and they serve to highlight the importance of improved provider training and compliance with established treatment guidelines. By overcoming such adversity, GI oncologists are able to significantly improve the quality of life for patients, demonstrating that there is more to whole-person care than simply curing the cancer. Moreover, future studies also identify the significance of immunotherapy in GI oncology, particularly in immune-related adverse events (irAEs) management.

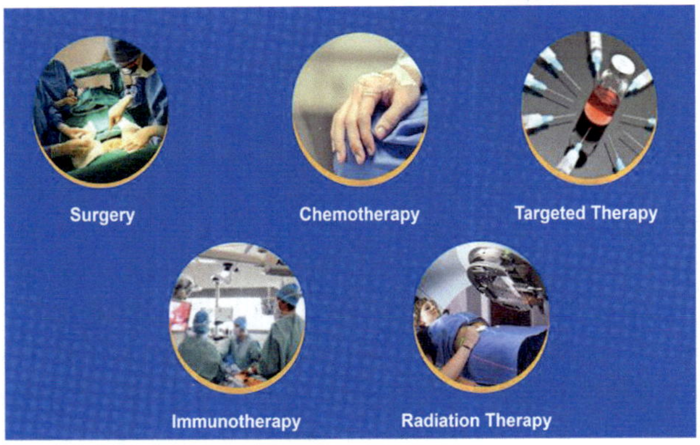

Figure 14.2. Importance of GI oncology in cancer treatment.

Source: https://actchealth.com/images/treatment/stomach-treat.png.

These treatments, like immune checkpoint inhibitors, have revolutionized the treatment strategy but present a unique set of issues, among them gastrointestinal toxicities that pose considerable risks to patient health. The complexity of treating these irAEs mandates an important understanding of their mechanisms, which typically resemble the immunologic responses those treatments attempt to exploit (Puzanov et al., 2017). Therefore, optimal management of such events is based on a proactive, interdisciplinary strategy focused on the early detection and proper interventions. As more is learned about these new therapies, it becomes increasingly important for GI oncologists to be leaders in cancer treatment technology, maximizing therapeutic advantages over possible risks and improving patient care outcomes in the field of GI oncology (Figure 14.2).

Overview of Gastrointestinal Cancers

Gastrointestinal (GI) cancers include a heterogenous group of malignancies , such as esophageal carcinoma, gastric carcinoma, pancreatic cancer, liver cancer, and colon cancer, all having characteristic features, risk factors, and management modalities. The major problem with these cancers is their frequent late diagnosis, which is mostly because of the gradual course of presentation of symptoms. For instance, pancreatic cancer, with its historically dismal prognosis, usually presents clinically only late in its course, a five-year survival rate of less than 10% being the rule in most instances. This tardy presentation emphasizes the need for greater awareness and screening tests that can lead to early discovery, ultimately providing improved patient results. In addition, the frequent occurrence of lifestyle risk factors , such as obesity and smoking, necessitates that public health interventions be used to stem the prevalence of GI cancers. The complex biology of GI tumors often enables the treatment protocols often to be challenging, thus requiring multidisciplinary management, tailoring the treatment regimens to the individual patient profile. Particularly for pancreatic neuroendocrine neoplasms, there are specialized diagnostic and treatment needs that require coordination among providers. These tumors are a rare type of pancreatic cancer with distinct biochemical markers, which need specialized imaging modalities and potential surgery that is often more challenging than for other cancers. The GI oncology environment is shaped by ongoing research efforts to establish the effectiveness of novel treatment approaches and optimization of proven therapy, spurring the development of patient-centered models considering the particular features of each oncological condition (Caplin et al., 2017). Research is currently directed at the prophylactic function in reducing GI cancer risk, with specific focus on the use of aspirin. Research indicates that aspirin will have protective effects against certain types of cancer, with effects being typically only evident after long exposure. Longitudinal findings indicate that patients who are taking aspirin consistently can have a relative reduction in incidence and total cancer mortality, particularly in those with high-risk status. But the benefits must be weighed against the potential side effects, including gastrointestinal bleeding, which in some cases can be marked, especially in elderly patients. The implication of these findings raises questions regarding individualized aspirin therapy in resections and in primary prevention in general against GI cancers, emphasizing patient education on risks and benefits of these drug therapies (Algra et al., 2014) (Figure 14.3).

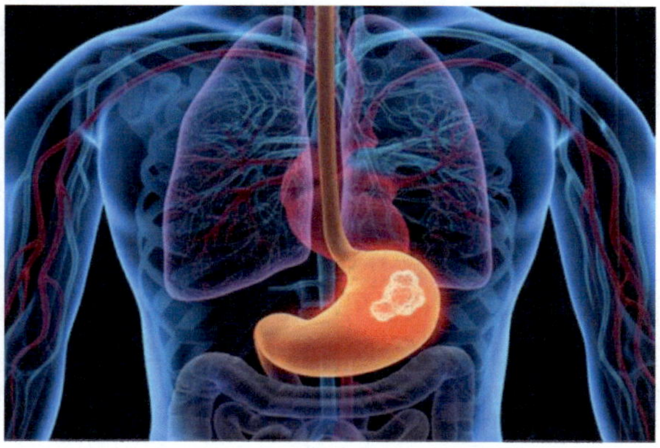

Figure 14.3. Overview of gastrointestinal cancers.

Source: https://external-content.duckduckgo.com/iu/?u=https%3A%2F%2Ftse3.mm.bing.net%2Fth%3Fid%3DOIP.JtP2l_xwQskCuRZTtNl2IQHaE3%26pid%3DApi&f=1&ipt=a09f0276b4ec8e01609c994a2687c9a13219cda28ee86332f6b28222b6b0b5af.

14.1. Types of Gastrointestinal Cancers

Gastrointestinal tumors are a series of tumors found along the digestive tract, from the esophagus to the rectum. Among them, one of the most prevalent is colorectal cancer, which presents as an abnormal growth in the colon or rectum. The risk factors include age, diet, and hereditary predisposition, so early detection is required in order to increase the survival rates. Relevantly, newer innovations in screening methods, for example, colonoscopy, have enabled earlier diagnosis, which is particularly significant given that late occurring cancers of colorectal cancers have limited modes of treatment. Besides colorectal cancer, other important forms of gastrointestinal cancers are those of the esophagus and stomach, both of which have unique risk factors, presenting symptoms, and issues of prognostication, which again reflect the heterogeneity of GI cancers. The heterogeneity of gastrointestinal cancers extends to rarer forms, like pancreatic and liver cancer, both well-known to be aggressively malignant and prognostically unfavorable. Pancreatic cancer, for instance, is usually asymptomatic until later in its course, leading to late diagnosis at less curable, more advanced stages. Risk factors for pancreatic cancer include smoking, obesity, and chronic pancreatitis, and so efficient early detection difficult. Parallel to this is liver cancer, or hepatocellular carcinoma, which often attends chronic viral hepatitis and cirrhosis, making treatment complicated by underlying liver pathology. Information shows that the median survival rate for these malignant tumors remains dismal, and continued investigation into biomarkers as well as novel treatments is necessary to further improve patient outcomes. Understanding of the characteristic biological behavior of these tumors can be used to guide therapy, illustrating the complexity inherent in

GI oncology. In addition to chemotherapeutic and surgical treatment, the emerging role of liquid biopsies in gastrointestinal cancer is a fascinating domain of advancement in this area. Studies have pointed out that an analysis of circulating tumor DNA may be revealing about the dynamics of the tumor, potentially influencing the treatment. For instance, research evidence indicates that patients with elevated levels of %ctDNA have a greater risk of worse overall survival compared to patients with low levels, thereby qualifying ctDNA as a potential prognostic marker of such cancers. Furthermore, the direct positive correlation between the number of alterations in ctDNA and survival underscores the need for using these new diagnostic tools in practice. By using such approaches, medical practitioners are able to more suitably tailor treatment strategies and monitor disease progression, generally enhancing general management practices for gastrointestinal cancers (Aizer et al., 2019; Goodman et al., 2020) (Figure 14.4).

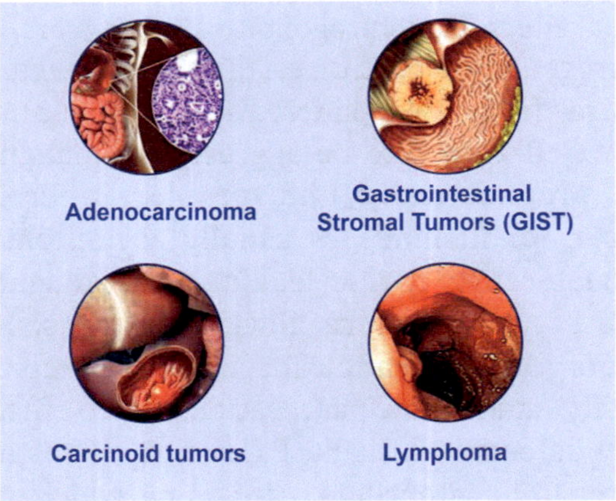

Figure 14.4. Types of gastrointestinal cancers.

Source: https://www.drsanjaysharmacancer.com/static/images/footer-services/stomach-cancer/types.jpg.

14.1.1. Esophageal Cancer

Esophageal cancer remains one of the more virulent cancers within the group of GI cancers, with the feature of very high morbidity and mortality. It usually arises from the epithelial lining of the esophagus and generally belongs to two broad categories: squamous cell carcinoma and adenocarcinoma. Epidemiological research has revealed striking geographical differences in the prevalence of these subtypes, with adenocarcinoma common in Western nations but squamous cell carcinoma being more prevalent in Asia and Africa. Risk factors for esophageal cancer are smoking, heavy alcohol intake, obesity, and the presence of gastroesophageal reflux disease (GERD), which in turn causes Barretts esophagus, a precursor lesion to adenocarcinoma. As the disease is stealthy and not easily diagnosed in its early stages, detection by the time advanced stages set in is common, hence leading to early treatment once the disease has progressed. The prognosis for patients diagnosed with esophageal cancer is quite variable depending on several factors , such as tumor stage, location, and histological type. In the past, the overall survival rate for advanced esophageal cancer has been low, usually estimated below 20% at five years after diagnosis. Worthy of mention is that evidence of distant metastases greatly reduces survival probabilities; metastatic patients have a much shorter median survival compared to their non-metastatic counterparts. A recent paper utilizing Diagnosis-Specific Graded Prognostic Assessment (DS-GPA) for gastrointestinal cancers provides helpful information regarding survival estimates in patients with brain metastases secondary to GI malignancies, e.g., esophageal cancer. The updated GI-GPA has identified influential prognostic factors, such as Karnofsky Performance Status and extracranial metastasis, that are available to enhance clinical decision-making regarding treatment selection and palliative care strategies (Aizer et al., 2019). Enhanced therapeutic options for esophageal cancer have become more evident, encompassing non-surgical and surgical interventions. Surgical resection remains the cornerstone for potentially curative therapy, especially in early disease, but with significant risks and patient selection. In patients for whom surgery is not possible, multimodal approaches with neoadjuvant chemotherapy and radiation are commonly employed to improve outcomes. As discussed within comparative analyses of radiation therapy treatment plans, techniques , such as hybrid arc therapy and volumetric-modulated arc therapy are demonstrating positive dosimetric results, which can enhance patient safety in addition to enhanced effectiveness of cancer control (Gunn et al., 2018). Additional research into novel therapeutic agents, immunotherapies, and targeted therapies is central to the optimization of the overall treatment landscape for esophageal cancer and offering hope to patients facing this devious diagnosis.

14.1.2. Gastric (Stomach) Cancer

The heavy burden of gastric cancer in the spectrum of gastrointestinal oncology cannot be overstated, since it is still the second most prevalent malignancy in the world despite notable declines in incidence, especially in more developed countries. A review of gastric cancer cases from Bugando Medical Centre highlights the grim reality in regions , such as northwestern Tanzania, where gastric cancer comprised 4.5% of the total malignancies in the period between 2007 and 2011. The findings yield a male-to-female ratio of 2.9:1 and a median patient age of 52 years, which highlights demographic trends deserving further study. Above all, the majority of patients present with extensive disease, rendering the possibility and prognosis of treatment difficult, and underscoring the importance of understanding local epidemiological patterns to tailor interventions that may enhance early detection patterns and outcomes of treatment in high-risk areas (Mabula et al., 2012). Going further in clinicopathological patterns of gastric cancer, it is certain that presentation with advanced staging on diagnosis is more frequent. The quoted retrospective study reveals that an astonishing 92.1% of the patients arrived at the clinic with Stage III or IV disease, and both lymph node and distant metastases signs were present in nearly 32% and 29% of cases, respectively. The observation not only emphasizes the aggressive nature of gastric adenocarcinoma but also reflects systemic breakdowns in the early detection and availability of healthcare. Given the fact that the antrum is most frequently involved, along with the advanced disease's high complication rate to which gastric cancer is prone, there is a strong reason for new approaches to screening and risk factor education for gastric cancer (Mabula et al., 2012).

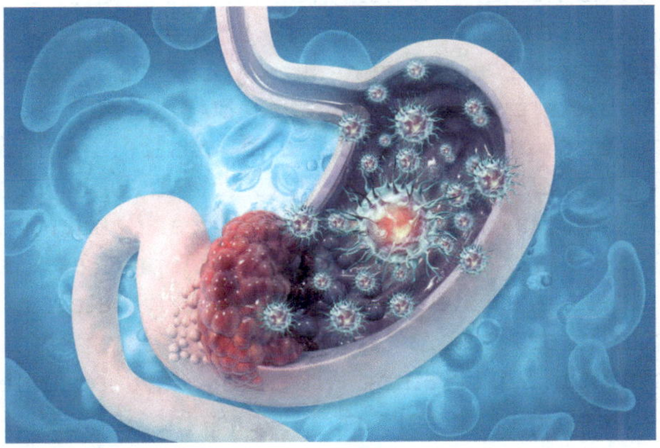

Figure 14.5. Gastric (stomach) cancer.

Source: https://www.toplinemd.com/omar-rashid/wp-content/uploads/sites/132/2022/08/When-to-Worry-About-Stomach-Cancer-What-is-It.jpg.

The management and treatment of gastric cancer reflect tremendous difficulties, most evident in outcomes of surgical treatment and the limited efficacy of adjunct treatments , such as radiotherapy and chemotherapy. Among 232 patients who were evaluated, a high number of 96.1% of the patients were operated on in the form of gastro-jejunostomy, with a majority, but postoperative mortality and complication rates reached alarming levels of 37.1% and 18.1%, respectively. Five-year survival was low at 6.9%, which was also a function of the unfavorable prognosis with delayed presentation. Poor outcome predictors were the stage of the tumor and metastasis at the time of diagnosis, necessitating more focus on public health initiatives for awareness creation and improving access to health centers for early detection and treatment (Mabula et al., 2012). All these initiatives are important in alleviating the load of gastric cancer among vulnerable groups (Figure 14.5).

14.1.3. Colorectal Cancer

Colorectal cancer (CRC) remains a significant public health problem, ranking as one of the leading cancer-related morbidity and mortality worldwide. Pathogenesis of CRC is overall typified by complex interactions between genetic predisposition and environmental factors, eventually leading to various subtypes of cancers with varying biological behaviors. Adenomatous polyp to malignancy progression underscores the importance of early detection and intervention. Since CRC has nonspecific symptoms, screening programs have become increasingly important in reducing incidence rates. Current guidelines advise periodic screening in average-risk patients starting at age 45 and can aid in early detection of precancerous lesions and improve outcomes by allowing early treatment interventions. The treatment strategy for CRC has also seen significant changes, particularly in the staging and metastasis. Patients with synchronous liver metastases are subjected to complex decisions in management. A new network meta-analysis compared treatment options , such as the bowel-first approach, simultaneous resection, and the liver-first approach between patients with colorectal cancer and synchronous liver metastases (Berardi et al., 2020). Postoperative complications, rates of survival, and treatment completion were among the outcomes included to determine the best option. Notably, while the liver-first approach may be suitable in patients with more extensive metastatic disease, completion rates as well as long-term survival were better with the bowel-first approach, highlighting the necessity of patient-specific treatment protocols. Apart from the surgical method, the evolution of targeted therapies has revolutionized the management of metastatic CRC. Therapy with antibodies , such as bevacizumab, which inhibits vascular endothelial growth factor, has been proven to achieve dramatic improvements in both progression-free and overall survival when added to conventional chemotherapy regimens (Heinemann et al., 2010). Such drugs applied to therapeutic protocols represent a growing trend towards the utilization of molecular pathways for therapeutic targeting. With awareness that biomarkers, in this case, K-ras mutations, influence treatment response, clinicians are increasingly faced with delivering therapies on an individualized basis. As ongoing discoveries further elucidate the nuances of CRC, the integration of new agents and approaches will likely remain instrumental in maximizing outcomes and patient survival within GI oncology practice.

14.2. Risk Factors for GI Cancers

The etiology of GI cancers is multifactorial, with numerous risk factors that significantly enhance the risk of malignant transformation within the gastrointestinal tract. Of these, lifestyle measures , such as obesity, smoking, and alcohol play pivotal roles. Metabolic-associated steatotic liver disease (MASLD) has also been recognized as a significant risk factor, particularly in obese patients, as it results in a pro-inflammatory condition that is conducive to cancer formation. Research has established that MASLD patients are at greater risk for hormone-sensitive and GI malignancies, evincing the imperative role of obesity in these cancer pathogeneses. Bariatric surgery has been proposed as a potential ameliorating process, suggesting that weight loss and metabolic normalization can prevent the oncogenic risks of MASLD and related co-morbidities (Mukherjee et al., 2025). Also, the interaction between genetic predisposition and environmental exposures must be taken into consideration when balancing GI cancer risk factors. Certain inherited syndromes, such as Lynch syndrome and familial adenomatous polyposis, greatly increase a person's susceptibility to colorectal and other GI cancers. These genetic mutations need heightened surveillance along with preventive interventions in the at-risk population. Environmental aspects like dietary lifestyle and the consumption of processed meat have also been linked to a high risk for GI cancers. It is noted in epidemiology that excessive fat intake and a poor fiber diet have negative impacts, with the findings established for higher cases of colorectal cancer. It is essential to understand these interrelated factors to evaluate the risk and develop prevention programs for the targeted groups (Mukherjee et al., 2025). Along with genetic and lifestyle influences, the occurrence of chronic inflammation within the gut is a significant risk factor for cancer development. Conditions , such as inflammatory bowel disease (IBD) and chronic gastritis provide a field favorable to malignant change by the maintenance of inflammation. Patients with long-standing IBD are at risk for increased development of colorectal carcinoma, particularly with extensive colonic involvement. Moreover, *Helicobacter pylori* infection has been linked to the development of gastric cancer, which reflects the relationship between infectious agents and oncogenesis. The data emphasize the importance of treating underlying conditions of inflammation as a method for reducing the risk of GI cancers, where multimodal approaches to integrated care aimed at controlling inflammation could be beneficial in cancer prevention (Tounkara et al., 2025) (Figure 14.6).

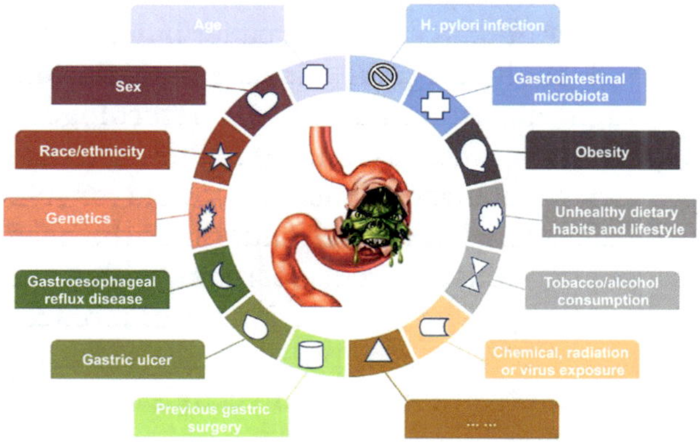

Figure 14.6. Risk factors for GI cancers.

Source: https://f6publishing.blob.core.windows.net/bfd8fe9d-550a-4856-ae2a-ab2e36ef26b4/WJG-29-2452-g005.png.

14.2.1. Genetic Predispositions

Genetic predispositions form the backbone of the field of gastrointestinal (GI) oncology, more particularly in connection with the etiology and behavior of various malignancies. The presence of specific genetic variants can influence an individual's predisposition to cancers , such as colorectal cancer (CRC) and other GI cancers. Genetic studies have demonstrated that inherited mutations can lead to cancer-threatening disorders like Lynch syndrome and familial adenomatous polyposis (FAP), with a close association with CRC. Such genetic disorders facilitate a better understanding of personalized medicine approaches, as those patients with identifiable genetic susceptibility can be managed with tailor-made screening regimens and specific therapy. Thus, the discovery of such genetic markers becomes important not only to enhance patient care but also to inform public health policies that assist in reducing overall cancer risk in populations at risk for some genetic susceptibility. With continuing research, the complexities of genetic susceptibility become more evident. For instance, recent research on the genetic origins of autism spectrum disorder (ASD) and its association with cancer susceptibility illustrates the extent to which genetic variations can have broader implications beyond their original disease association. Through an examination of heterologous populations , such as the Vietnamese, where primary genetic variations responsible for ASD were discovered, it further underlines the need to consider genetic predispositions within the context of geographic and ethnic differences (Bui et al., 2020). Such studies can reveal novel genetic contributors and mechanisms to GI cancer, enhancing the knowledge of how these types of genetic traits lead to an elevated risk of cancer in a particular population or age group. By combining this information, researchers are better positioned to comprehend the genetic influences that define GI oncology.

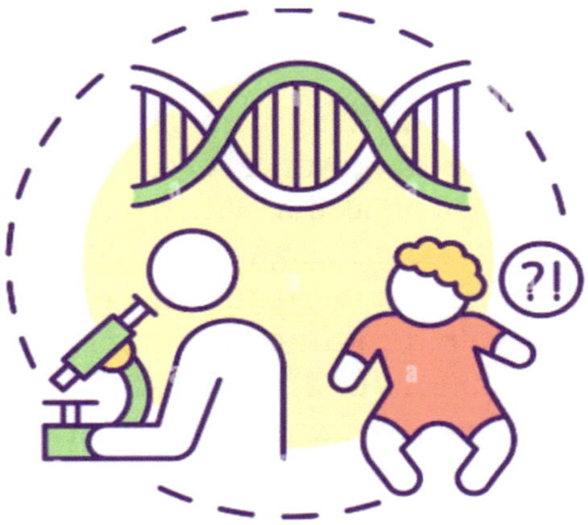

Figure 14.7. Genetic predispositions.

Source: https://c8.alamy.com/comp/2DDP9BN/genetic-predisposition-concept-icon-2DDP9BN.jpg.

Further emphasizing the role of genetic predispositions in GI oncology, the epidemiology of colorectal cancer presents a clear model for how such factors would likely be manifest in various populations. For countries , such as Pakistan, genetic predispositions to CRC, combined with lifestyle and environmental exposures, represent large public health burdens. Studies show that CRC incidence is increasing in younger age groups, which is alarming and suggests a complex interplay of genetic and epigenetic factors (Abbas et al., 2023). With the growing understanding of genetic and molecular processes, like CpG Island Methylator Phenotype (CIMP), Chromosomal Instability (CIN), and Microsatellite Instability (MSI), it becomes crucial to explain how these determinants of genetics interact with lifestyle behaviors to have an impact on cancer initiation. This multifactorial nature of cancer underscores the need for continued research into genetic susceptibility in specific populations, ultimately enabling the application of improved prevention, diagnosis, and treatment strategies in conformity with the individualized genetic composition of diverse groups of patients (Figure 14.7).

14.2.2. Lifestyle Factors (Diet, Smoking, Alcohol)

The interaction of lifestyle determinants with the risk of gastrointestinal (GI) cancers is a significant area of study in GI oncology. Nutrition, for example, is a critical factor in cancer susceptibility, particularly in association with fat consumption. Research has shown that excessive saturated fat intake has been associated with an elevated risk of certain lung cancers, especially in current smokers, indicating a synergistic interaction between the diet and smoking (Yang et al., 2017). In contrast, increased consumption of polyunsaturated fat has been implicated in reducing the risk of lung cancer, highlighting the role of food composition in cancer prevention. This correlation calls for food intervention that will provide healthier diets in hopes of minimizing cancer risks to vulnerable populations. In addition to diet, smoking is one of the most powerful risk factors for the development of various gastrointestinal cancers. The carcinogenic potential of tobacco has been well known for many years, with a definitive association between smoking and elevated risk of gastric and esophageal cancer.

Smoking not only introduces harmful chemicals into the body but may also enhance the effect of diet. For example, smokers who consume high intakes of saturated fat have doubled the risk of developing lung cancer compared to non-smokers, illustrating how lifestyle determinants collectively can alter cancer risks (Yang et al., 2017). This interaction calls for an integrated reaction to public health measures towards smoking abstinence, especially among high-fat-diet-consuming populations. Moreover, one should not overlook the contribution alcohol consumption plays in oncology of the GI tract. Chronic alcohol consumption has been known to be a significant risk factor for cancers of different types, including liver and esophageal cancers. Alcohol can also be a solvent for other carcinogens, leading to enhanced absorption and effect on the gastrointestinal system. Further studies also indicate that non-smokers with regular low levels of alcohol intake have lower risks for smoking- and diet-related cancers. This reaffirms the importance of promoting moderate alcohol consumption along with diet and cessation of smoking as multiple-factor approaches in the fight against GI cancers. Through the integration of lifestyle modifications, public health initiatives are able to foster an active response towards GI oncology via prevention rather than treatment alone.

14.2.3. Environmental Influences

The interconnection between environmental issues and gastrointestinal (GI) oncology is a critical area of study, particularly as we attempt to understand the interconnected variables in the development of cancer. Several research studies have suggested that diet and lifestyle play significant roles in the development of GI cancers. This does not only involve processed foods and consumption of fats, but also exposure to toxins. Striking evidence from the World Health Organization indicates that lifestyle factors are responsible for a large proportion of cancer cases, pointing out that environmental carcinogenic agents can combine with genetic factors to elevate cancer risk. Resolution of lifestyle conditions requires a coordinated public health response to cancer risk reduction through education and policy reforms leading to healthier lifestyles. Chemical exposures, including pesticides, heavy metals, and industrial chemicals, also contribute to the environmental complexity of GI cancers. Scientific evidence indicates that most of the carcinogenic effect results from low-dose exposure to chemicals with the ability to synergistically interact and promote cancer growth. In testing 85 chemicals, none of them showed explicit dose-response thresholds, but the majority of them produced effects with low doses, which implies that cumulative exposure could cause carcinogenic effects. Such an observation with carcinogenesis supports emerging knowledge that environmental exposures combined with genetic susceptibility can enhance the hazard for GI malignancy development. This calls for reworking existing paradigms, for instance, the World Health Organization's Mode of Action, to better incorporate the complexity of modern environmental exposures into the realm of cancer biology (Goodson et al., 2015). In addition, it becomes increasingly crucial to put research effort into elucidating how different environmental exposures play out in interact with one another in biological systems. The hazard of chemical mixtures to cause adverse effects also renders this an area ripe for investigation. Because differences in exposures to environmental carcinogens usually reflect disparities in overall socioeconomic status, prevention strategies must likewise reverse these disparities. Enhanced research techniques, including long-term epidemiologic studies and in vitro studies of chemical mixtures, would more accurately explain how environmental factors are involved in GI cancers. Lastly, learning about these environmental factors not only unravels the etiology of GI malignancies but also prompts the institute of public health measures aiming to reduce exposure to harmful substances, potentially reducing the number of GI cancers in the population (Focal Spot, Fall/ Winter 2010/2011) (Figure 14.8).

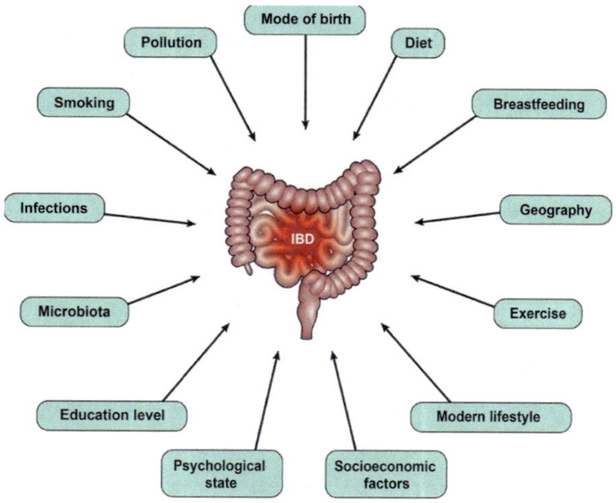

Figure 14.8. Between environmental influences and gastrointestinal (GI).

Source: https://media.springernature.com/full/springer-static/image/art%3A10.1038%2Fnrgastro.2017.136/MediaObjects/41575_2018_Article_BFnrgastro2017136_Fig1_HTML.jpg.

14.3. Symptoms and Diagnosis

Early detection of gastrointestinal cancers, e.g., gastric cancer, to a great extent depends on the identification of symptoms, which are themselves nonspecific and indeterminate in nature. The patients usually present with nonspecific gastrointestinal symptoms , such as abdominal pain, weight loss, and chronic dyspepsia, further complicating the diagnosis. Studies have illustrated that a significant number of patients, particularly in underserved regions, will report late into the progression of their disease, as symptoms can initially be mistaken for being caused by less serious conditions. Early gastric cancer also presents with minimal manifestations that can easily be belittled, prompting a pressing need for greater awareness about these manifestations among both patients and medical professionals. This lack of awareness is the causative agent for the delay in diagnoses, ratifying the importance of education in maximizing outcomes in GI oncology (Brém et al., 2020). Cancer of the gastrointestinal tract diagnosis encompasses a variety of modalities, from imaging tests to endoscopic examinations. While laboratory tests will provide information independently, ultimate diagnosis often relies on histopathological examination through biopsy. For instance, the endoscopy not only assists in visualizing the gastrointestinal tract lining but also directs biopsy, resulting in a more accurate diagnosis. Emerging advances in imaging technology , such as computed tomography (CT) and magnetic resonance imaging (MRI), have significantly enhanced tumor detection as well as assessment of extent. Furthermore, biomarker testing has emerged as a promising addition to the diagnostic arsenal in favor of tailored therapy modalities. The convergence of these diagnostic approaches not only guarantees timely intervention but also maximizes the understanding of cancer staging, which is fundamental for setting the treatment plan (Brém et al., 2020). Early diagnosis in GI cancer is essential but remains hampered by numerous factors, primarily socioeconomic limitations and lack of access to healthcare. Advanced cancer is more prevalent with presentation in resource-poor settings since screening programs are not in place, and primary care physicians have a lower index of suspicion. There is evidence that gastric cancer in certain areas, like northwestern Tanzania, exhibits a rising trend of being diagnosed at an early age and at an advanced stage, emphasizing the need for increased screening interventions and public health to raise awareness (Mabula et al., 2012). In addition to this, complications stemming from advanced disease also complicate management and treatment, typically generating poorer prognoses compared to detection at an early stage. Therefore, determination of these systemic defects is necessary in achieving the optimal diagnosis and ultimately optimizing the outcome for gastrointestinal cancer patients.

14.3.1. Common Symptoms of GI Cancers

In gastrointestinal (GI) oncology practice, the recognition of classic symptoms of GI cancer is a key element for timely diagnosis and effective intervention. Patients will have nonspecific symptoms of abdominal pain, weight loss, and change in bowel habits, which will lead to diagnostic delay. Pain in the abdomen is a frequent complaint and may be variable in quality and localization, complicating the clinical presentation. Other dangerous symptoms include gastrointestinal hemorrhage, either overt through hematochezia or occult through occult blood testing, and dysphagia, which is characterized by the inability to swallow. Such symptoms, while prevalent in the majority of GI cancers , such as gastric and colorectal cancer, can be produced by benign conditions, and therefore, stringent investigation has to be done to discern between malignancies and other gastrointestinal illnesses. Clinicians must remain alert to recognize common symptoms of GI cancers, since early diagnosis influences patient outcomes. For instance, gastric cancer patients complain of decreased appetite and early satiety, resulting in unintentional weight loss—a sign that warrants further investigation. In addition, jaundice presentation may be indicative of biliary obstruction or metastasis to the liver in pancreatic cancers. It should be noted that most of the patients are diagnosed late in the course of the disease, with many presenting late because such symptoms evolve insidiously and hence keep the patients beyond the window period for cure. In localities with limited access to medical centers, presentation at the advanced stages is especially prevalent, emphasizing the necessity of creating awareness of GI cancer symptoms not just among clinicians but also the public (Mabula et al., 2012). Furthermore, patients with GI cancer may have systemic symptoms , such as fatigue, anemia, and striking generalized changes, which can reduce quality of life. The presence of metastasis has a tendency to introduce complications that worsen the clinical state. For instance, liver metastasis patients can develop ascites and thus abdominal distension and pain, and patients with end-stage cancers of the gastrointestinal tract can be malnourished due to impaired digestion and absorption. Recognition of the spectrum of symptoms seen in GI malignancies can potentially initiate early referral to diagnostic evaluations, such as imaging and endoscopic evaluations, thereby facilitating appropriate treatment interventions. Moreover, being current with newly arising prognostic factors, as discussed within current literature, can assist in improving clinicians' prognostic capability in patients and tailoring approaches in the context of advanced symptomatology and disease stage (Aizer et al., 2019) (Figure 14.9).

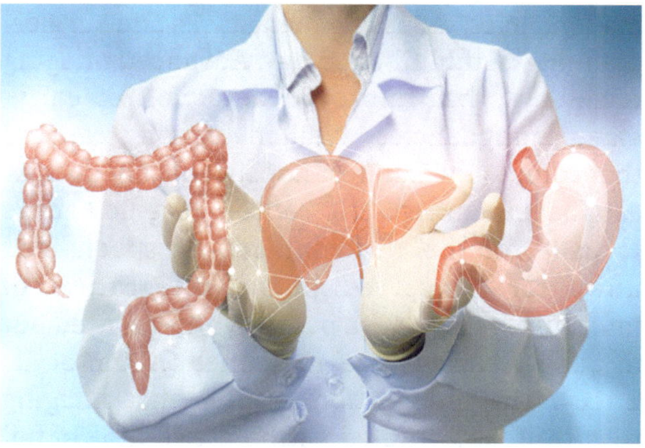

Figure 14.9. Common symptoms of GI cancers.

Source: https://www.yashodahealthcare.com/blogs/wp-content/uploads/2021/07/gastrointestinal-cancers.jpeg.

14.3.2. Diagnostic Procedures (Endoscopy, Imaging)

Application of diagnostic methods, particularly imaging and endoscopy, forms the cornerstone of GI oncology practice and significantly enhances cancer detection and treatment accuracy. Endoscopic techniques allow for direct visualization of the GI tract, such that lesions can be seen, which could otherwise not be detected by other imaging modalities. With advancements in technology, modalities , such as endoscopic retrograde cholangiopancreatography (ERCP) are now essential, especially in diagnosing conditions , such as annular pancreas, wherein research indicates high technical success of ERCP in patients with pancreatic abnormalities (Easler et al., 2019). As a result, endoscopy not only enables diagnosis but also permits therapeutic maneuvers, optimizing patient care through early decision-making based on unambiguous visual information. Imaging modalities like computed tomography (CT) and magnetic resonance imaging (MRI) complement endoscopic techniques by providing a holistic picture of the abdominal cavity and detecting tumors at various stages of growth. These modalities play a significant role in staging malignancies, assessing metastasis, and surgical planning within GI oncology. Advanced imaging technology has improved detection of early-stage malignancies, vital in treating cancers that commonly manifest nonspecifically, such as esophageal and gastric cancer. Text nowadays focuses on the development of specialized units for cancer with the integration of multidisciplinary care pathways, as pointed out in quality cancer care guidelines (Allum et al., 2018). This integration assures that imaging results are interpreted within the context of full patient assessments, leading to more effective, individualized treatment planning. Moreover, the performance of these diagnostic tests is not only based on technical proficiency but also on adherence to quality assurance principles to ensure enhanced patient safety and outcomes of care. As has come to be discovered in studies focused on endoscopic findings in patients with conditions like annular pancreas, the conditions under which these procedures are performed have a direct influence on success rates and patient satisfaction (Easler et al., 2019). Quality improvement in GI oncology includes developing guidelines for endoscopic and imaging approaches that prioritize patient-centered care. By ensuring that oncology practitioners remain well versed with the latest knowledge and practices, the profession can realize its potential in providing high-standard oncology treatment with immense impact on early detection, correct diagnosis, and subsequent management of gastrointestinal cancers (Allum et al., 2018).

14.3.3. Importance of Early Detection

In the case of gastrointestinal (GI) oncology, the necessity of early detection cannot be overstated. Early detection of cancers improves the prospects of treatment, as early-stage tumors are more amenable to therapy. Due to advances in technology and methodology, various biomarkers have been identified that can potentially facilitate early diagnosis. For instance, clinical proteomics has proven to be a promising avenue for the discovery of biomarkers, and it has spawned more than 130 investigative studies targeted towards GI oncology that have identified candidate markers in serum, GI secretions, or tumor tissue. However, these advances notwithstanding, the clinical relevance of these studies remains limited, suggesting the need for continued refinement in establishing proteomic findings to be suitable for useful early-cancer detection tools (Emadali et al., 2008). This serves to reinforce the calls for ongoing research and collaboration among the oncology community to facilitate the full potential of these breakthroughs. Liquid biopsies have also revolutionized the area of early detection in GI oncology. Liquid biopsies entail examining circulating tumor DNA (ctDNA) of whole blood samples, and from these, clinicians can gain a lot regarding the presence and activity of tumors without the need for invasive tests. Studies have indicated that there is an association between ctDNA percent and survival rates overall; in other words, those with elevated ctDNA have poorer outcomes. For example, patients who have a 5% or more elevated ctDNA level of ctDNA have exhibited significantly decreased overall survival compared to patients with lower levels (Goodman et al., 2020). The association of ctDNA with tumor burden highlights the use of liquid biopsies as diagnostic agents not just for cancer detection but also for treatment response and recurrences, with early detection being a fundamental part of individualized oncology treatment.

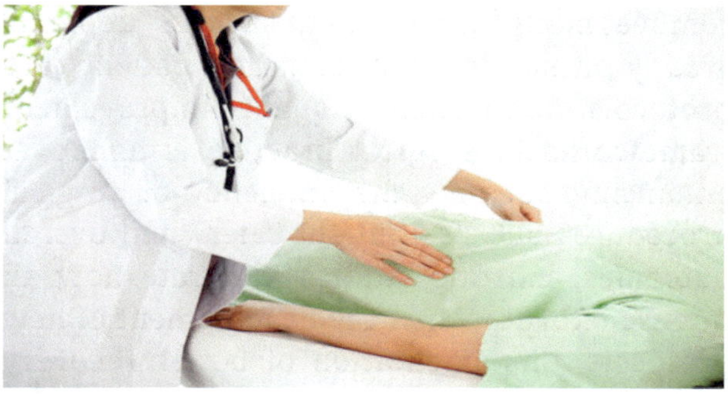

Figure 14.10. Importance of early detection.

Source: https://oncologynews.com.au/wp-content/uploads/gastrointestinal-fistula_thumb-1-732x549-1-702x336.jpeg.

Last but not least, early detection in GI oncology is a broader aim to improve patient outcomes by means of intensive medical practice. Detection of gastrointestinal cancers at an early stage inevitably provides a higher number of treatment options and enhances the likelihood of positive outcomes. The integration of advanced technologies, such as proteomics and liquid biopsies, is the most significant step towards achieving it. While the way ahead will involve addressing challenges in translating research into practice, ongoing commitment to early detection is critical. By ongoing investment in research and clinical trials, the medical community can realize the promise of these new diagnostic technologies, on the way to an age when GI cancers can be diagnosed and treated more effectively at their earliest presentation, and ultimately save lives and improve the quality of care in oncology (Figure 14.10).

14.4. Treatment Options

Treatment in gastrointestinal (GI) cancer is very diverse based on the specific type and stage of the cancer, as well as on individual patient characteristics. Standard surgery continues to be a cornerstone, particularly for localized esophageal, gastric, and colonic tumors. The operations can range from resection of the tumor to more extensive procedures , such as gastrectomy or colectomy. However, the course of cancer may undermine surgery, and other methods must then be utilized , such as radiation therapy and chemotherapy. Hypofractionated radiotherapy has offered a good alternative to certain GI cancers, with clinical trials indicating similar effectiveness to conventionally fractionated regimens but varying patient tolerance and patterns of toxicity. There is a growing consensus that multimodal treatment combinations would enhance the effectiveness of treatment and the alleviation of ensuing adverse effects borne by the patients. Chemotherapy is another important treatment modality in GI oncology, often utilized either as an initial intervention or adjuvant therapy after surgery. Cytotoxics , such as fluorouracil, oxaliplatin, and irinotecan have been stalwarts of colorectal cancer treatment, used extensively as combination regimens to maximize patient benefit. Targeted therapies and immunotherapies have also stretched the treatment era, with drugs intended to block cancer hallmarks in cancer cells or activate the immune system against cancer cells. For example, in advanced gastric cancer, the addition of trastuzumab has revolutionized treatment in this disease in patients with HER2-positive disease. But selection of chemotherapy drugs must also consider the cancer subtype and molecular markers, proving the necessity for personalized treatment that considers patient profiles and tumor biology. Development of radiation technology over the recent past also has an important contribution to make to the new paradigms of treatment in GI oncology. Technologies like stereotactic body radiation therapy (SBRT) and advanced multileaf collimator (MLC) technology have improved the accuracy of radiation delivery to tumors with sparing of the surrounding normal tissues.

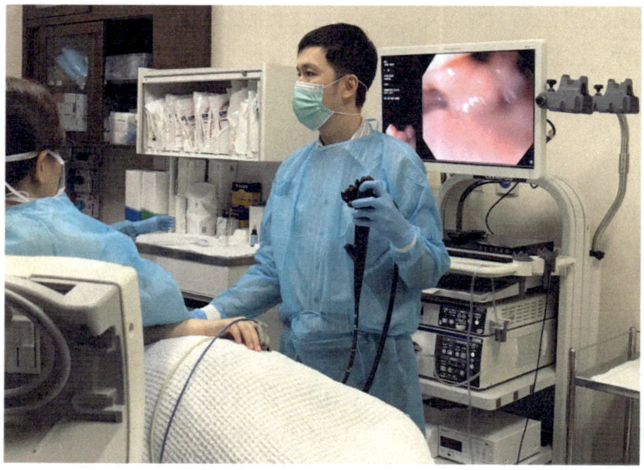

Figure 4.11. Gastrointestinal (GI) oncology treatment options vary significantly depending.

Source: https://aliveomedical.com/wp-content/uploads/2020/02/IMG_7074.jpg.

These new technologies have been demonstrated to enhance conformity of dose and decrease low-dose spill to healthy organs, particularly for non-small cell lung cancer and other thoracic cancers involving the GI tract. Moreover, studies have shown that the dosimetric precision of dual-layer MLC systems can potentially have a significant impact on treatment efficacy and safety, particularly for patients presenting with multifocal or complex tumor patterns and more than one target. Continuous monitoring of the effectiveness and safety of treatment modalities as these evolve will be of vital importance in directing the course of GI oncology in the future, ensuring that customized treatment options are able to maximize curative benefits while overcoming the hurdles posed by individual cases (Figure 14.11).

14.4.1. Surgical Interventions

Surgery is an integral component of treatment for gastrointestinal oncology, particularly for localized tumors that can be resected successfully. Colectomies and pancreatoduodenectomies are some of the surgical interventions required to remove malignancies, and success depends greatly on surgical precision and patient care protocols. Application of quality improvement frameworks in surgical practice is aimed at enhancing not only the efficiency of surgical procedures but also patient safety and overall outcomes. Existing studies illustrate how an intense effort towards the development of new protocols, implementation of better recovery after surgery (ERAS) procedures, and data analysis can enormously enhance gastrointestinal surgical care. These QI projects play a significant role, particularly in achieving the distribution of surgical interventions among various subfields in which adult and spine surgeries are the undisputed favourites according to existing literature (Madan et al., 2025). As surgical techniques are advancing, minimally invasive surgery is becoming the first choice in gastrointestinal oncology. Techniques , such as laparoscopic surgery and robotic surgery have demonstrated attractive advantages in terms of shorter hospital stays and reduced postoperative complications. McKeown's minimally invasive oesophagectomy is an example that provides new approaches that minimize the risks usually associated with more destructive traditional techniques. But operative teams must be aware of potential intraoperative complications , such as iatrogenic tracheobronchial injury (TBI), which, while infrequent, can have severe implications if not immediately addressed.

Raised awareness and established management principles are significant because early diagnosis and treatment can greatly improve patient outcomes and reduce the impact of such complications on postoperative recovery (Gill et al., 2025). The integration of advanced diagnostic and monitoring technology into surgical oncology also contributes significantly to increased patient outcomes. For example, the application of bronchoscopy and advanced imaging strategies in the diagnosis of such complications as TBI in minimally invasive surgery reflects how technology can enable more efficient surgical operations. By guaranteeing that surgical teams are able to identify and treat complications early, opportunities for adverse outcomes are significantly minimized. Moreover, ongoing studies on surgery methods and technologies will stimulate the development of best practices that can be disseminated across various GI cancer procedures. This cycle of learning and iterative improvement in process standards underscores the importance of an end-to-end surgery approach, with technology and methodology progress always being aimed at patient safety and optimizing recovery in gastrointestinal oncology (Gill et al., 2025; Madan et al., 2025).

14.4.2. Chemotherapy and Radiation Therapy

The synergy between radiation therapy and chemotherapy in GI oncology is a cornerstone of treatment in several cancers with disproportionate preponderance in the digestive tract. Chemotherapy has emerged as a valuable cancer modality, particularly in situations where surgery cannot be performed or in the event of an incomplete resection. Drugs , such as carboplatin and doxorubicin have been central to the treatment of cancers, with studies indicating that specific protocols could maximize the patient's outcome and minimize AEs (Burton et al., 2014). How well chemotherapy may be employed to maximize survival times is generally placed against the side effects that this yields, and thus the reasons why appropriate protocols need to be selected in relation to the particular demands of each patient. Radiation therapy complements chemotherapy with targeted therapy to destroy cancer cells while sparing the adjacent normal tissue. This modality has a special place in GI oncology, where tumors can be located in a strategic position. Radiation therapy challenges are manifold, such as those of oral complications like dental caries and periodontal disease.

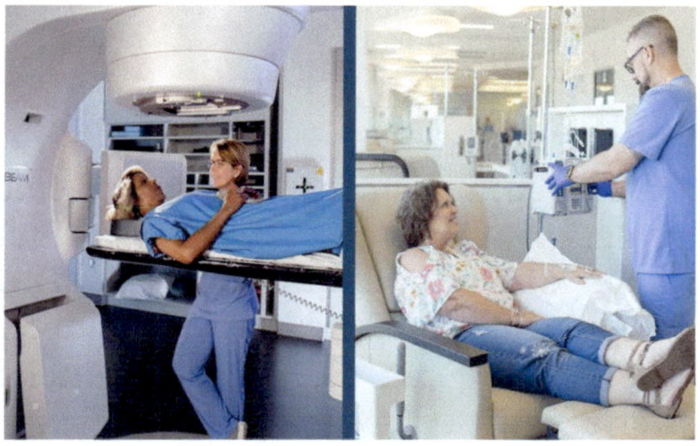

Figure 14.12. Chemotherapy and radiation therapy within the realm of gastrointestinal (GI) oncology.

Source: https://www.carti.com/app/uploads/2020/11/CAR0820-005-Radiation-vs-Chemotherapy-Blog-Image-1024x597.jpg.

A systematic review found patients following radiation therapy to have immensely higher dental issues, with the weighted overall prevalence of dental caries coming in at 28.1% (Hodgson et al., 2010). It points toward the requirement of patient management standards that not only detect cancer treatment but also actively address secondary effects arising from treatments. Concurrent administration of chemotherapy and radiation therapy tends to offer synergistic effects that enhance therapeutic efficacy in GI oncology. The risk of increased toxicity does, however, call for a cautious approach to patient management. As an example, toxicities , such as mucositis and infections are complications of therapy, as is illustrated by the reported 5.8% incidence of dental infections in chemotherapy patients (Hodgson et al., 2010). Thus, preventive interventions , such as the use of fluoride rinses and regular dental assessment should be incorporated in order to limit such risks. Overall, the successful application of chemotherapy and radiation therapy in GI oncology is primarily subject to an integrated approach that takes into account both cancer eradication and preserving patients' overall health and wellness (Figure 14.12).

14.4.3. Targeted Therapies and Immunotherapy

The therapeutic landscape in GI oncology is revolutionized by the advent of targeted therapies and immunotherapy, presenting novel opportunities for improving outcomes in patients. Targeted therapies are intended to interfere with specific molecular targets involved in cancer cell development and growth. To illustrate, in the treatment of esophageal cancer (EC), anti-programmed death-ligand 1 (PD-L1) inhibitors have drawn much attention. PD-L1 inhibitors nivolumab and pembrolizumab were recently approved for first-line treatment based on promising evidence from clinical trials , such as CheckMate 648 and KEYNOTE-590. These clinical trials emphasize the relevance of immunotherapy in enhancing immunity against cancer cells, hence enhancing survival rates and effectiveness of treatment regimes in advanced EC (Bone et al., 2025). Furthermore, the treatment of gastrointestinal cancers has also been transformed by immunotherapy, through takes advantage of the body's immune system to identify and destroy cancer cells. The application of immune checkpoint inhibitors, including PD-1 and PD-L1 blockers, has been successful, particularly in instances where there is high PD-L1 expression. However, as discussed in recent clinic debates, PD-L1 status was recognized as a less major parameter in treatment choice than other signs, such as tumor histology and ECOG performance status. This finding hints at a complex interaction among molecular markers and other clinical parameters in determining response to therapy. The more advanced understanding of immune responses in GI oncology needs to be translated into practice in the clinic by way of greater educational activity aimed at oncologists to keep them appropriately informed about current treatment data and patient management strategies (Bone et al., 2025). In addition to immunotherapy, targeted therapies have considerably contributed to the armamentarium at the disposal of GI oncologists. These therapies are designed to target cancer cells selectively with a reduced effect on normal tissues, thereby reducing side effects typically encountered with conventional therapies. For example, the inclusion of molecular testing, assisting in the detection of specific genetic mutations, enhances the ability to individualize therapy more effectively. As has been noted in lung cancer using targeted therapies focusing on such pathways as EGFR and FGFR1, the same is being explored in GI cancer. These advances underscore the importance of not only defining successful treatment regimens but also the attendant challenges, such as immune resistance and the genomic heterogeneity of tumors, that impede treatment effectiveness. Studies in these areas continue to examine mechanisms in greater detail and bridge targeted therapies with immunotherapy as a possible approach against treatment-refractory subsets of GI cancer.

14.5. Advances in Research

Genomics breakthroughs have transformed the field of gastrointestinal oncology, and it has opened new horizons for targeted therapy personalized to the tumor characteristics. The application of extensive genomic profiling has come into prominence because it allows us to identify some mutations in tumors. This strategy has been very promising for finding actionable genetic alterations that will ultimately translate into precision medicine interventions. For example, a trial on heterogeneous and challenging-to-treat cancer types in patients detected that 96% of tumors examined contained at least one significant genomic mutation that can be used to design personalized treatment strategies. This shift toward genomically guided therapy highlights the necessity of integrating the application of genomic data into the clinic to enhance the efficacy of treatment protocols for gastrointestinal cancers, which have multicomponent genetic foundations. Multidisciplinary molecular tumor boards have also facilitated translation of genomic findings to practice. They are an important forum where experts collectively review the findings from genomic sequencing, and the clinical actionability and feasibility of the suggested treatment are debated. In an important trial, extensive profiling provided actionable recommendations for clinical care in approximately 35% of patients, which reflects the potential for radical alteration of treatment regimens on the basis of genomics. But there are obstacles, chiefly to the availability of experimental treatments and patients' clinical status. This challenge must be resolved to maximize the benefit of genomic profiling in GI oncology so that emerging biomarkers offer rational, life-saving therapy to patients who are facing rare or aggressive cancer. Also, continuing advances in sequencing technology promise to expand our understanding of the molecular basis of gastrointestinal cancer. With advancing studies, there is a growing need for emphasis on serial and early genomic testing to achieve maximization of patient benefit. This practice will enable timely adjustment of therapeutic approaches and optimal monitoring of developing resistance patterns. Further, greater access to early-stage clinical trials and targeted therapies is required to expand treatment strategies, particularly for patients with less common types of cancer. By identifying significant determinants impacting the actionability of genomic results, researchers and clinicians would be able to synergize and maximize therapeutic planning, thereby enhancing clinical outcomes and, ultimately, shaping the destiny of the future of GI cancer. (Focal Spot, Fall/Winter 2010/2011; Aisner et al., 2016) (Figure 14.13).

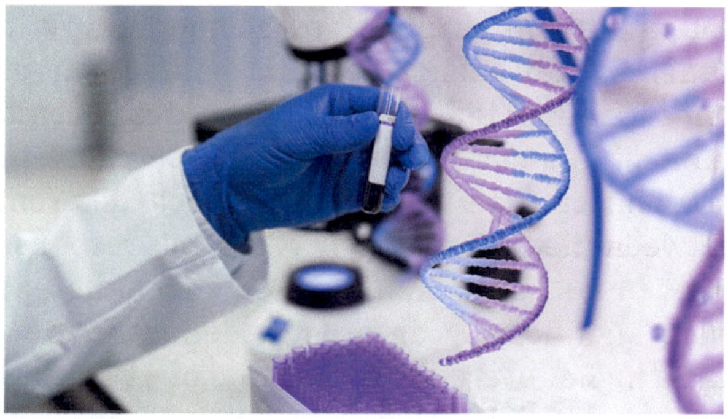

Figure 14.13. Advancements in genomic research.

Source: https://www.fomatmedical.com/wp-content/uploads/2023/10/dna-doctor-does-lab-tests-1400x788.jpg.

14.5.1. Recent Breakthroughs in GI Oncology

Current developments in gastrointestinal (GI) oncology have greatly enhanced the diagnosis and management of complex malignancies largely through advancements in targeted therapies and immunotherapy. The intersection of precision medicine, whereby therapy is tailored to the genetic makeup of the patient, has evolved into a game-changing approach in GI cancer treatment. For instance, emerging genomic sequencing technologies allow oncologists to target specific mutations that inform decisions on treatment, enabling them to select drugs most likely to succeed in a given individual patient. This paradigm shift not only maximizes treatment response but also decreases the side effects of traditional chemotherapy regimens. Consequently, precision oncology keeps widening the doors to even more personalized therapy modalities, holding potential for increased survival and quality of life in GI cancer patients. In addition to precision medicine, newer research puts a strong focus on the role of histological subtypes in predicting treatment outcome in esophageal cancers. It has been demonstrated in clinical studies that there are minor differences in survival and treatment response to chemotherapy in patients with adenocarcinoma and squamous cell carcinoma (SCC) of the esophagus. Overall survival in a pooled analysis of three phase III randomized trials was not appreciably different between the two histologic types, but response rates to fluoropyrimidine-based chemotherapy were significantly different. Adenocarcinoma had a higher overall response rate of 44% when compared to 33% for SCC and hence emphasizes the necessity for SCC-specific treatments to enhance patient outcomes (Chau et al., 2017). This new recognition of histological impact on response to therapy is valuable to make treatment more individualized and ultimately contribute to enhancing treatment efficacy in clinical care. Immunotherapy's role in GI cancer is also being revolutionized. Checkpoint inhibitors, now at the forefront of cancer treatment in various cancers, are increasingly being explored extensively in GI malignancies like gastric and colorectal cancers. The therapeutic activity of checkpoint inhibitors against the immune system has come with extremely promising results, particularly in patients with microsatellite instability-high (MSI-H) tumors, with superior clinical responses. These advances are in the direction of shifting toward the integration of immunotherapeutic interventions as part of the standard of care for select GI malignancies, from a blanket treatment approach to one that is accommodative of the cancer's biological characteristics. Although future clinical trials are directed towards maximizing and expanding the indications of immunotherapy in GI cancer, expectations of improved survival and control of the disease continue to grow, with this representing a landmark in the therapy profile of gastrointestinal cancers (Focal Spot, Fall/Winter 2010/2011. Bernard Becker Medical Library Archives. Washington University School of Medicine, Saint Louis, Missouri).

14.5.2. Clinical Trials and Their Significance

Clinical trials are the cornerstones of advancements in gastrointestinal (GI) cancer, a systematic process of evaluating new treatment plans and refining therapeutic regimens. Clinical trials have a critical function in determining the efficacy as well as the safety of new agents to treat various GI cancers, such as colorectal and pancreatic cancers. With well-controlled trials, researchers can make informed comparisons among new treatments and standard care alternatives so that choices are based upon objective facts. The contrast in professional opinion on the application of hypofractionated radiation regimens by North American genitourinary specialists, as noted by recent surveys, underlines the ongoing need for strong clinical trials to underpin practice guidelines and optimize patient-centered management of problematic conditions like prostate cancer. The data acquired through such trials then feedback into clinical practice guidelines and guide future oncology treatment strategies (Chen et al., 2019). Furthermore, clinical trials not only facilitate the study of therapeutic effectiveness but also provide informative results on the safety profiles of emerging drugs. In GI cancer, the addition of agents like bevacizumab to established chemotherapy regimens is the essence of the potential therapeutic benefit that new combinations can bring to patient outcomes. Studies have consistently shown that adding bevacizumab to irinotecan therapy significantly increases progression-free and overall survival in metastatic colon cancer patients (Heinemann et al., 2010). Such findings are significant not only because they reflect improving clinical outcomes but also because they result in a more informed understanding of the mechanisms of tumor growth and drug resistance. This knowledge facilitates the development of more efficacious treatment regimens based on the unique characteristics of each tumor, a step toward personalized medicine. In addition to their influence on the care of individual patients, the value of clinical trials in GI oncology also lies in that they are beginning to push open doors to sea changes in public health policy and accessibility of cancer care. By adhering to rigorous scientific protocols, these trials yield robust evidence that can guide treatment algorithms and reimbursement and, ultimately, the way therapies are delivered in the clinical setting.

The approximate even division among specialists regarding hypofractionated EBRT for prostate cancer means there will be a continued need for study and trials to answer uncertainty and establish new standards of care in oncology. In addition, patient-oriented decision-making is encouraged by these trials so that patients' needs and unique circumstances are considered when developing treatment. In this manner, clinical trials thus play an irreplaceable part not just in enhancing individualized care for the patient but also in shaping the general oncology treatment paradigms (Figure 14.14).

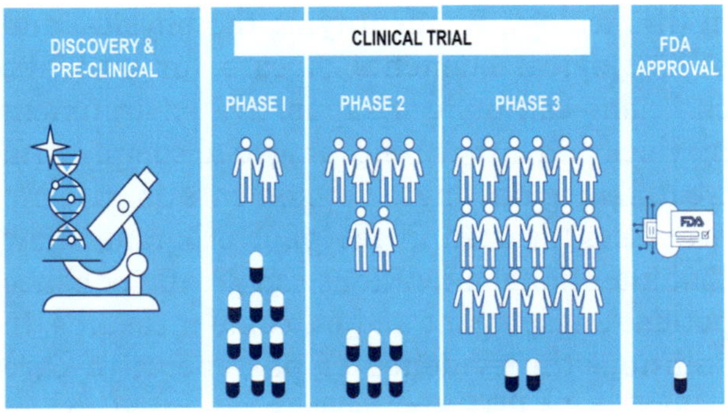

Figure 14.14. Clinical trials and their significance.

Source: https://i.ibb.co/k46pCj6/clinical-trials-process.png.

14.5.3. Future Directions in GI Cancer Research

The landscape of GI cancer research is evolving at an unprecedented pace, with future horizons holding the promise of new methods for diagnosing and treating cancer. Novel technologies , such as liquid biopsies offer a non-invasive means to detect circulating tumor DNA and analyze tumor heterogeneity and hence allow real-time assessment of therapeutic responses. This shift towards personalized medicine is essential as it potentially allows more effective and better-targeted treatment strategies. In addition, advances in imaging technologies, including positron emission tomography (PET) and magnetic resonance imaging (MRI), are enhancing the accuracy of tumor staging and localization, with a potential for improved outcomes for patients. Continuing studies toward biomarkers for early detection and prognostic application will be a key driver for future research and clinical practice in GI oncology, with the long-term aim of reducing mortality from these cancers. The use of immunotherapy in the treatment strategy of GI cancers is arguably the most encouraging research direction to pursue. In recent studies, the use of immune checkpoint inhibitors for a variety of GI tumors has been made possible, and most agree that they show potential to increase overall survival rates. A comprehensive knowledge of the tumor microenvironment and the immune evasion factors is necessary to precision-improve immunotherapy strategies. Additional studies need to be carried out in order to establish predictive biomarkers that can help in the selection of those patients who will most benefit from such therapies. Additionally, integrating immunotherapies with standard treatments, like chemotherapy or targeted therapies, could improve therapy efficacy. As scientists continue to unravel the complexities of GI cancer immunology, the prospect of converting such cancers into a chronic disease that can be treated becomes increasingly possible, and hence ongoing investment in the discipline ever more critical. The addition of novel agents, as exemplified by the use of monoclonal antibodies , such as bevacizumab, forms the key to further developing therapy for GI cancers. Bevacizumab is demonstrated to be highly effective with irinotecan to treat metastatic colorectal cancer, highlighting the significance of targeted therapies in patient survival (Heinemann et al., 2010). However, ongoing research must tackle mechanisms of acquired resistance that can occur over time. Research into combination therapy with bevacizumab and other agents might enhance treatment response and management of adverse effects. Also, clinical trials that assess novel combinations of efficacy and safety in heterogeneous populations of patients are important in developing treatment approaches for multidisciplinary care. With encouraging outcomes from ongoing trials, further advancements in the treatment of GI cancer will most likely lead to more specific and effective therapies, which promise better results in the future.

14.6. Patient Care and Support

Excellent patient care and assistance in the practice of GI oncology demand complete knowledge of the multifaceted issues faced by patients through their cancer care journey. The integration of tobacco treatment into the cancer treatment protocol, and more significantly, into oncology clinics, is one such element. A pilot study in the Stanford Cancer Center highlights the necessity to address smoking cessation as part of an integrated patient management approach. Precedent experience in the Head and Neck Oncology Clinic identified high rates of smoking in patients, but extremely low usage of cessation programs. Streamlining the referral process and integrating treatment services into routine care delivered by the clinic resulted in dramatic improvement, including greater screening and participation rates. This figure emphasizes that personalized interventions can enhance patient outcomes, particularly in high-risk patients, thereby emphasizing the important contribution of patient support systems in GI oncology. The patient support is not just confined to psychology; it has to incorporate intense medical management, particularly in complex treatment scenarios , such as intraperitoneal photodynamic therapy (IP PDT) following surgical debulking. According to research, patients who have had this operation are likely to develop a systemic capillary-leak syndrome, which results in severe perioperative complications and calls for prolonged postoperative management. One study depicted that such patients have high percentages of respiratory distress, infection, and complications requiring intensive monitoring and treatment. The findings bring out the necessity for preemptive and reactive care measures that not only take care of direct surgical risks but also facilitate recovery in the long term. Care teams must be equipped to manage the needs of postoperative care, thus allowing patients to receive individualized supportive care that is responsive to unique treatment outcomes and healthcare needs (Gali et al., 2020). The integration of holistic models of care is essential in enhancing the care experience of patients in GI oncology. By identifying the physical and psychological elements of care for patients, clinicians can build a supportive environment in which patients are encouraged to comply with treatment guidelines. Refinements in referral processes, as seen in the pilot program, show that intentional alterations can greatly enhance patient engagement and outcome measures. In addition, the evidence of postoperative care following IP PDT emphasizes the provision of continuous support even in acute care settings. Understanding the complexity of GI oncology patients' needs supports more effective care strategies, ultimately translating into better patient experiences and improved treatment outcomes (Canter et al., 2003; Gali et al., 2020). It not only preserves the quality of life but also empowers patients to take control of their journey to recovery (Figure 14.15).

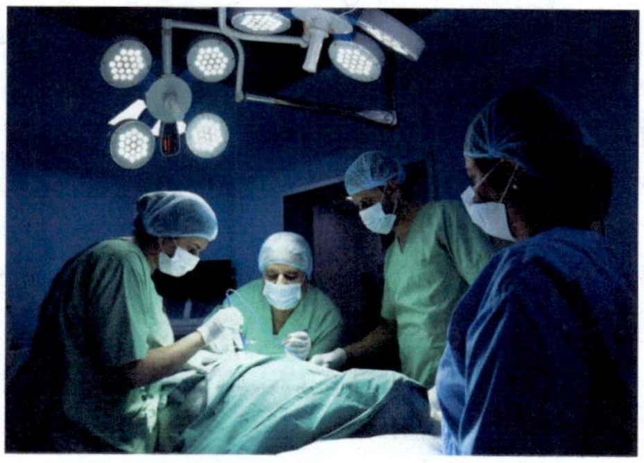

Figure 14.15. Effective patient care and support within the field of GI oncology is necessary.

Source: https://www.medanta.org/storage/speciality-contents/January2024/PtyTd56xSsA2EJlsa0RjuoVftwmiJi-metac2h1dHRlcnN0b2NrXzIzMTM4MTkyMDUgKDEpLmpwZw==-.jpg.

14.6.1. Importance of Multidisciplinary Care

In GI oncology, multidisciplinary care is critical to optimizing patient outcomes and enhancing the overall quality of life. Because gastrointestinal cancer is so multifaceted and intricate, patients generally require an assortment of services that extend beyond the typical provision of medical treatment. An interdisciplinary strategy, including surgeons, medical oncologists, radiation oncologists, nutritionists, palliative medicine specialists, and mental health clinicians, ensures that patients are provided with holistic care based on their individual needs. This blending of specialties not only maximizes symptom control but also allows prompt intervention on psychosocial and nutritional aspects, which are important in controlling side effects of intense cancer therapies. Early referral to palliative care, a topic discussed in current research, resolves the issue of enhanced patient experience and survival if all aspects of care are properly coordinated (Konstantis et al., 2025). Current evidence also indicates that the employment of multidisciplinary teams (MDTs) in GI oncology can bring significant improvement in treatment pathways and patient engagement. MDTs enable the free exchange of information between healthcare practitioners and thereby enable an environment where treatment options are thoroughly analyzed based on a convergence of expertise. This team-based model enables patients not only to be cured of the cancer but also to be guided through its attendant physical and emotional burdens. By addressing all the processes of cancer management, which include everything from surgical interventions to palliative care, MDTs can potentially enhance clinical decision-making as well as embrace a holistic approach towards treatment. Research emphasizes that if healthcare professionals work together, they are better positioned to ensure patient-centered care consistent with guidelines and thus maximize clinical outcomes (Al-Jawaldeh et al., 2025). Moreover, care's multidisciplinary nature in GI oncology is not confined to immediate management; it is also pivotal in planning survivorship and handling the complexities of long-term care. Those with cancers of the gastrointestinal system typically present with unique challenges, such as the need for specialist dietetic care and psychological counseling throughout their treatment pathway. In an integrated survivorship plan, coordinated care has proven to minimize late effects of treatment, minimize the risk of recurrence, and maximize patients' psychosocial well-being. Policies that encourage education among clinicians on the importance of multidisciplinary practice, particularly in nutritional, psychological, and palliative care, have been observed to boost health systems. Addressing these elements of cancer care ensures that all patients receive not only survival-focused care but also the support needed to thrive after their cancer diagnosis (Konstantis et al., 2025).

14.6.2. Psychological Support for Patients

Psychological care for GI oncology patients is important in enhancing the overall treatment and quality of life. With the issues of their diagnosis, issues that also test them daily, like intrusive thoughts and unnecessary emotional distress, offering effective mental health services becomes necessary. Studies demonstrate that psychological distress is present in patients with all cancer diagnoses and that anxiety and depression are significant comorbidities. Addressing these psychological concerns via support services has the potential to reduce symptoms and improve attitudes toward treatment and recovery. Good psychological care not only assists patients in dealing with their emotional response but also allows them to become a part of their own healthcare process, building their resilience against this overwhelming experience. The importance of individualized psychological treatments cannot be overemphasized since they can play a significant role in developing a harmonious atmosphere. Recent research identifies the connection between all dimensions of social support and cancer patients' mental health outcomes. Specifically, emotional, concrete, and affectionate support significantly determines a patient's experience of intrusive thoughts in illnesses , such as GI oncology. Supported patients are likely to have lower psychological distress, emphasizing the role of community and family involvement in the recovery process. Interventions that fortify these support systems, either through official family meetings, support groups, or therapy, can also significantly reduce isolation and helplessness, inducing improved psychological well-being along with physical care. Furthermore, the addition of psychological support to standard care regimens for GI oncology patients provides an interdisciplinary approach towards integral treatment. For instance, interventions that not only address physical aspects of treatment but also coping strategies for dealing with psychological distress will be more likely to have higher patient adherence and satisfaction. Because patients are likely to face emotional difficulties presented by intrusive illness-related thoughts, providing coping strategies founded on psychological support can truly optimize their overall treatment outcome. Training of health providers in the importance of mental health care and encouragement of their capacity to recognize the indicators of distress can provide the gateway to greater patient outcomes. In this regard, the inclusion of psychological support measures in GI oncology initiatives is fundamental to facilitating more complete care and ensuring improved recovery processes for patients who experience the dual jeopardy of a cancer diagnosis and its psychological consequences (Figure 14.16).

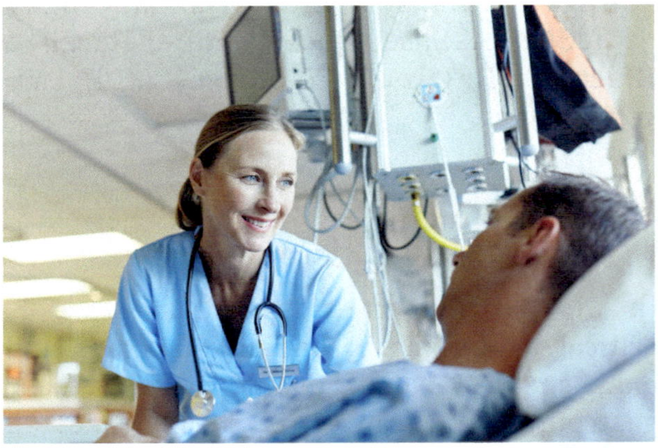

Figure 14.16. Psychological support for patients.

Source: https://www.oncologynurseadvisor.com/wp-content/uploads/sites/13/2019/02/surgeryg493216413_1527923.jpg.

14.6.3. Nutritional Considerations During Treatment

Proper nutrition management is part of the care of GI cancers, as patients have unusual issues that can impact their health and treatment outcome. Cancer cachexia, malnourishment, and therapy side effects in the guise of surgery, chemotherapy, and radiotherapy can result in unintended weight loss and alterations in metabolic processes. These issues necessitate an individualized nutritional therapy that takes into account the unique requirements of each patient to ensure that they receive adequate caloric intake and necessary nutrients. The holistic approach to addressing nutrition not only seeks to provide relief for symptoms but also enhances the patient's quality of life, thereby emerging as a critical component in the overall treatment strategy for GI malignancies (Antolino et al., 2017). Throughout the course of treatment, one must consider individualized dietary maneuvers that may enhance tolerance to treatment and decrease side effects. Patients undergoing chemotherapy, for example, may experience nausea, vomiting, or alterations in taste, which require adjustment in food selection and preparation to optimize palatability and adherence. Integrative medicine ideas can help in that respect by employing complementary strategies , such as acupuncture, herbal supplements, and diet changes, that can provide symptomatic relief during treatment sessions (Staff et al., 2006). These interventions can make the environment more supportive for healing, so the patients are in a better position to cope with the physical and psychological burdens of cancer. Close tracking of nutritional status throughout treatment is also important, with weight and nutrient alterations indicating the need for changes in dietary guidance. Regular assessment by healthcare providers—, such as dietitians with oncology specialty training, can permit deficits to be identified and interventions implemented in a timely fashion. Also, the involvement of a multidisciplinary team of professionals elevates the care of not only nutritional needs but also of psychosocial support, again emphasizing the benefit of addressing the whole patient and not only the cancer. Lastly, a holistic nutritional plan that is specifically tailored to address the particularities of GI oncology can contribute significantly towards influencing recovery and long-term survival (Antolino et al., 2017).

CLOSER LOOK

INCLUDING THE ESOPHAGUS:

The esophagus is a muscular, tubular organ that connects the throat to the stomach, serving as a critical conduit for food and liquid. A closer look at the esophagus reveals its complex structure, coordinated function, and its role in both digestive health and disease. Understanding the esophagus is essential for evaluating symptoms such as difficulty swallowing, chest pain, or acid reflux, as well as for guiding diagnostic and therapeutic interventions. Structurally, the esophagus consists of several layers: the mucosa, submucosa, muscularis propria, and adventitia. Its mucosal lining is stratified squamous epithelium, which provides protection against mechanical and chemical stress. Beneath this, smooth and skeletal muscle fibers coordinate peristaltic movements, propelling swallowed food toward the stomach. The esophagus also contains sphincters at its upper and lower ends—the upper esophageal sphincter (UES) and the lower esophageal sphincter (LES)—which regulate entry and prevent backflow, maintaining unidirectional movement.

Functionally, the esophagus plays a central role in swallowing and reflux prevention. Swallowing is a highly coordinated process involving voluntary and involuntary phases, requiring precise timing between the oropharyngeal muscles and esophageal peristalsis. The LES acts as a barrier against gastric contents, protecting the mucosa from acid and digestive enzymes. Dysfunction of these mechanisms can lead to clinical conditions such as gastroesophageal reflux disease (GERD), dysphagia, or esophageal motility disorders.

A pathological conditions involving the esophagus highlights its vulnerability. Chronic acid exposure can cause esophagitis, Barrett's esophagus, or increase the risk of esophageal adenocarcinoma. Structural abnormalities, including strictures, webs, or rings, can impede swallowing, while motility disorders like achalasia or diffuse esophageal spasm disrupt peristaltic coordination. Additionally, infections, autoimmune diseases, and medication-induced injuries can compromise the integrity of the esophageal lining. Diagnostic approaches to esophageal disorders include endoscopy, esophageal manometry, pH monitoring, and imaging studies. These tools assess structural integrity, motility, acid exposure, and mucosal health. Management strategies vary from lifestyle modifications—such as dietary adjustments and positional therapy—to pharmacological interventions, including proton pump inhibitors, or procedural options like dilation or surgical repair.

A closer examination of the esophagus underscores its importance beyond a simple food conduit. Its structure, function, and susceptibility to disease make it a focal point for gastrointestinal health. Maintaining esophageal integrity through preventive measures, early diagnosis, and targeted therapy is critical for ensuring optimal digestive function and overall well-being.

SUMMARY

In summary, cutting-edge gastrointestinal oncology reflects a multidisciplinary view of the relationship between chronic inflammation and cancer development. Ailments like GERD, BE, and inflammatory bowel diseases are basically based on inflammation as an essential force behind tumorigenesis. Oxidative stress consequent to these chronic conditions is a major contributor to genetic damage that precedes cancer. Thus, there is a pressing need for more research and new models to more accurately expose these mechanisms. With the development of three-dimensional human cell and tissue culture systems that mimic in vivo conditions, scientists can gain valuable insights into disease progression and correctly evaluate therapeutic strategies. These advances create the opportunity for improved patient results in GI oncology, and especially with regard to chronic inflammatory disorders (Hartman et al., 2013). Also emphasized by the cachexia implications of pancreatic cancer is the supreme complexity of the management of GI malignancies. Characterized by significant loss of muscle and fat tissue, cancer cachexia complicates treatment and lowers the quality of life of patients. In the spectrum of oncology, treatment of this multifactorial syndrome requires an integrative understanding of its pathophysiology and the convergence of nutritional support with pharmacologic treatment. Effective management will thus have to transcend traditional oncology practice, recognizing cachexia as a central consequence of tumor disruption in the body's metabolic activity. This extended approach not only can improve patient care but also identifies the interconnectedness of the different issues that are presented in GI oncology. By employing innovative clinical practices and research models, we can best combat these comorbid conditions (Hendifar et al., 2014). Ultimately, GI oncology's future will rely on a multidisciplinary paradigm that incorporates state-of-the-art research, innovative treatment approaches, and overall patient care. As specialties work together, particularly in mechanisms of inflammatory diseases and modalities of cancer therapy, the medical community can gain a better grasp of the various pathways to GI cancer. Sustained efforts toward developing patient-oriented models of care, together with prioritization of inflammation and cachexia, are important for improving overall therapeutic effectiveness. With continued research, it is important to have a continued focus on the exploration of new strategies aimed at both disease and its debilitating complications in patients. In doing so, the art of GI oncology can aspire not only to prolong life but ultimately give patients with these challenging diseases a better quality of life.

GI oncology as a field has evolved rapidly, providing critical insights into the molecular underpinnings of the majority of gastrointestinal cancers. A notable milestone here includes the TCGA revelations that prodded the multifactorial origins of cancers , such as glioblastomas, where chromosomal defects, gene mutations, and epigenetic alterations come together to facilitate tumorigenesis. For GI cancers as well, such aberrations provide a paradigm for comprehension of not just the biological basis of neoplasia, but also of potential therapeutic targets. Remarkably, key gene analyses , such as those directed against ERBB2, NF1, and TP53, teach us the manner in which such molecular changes predict clinical outcome and therapy response, thereby accentuating the value of genomic studies in the refinement of diagnostic and therapeutic strategies in GI oncology (Network, 2008). A second important research area involves the role of environmental exposures in the etiology and development of gastrointestinal cancers. Evidence indicates that lifestyle and environmental exposures account for a significant proportion of cancer occurrence, with estimates suggesting that toxins are responsible for 7% to 19% of cancer worldwide. These conclusions highlight the imperative of a further exact understanding of how chemical exposures at low doses interact synergistically to disrupt cellular functions, leading to carcinogenesis in sensitive organs like the gastrointestinal tract. The complexities of interactions call for further studies into the interactions of environmental toxins and the impact that the interactions of these toxins may have on cancer prevention as well as cancer treatment paradigms. Therefore, this information can inform public health interventions to reverse exposure to carcinogenic chemicals and thus lower the incidence of GI cancers (Goodson et al., 2015). Furthermore, integration of molecular data derived from genomic studies with environmental data can provide pathways for personalized therapy in GI cancers. As researchers identify the individual genetic alterations involved in different gastrointestinal cancers, clinicians can personalize treatment regimens based on the individual genetic profile of a patient and exposure status. This paradigm shift not only enhances the specificity of cancer treatment but also informs risk stratification and screening algorithms such that preventive measures are targeted to high-risk groups. Lastly, the interaction among the genetic, environmental, and lifestyle factors reflects the intricate topography of GI oncology, signaling the importance of a multidisciplinary approach that combines molecular biology, epidemiology, and clinical practice to create cancer care and improve patient care.

References

1. Goodson, W. H., 3rd, Lowe, L., Carpenter, D. O., Gilbertson, M., Manaf Ali, A., Lopez de Cerain Salsamendi, A., Lasfar, A., Carnero, A., Azqueta, A., Amedei, A., Charles, A. K., Collins, A. R., Ward, A., Salzberg, A. C., Colacci, A., Olsen, A. K., Berg, A., Barclay, B. J., Zhou, B. P., Blanco-Aparicio, C., ... Hu, Z. (2015). Assessing the carcinogenic potential of low-dose exposures to chemical mixtures in the environment: the challenge ahead. *Carcinogenesis, 36 Suppl 1*(Suppl 1), S254–S296. https://doi.org/10.1093/carcin/bgv039(accessed on 16th July 2025).
2. Abbas, A., Hameed, A., Khaliq, R. Z., Tahir, F., et al. (2023). *Colorectal Cancer in Pakistan: Genetic, Molecular, and Epidemiological Perspectives.* https://core.ac.uk/download/618235908.pdf (accessed on 16th July 2025).
3. Puzanov, I., Diab, A., Abdallah, K., Bingham, C. O., 3rd, Brogdon, C., Dadu, R., Hamad, L., Kim, S., Lacouture, M. E., LeBoeuf, N. R., Lenihan, D., Onofrei, C., Shannon, V., Sharma, R., Silk, A. W., Skondra, D., Suarez-Almazor, M. E., Wang, Y., Wiley, K., Kaufman, H. L., ... Society for Immunotherapy of Cancer Toxicity Management Working Group (2017). Managing toxicities associated with immune checkpoint inhibitors: consensus recommendations from the Society for Immunotherapy of Cancer (SITC) Toxicity Management Working Group. *Journal for immunotherapy of cancer, 5*(1), 95. https://doi.org/10.1186/s40425-017-0300-z (accessed on 16th July 2025).
4. Abdel-Azim, H., Abraham, A., Diaz, M. A., Dandoy, C., et al. (2017). *Outcomes following autologous hematopoietic stem cell transplant for patients with relapsed Wilms' tumor: A CIBMTR retrospective analysis.* https://core.ac.uk/download/323071219.pdf (accessed on 16th July 2025).
5. Aisner, J., Ali, S. M., Belyi, V., Bertino, J., et al. (2016). *Clinical actionability of comprehensive genomic profiling for management of rare or refractory cancers.* https://core.ac.uk/download/80790389.pdf (accessed on 16th July 2025).
6. Aizer, A., Aoyama, H., Attia, A., Beal, K., et al. (2019). *Estimating survival in patients with gastrointestinal cancers and brain metastases: An update of the graded prognostic assessment for gastrointestinal cancers (GI-GPA).* https://core.ac.uk/download/323062848.pdf (accessed on 16th July 2025).
7. Algra, T., Baigent, C., Baron, J. A., Bosetti, C., Burn, J., Cai, X., et al. (2014). *Estimates of benefits and harms of prophylactic use of aspirin in the general population.* https://core.ac.uk/download/46665961.pdf (accessed on 16th July 2025).
8. Al-Jawaldeh, A., Hammerich, A., Aldayel, F. A., Troisi, G., Al-Jawaldeh, H., Aguenaou, H., Alsawahli, H., et al. (2025). A review on the multidisciplinary approach for cancer management in the Eastern Mediterranean Region: A focus on nutritional, lifestyle and supportive care. *International Journal of Environmental Research and Public Health, 22.* https://www.semanticscholar.org/paper/dae4108a4559a6f12f8fd0d2731551fef2657413 (accessed on 16th July 2025).
9. Allum, W., Lordick, F., Alsina, M., Andritsch, E., Ba-Ssalamah, A., Beishon, M., Braga, M., Caballero, C., Carneiro, F., Cassinello, F., Dekker, J. W., Delgado-Bolton, R., Haustermans, K., Henning, G., Hutter, B., Lövey, J., Netíková, I. Š., Obermannová, R., Oberst, S., Rostoft, S., ...

Naredi, P. (2018). ECCO essential requirements for quality cancer care: Oesophageal and gastric cancer. *Critical reviews in oncology/hematology, 122,* 179–193. https://doi.org/10.1016/j.critrevonc.2017.12.019(accessed on 16th July 2025).

10. Almar, E., Arveux, P., Autelitano, M., Baldi, I., Bara, S., Barchielli, A., Benfatto, L., et al. (2019). *Treatment challenges in and outside a specialist network setting: Pancreatic neuroendocrine tumors.* https://core.ac.uk/download/287859188.pdf (accessed on 16th July 2025).
11. Alonso-Basanta, M., Dong, L., Irmen, P., Li, Y., et al. (2019). *Dosimetric performance and planning/delivery efficiency of a dual-layer stacked and staggered MLC on treating multiple small targets: A planning study based on single-isocenter multi-target stereotactic radiosurgery (SRS) to brain metastases.* https://core.ac.uk/download/213445703.pdf (accessed on 16th July 2025).
12. Antolino, L., Aurello, P., D'Angelo, F., Giulitti, A., et al. (2017). *Follow-up after curative resection for gastric cancer: Is it time to tailor it?* https://core.ac.uk/download/132156762.pdf (accessed on 16th July 2025).
13. Yang, J. J., Yu, D., Takata, Y., Smith-Warner, S. A., Blot, W., White, E., Robien, K., Park, Y., Xiang, Y. B., Sinha, R., Lazovich, D., Stampfer, M., Tumino, R., Aune, D., Overvad, K., Liao, L., Zhang, X., Gao, Y. T., Johansson, M., Willett, W., ... Shu, X. O. (2017). Dietary Fat Intake and Lung Cancer Risk: A Pooled Analysis. *Journal of clinical oncology : official journal of the American Society of Clinical Oncology, 35*(26), 3055–3064. https://doi.org/10.1200/JCO.2017.73.3329Baumann, B. C., Fischer-Valuck, B. W., Gay, H. A., Michalski, J. M., et al. (2019). *A brief review of low-dose rate (LDR) and high-dose rate (HDR) brachytherapy boost for high-risk prostate.* https://core.ac.uk/download/286537376.pdf (accessed on 16th July 2025).
14. Berardi, G., Ceelen, W., Ghiasloo, M., Pavlenko, M., et al. (2020). *Surgical treatment of stage IV colorectal cancer with synchronous liver metastases: A systematic review and network meta-analysis.*
15. Bone, R. N., Nwotchouang, B., Moffett, N., Jeune-Smith, Y., & Feinberg, B. (2025). Influence of data review on community physicians' treatment preferences in frontline esophageal cancer (EC). *Journal of Clinical Oncology.* https://www.semanticscholar.org/paper/7aaa2e903b29a307187575a27702c74fd3827c4b (accessed on 16th July 2025).
16. Hartman, K. G., Bortner, J. D., Falk, G. W., Yu, J., Martín, M. G., Rustgi, A. K., & Lynch, J. P. (2013). Modeling inflammation and oxidative stress in gastrointestinal disease development using novel organotypic culture systems. *Stem cell research & therapy, 4 Suppl 1*(Suppl 1), S5. https://doi.org/10.1186/scrt366(accessed on 16th July 2025).
17. Brém, E., Koyfman, A., & Long, B. J. (2020). *Oncologic Emergencies: Immune-Based Cancer Therapies and Complications.* https://core.ac.uk/download/305124082.pdf (accessed on 16th July 2025).
18. Bui, H. T. P., Dao, L. T. M., Do, D. H., Ha, T. T., et al. (2020). *Genetic landscape of autism spectrum disorder in Vietnamese children.* https://core.ac.uk/download/293755065.pdf (accessed on 16th July 2025).
19. Burton, J. H., Lana, S. E., Selmic, L. E., Thamm, D. H., et al. (2014). *Comparison of carboplatin and doxorubicin-based chemotherapy protocols in 470 dogs after amputation for treatment of appendicular osteosarcoma.* https://core.ac.uk/download/323071710.pdf (accessed on 16th July 2025).

20. Cancer Genome Atlas Research Network. (2008). *Comprehensive genomic characterization defines human glioblastoma genes and core pathways.* https://core.ac.uk/download/323062204.pdf (accessed on 16th July 2025).

21. Canter, R. J., Fraker, D. L., Glatstein, E. J., Hahn, S. M., et al. (2003). I*ntraperitoneal photodynamic therapy causes a capillary-leak syndrome.* https://core.ac.uk/download/323068075.pdf (accessed on 16th July 2025).

22. Caplin, M., Falconi, M., Fusai, G. K., Lykoudis, P. M., et al. (2017). *Treatment challenges in and outside a specialist network setting: Pancreatic neuroendocrine tumors.* https://core.ac.uk/download/168403284.pdf (accessed on 16th July 2025).

23. Mabula, J. B., McHembe, M. D., Koy, M., Chalya, P. L., Massaga, F., Rambau, P. F., Masalu, N., & Jaka, H. (2012). Gastric cancer at a university teaching hospital in northwestern Tanzania: a retrospective review of 232 cases. *World journal of surgical oncology, 10*, 257. https://doi.org/10.1186/1477-7819-10-257(accessed on 16th July 2025).

24. Chau, I., Cunningham, D., Davidson, M., Hickish, T., et al. (2017). *Impact of tumor histological subtype on chemotherapy outcome in advanced oesophageal cancer.* https://core.ac.uk/download/96655240.pdf (accessed on 16th July 2025).

25. Chen, Q., Zheng, X., Cheng, W., & Li, J. (2024). Landscape of targeted therapies for lung squamous cell carcinoma. *Frontiers in Oncology, 14.* https://www.semanticscholar.org/paper/0755b28acb3dd532c8bea77b4b995d657c2e509e (accessed on 16th July 2025).

26. Chen, Y., Degnin, C., Hung, A. Y., McClelland, M., et al. (2019). *Is moderate hypofractionation accepted as a new standard of care in North America for prostate cancer patients treated with external beam radiotherapy? Survey of genitourinary expert radiation oncologists.* https://core.ac.uk/download/228066084.pdf (accessed on 16th July 2025).

27. Clinic Staff. (2006). *Integrative Medicine Approach to Colon Cancer.* https://core.ac.uk/download/46965740.pdf (accessed on 16th July 2025).

28. den Hoed, C. M., & Kuipers, E. J. (2016). *Gastric Cancer: How Can We Reduce the Incidence of This Disease?* https://core.ac.uk/download/154410385.pdf (accessed on 16th July 2025).

29. Easler, J. J., El Hajj, I. I., Fogel, E. L., Gromski, M. A., et al. (2019). *Annular pancreas: Endoscopic and pancreatographic findings from a tertiary referral ERCP center.* https://core.ac.uk/download/227054194.pdf (accessed on 16th July 2025).

30. Emadali, A., Gorg, A., Schmidt, A., Polley, A. C., Feldman, A. L., Rodriguez-Pineiro, A. M., Salzano, A. M., et al. (2008). *The Current State of Proteomics in GI Oncology.* https://core.ac.uk/download/pdf/8531789.pdf (accessed on 16th July 2025).

31. Escalera, C., Nápoles, A. M., Ortiz, C., Santoyo-Olsson, J., et al. (2019). *Social support as a moderator in the relationship between intrusive thoughts and anxiety among Spanish-speaking Latinas with breast cancer.* https://core.ac.uk/download/323063219.pdf (accessed on 16th July 2025).

32. Gali, K., Pike, B., Kendra, M. S., Tran, C., Fielding-Singh, P., Jimenez, K., Mirkin, R., & Prochaska, J. J. (2020). Integration of Tobacco Treatment Services into Cancer Care at Stanford. *International journal of environmental research and public health, 17*(6), 2101. https://doi.org/10.3390/ijerph17062101(accessed on 16th July 2025).

33. Fsadni, C. J. (2015). *A study on the management of corticosteroid side effects in cancer patients.* https://core.ac.uk/download/46603767.pdf (accessed on 16th July 2025).

34. Gill, T., Loo, G. H., Muthkumaran, G., & Kosai, N. (2025). Posterior membranous tracheal injury during McKeown oesophagectomy: A case report with literature review. *Frontiers in Oncology, 15.* https://www.semanticscholar.org/paper/fa38a1788acf5808ac16dfab56fef8b028487380 (accessed on 16th July 2025).

35. Goodman, A., Khagi, Y., Kurzrock, R., Riviere, I., et al. (2020). *Total number of alterations in liquid biopsies is an independent predictor of survival in patients with advanced cancers.* https://core.ac.uk/download/322493964.pdf (accessed on 16th July 2025).

36. Gunn, V., Li, J., Lui, H., Shi, W., et al. (2018). *Evaluation of hybrid arc and volumetric-modulated arc therapy treatment plans for fractionated stereotactic intracranial radiotherapy.* https://core.ac.uk/download/213444217.pdf (accessed on 16th July 2025).

37. Heinemann, V., & Hoff, P. M. (2010). *Bevacizumab plus irinotecan-based regimens in the treatment of metastatic colorectal cancer.* https://core.ac.uk/download/16432399.pdf (accessed on 16th July 2025).

38. Hendifar, A. E., Tan, C. R., Jamil, L., Nissen, N., Yaffee, P., Tuli, R., et al. (2014). *Pancreatic cancer cachexia: A review of mechanisms and therapeutics.* https://core.ac.uk/download/323077283.pdf (accessed on 16th July 2025).

39. Hodgson, B. D., Hong, C. H. L., Spijkervet, F. K. L., Napeñas, J. J., Elting, L. S., Brennan, M. T., Stokman, M. A., et al. (2010). *A Systematic Review of Dental Disease in Patients Undergoing Cancer Therapy.* https://core.ac.uk/download/213086305.pdf (accessed on 16th July 2025).

40. Konstantis, A., Paraskeva, M., Avgoustidi, M., Kiagia, M., Kounnis, V., Rovithi, M., Alexaki, M., et al. (2025). The implementation of palliative care in Greece: A position paper by the Palliative Care Working Group of the Hellenic Society of Medical Oncology (HeSMO). *Forum of Clinical Oncology, 0.* https://www.semanticscholar.org/paper/af70ab4533ec340b1a6ebfdda5cded6ca2785899 (accessed on 16th July 2025).

41. Mukherjee, D., Alqahtani, S. A., & Krishnan, A. (2025). Bariatric surgery and risk of gastrointestinal and hormone-sensitive cancers in patients with metabolic-associated steatotic liver disease and obesity: A multicenter matched cohort study. *Journal of Clinical Oncology.* https://www.semanticscholar.org/paper/7e54a3c3c8befbd4410ca0441fe189c831a77daf (accessed on 16th July 2025).

42. Focal Spot, Fall/Winter 2010/2011. Bernard Becker Medical Library Archives. Washington University School of Medicine, Saint Louis, Missouri(accessed on 16th July 2025).

43. Tounkara, F., Sara, A., Thanikachalam, K., Noonan, A. M., Mittra, A., Malalur, P., Jin, N., et al. (2025). Predicting immune-related adverse events (irAE) in gastrointestinal malignancies (GI-M): Tumor-specific risk factors (TS-RF), hematological markers (HM), and clinical outcomes. *Journal of Clinical Oncology.* https://www.semanticscholar.org/paper/d8f7723a2c15e181bde17c86fcf38731ef8bb8d7 (accessed on 16th July 2025).

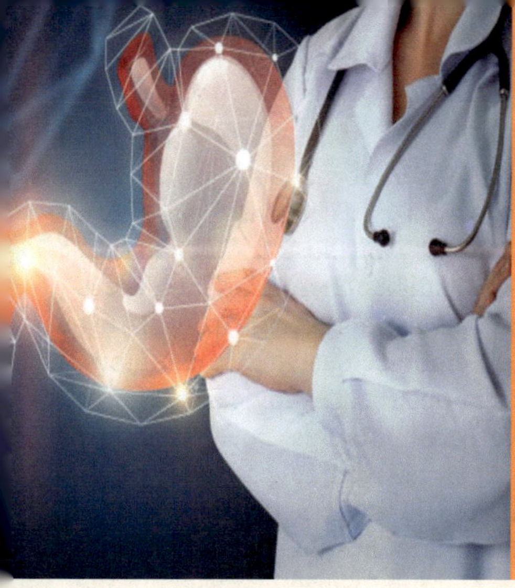

Chapter 15

ADVANCES AND FUTURE TRENDS IN GASTROENTEROLOGY

Contents

Introduction

Over the past few decades, gastroenterology has seen incredible progress facilitated by advances in technology as well as a better comprehension of the multifaceted interactions in the human body. Scientists have more and more recognized the central role played by the gut microbiome in shaping gastrointestinal health, giving rise to seminal findings about digestive disorders and their pathophysiology. By illuminating the vast array of metabolites synthesized by gut bacteria, scientists have begun to link such metabolites to a vast array of physiological processes far beyond the gut. Such studies not only increase our understanding of conditions associated with aging and obesity but also provide opportunities for new therapeutic strategies for manipulating the gut microbiome to maximize health. This convergence of gastroenterology and microbiology is pushing the field into a future in which the targeted interventions may totally transform patient care and treatment modalities (Fogelson et al., 2023). Furthermore, as conventional therapeutic practices are facing limitations, especially in treating infections , such as Helicobacter pylori, the gastroenterological landscape is changing very fast. The shift away from considering peptic ulcers to be chronic illnesses and toward single events is an example, reflecting a strong shift away from past treatment practices. New guidelines now encourage aggressive treatment and testing, particularly in those at high risk of gastric cancer, reflecting an urgent need for widespread public health interventions. Increasing incidences of resistance to antimicrobials have also complicated matters, necessitating a redesign of existing treatment guidelines. These developments underscore the imperative to embrace sustainable antibiotic stewardship measures that are essential as we navigate the complexity of gastroenterological treatment in this changing world (Yi-Lee et al., 2022). As this field continues to evolve, future gastroenterological trends will revolve around precision medicine, with therapy approaches tailored to patient profiles that are individualized based on their unique microbiomes and genetic setups. The addition of new diagnostic technologies, such as metagenomics and personalized metabolomics, has the promise to shed light on diet, intestinal health, and overall well-being. Furthermore, the more the world learns about the interconnections between intestinal health and overall disease, interdisciplinary approaches are going to become more popular, further solidifying the necessity for collaboration between healthcare providers across specialties. These developments do not simply hold the potential for advancing the standard of care in gastroenterology but also provide wide fields of investigation, promising to bring to an end the thousands of issues that still persist in this rapidly evolving field (Figure 15.1).

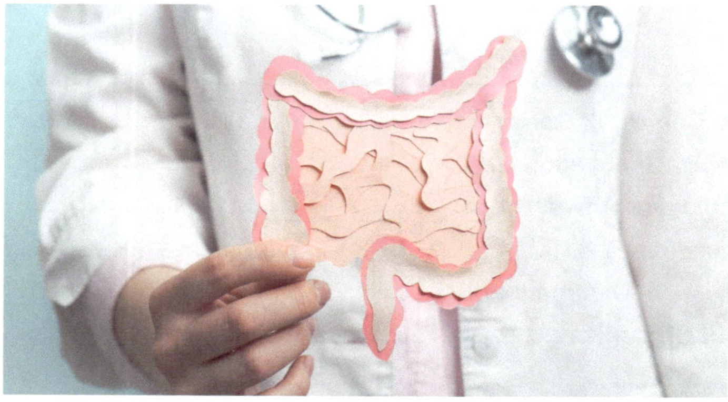

Figure 15.1. Advances and future trends in gastroenterology.

Source: https://www.healixhospitals.com/tinyimages/Gastroenterlogy-Healix%20Hospitals.jpg.

Definition of Gastroenterology

The intricate interaction between many bodily biological systems emphasizes the complexity of gastroenterology, an important medical specialty that is dedicated to investigating, diagnosing, and treating gastrointestinal illness. Not only does gastroenterology encompass the esophagus, stomach, and intestines, but also accessory organs , such as the liver, pancreas, and gallbladder. With the varied role of the organs involved in the process of digestion and absorption, gastroenterology plays a crucial role in handling how malfunctions in the processes associated with these systems can lead to grave medical issues. Recent advances in microbial biology and neuroscience have led to the gut-brain axis becoming a prominent issue, with a focus on the need for new models to accommodate the dynamic interactions between gut health and overall well-being and, by extension, refocus some of the gastroenterology attention onto an integrated approach to states of health and disease (Morar & Skorburg, 2018). The continued growth of gastroenterology reflects broader trends in the practice of medicine, particularly the reaction to emerging public health needs. Over the past decades, there has been a considerable move away from an entirely hospital-based approach towards one that values the delivery of community-based services and prevention. This change recognizes the significance of lifestyle and behavioral risk factors in gastrointestinal disease, realizing that illnesses , such as obesity, inflammatory bowel disease, and colorectal cancer are increasingly linked with societal alterations in diet and physical activity. As a case in point in the work of medical specialists like Sir Kenneth Calman, the evolution of technology has played a pivotal role in improving diagnostic and therapeutic approaches in gastroenterology, ultimately determining patient outcomes (Bergman et al., 2018). Additionally, gastroenterology studies are increasingly being informed by an integrated understanding of microbiomes and their significance in gastrointestinal health. The latest research emphasizes the pivotal role played by gut microbiota in the modulation not only of gastrointestinal diseases but also of overall health conditions, including metabolic syndrome and mental disease. Consequently, the integration of microbiological principles with gastroenterological practice is providing the potential for novel therapeutic strategies, such as fecal microbiota transplantation and tailored diets. These advancements further put pressure on the promise of new therapies alongside the emphasis on interdisciplinarity in gastroenterology, nutrition, and public health. As the profession develops and advances, its definition will further reflect these advancements, ultimately constituting a more integrated and effective way of addressing digestive health (Morar & Skorburg, 2018).

Importance of Advancements in the Field

Complexity in gastroenterological diseases necessitates ongoing advancement in medical science and technological progress, and thus, it is necessary to keep conducting research in this field. The developing understanding of diseases , such as necrotizing enterocolitis (NEC) has given rise to greater awareness of the intricate relationship between intestinal microbiota and mucosal immunity. Current studies have identified critical mechanisms in disease pathogenesis, including a role for cytokines and immune cells. This information is crucial not only for explaining the pathogenesis of NEC but also for the identification of candidate therapeutic targets that could vastly enhance patient outcomes. By advancing at the cellular level of intestinal epithelium, advances in the understanding of NEC not only bring with them potential for enhanced treatments but also improve our general grasp of gut health and prevention of disease, thus advancing the field in significant ways (Bolock et al., 2017). For the treatment of vascular lower GI bleeding, advances have transformed clinical practice on a grand scale. Enhanced endoscopic techniques, such as high-definition vision and narrow-band imaging, have contributed to increased diagnostic yield and therapeutic effectiveness. These technologies provide more targeted interventions, which are critical for reducing patient morbidity from bleeding events. Concurrently, advancements in angiographic methods, such as computed tomographic angiography (CTA) and superselective embolization, provide valuable alternatives for managing bleeding in patients where endoscopy may not be sufficient. The ability to utilize both endoscopic and angiographic modalities represents a treatment decision milestone, leading ultimately to an individualized modality that considers personal patient parameters. The marriage of these technologies is evidence of the overriding importance of innovations in improving results and guiding clinical practice in the field of gastroenterology (Alomair, 2024). In addition, the future of gastroenterology is also projected to be shaped by technologies that integrate artificial intelligence and machine learning into practice. These are anticipated to improve decision-making processes by scrutinizing enormous amounts of data at rates quicker than human practitioners. For example, AI algorithms may assist in identifying faint patterns on imaging studies, which can offer diagnostic insights that may otherwise be left undetected. Simultaneously, the development of novel embolic agents and hybrid treatment strategies can also reshape the treatment of advanced conditions with personalized therapies that appeal to some patients' interests. With more investigations conducted to unravel the complexities of gastrointestinal disease, the trends are pointing towards an increasingly collaborative and technology-assisted approach. These advances not only represent progress in gastroenterology but also signal the importance of interdisciplinary collaboration for the enhancement of patient care across the healthcare continuum (Bolock et al., 2017; Alomair, 2024) (Figure 15.2).

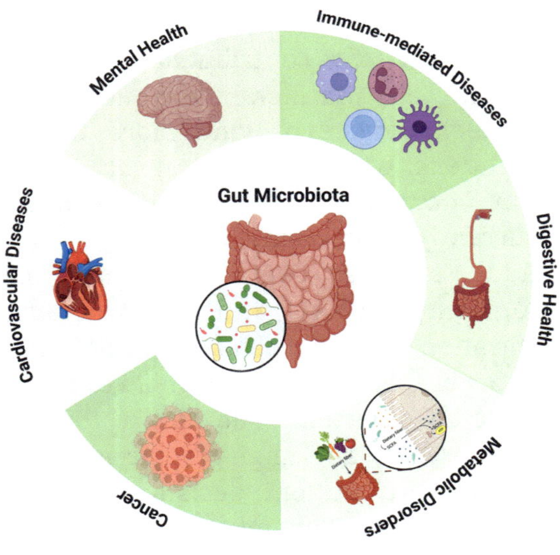

Figure 15.2. Importance of advancements in the field.

Source: Yaqub MO, Jain A, Joseph CE, Edison LK. Microbiome-Driven Therapeutics: From Gut Health to Precision Medicine. *Gastrointestinal Disorders*. 2025; 7(1):7. https://doi.org/10.3390/gidisord7010007

15.1. Historical Context of Gastroenterology

Emerging from a rich cultural weave of medical mythology, gastroenterology has, over the decades, been influenced by major breakthroughs that enunciate evolution in science and technology as much as in medicine. Gastrointestinal disorders were generally rationalized in the past in terms of mystical or humoral imbalances, denying optimized effectiveness in management. With the rise of the Enlightenment, empirical observation and the scientific approach began to find momentum. Early gastroenterological practices were founded by Thomas Willis and Giovanni Maria Lancisi, who provided basic insights into disorders in the digestive system. Dissection-driven advances in anatomy slowly revealed the pathophysiology underlying gastrointestinal diseases. The 19th century witnessed the discovery of a range of diagnostic devices, opening doors to contemporary gastroenterology. This historical progress not only represents an extension of the understanding of gastrointestinal pathologies but also indicates the ceaseless search for new therapies that characterizes the field in the modern era. With the course of development of the 20th century, fundamental advancements in the biomedical sciences transformed gastroenterology from an emerging specialty to a cornerstone of internal medicine. The introduction of endoscopy redefined diagnostics, allowing physicians to look directly into the gastrointestinal tract and perform interventional treatments. These advances broadened the options for treating peptic ulcers and gastrointestinal bleeding and numerous other disorders. Furthermore, the advent of microbiology uncovered the intricate dance between gut flora and health in general and threw the gut into the limelight as a key player among systemic diseases. Furthermore, preventive and curative public health programs for liver diseases represented a milestone in the historical background of gastroenterology, particularly in pediatric cases in which early-stage diagnosis is complicated, as emphasized by growing warnings against chronic liver diseases in children, which have the potential to be harbingers of adult ailments like cirrhosis and hepatocellular carcinoma (Della Corte et al., 2016). Today, the practice of gastroenterology continues to evolve at a rapid pace, driven by new research and an expanding understanding of molecular and genetic pathogenic pathways of gastrointestinal disorders. The advent of direct-acting antivirals (DAAs) for the management of hepatitis C is one of the most impressive advances of recent years, which has opened a positive horizon for obtaining high cure rates with fewer side effects compared to traditional regimens. The challenge does persist, however, in moving universal access to these emerging therapies, particularly for underrepresented groups, such as those of Native American descent, where genetic markers may predict the effectiveness of treatment (Trinks et al., 2017). These innovations show the ongoing dialogue between past and future in gastroenterology, which shows the need to integrate lessons regarding how to overcome obstacles and achieve breakthroughs in the past into future studies and treatment strategies.

15.1.1. Early Practices and Discoveries

The origins of modern gastroenterology are steeped in a rich legacy of early medical science and discovery that provided the foundation for continued progress. Concepts of gastrointestinal illnesses in the earliest days were apt to arise from observation of symptoms and primitive forms of therapy, with clinicians relying heavily on herbal remedies and dietary modifications. This method of trial and error, even limited by the quality of science at that time, laid the groundwork for further research. With the changing centuries, the advent of techniques , such as endoscopy transformed this branch of medicine to enable the visualization of interior organs directly. As the instrumentation and machinery improved, so did the methods used to cut into complex gastrointestinal illnesses, encouraging more targeted forms of therapy. The initial practices, as such, not only shed light upon the character of gastrointestinal disease but also directed the ongoing development of diagnosis and treatment models that continue to evolve to this day. The research trajectory of gastrointestinal development has also been closely interwoven with the major discoveries concerning pathogens and their role in digestive disease. The identification of *Helicobacter pylori*, in particular, was particularly seminal, standing gastronomy on its head and rendering peptic ulcer disease a very different entity. Stress and lifestyle were first to be blamed for the ulcers, but were refocused by elucidation of the presence of *H. pyloris* in the gastric mucosa as a microbiological cause. This paradigm shift emphasized the call for antimicrobial intervention, paving the way for more aggressive diagnostic practices and intervention planning. The result was population-level screening activities increasing in response to increased gastric cancer incidence across various nations, reflecting growing knowledge of the cause of the disease and the call for preventive measures. H. has been researched. Poky infection demonstrates how initial discoveries can have the ability to initiate paradigm shifts in gastroenterology practice, serving as the stage for future breakthroughs. Furthermore, the new science of artificial intelligence can potentially redefine the landscape of gastroenterology, riding on initial discoveries that have developed it. As noted, modern drug discovery processes rely increasingly on sophisticated algorithms and machine learning, which enhance therapeutic candidate identification speed and precision. This revolution is a world away from the yesteryear models, where drug making was a laborious and costly process that exceeded a decade to complete. Current trends point to the fact that, using big data sets and advanced computing capabilities, gastroenterology can not only accelerate the development of new drugs but also refine existing treatment protocols. The implications of these advancements are monumental, with the potential to improve patient care with increased specialization and efficiency of treatment. The early habits and results, thus, are less a historical account but also a catalyst for future innovations within the field of gastroenterology to shape the course of future trends and technologies (Figure 15.3).

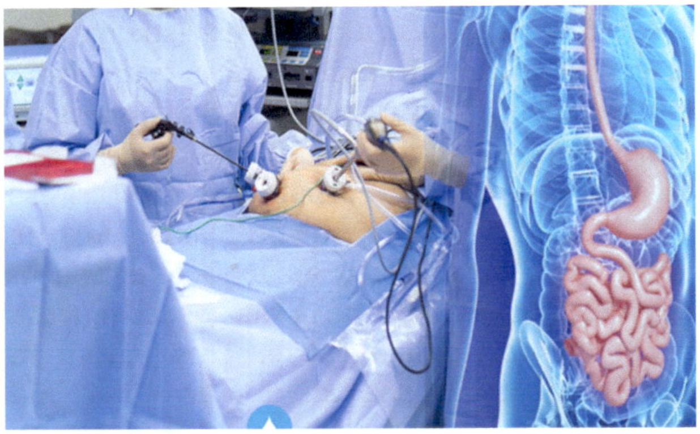

Figure 15.3. Early practices and discoveries of modern gastroenterology.

Source: https://ilshospitals.com/blog/wp-content/uploads/2020/10/gastroenterology-banner.jpg.

15.1.2. Evolution of Diagnostic Techniques

Advances in diagnostic techniques have extensively transformed the field of gastroenterology, addressing the age-old problems associated with the diagnosis and treatment of gastrointestinal disorders. Previously, invasive techniques , such as endoscopies and biopsies were at the core of diagnostics; these were traditionally risky for patients and were also limited in application. Over time, technologies like non-invasive imaging modalities like ultrasound, magnetic resonance imaging (MRI), and computed tomography (CT) scans have proved to be useful weapons. They provide visualization of the gastrointestinal tract and the surrounding organs in more detail, paving the way for earlier and more accurate diagnoses. Thus, these non-invasive approaches have been incorporated into clinical practice, useful for the detection of diseases ranging from liver conditions to gastrointestinal cancers, thereby improving patient care and allowing early interventions. Besides, the stimulus for diagnostic innovation has also been technological advancements in the field of molecular biology and genomics, which have made possible the evolution of precision medicine in gastroenterology. Techniques , such as liquid biopsies and advanced biomarker analysis are revolutionizing the path of diagnosing and monitoring gastrointestinal diseases. For instance, understanding the molecular and genetic etiology of conditions , such as chronic liver diseases has uncovered new diagnostic pathways that enable the diagnosis of the disease in a previously undetected phase. As is highlighted in the recent literature, these new developments not only improve diagnostic accuracy but also provide leads on treatment customized for the patient. This personalized approach has huge possibilities for addressing multifactorial disease, a paradigm shift towards precision treatments that could adapt to the specific needs of patients with gastrointestinal disorders (Della Corte et al., 2016). Converting from standardized systems like the Liver Imaging Reporting and Data System (LI-RADS) also becomes a necessity in diagnostic technology, particularly in the detection of hepatocellular carcinoma (HCC). LI-RADS aims to improve radiologists' consistency in interpretation, thereby enhancing clinical decision-making regarding the management of liver disease. These sequential updates reflect a commitment to excellence in diagnostic imaging that is long-standing, with the resultant criteria used for the assessment of liver lesions being ever relevant and scientifically sound (Elsayes et al., 2017). As gastroenterology progresses, such systems of structured reporting will become increasingly crucial in rebuffing the complexities of the diagnosis of liver disease, eventually decreasing variation and providing high-quality patient care. Such a progression demonstrates gastroenterology's capacity to rapidly adapt and develop in reaction to emergent challenges, making possible an increasingly accurate and accessible diagnostic process in the future.

15.1.3. Milestones in Treatment Options

The therapeutic history in gastroenterology has been marked by significant milestones that highlight progress in medical technology and science. Over the past few decades, understanding various gastrointestinal diseases has become more profound, and this has resulted in therapeutic advancements aimed at improving patient outcomes. New understanding of the pathogenesis of liver disease, particularly among children, has contributed significantly. Through the identification of mechanisms underlying these disorders, scientists have developed new therapeutic targets, and the ability to treat diseases previously untreatable has increased.

The traditional approaches, often symptomatic relief-oriented, have since been augmented with treatments aimed at disease modification and, in some cases, cure, and consequently, management approaches in pediatric gastroenterology have been modified (Della Corte et al., 2016). In viral hepatitis, major strides have been made, most importantly in the treatment of hepatitis C virus (HCV) infection. The introduction of direct-acting antiviral drugs (DAAs) has revolutionized treatment regimens with excellent cure rates and an improved side effect profile compared to previous regimens. This is not only a win for the drug industry but a paradigm shift towards personalized therapy. An understanding of host genetic markers has opened doors in the sense of variation in treatment efficacy, and evidence has been forthcoming towards the potential of personalized therapy based on individual genetic profiles. Still, there would seem to remain much to be overcome in light of such advances, in particular where economic factors limit DAAs' access. The integration of pharmacogenomic testing could thus be critical in the sense of prioritizing treatment in underprivileged populations (Trinks et al., 2017). Looking ahead, the art of gastroenterology treatment will likely continue to evolve with the foundation of new research and technological advances. New technologies, such as gene therapy and advanced endoscopic therapy, will provide yet another level of therapeutic capability for practitioners to employ. Additionally, the increasing emphasis placed upon interdisciplinary treatments involving diet, microbiome, and patient education addresses an integrated model of gastroenterological health. Technological advances in telemedicine and remote monitoring will allow greater patient involvement and adherence to treatment protocols, with possible therapeutic efficacy. Moving ahead on the basis of achievements till date, the future of gastroenterology promises more substantial patient gains through emphasis on continuous evolution and modification of treatment modes (Figure 15.4).

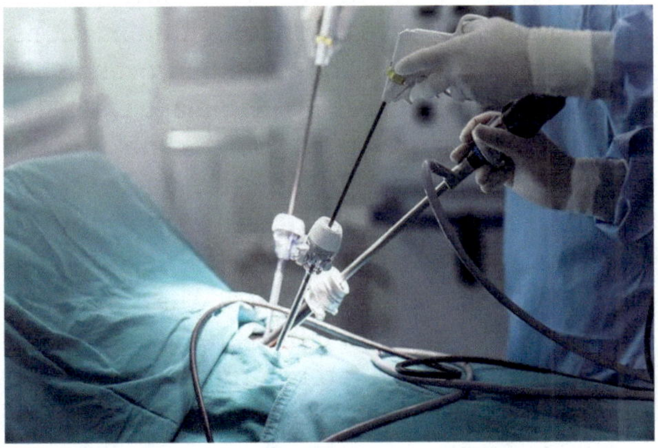

Figure 15.4. Milestones in treatment options.

Source: https://ntxsurgical.com/wp-content/uploads/2023/09/Screenshot-2023-09-16-182907.png.

15.2. Technological Innovations

In gastroenterology, the confluence of technological developments has radically transformed diagnostic and treatment methods to unprecedented levels of patient care. Some of these technologies are the use of artificial intelligence (AI) for image interpretation of complex imaging data, to speed up and intensify diagnosis. New technologies , such as endoscopic ultrasound and capsule endoscopy, are transformed by AI algorithms that scan for abnormalities with an accuracy unimaginable to the human eye. Besides, the use of machine learning makes it easier to identify patterns from large datasets and enhance predictability in gastroenterology. Besides accelerating workflows, this innovation also reduces the cognitive burden for healthcare professionals, hence leaving more time for patient-centered practice and clinical interaction. Aside from imaging technology, the advent of generative AI and large language models (LLMs) implies a revolution in gastroenterology information management. These technologies possess revolutionary potential to streamline patient data management, treatment recommendations, and even clinical decision-making processes. As noted, LLMs like ChatGPT can manage extensive medical literature that assists physicians in keeping abreast of the latest research and therapeutic approaches. However, the integration of such technologies necessitates a well-established framework that includes coordination among clinicians, technology developers, and regulatory ethicists to ensure the effective and ethical employment of AI tools in clinical care. By promoting a collaborative approach, the gastroenterology practice can implement these advances to maximize the quality and efficiency of care. The benefit of these technological innovations extends beyond immediate clinical application; it also facilitates long-term innovation in personalized medicine in gastroenterology. By leveraging data analytics and biomarker discovery, physicians can tailor treatment to patients and achieve maximized outcomes as well as patient satisfaction.

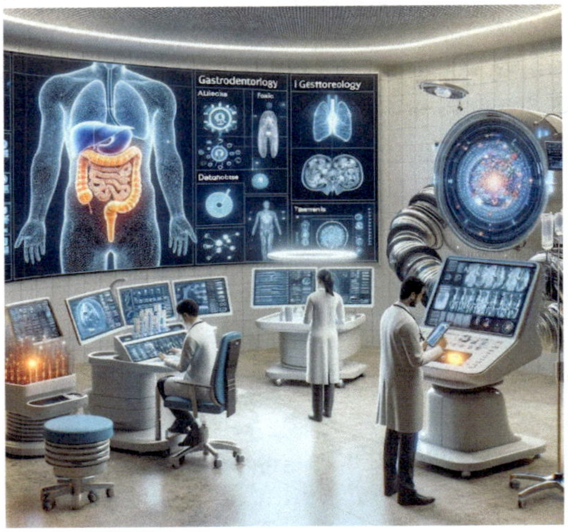

Figure 15.5. Technological innovations in gastroenterology.

Source: https://blogger.googleusercontent.com/img/b/R29vZ2xl/AVvXsEgNt5tAGn5rRRtds42gq7S-M69SkvTNd4qPUat4hdQ7yefJkevbTFxf-iRh4tlzXyAF8FgjpSUz0TWTNDidTn5ye9BkW95RtoY2-w7oz6J2JA1k1HZ5f9ZtijQlxdavGmsaK0mNe7oEpyoDeqWhWUi7dy0cRKQLUta0wTauPE4SOzVm5mF6q8O3NvEg6oo/w640-h640-rw/DALL%C2%B7E%202024-03-08%2004.51.14%20-%20The%20image%20should%20depict%20the%20transformative%20impact%20of%20Artificial%20Intelligence%20(AI)%20in%20gastroenterology%20as%20seen%20in%202024.%20Envision%20a%20state-of-the-art%20gas.webp.

In addition, as the field progresses, it is essential to address significant ethical and legal concerns regarding AI and data technologies. Exploring these elements ensures that innovations are implemented equitably and responsibly. As gastroenterology continues to progress, embracing these technological advancements will be key to shaping future trends and improving patient care in general, ultimately being a manifestation of an ideology of innovation that will define the field for decades to come (Figure 15.5).

15.2.1. Role of Endoscopy in Diagnosis and Treatment

Improvement in endoscopic techniques has significantly enhanced diagnostic capability in gastroenterology, particularly in detecting and treating pancreatic cystic lesions. With advancing imaging technology, it has become more frequent to detect such cysts; however, it remains a complex task for doctors to identify which of these lesions harbor malignant potential. Recent studies have delineated the significant role of endoscopic ultrasound-guided interventions. Especially, endoscopic ultrasound (EUS) allows for the precise evaluation of cystic lesions, after which characterization can be done through fine-needle aspiration and cytological study. With this rapid and minimally invasive technique, therapeutic decisions can be made to guide proper interventions based on each patient's risk profile, preventing unnecessary surgical procedures. Endoscopic techniques also have a paradigm-changing effect on therapeutic management, particularly in neoplastic pancreatic cysts. Traditional surgical interventions carry important risks, with substantial morbidity for pancreatic resections. Techniques for EUS-guided chemoablation have evolved as a novel intervention balancing efficacy with an acceptable safety profile. Non-alcohol-based cocktails of chemoablation have recently been demonstrated to produce effective ablation of cystic lesions without the dangers of alcohol use, such as pancreatitis. The development and growth of such techniques suggest a bright future for EUS in the diagnosis and therapy of pancreatic disease, expanding gastroenterology's therapeutic domain. Further evidence in support of endoscopy in managing the gastrointestinal tract is provided by newly developing data on SCN. As studies reveal, most SCN patients are asymptomatic, resulting in a delay in proper intervention. Under such conditions, endoscopic surveillance has the potential to facilitate active monitoring of cyst growth and tracking of malignant transformation. Evidence of low rates of SCNs growth supports observational, conservative management in the majority of patients, with endoscopy still playing a crucial role for those who require definitive diagnosis or therapies. The management of SCN emphasizes the flexibility of endoscopic therapy, reflective of a broader trend in gastroenterology towards minimizing invasiveness and maximizing patient-oriented therapies with a focus on patient outcomes and safety.

15.2.2. Advancements in Imaging Techniques

The evolution of imaging techniques in gastroenterology has revolutionized the diagnosis and management scenario in gastrointestinal disease. Although problems persist with accuracy in diagnosing conditions due to superimposed symptoms and silent disease presentation of disorders, advances , such as high-resolution ultrasonography and magnetic resonance imaging (MRI) are proving to be priceless. These technologies not only improve the visualization of anatomical structures but also improve functional assessment, such that subtle pathophysiologic changes can be distinguished by clinicians. Improved imaging quality is capable of detecting liver diseases earlier, as a study demonstrates in improved imaging modalities improve understanding of chronic liver disease in children and result in more suitable therapeutic interventions (Della Corte et al., 2016). The use of these new modalities in standard diagnostic schemes is a clear indication of the trend towards precision medicine, eventually improving patient outcomes in gastroenterology. Aside from structural abnormality detection, the role of imaging also covers therapeutic response and disease progression evaluation. Functional imaging approaches, including nuclear medicine techniques and advanced MRI protocols, have opened new aspects in evaluating gastrointestinal motility and perfusion. This non-invasive ability to evaluate parameters of function is particularly significant in conditions with a dysmotility pattern, such as IBS. When dealing with the neuro-gastrointestinal axis, novel imaging modalities provide information regarding visceral message processing by the brain and also emphasize the complexity of gastroenterological disorders (Aziz et al., 2019). By employing such advanced imaging techniques, clinicians can better tailor treatment methods based on individual disease characteristics, and this is a step along the way to the ultimate goal of personalized patient management. Ultimately, the future of gastroenterology imaging will be shaped by technological progress and interdisciplinarity.

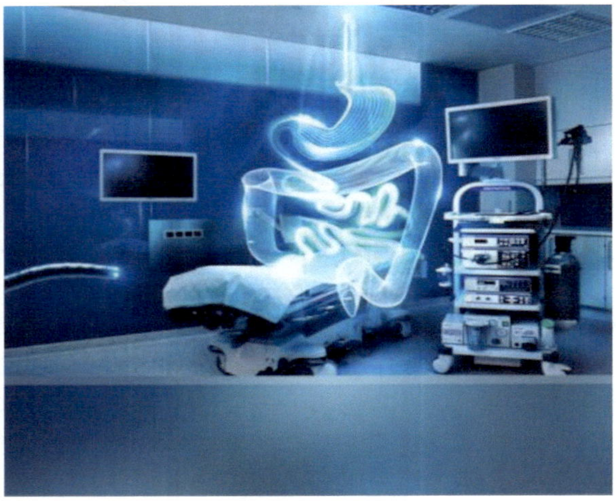

Figure 15.6. Advancements in imaging techniques of imaging techniques within gastroenterology

Source: https://bimedis.com/latest-news/showimg/574_02_olympus_nbi_1170-1180jpg.jpg/400.

Progress in multi-modal imaging techniques that combine different methodologies, e.g., merging endoscopy with advanced imaging modalities, is of huge promise to elucidate gastrointestinal pathology. In addition, the creation of standardized data acquisition protocols and sharing policies among research consortia will enable enhanced capacity in the form of processing large datasets to detect disease signatures and stratify patients by treatment response. This collaborative momentum will enable a better comprehension of the intricate crosstalk among the brain, gut, and microbiome, and deliver the base for paradigm-shifting findings in diagnostic sensitivity and therapeutic effectiveness. Fostering innovation in imaging serves not only clinical application but also directs future research priorities in gastroenterology and underscores the need for continuing investment in technology advancement (Figure 15.6).

15.2.3. Development of Minimally Invasive Surgical Procedures

The advancement in minimally invasive surgical methods has transformed the practice of gastroenterology, particularly the management of complex conditions , such as pancreatic cysts. With an ageing population and advanced imaging technologies becoming increasingly prevalent, the incidence of pancreatic cystic lesions has grown, necessitating effective management strategies. The traditional surgery, in terms of high morbidity, is being substituted with techniques , such as endoscopic ultrasound-guided chemoablation. This new approach holds potential for the management of neoplastic cysts with low risk of complications, as reported in recent studies highlighting the effectiveness of non-alcohol-based ablation techniques. These advances underscore a general trend toward less invasive alternatives with improved patient safety and prognosis and address the pressing requirement for effective handling of conditions that can evolve into pancreatic cancer, which has a notoriously bleak prognosis (Moyer et al., 2019). Robotic technology has appeared in the area of gastrointestinal surgery with significance, as it has the capability to enhance dexterity and precision during operations. Especially, the application of robotic-assisted total gastrectomy is a great example of development in that line. The Parisi Technique, applied at the reconstruction stage of surgery, has been showing promising results regarding minimal blood loss and reduced hospital stay. Results showing no conversions to open procedure and rapid return to firm diet confirm the safety and efficacy of these minimally invasive procedures.

These advances not only improve patient surgical results but also identify the worth of individually suited surgical methods for each patient's needs. These developments signal a shift in surgical ethos towards surgery with increased focus on patient recovery and overall care quality (Cirocchi et al., 2017). Evolution of minimally invasive techniques in gastroenterology is one aspect of a broader commitment to optimizing outcomes with minimal distress for the patient. As progress evolves, integration of advanced technologies, such as laparoscopic and robotic systems, propels this shift in paradigm. Surgeons are adopting these techniques to perform intricate procedures otherwise necessitating extensive cuts, thereby providing quick recovery times and minimum postoperative pain. Future trends predict that further research and development will allow even greater precision in surgical intervention, which will allow for intricate procedures suited for the management of complex gut problems without compromising the benefits of minimally invasive surgeries. With the ever-increasing developments in the specialty, the continued advancement of such surgical techniques will be of profound importance to future gastroenterological practice, ensuring better patient care and long-term success.

15.3. Pharmacological Advances

Recent pharmacotherapy innovations have significantly impacted the management of most gastrointestinal illnesses, representing a paradigm shift towards individualized therapy. The development of biologic drugs, particularly monoclonal antibodies, has revolutionized the treatment model of conditions , such as IBD and IBS. These medications are engineered to work through specific mechanisms of inflammation, therefore evading the typical systemic adverse effects of traditional treatments. Besides, the emergence of small molecules as oral medications presents an opportunity for increased compliance and lifestyle adaptation on the part of the patient, rescuing the practical problems related to most of these patients' chronic gastrointestinal disorders. Ongoing research continues on enhancing these medicines with optimum efficacy and safety profiles, indicative of the pivotal contribution that pharmacological advances have in enhancing the quality of life for the patients afflicted by such incapacitating disorders. Other than the aforementioned biologic agents, advances in the field of pharmacogenomics have also transformed gastroenterology. By uncovering the genetic determinants that cause drug metabolism and response, clinicians now can tailor treatment according to their patients' genetic makeup. This focused approach is aimed at minimizing side effects and maximizing drug effectiveness, maximally treating conditions , such as gastroesophageal reflux disease (GERD) and peptic ulcer disease. New evidence indicates that specific genetic markers can predict a patient's reaction to proton pump inhibitors or H2 receptor blockers, transforming the practice of drug prescribing. With increasing pharmacogenomic research, its use in practice will enhance therapeutic effectiveness and eventually be a more precise and personalized approach to gastrointestinal therapy. In addition, new discoveries of therapy agents are continually developing gastroenterological pharmacotherapy. Active clinical trials are eagerly investigating the therapeutic value of drugs targeting the gut microbiome as a treatment for various ailments, including metabolic syndrome and obesity. Such drugs are a novel approach, recognizing the intricate tie-in between gut health and overall metabolic well-being. As demonstrated by recent research on fecal microbiota transplantation, the promise of microbiome-targeting therapies will revolutionize gastrointestinal therapeutics. Moreover, with advancing clinical guidelines, such as management guidelines on transjugular intrahepatic portosystemic stent-shunt (TIPSS) (Tripathi et al., 2020), will ensure that the progress in pharmacology aligns with holistic approaches to patient care, as per an innovative trajectory for gastroenterology in the future (Figure 15.7).

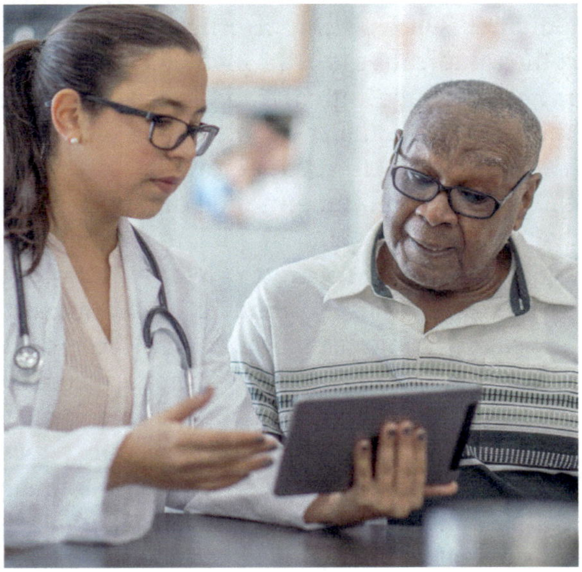

Figure 15.7. Pharmacological advances and developments in therapies.

Source: https://www.gerascentre.ca/wp-content/uploads/2022/09/Untitled-design-6.png.

15.3.1. New Medications for Inflammatory Bowel Disease

With the evolving gastroenterology, novel treatment approaches for inflammatory bowel disease (IBD) are emerging with extremely promising implications on patient management and care. Ongoing research has focused on biologic therapies targeting specific elements of the immune system, such as tumor necrosis factor-alpha (TNF-α) inhibitors, that have revolutionized treatment in Crohn's disease and ulcerative colitis. These medications have worked to induce and maintain remission in most patients and reduce their symptoms and improve their quality of life. The complexities of IBD, however, necessitate continuous development, and research into novel biological drugs that are more tailored to treatment options follows. Through the elucidation of IBD pathogenesis at the molecular level, such progress holds the potential to streamline the current therapy protocol, eventually resulting in better patient outcomes for those dealing with these chronic diseases. Additionally, there has been interest in the potential role that micronutrients, specifically biotin, can play in treating IBD in recent research. Research indicates that biotin deficiency could worsen colitis symptoms and negatively affect the gastrointestinal system. New preclinical models have shown that high-dose biotin supplementation not only delays the onset of colitis but also decreases its severity and duration. Specifically, studies indicate that biotin administration can maintain remission by reducing the expression of inflammatory cytokines and preserving the integrity of the intestinal barrier, primarily by blocking the nuclear factor kappa-light-chain-enhancer of activated B cells (NF-κB) pathway. This direction of research in nutritional therapy is a crucial step towards integrative IBD management, with drug therapy complemented by dietary therapy, culminating in holistic treatment protocols. As the pathogenesis of IBD is better understood, the prospects for drug development are excellent, with attention turning to patient-oriented, individualized drugs. The function of growing pharmacogenomics is likely to be determinant, as genetic testing will allow drug responses in patients to be predicted. Through the association of genetic markers with medication efficacy, doctors will be able to optimize therapy while limiting the risk of adverse side effects. Furthermore, ongoing clinical trials are needed to establish the effectiveness of new treatments and define their long-term safety profiles. Considered in this light, the future of IBD treatment is poised to be revolutionized toward improved patient outcomes and potentially a more holistic approach to therapeutic intervention in gastroenterology.

15.3.2. Innovations in Liver Disease Management

One of the primary drivers of the advancement of gastroenterology is the integration of emerging technologies and techniques to better manage liver disease. The introduction of non-invasive diagnostic technology in the form of elastography and imaging technologies has revolutionized the monitoring of the development of liver fibrosis and cirrhosis. These technologies reduce the occurrence of invasive biopsies on the liver, enabling clinicians to assess patients with greater safety and comfort. Also, biomarker identification and genetic profiling are now core components of individualized treatment for liver diseases, offering a more personalized approach that enhances therapeutic response and minimizes side effects. New therapies, such as direct-acting antivirals for the treatment of hepatitis C, demonstrate the trend towards efficacious and targeted management strategies with an emphasis on patient-focused care while addressing the complex conditions effectively. Moreover, research on regenerative medicine has great promise for the future of the treatment of liver disease, particularly for liver transplantation and recovery. Stem cell therapy is being evaluated as an extremely good candidate for the regeneration of damaged liver tissue and the recovery of function in patients with extremely severe liver disease. The use of induced pluripotent stem cells (iPSCs) is a breakthrough approach, as the cells possess infinite replication capacity and can develop into working hepatocytes. Advances in bioprinting technology also seek to create liver tissue constructs that will serve as substitutes for damaged areas or temporary support for failing livers and, ultimately, enhance transplant success. These advances not only add to the therapeutic armamentarium but also provide the basis for less dependency on donor organs in the immediate future, with an extremely grim shortage of transplants being addressed. In the field of pharmacologic innovation, the use of newer drugs for the treatment of liver disease has been progressing very actively.

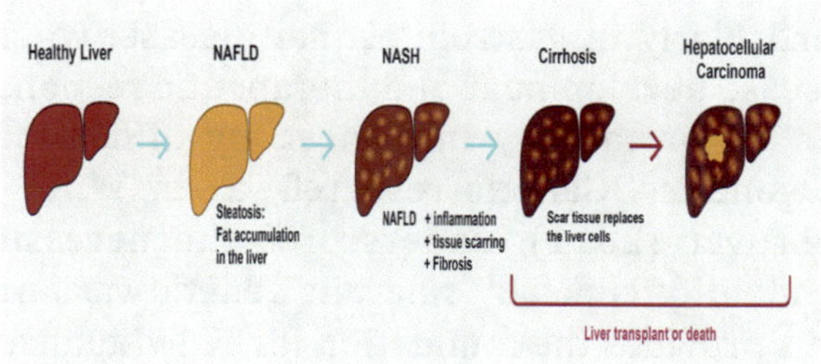

Figure 15.8. Innovations in liver disease management.

Source: https://cn-bio.com/wp-content/uploads/2019/05/CN-Bio-NASH-Schematic-2019-web-1080x350.png.

For example, a growing understanding of the pathophysiology of non-alcoholic fatty liver disease (NAFLD) has led to the development of varied molecules targeting root mechanisms , such as inflammation and fibrosis. The novel drugs are intended to offer improved treatment options for patients who previously had little available to them. In addition, current clinical trials are assessing the long-term safety and effectiveness of these novel drugs, which would revolutionize the treatment of chronic liver diseases , such as cirrhosis and hepatitis. Implementation of these innovations, along with evidence-based therapies as outlined in the recent guidelines (Fujita et al., 2023), enhances the role of gastroenterologists in directing treatment and optimizing patient outcomes in an increasingly complex therapy setting (Figure 15.8).

15.3.3. Role of Personalized Medicine in Gastroenterology

The evolving context of individualized medicine in gastroenterology is characterized by the shift towards precision diagnosis that encompasses both microbial and genetic dimensions. As medicine evolves away from the "one size fits all" mode, the need to integrate full-genome genetic profiling into practice grows and grows. This is a key component of treatment planning, particularly in gastrointestinal disease, where disease development and therapeutic response can be profoundly influenced by differences in genetics. Genetic research, as in Wiita & Schrijver (2011), underscores the necessity to identify clinically relevant genetic variants. This provides the foundation for individualized therapy that optimizes patient outcome, optimizing drug efficacy while minimizing side effects. The consequences for clinical practice routine assessment are evident, suggesting the need for widespread application of high-throughput analysis technologies that allow gastroenterologists to make evidence-based choices in clinical practice. With genetic findings to rely on, the role of the gut microbiota adds additional dimensions to individualized medicine in gastroenterology. The intricate dynamics between gut microbiota and gastrointestinal well-being have garnered significant attention, particularly in reference to long-term illnesses like nonalcoholic fatty liver disease (NAFLD). The possibility of microbiome modulation with diet or therapeutic interventions holds revolutionary potential for individualized treatment protocols. As Sharpton et al. (2019) state, next-generation sequencing technologies have enabled the unravelling of the complex intricacies and functional gene content of gut microbiota. These developments not only enhance our understanding of the microbial determinants of disease but also open up new ways for the creation of personalized treatment protocols. By designing therapies in accordance with the specific microbiome patterns in patients, gastroenterologists can potentially correct dysbiosis and improve the effectiveness of therapy for a large spectrum of gastrointestinal diseases. Beyond the direct clinical intervention, the extension of personalized medicine to gastroenterology includes long-term patient management and prevention as well. The addition of pharmacogenomic testing allows for the identification of those patients who are likely to benefit by particular therapies based on the genetic variation of the patient and thus enables individualized therapy in relation to their response. This not only maximizes the therapeutic outcome but also minimizes the risk burden resulting from conventional methods of treatment. The concerns put forth in Wiita & Schrijver (2011), including the rapid speed of our ability to detect genetic variants versus our ability to interpret them clinically, necessitate ongoing education and protocol development among the medical community. In the future use of personalized medicine in gastroenterology, patient care will be more proactive and information-driven and ultimately be in favor of patients suffering from gastrointestinal illnesses by improving the quality of their lives.

15.4. Microbiome Research

The comprehension of the structure and function of the human microbiome has emerged as the core of interest in gastroenterology. The microbiome, composed of trillions of microbes residing in the gut, plays a crucial role in maintaining gastrointestinal health and regulating systemic physiological function. Recent advances in microbial genomics and metagenomics have enabled the portrayal of intricate dynamics between host physiology and gut microbiota. This knowledge is especially relevant in the context of the rising prevalence of diseases , such as non-alcoholic fatty liver disease (NAFLD) and inflammatory bowel disease (IBD). Knowing the microbiome's function in controlling inflammation and metabolism enlightens us about possible therapeutic avenues. The challenge is to translate this information into the clinic, bridging the gap between microbiome research and personalized therapeutic strategies (Heyens et al., 2021). Moreover, the shift of microbiome science to precision medicine holds the promise to transform gastroenterological practice. The shift to a patient-centric approach necessitates an integrated appreciation for genetic, environmental, and microbial determinants of health consequences. According to literature, the identification of characterized microbial signatures has begun to be used in the diagnosis and treatment of various gastrointestinal disorders, including dysbiosis and associated complications. Techniques , such as state-of-the-art metabolic profiling and deep clinical phenotyping allow the construction of causal associations between the microbiota community and the disease pathology. The evolving precision medicine environment accentuates the requirement to harness novel data and technologies to inform clinical decision-making and maximize the effectiveness of treatment (Seyhan & Carini, 2019). To realize the full potential of microbiome research, current challenges must be addressed, most importantly in interpreting data and applying it in the clinic. The enormous amount of genomic and metabolomic data requires sophisticated computational approaches like artificial intelligence and machine learning to summarize conclusions and enhance diagnostic insight. Besides, as the field develops further, the necessity for robust standardized procedures for microbiome sampling and analysis arises so that it can be translated across studies. Ethical concerns of microbiome-based treatments are also worthy of examination because personalized treatments can have variable health impacts in diverse populations. Lastly, the incorporation of microbiome science into gastroenterology will revolutionize disease therapy and enable precision medicine that is a match for each patient's specific needs (Seyhan & Carini, 2019; Heyens et al., 2021).

15.4.1. Understanding the Gut Microbiome

Recent gastroenterology research continues to emphasize the complicated interplay between the gut microbiome and various metabolic processes of the human body. These complicated microbial communities, positioned within the digestive tract, produce a wide array of metabolites that have the capacity to significantly influence host physiology. A good example of such a metabolite is bile acid and short-chain fatty acid, which have been identified to shape everything from metabolic health to aging. Exploring the pathways through which gut-derived metabolites interact with host tissues presents an exciting avenue for progressing therapeutic strategies. It has been indicated in recent studies that by manipulating the gut microbiota, medical professionals would be able to successfully prevent disease or promote improved health outcomes and thereby usher in a future where microbial treatments are the bedrock of gastrointestinal treatment approaches. This revised perception of the gut microbiome suggests a shift towards understanding how it has a role not just as a digestive aid, but as an active player in larger health dynamics (Fogelson et al., 2023). The gut microbiome also has critical relevance to treating chronic illnesses , such as non-alcoholic fatty liver disease (NAFLD). A predicted global rise in the prevalence of NAFLD underscores the need for effective diagnostic and treatment methods, such as the disease progresses undetected from steatosis to severe types like non-alcoholic steatohepatitis (NASH). The connection between gut microbiota composition and liver health has triggered investigations into how microbial balance impacts liver inflammation and fibrosis. The current diagnostic methods lag behind, remaining largely based on invasive biopsies that do not account for the asymptomatic course of disease progression. Non-invasive diagnostic methods are increasingly popular, integrating metabolic profiling of gut-derived metabolites in the identification and monitoring of the stages of NAFLD effectively. Further elucidation of such correlations between gut microbiota and liver pathology has the potential to transform clinical practices in gastroenterology in the future (Heyens et al., 2021).

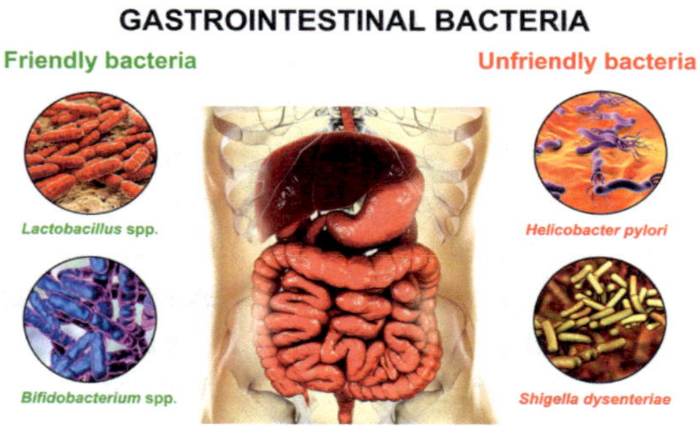

Figure 15.9. Understanding the gut microbiome research in gastroenterology.

Source: https://sanctuaryfunctionalmedicine.com/wp-content/uploads/2020/08/04_S04A_microbiomeGI_shutterstock_1027579135-2048x1300.jpg.

Last but not least, the gut microbiome's function is not restricted to metabolic disorders but reaches across other aspects of health, opening up its potential to play a significant role in disease states previously not considered associated with gastrointestinal status. Evidence suggests the gut microbiome can influence neurological conditions, therefore refuting what was previously assumed regarding the gut-brain axis. Advances in this field are not only illuminating how these microbiota influence mental function but also offer paths through which alterations in gut health could influence mental health. As scientists continue to dissect the gut microbiome's complexity, integration of microbiome analysis into broader diagnostics may unlock new preventative strategies or treatments for a range of illnesses. In this possibility, gastroenterology stands at the threshold of a revolution that could reshape paradigms for disease and health therapy (Fogelson et al., 2023) (Figure 15.9).

15.4.2. Impact of Microbiome on Gastrointestinal Health

The interaction of the gut microbiome with human health is a new entity that has attracted lots of attention in gastroenterology. New advancements in genomic and metabolomic technologies have recently shown the complex nature of microbial communities in the gastrointestinal tract. The intestinal microbiome plays a crucial role in digestion and nutrient absorption and also influences immune processes. Microbiota imbalances or dysbiosis have been implicated in many gastrointestinal diseases, including inflammatory bowel disease (IBD) and irritable bowel syndrome (IBS). More understanding of the mechanisms through which alterations in the microbiome modulate intestinal health is required for the development of targeted therapies that might restore the equilibrium of microbiota and alleviate symptoms of these chronic conditions. Thus, studies into microbial communities and their functional gene content remain the key focus of developing gastroenterology as a science. Current research to determine how microbes influence host physiology is unlocking new therapeutic avenues. The introduction of probiotics, prebiotics, and fecal microbiota transplantation (FMT) demonstrates potential means to restore microbial homeostasis. Live and beneficial probiotics are live, beneficial bacteria that have been promising in modulating the gut flora and in alleviating symptoms of gastrointestinal diseases. Additionally, dietary treatment research, aimed at enriching or enriching the gut microbiome, is ongoing. Such strategies can boost the production of bioactive metabolites that are required for gut health. By boosting a healthy balance of microbiome, these treatments may enhance orthodox medical treatments, bridging a more holistic management of gastrointestinal health. Consequently, the present studies and clinical trials hold promise for meaningful evidence regarding microbial therapy potential in treating gastrointestinal disease.

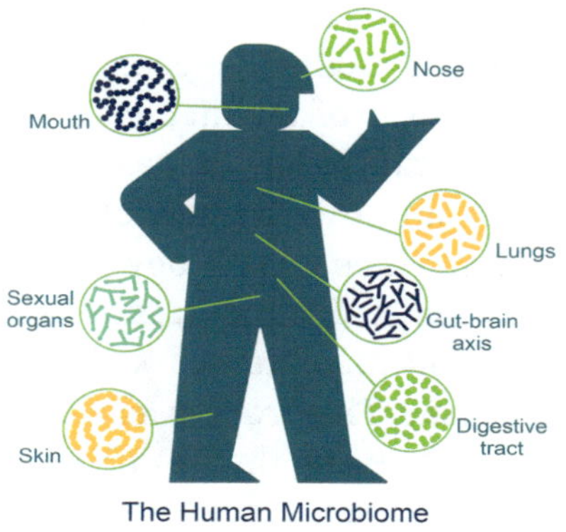

Figure 15.10. Impact of microbiome on gastrointestinal health.

Source: https://khni.kerry.com/wp-content/uploads/2022/10/Human-microbiome-1.png.

The relationship between microbiome diversity and the development of chronic gastrointestinal diseases has also been indicated in studies directed toward single diseases. For instance, NAFLD has been shown to be linked to dysbiosis, suggestive of the microbiome's potential role in its pathogenesis. It has been shown that the gut microbiome harbors a rich repertoire of functional genes many times larger than that of the human genome, which can be used to support intricate metabolic functions with health implications. Microbial metabolism production of bioactive compounds, may influence local and systemic inflammation, thereby leading to disease development under imbalances. Techniques involving large-scale data collection, such as citizen-science initiatives like the American Gut Project, can significantly advance our understanding of such relationships. By the convergence of various methodologies, researchers are able to explain how microbiome dynamics affect gastrointestinal health and establish new avenues for prevention and treatment of concurrent diseases to further enhance prospective future progress in gastroenterology (McDonald et al., 2015; Sharpton et al., 2019) (Figure 15.10).

15.4.3. Future Therapies Targeting the Microbiome

Recent advances in microbiome research have uncovered its vast influence on many medical disorders, notably in gastroenterology. The connection emphasizes the potential of curative therapy that adjusts the makeup of the microbiota to enhance patient outcomes. Attention has further been concentrated on employing new approaches , such as probiotics, prebiotics, and fecal microbiota transplantation (FMT), to modify dysbiotic gut microbiomes. Through sensitive modulation, these treatments can restore a normal microbiota, enhancing digestive health and alleviating the effects of gastrointestinal diseases , such as irritable bowel syndrome and inflammatory bowel disease. Moreover, as diagnostic modalities evolve, clinicians will increasingly be able to provide personalized microbiome-directed therapy, addressing specific microbial signatures present in each patient, thereby transforming treatment approaches to gastroenterology. The field of oncology, including as it relates to prostate cancer, has also witnessed growing interest in the establishment of microbiome-targeting therapy. There is an indication that specific communities of microbes may have a profound impact on tumor formation and treatment response, and therefore inform therapeutic decision-making. For instance, studies demonstrate that particular genera within cancerous tissues are correlated with enhanced inflammation and immune modification that can predispose to oncogenesis within the prostate microenvironment (Pei et al., 2025). Deciphering such microbiome-cancer interactions can lead to novel interventions that purposefully modulate microbial communities, possibly improving resistance to conventional therapies , such as androgen deprivation therapy. With ever more insight into the nuanced interaction between microbiome and cancer biology, therapies may emerge in the future that leverage these connections to provide integrative, individualized treatment protocols for patients with cancer. As microbiome and gut health studies progress, the incorporation of artificial intelligence (AI) into therapies targeting the microbiome is an area for personalized gastroenterology medicine. AI systems can review massive datasets from microbiome profiling to better understand microbial interactions and their effects on human health. By classifying microbial properties and predicting the response of the patient to the treatments, third-generation microbiome interventions that are better and also tailored to the patient's individual physiological needs can be developed (Manrique et al., 2024). The significance of leveraging technology innovation along with microbiome science is a paradigm shift in control of chronic disease, ultimately leading to new therapeutic approaches that maximize quality of life for patients with gastrointestinal disorders.

15.5. Telemedicine in Gastroenterology

The expansion of telemedicine has revolutionized several aspects of health care provision, enabling new methods of patient encounter and treatment. Telemedicine in gastroenterology as a specialty enables efficient communication between patients and providers, particularly in instances requiring diligent follow-up, such as inflammatory bowel diseases and liver illnesses. Telemedicine, in addition to enhancing access for rural or remote-area patients, addresses continuity-of-care issues. The ability to transmit electronic medical data across distance, as the HCAB (2003) conceptualizes it, allows clinicians to deliver quality care without geographical boundaries. These characteristics feature telemedicine's ability to revolutionize the field, facilitating timely intervention and patient participation and with the potential to adapt to various clinical situations and patient preferences, leading to improved health outcomes. In particular, teleconsultation, one of the key features of telemedicine, has caught on because it can facilitate real-time, remote interaction among gastroenterologists and patients. Using video technology, physicians can assess symptoms, discuss treatment options, and monitor chronic illnesses without the need for in-office visits. The process has been found to work, especially during the COVID-19 pandemic, when in-person consultations were troublesome due to safety measures and social distancing policies. Research indicates that teleconsultation allows for the progressive development of health professionals' roles to a considerable degree, significantly enhancing their therapeutic interaction and clinical assessment capabilities in spite of physical distance. Outcomes of studies on registered nurses' experience of teleconsultation exhibit a complex interaction of operational and clinical factors affecting the efficacy of remote interactions, necessitating the use of some strategies to increase the impact of telemedicine for gastroenterology (Barrett, 2017). The application of telemedicine goes beyond direct patient contact to influence overall gastroenterology care delivery in hospitals and healthcare systems. Telemedicine has the potential to alleviate pressure on healthcare facilities with large patient volumes and long waiting periods for in-person visits. In addition, the modality allows patients to engage in self-care and patient empowerment through greater active participation in monitoring health and managing symptoms. With telemedicine increasingly being adopted by gastroenterologists, there is the possibility to include digital platforms that allow for remote monitoring of patients via wearable devices and mobile health applications. These technologies signal the dawn of an era of personalized treatment, whose modalities are tailored to individual needs and greater patient participation. Therefore, the ongoing use of technology in gastroenterology reflects a very fundamental shift towards more efficient, accessible, and patient-centered healthcare delivery (Oliai, 2005) (Figure 15.11).

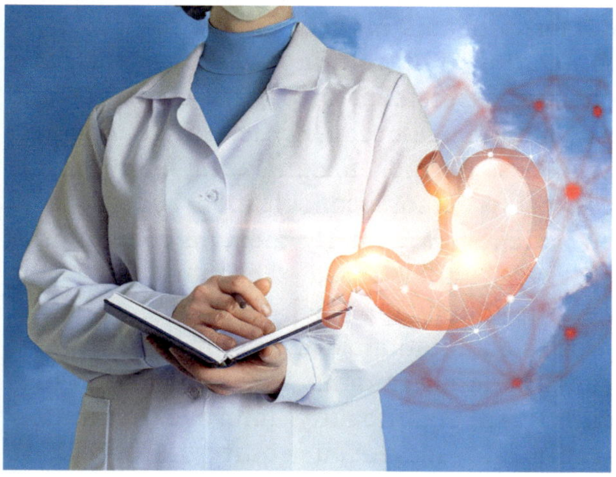

Figure 15.11. Telemedicine in gastroenterology.

Source: https://borderlessaccess.com/blog/wp-content/uploads/2024/08/telemedicine-in-gastroenterology-care.webp.

15.5.1. Rise of Telehealth Services

The integration of telemedicine services into the health sector is a considerable advancement, particularly in gastroenterology. While medical practitioners grapple with problems associated with infectious diseases, such as the recent COVID-19 pandemic, telemedicine has emerged as a vital substitute for personal consultations. Telemedicine services allow patients to receive medical counsel, triage, and follow-up without physical contact, thereby decreasing the risk of the spread of viruses. With technological advances in communication and rising acceptability among clinicians and patients alike, telehealth has proven to be a key tool to control gastrointestinal diseases that often require constant monitoring. This shift not only represents adaptability within the health infrastructure but also provides the possibility for better patient engagement and continuity of care in emergencies that limit access to traditional healthcare. In addition, telehealth benefits extend beyond convenience; they offer access to specialist gastroenterological services to the underprivileged communities. Many gastroenterology patients reside in distant or rural areas where specialty health care may be in short supply. Telehealth services bridge the gap by connecting such patients with competent gastroenterologists, paving the way for timely interventions and better health results later on. As highlighted by recent studies, telehealth can reduce travel burdens, reduce waiting times, and optimize the use of existing resources in busy clinical environments. Integration of remote care into traditional care models can effectively enhance patient satisfaction and adherence to treatment, particularly in long-term diseases that necessitate regular follow-ups. This change represents a proactive approach to the provision of health care, highlighting the significance of telehealth services in enhancing accessibility and efficiency in patients' care. Notably, while telehealth has numerous advantages, it also raises important discussions regarding its usage in gastroenterology. Evidently, as noted, the adoption of telehealth is partly hampered by data privacy concerns, patients' level of digital literacy, and the quality of remote consultations in general. Despite breakthroughs , such as robotic gastroscopes and artificial intelligence diagnostics (Marlicz et al., 2020), there remain constraints in terms of bodily examination of patients and the ability to perform certain procedures remotely. Gastroenterology, therefore, will need to reconcile telehealth with in-person care to offer comprehensive treatment without the risks associated with poor or inapt teleconsultations. The experience gained during the pandemic has highlighted both the promise and pitfalls of telehealth, and it paved the way to an era when hybrid models of care will be the norm. To plan ahead, continued investment in technology and education will be needed in order to fill these gaps and maximize the advantages of telehealth in the specialty.

15.5.2. Benefits and Challenges of Remote Consultations

Evolutionary technologies keep transforming the landscape of gastroenterology, with a majority of the effects being felt in the region of patient consultations. Telemedicine has created a state-of-the-art platform to enhance patient care through increased accessibility and convenience for patients who may face geographical or physical barriers. For rural or remote patients, the ability to access healthcare providers through telehealth can become a determining factor in eliminating the burdens of travel as well as its accompanying cost. Moreover, synchronous video consultations in real time provide an immediate method of communication, with patients and clinicians both able to communicate in real time with each other. Such an interactive process not only provides a sense of connection but also allows for concerns to be communicated more accurately, possibly resulting in faster diagnoses and individually suitable treatment pathways (Bywood et al., 2013). The incorporation of remote consultations represents a significant move towards universal delivery of gastroenterology care. But with these benefits, several hindrances lie in the practice of remote consultations. Among them is the likelihood of technological disadvantages that can exclude certain patient groups, particularly elderly individuals who may not be well-acquainted with computer platforms. Apart from this, the quality of care rendered through remote access is at times unreliable, contingent upon the efficiency of the technology used and the physician's and patient's level of acquaintance with telehealth facilities. In the absence of personal interactions, certain subtleties of patient-provider communication may get lost, so that it is challenging to observe the entire range of symptoms and issues a patient may exhibit under normal circumstances. Therefore, although remote consultations offer exciting options for the delivery of medical services, the necessity for strong training and infrastructure support to facilitate effective communication and service delivery cannot be overemphasized (Oliai, 2005). In the future, remote gastroenterology consultations will be contingent on solutions to the merits and demerits of this model. While clinicians keep innovating and refining telemedicine care, ongoing assessment of patient outcomes and satisfaction will become crucial in guiding best practices. Further, making technology usable can make remote consultation accessible to all patients, particularly those in communities that are underserved. Through embracing an integrated approach that acknowledges probable limitations while tapping into remote consultation strengths, the gastroenterology clinic can significantly improve, ultimately leading to increased equity in access to healthcare and improved patient outcomes. As remote technology becomes more popularly utilized, acknowledging its impact on clinical effectiveness will be essential to the future of patient care in gastroenterology.

15.5.3. Future Implications for Patient Care

The gastroenterology scene is poised to see revolutionary changes that will undoubtedly affect patient care in the coming years. Technologies , such as artificial intelligence and machine learning are revolutionizing diagnostic tests, which enable more precise evaluations of gastrointestinal disease. While algorithms sort through vast amounts of clinical data, they can pick up patterns that might otherwise escape human providers. This move towards technologically aided diagnostics enables gastroenterologists to customize interventions better, so that interventions specifically match the conditions of individual patients. Additionally, the use of telemedicine allows the reach of specialist care, especially for those in remote regions, and can help close healthcare disparities. These emerging trends signal a future not only where patient care is more efficient but also more equitable, addressing the needs of individuals and healthcare disparities identified by Bergman et al. (2018). Yet another important consideration molding the future of patient care in gastroenterology is increasing attention to preventive medicine and lifestyle modification. The recognition of lifestyle determinants as central drivers of gastrointestinal health is revolutionizing how providers approach treatment. Practitioners are increasingly having diet, exercise, and other non-pharmacologic interventions as core components of treatment plans. With growing awareness in the public eye, the patient is becoming an engaged actor in healthcare, seeking information about the role of lifestyle in gastrointestinal health. This paradigm will necessitate a rethinking of traditional clinical training, such that the future generation of gastroenterologists will have learned how to campaign for holistic changes in their patients' lifestyle. Such programmes will eventually not only improve individual outcomes for health but could potentially decrease the system burden overall, as evidenced by trends in trends of service use indicating an orientation towards preventative care (Bergman et al. 2018). In the future, the addition of personalized medicine is a paradigm that will redefine patient care in gastroenterology. As genomic research increasingly untangles the complexity of gastrointestinal diseases, targeted therapeutic strategies are now becoming feasible. The ability to stratify patients based on genetic markers can foretell a new era in which treatments are not just customized by symptomatic presentation but by personal genetic profiles, thus optimizing efficacy and minimizing side effects. Further, such advances can guide the development of targeted treatments for specific subtypes of disease, which is particularly valuable in conditions like inflammatory bowel disease and colorectal cancer. This trend towards more personalized style is a function of a new paradigm in patient care that not only entails the treatment of illness but also holistic regard for the distinctive contexts of individual patients, potentially replotting the chart of gastroenterological practice for many years to come (Figure 15.12).

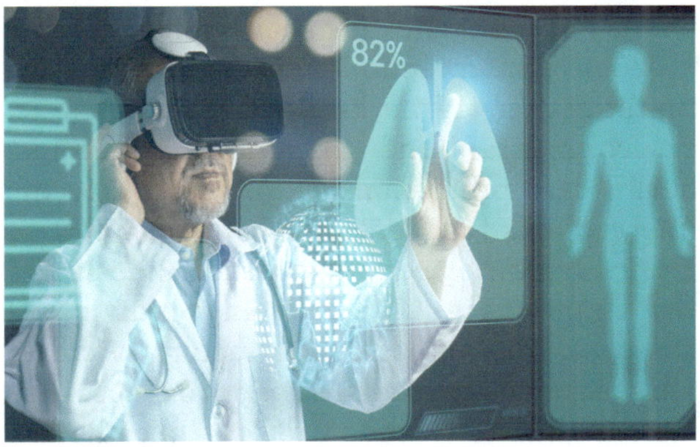

Figure 15.12. Future implications for patient care.

Source: https://cloudwars.com/wp-content/uploads/2022/02/Metaverse-Healthcare.jpg.

15.6. Preventive Strategies

Preventive interventions in gastroenterology have taken center stage as clinicians seek to abate the increasing burdens of many gastrointestinal disorders. Diverticular disease, acute diverticulitis (AD), has taken significant attention in recent years, with a significant economic burden, particularly with the increasing population aging. Evidence indicates that the population is experiencing increasing hospitalization due to AD, especially in the young and in women. Focus on preventative measures is thus essential with the advancement in understanding the pathophysiology of the conditions. In spite of attempts at defining risk factors and preventive interventions, there has been limited success with current interventions, including the administration of rifaximin or probiotics for primary and secondary prevention (Severiet al., 2018). This suggests an urgent necessity for more research and targeted interventions to be applied effectively towards preventing the occurrence and recurrence of AD in different patient populations. The multimodal etiology of acute diverticulitis points out the challenge of developing effective preventive interventions worthy of extensive investigation. With knowledge of genetic, environmental, and lifestyle interactions, health care professionals can design specific interventions that consider the unique patient factors. A growing body of evidence underscores the importance of stratifying individuals based on some predisposing factors to create personalized therapeutic approaches. For instance, lifestyle modification, like dietary modification and the intake of more fiber, might take precedence in order to decrease the risk of AD events. Moreover, the paradigm shift towards outpatient management of uncomplicated cases has alleviated the costs of healthcare, thus providing a potential avenue for preventive care interventions (Severiet al., 2018). Overall, a closer examination of the determinants of medical intervention can lead to new paradigms for prevention in gastroenterology. Preventive interventions extend beyond the setting of diverticulitis to the general setting of gastrointestinal well-being. The Department of Veterans Affairs (VA) is one model for an active approach focused on the health of returning veterans from recent wars. Investigators are exploring various means of enhancing the delivery and integration of health care for this population and ultimately reintroduction to normal living. Such initiatives rely not only on dealing with situations as they arise but even promoting wellness through preventive systems of health care. In gastroenterology, the use of the same paradigms could lead to advances in preventive medicine, for instance, screening and disease prevention programs against conditions like colorectal cancer. As more research continues to be conducted in these directions, the future trends in gastroenterology could have promising prospects of providing more new avenues towards enhancing patient outcomes through efficient preventive intervention.

15.6.1. Importance of Screening and Early Detection

The gastroenterologic scenario has radically altered, particularly with respect to screening and early diagnosis, which are vital in improving patient outcomes. Early diagnosis of gastrointestinal diseases, for instance, gastric cancer, is a prime influence on raising the effectiveness of treatment and survival. The malignant nature of such diseases as gastric cancer has the propensity to come up with later-stage diagnoses, thus the lack of therapeutic options and unfavourable prognoses. Here, novel screening technologies, such as the identification of molecular biomarkers , such as miR-21 and miR-106, open up encouraging avenues for non-invasive diagnostic assays that can alter the course from traditional invasive methods to more efficient, patient-friendly strategies. These new detection technologies enable clinicians to potentially improve prognosis in high-risk populations and reduce late-stage diagnosis-related morbidity (Altamemi et al., 2020). Moreover, the inclusion of immunodiagnostic innovation has increased the sensitivity and effectiveness of screening processes in gastroenterology. New immunoassay formats enable the detection of many gastrointestinal illnesses in an expanding array of biological samples, extending beyond typical serum analysis to early diagnosis. It is particularly significant, particularly for gastrointestinal cancers that do so clandestinely, often evading clinical recognition until late in their course. With the ever-changing immunodiagnostic industry, it is crucial that gastroenterologists keep abreast of these developments so that they can incorporate them competently in practice. Facilitating greater access to these new screening equipment will also contribute towards early diagnosis and enhance the process of patient care as a whole in gastroenterology (Velikova, 2018).

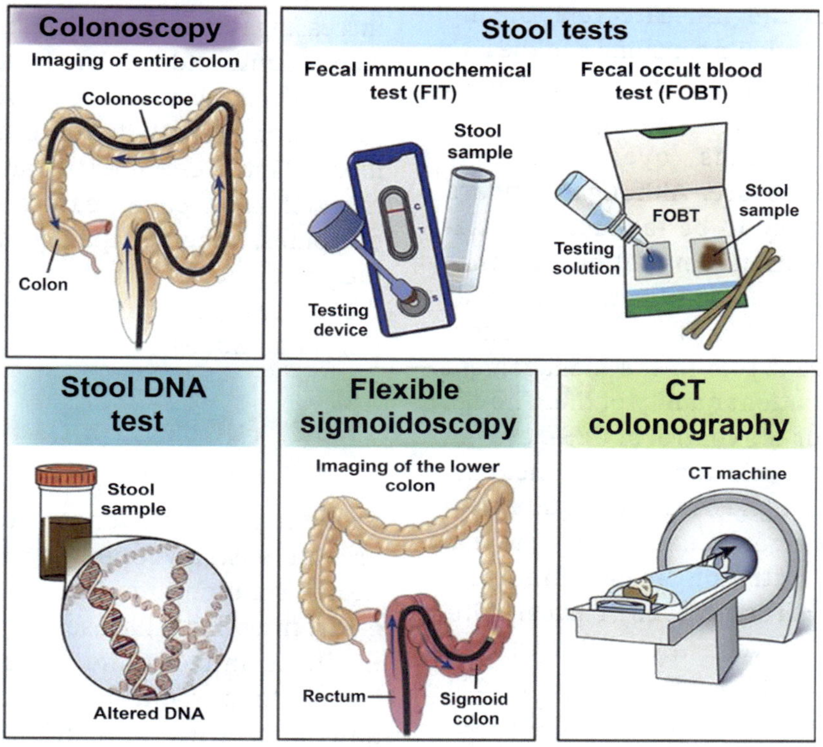

Figure 15.13. Importance of screening and early detection landscape of gastroenterology.

Source: https://els-jbs-prod-cdn.jbs.elsevierhealth.com/cms/attachment/a5a960eb-5bb7-44ab-906c-99043ae300dc/gr1_lrg.jpg.

The impact of successful screening regimens extends beyond results for individual patients; it also has implications for public health at the population level. High early detection rates can generate lower healthcare costs in the long term by minimizing the need for complex, invasive therapy that is too often connected with late disease stages. Furthermore, the implementation of organized screening programs could enable intervention at an earlier stage within high-risk groups with a resulting decrease in disease prevalence. These preventive strategies are particularly valuable in gastroenterology, where disparities in access to medical care often hinder timely diagnosis and treatment. Through the promotion of a culture of prevention and early detection, the future of gastroenterology is promising, with much room for improvement in health outcomes on both an individual and population level (Altamemi et al., 2020) (Figure 15.13).

15.6.2. Role of Diet and Lifestyle Modifications

The contribution of food choices and lifestyle modifications towards the management of gastrointestinal disease cannot be overestimated, particularly as the medical community continues to explore alternative treatment strategies. Recent evidence suggests the intricate relationship between the foods patients consume and the risk of developing conditions like gastroesophageal reflux disease (GERD), characterized by troublesome symptoms overwhelmingly blamed on acid exposure. Although standard therapy is more likely to be founded on acid-suppressive medications, mounting evidence suggests that lifestyle modification, such as reduced sugar and more fiber consumption, can play a significant role in the management of symptoms and patient quality of life. Though dietary practices for the control of GERD are not completely explained, clarification of functional food components emphasizes the requirement for stronger explicit guidelines and educational programming in nutrition as an important avenue to control (Herdiana, 2023). Furthermore, the relationship between diet, lifestyle, and gut microbiota has increased in significance, particularly for gastroenterological well-being. A healthy gut microbiome is important for the effectiveness of digestion and regulation of metabolic functions, further reinforcing the significance of gut health in preventing many diseases, including cardiometabolic disease. Diet composition and early nutrition may have significant impacts on gut microbiota, with the suggestion that interventions initiated early in life may be beneficial in the long term. Current knowledge in microbiome science reveals that diet and lifestyle modifications can affect microbial diversity, which in turn affects host metabolic activities. Thus, these dynamics need to be known to construct strategic dietary recommendations that could mitigate the risk of diseases linked to gut dysbiosis (Gabriel & Ferguson, 2023). In conclusion, although gastroenterology progress puts more emphasis on a patient-oriented approach to treatment, importance is placed on diet and lifestyle adjustments. One needs to move forward towards integrating nutritional guidance and personalized eating plans into clinical practice in an effort to establish more effective modalities of treatment for gastrointestinal disease. With increasing research into the impact of some food constituents and lifestyle factors on gut health, more effective care will be provided by healthcare practitioners involving both medical and lifestyle interventions. Ultimately, implementing these changes could lead to improved patient outcomes, improved quality of life, and reduced the prevalence of gastrointestinal disease within the general public (Gabriel & Ferguson, 2023; Herdiana, 2023).

15.6.3. Future Trends in Preventive Gastroenterology

Preventive gastroenterology innovations are increasingly opening the door for new health solutions to stave off the incidence of gastrointestinal diseases. Uptake of genomic medicine into routine screening practices is ripe with possibilities, as testing for genes and analyzing biomarkers could enable early diagnosis of susceptibility to diseases , such as colorectal cancer and inflammatory bowel disease. This targeted approach can offer individualized lifestyle interventions and monitoring regimens, maximizing the effectiveness of prevention programs. Furthermore, new non-invasive screening technologies , such as stool DNA testing and advanced imaging modalities, are revolutionizing preventive medicine. Implementation of these approaches not only enhances compliance in patients but also maximizes outcomes in high-risk populations, potentially reducing healthcare spending on late-stage interventions. On a similarly pivotal point, public health programs themselves are being fundamentally reoriented to fill preventive gastroenterology lacunae, and most relevantly to the field of vaccine science. The constant threat of enteric pathogens that bear on gastrointestinal health, norovirus and *Helicobacter pylori,* being the most recently highlighted, makes the urgent necessity for innovative vaccines highly compelling. Preventive gastroenterology can be complemented by cross-disciplinary research methodologies focused on promoting vaccination coverage and interventions against vaccine hesitancy, especially in risk groups. Public health initiatives offering education regarding the crucial role of vaccines in disease prevention, along with engagement in primary care settings, will optimize the effect of these interventions. Through overcoming both educational and logistical challenges, future developments in preventive gastroenterology can shift toward expanded use and application of vaccination technologies to further decrease disease burden. Future technologies premised on artificial intelligence (AI) and machine learning are poised to radically change preventive gastroenterology through improved diagnostic performance and treatment personalization. These technologies offer considerable potential for the interpretation of large amounts of healthcare data, pattern recognition, and the prediction of disease risk based on one's health profile. Furthermore, AI-based platforms can assist in generating tailored diet and lifestyle guidance for preventing disorders like obesity and functional gastrointestinal disorders. Telemedicine, integrated with AI tools, facilitates continuous patient interaction and monitoring for preventive compliance. Enhanced through multidisciplinary partnership, such technologies foretell a new era of preventive gastroenterology for precision medicine and patient-oriented care, ultimately leading to improved public health outcomes in gastroenterology (Sekar et al., 2024; Garbarczyk et al., 2025) (Figure 15.14).

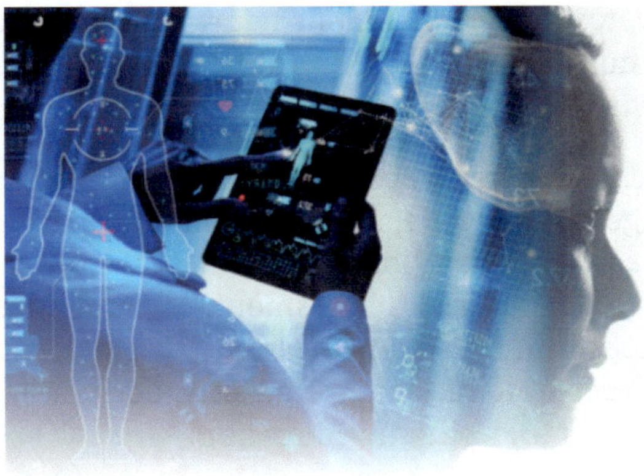

Figure 15.14. Future trends in preventive gastroenterology.

Source: https://blogs.bcm.edu/wp-content/uploads/2023/04/FUTURE-OF-MEDICINE-image-515x380.png.

CLOSER LOOK

TREATMENT RECOMMENDATIONS:

Treatment recommendations are evidence-based guidelines designed to optimize patient outcomes, minimize complications, and standardize care across healthcare settings. A closer look at these recommendations highlights their role in guiding clinical decisions, tailoring therapies to individual patient needs, and integrating preventive strategies with active treatment. Effective treatment recommendations consider disease severity, patient comorbidities, risk factors, and the latest clinical research. Individualized assessment is the foundation of treatment recommendations. Clinicians evaluate the patient's medical history, current health status, lifestyle factors, and potential contraindications before determining the appropriate intervention. For chronic conditions such as diabetes, hypertension, or heart disease, treatment recommendations include both pharmacologic and non-pharmacologic strategies, emphasizing lifestyle modifications like dietary changes, physical activity, stress management, and smoking cessation alongside medication management.

Pharmacological recommendations are guided by efficacy, safety, and patient-specific factors such as age, renal or hepatic function, and potential drug interactions. For example, in cardiovascular disease, clinicians may recommend statins, antihypertensives, or antiplatelet therapy based on individualized risk assessment. In infectious diseases, antibiotic choice is informed by pathogen susceptibility, resistance patterns, and patient tolerance. Adherence to prescribed therapy is critical, and recommendations often include strategies to improve compliance, such as simplified dosing regimens and patient education.

Procedural or surgical recommendations are considered when conservative measures are insufficient or when interventions can prevent complications. For instance, in gallbladder disease with recurrent attacks, cholecystectomy is recommended, while in advanced gastrointestinal cancers, endoscopic or surgical interventions may be advised alongside systemic therapies. Recommendations emphasize weighing potential benefits against procedural risks, recovery considerations, and patient preferences.

Lifestyle and supportive care are integral to comprehensive treatment recommendations. Nutritional guidance, physical rehabilitation, counseling, and psychosocial support enhance recovery, prevent relapse, and improve quality of life. For chronic or complex conditions, multidisciplinary approaches—integrating physicians, nurses, dietitians, therapists, and social workers—ensure that all aspects of patient care are addressed. Treatment recommendations are also dynamic, reflecting advances in medical research, evolving clinical guidelines, and emerging therapies. Evidence-based guidelines from professional organizations, clinical trials, and expert consensus help ensure that care remains current, effective, and safe.

Treatment recommendations demonstrates that they are more than prescriptive instructions—they are structured, evidence-informed pathways that guide individualized care. By combining medical expertise, patient-specific factors, and ongoing evaluation, treatment recommendations enhance outcomes, reduce complications, and support a proactive, patient-centered approach to health management.

If you want, I can create a version focused specifically on gastrointestinal or liver disease treatment recommendations for a more targeted clinical perspective.

SUMMARY

In reflecting on the remarkable progress in gastroenterology, it is essential to see both the gains achieved and the challenges ahead. Integration of state-of-the-art technology, such as artificial intelligence and new imaging techniques, has revolutionized diagnostic capability, with early recognition of gastrointestinal disease now possible. Through enhanced precision medicine, treatment protocols can be tailored on the basis of specific patient profiles, leading to better outcomes and fewer side effects. Since the major is always evolving, one should carefully follow the new developments to ensure maximum utilization of new ideas in practice. As a result of the complexity of gastrointestinal disease, upcoming trends must be embraced to improve patient experience and care, and in fact, major on the importance of massive training programs that equip health professionals with the information to utilize these developments in the right way. The future of gastroenterology is, however, not without its set of challenges. Socioeconomic determinants and health inequities will potentially hinder the equitable implementation of these advances. As research continues to uncover the intricate intersection of gut health and systemic illness, widespread awareness and medical adoption will be essential. This requires collaborative efforts by policymakers, practitioners, and researchers to make novel treatments and technologies available to all populations. Furthermore, the detrimental implications of weight stigma within health systems require urgent attention, as noted by researchers advocating for the eradication of clinical bias (Rubino et al., 2020). By resolving these system issues, we can build a culture that optimizes results in all patients with gastrointestinal diseases. At the conclusion of this discourse, the conclusion affirms the complementarity of innovation and accessibility in the future direction of gastroenterology. Through interaction between scientists and healthcare professionals in breaking down the complexity of the gastrointestinal tract, the commitment to build knowledge and patient care needs to be strong. This includes not just improving diagnostic and treatment strategies but also evidence-based practice to promote awareness and de-stigmatize gastrointestinal disorders. Disease complexity requires a multidisciplinary response, and in planning the future directions in this space, keeping patient care holistic at the core will be crucial. Contemporary appeals for improved medical training and policy reforms will shape the creation of a gastroenterological culture that can address new health challenges, with broad implications for world health (Sadowska et al., 2020).

Some innovative strategies have emerged in gastroenterology, namely the newer therapeutic modalities for an array of gastrointestinal (GI) conditions. Advances in biocompatible materials , such as hydrogels, revolutionized human–machine interfacing (HMI) in medicine. Not only are these materials mechanically flexible and responsive, but they also exhibit immense potential to be interfaced with biological tissues to enhance the efficiency of drug delivery and diagnostic devices. Further, advanced 3D/4D printing technologies also facilitate tailoring of hydrogel properties for optimizing their functions toward specific medical applications (Ullah et al., 2025). This new generation of materials reflects a shift in the approach of patient-centered therapeutic approaches involving technology in the monitoring and management of GI disorders, with the potential to provide improved patient outcomes. The article of gastroenterology has likewise experienced a transformative change in the finding and application of microbiome science. Case studies of the human microbiome have opened up new avenues to the explanation of intricate interactions and associations between microbial communities and gut health. As investigations illuminate the role of the microbiome in gastrointestinal illness, therapeutic interventions aimed at harnessing gut flora and modulating it through the use of probiotics or fecal microbiota transplantation are making clinical headway (Yang, 2007). Such approaches hold significant implications, particularly for conditions like irritable bowel syndrome and inflammatory bowel disease, where conventional therapies are suboptimal. Targeting the microbiome, they represent not only a new leap in therapeutic technology but also a broader trend toward the development of personalized medicine in gastroenterology. In addition, the integration of advanced technology into diagnostics has significantly enhanced the accuracy and efficiency of gastrointestinal disease diagnosis. Novel imaging technologies, such as capsule endoscopy and high-definition endoscopy, provide a unique visual interaction with the GI tract, allowing for earlier detection of conditions that were previously hard to diagnose. These technologies reduce the need for more invasive medical interventions and improve patient safety and comfort (Yang, 2007). In addition, a computer application for diagnosing imaging data through artificial intelligence enables practitioners to identify abnormalities with greater precision and speed. Such advances seem to be leading towards a way of more precise and preventive gastrointestinal treatment, suggesting the necessity for continuous innovation in attempts at enhanced diagnosis and treatment in the field.

References

1. Elsayes, K. M., Kielar, A. Z., Agrons, M. M., Szklaruk, J., Tang, A., Bashir, M. R., Mitchell, D. G., Do, R. K., Fowler, K. J., Chernyak, V., & Sirlin, C. B. (2017). Liver Imaging Reporting and Data System: an expert consensus statement. *Journal of hepatocellular carcinoma, 4*, 29–39. https://doi.org/10.2147/JHC.S125396(accessed on 16th July 2025).
2. Della Corte, C., Mosca, A., Vania, A., Alterio, A., Alisi, A., & Nobili, V. (2016). Pediatric liver diseases: current challenges and future perspectives. *Expert review of gastroenterology & hepatology, 10*(2), 255–265. https://doi.org/10.1586/17474124.2016.1129274 (accessed on 16th July 2025).
3. Alomair, O. A. (2024). *New trends in management of vascular lower GI bleeding between endoscopy and angiography: Literature review*. https://core.ac.uk/download/640070005.pdf (accessed on 16th July 2025).
4. Altamemi, I., Salim, R., & Muslim, O. T. (2020). *Circulating micro-RNA (106, 21) as biomarker for Helicobacter pylori associated gastric cancer*. https://www.semanticscholar.org/paper/e6dc29eeed51d0162442a588fcfb3f5b7423ed8b (accessed on 16th July 2025).
5. Severi, C., Carabotti, M., Cicenia, A., Pallotta, L., & Annibale, B. (2018). Recent advances in understanding and managing diverticulitis. *F1000Research, 7*, F1000 Faculty Rev-971. https://doi.org/10.12688/f1000research.14299.1 (accessed on 16th July 2025).
6. Aziz, Q., Borsook, D., Elsenbruch, S., Kilpatrick, L., et al. (2019). *Role of brain imaging in disorders of brain-gut interaction: A Rome Working Team Report*. https://core.ac.uk/download/323078713.pdf (accessed on 16th July 2025).
7. Barrett, D. (2017). Rethinking Presence: A Grounded Theory of Nurses and Teleconsultation. https://core.ac.uk/download/151161610.pdf (accessed on 16th July 2025).
8. Bergman, B. P., Laing, F., Chandler, A. S., & Calman, K. C. (2018). Witnessing history: a personal view of half a century in public health. *The journal of the Royal College of Physicians of Edinburgh, 48*(2), 181–191. https://doi.org/10.4997/JRCPE.2018.214(accessed on 16th July 2025).
9. Bolock, A. M., Good, M., & Hodzic, Z. (2017). *The role of mucosal immunity in the pathogenesis of necrotizing enterocolitis*. https://core.ac.uk/download/80495060.pdf (accessed on 16th July 2025).
10. Bywood P, Raven M, Butler C. (2013). Telehealth in primary health care settings within Australia and internationally. PHCRIS Policy Issue Review. Adelaide: Primary Health Care Research & Information Service(accessed on 16th July 2025).
11. Cahalan, M. D., Hwang, M., Nakasaki, M., Sabui, S., et al. (2020). *Biotin supplementation ameliorates murine colitis by preventing NF-κB activation*. https://core.ac.uk/download/323069628.pdf (accessed on 16th July 2025).
12. Trinks, J., Caputo, M., Hulaniuk, M. L., Corach, D., & Flichman, D. (2017). Hepatitis C virus pharmacogenomics in Latin American populations: implications in the era of direct-acting antivirals. *Pharmacogenomics and personalized medicine, 10*, 79–91. https://doi.org/10.2147/PGPM.S125452(accessed on 16th July 2025).

13. Chandra Sekar, P. K., Thomas, S. M., & Veerabathiran, R. (2024). The future of cervical cancer prevention: Advances in research and technology. *Exploration of Medicine*. https://www.semanticscholar.org/paper/55b221c3206ca27c0dca312d01887cbf6d442259 (accessed on 16th July 2025).

14. Cirocchi, R., D'Andrea, V., Desiderio, J., Gemini, A., et al. (2017). *New totally intracorporeal reconstructive approach after robotic total gastrectomy: Technical details and short-term outcomes*. https://core.ac.uk/download/98347731.pdf (accessed on 16th July 2025).

15. Marlicz, W., Ren, X., Robertson, A., Skonieczna-Żydecka, K., Łoniewski, I., Dario, P., Wang, S., Plevris, J. N., Koulaouzidis, A., & Ciuti, G. (2020). Frontiers of Robotic Gastroscopy: A Comprehensive Review of Robotic Gastroscopes and Technologies. *Cancers, 12*(10), 2775. https://doi.org/10.3390/cancers12102775(accessed on 16th July 2025).

16. McDonald, D., Hornig, M., Lozupone, C., Debelius, J., Gilbert, J. A., & Knight, R. (2015). Towards large-cohort comparative studies to define the factors influencing the gut microbial community structure of ASD patients. *Microbial ecology in health and disease, 26*, 26555. https://doi.org/10.3402/mehd.v26.26555(accessed on 16th July 2025).

17. Moyer, M. T., Maranki, J. L., & DeWitt, J. M. (2019). EUS-Guided Pancreatic Cyst Ablation: a Clinical and Technical Review. *Current gastroenterology reports, 21*(5), 19. https://doi.org/10.1007/s11894-019-0686-5(accessed on 16th July 2025).

18. Dunn, A., Shapiro, A., Liebman, E., & Pack, S. (2025). *Medical care expenditure indexes: A comparison of indexes using MarketScan and Pharmetrics data.* https://core.ac.uk/download/pdf/6786329.pdf (accessed on 16th July 2025).

19. Fogelson, K., Dorrestein, P. C., Zarrinpar, A., & Knight, R. (2023). The gut microbial bile acid modulation and its relevance to digestive health and diseases. *Gastroenterology, 164*, 1069–1085. https://doi.org/10.1053/j.gastro.2023.02.022 (accessed on 16th July 2025).

20. Fujita, N., Yasuda, I., Endo, I., Isayama, H., Iwashita, T., Ueki, T., Uemura, K., et al. (2023). Evidence-based clinical practice guidelines for cholelithiasis 2021. *Journal of Gastroenterology, 58*, 801–833. https://doi.org/10.1007/s00535-023-02014-6 (accessed on 16th July 2025).

21. Gabriel, C. L., & Ferguson, J. F. (2023). Gut microbiota and microbial metabolism in early risk of cardiometabolic disease. *Circulation Research, 132*, 1674–1691. https://doi.org/10.1161/circresaha.123.322055 (accessed on 16th July 2025).

22. Garbarczyk, W., Napieralska, A., Kapla, A., Černohorská, A., Bednarczyk, D., Białeta, J., Siembab, K., et al. (2025). Systematic review of pertussis: Trends, challenges, and advances in care and prevention. *Journal of Education, Health and Sport*. https://www.semanticscholar.org/paper/8b0188b60f5ccaadae8251b17ce7c0d15832165a (accessed on 16th July 2025).

23. Herdiana, Y. (2023). Functional food in relation to gastroesophageal reflux disease (GERD). *Nutrients, 15*, 3583–3583. https://doi.org/10.3390/nu15163583 (accessed on 16th July 2025).

24. Heyens, L., Busschots, D., Koek, G. H., Robaeys, G., & Francque, S. (2021). Liver fibrosis in non-alcoholic fatty liver disease: From liver biopsy to non-invasive biomarkers in diagnosis and treatment. *Frontiers in Medicine, 8*. https://doi.org/10.3389/fmed.2021.615978 (accessed on 16th July 2025).

25. Lee, Y. C., Dore, M. P., & Graham, D. Y. (2022). Diagnosis and treatment of *Helicobacter pylori* infection. *Annual Review of Medicine, 73*, 183–195. https://doi.org/10.1146/annurev-med-042220-020814 (accessed on 16th July 2025).

26. López-Chila, R., Llerena-Izquierdo, J., Sumba Nacipucha, N., & Cueva Estrada, J. (2023). Artificial intelligence in higher education: An analysis of existing bibliometrics. *Education Sciences, 14*, 47–47. https://doi.org/10.3390/educsci14010047 (accessed on 16th July 2025).
27. Sharpton, S. R., Yong, G. J. M., Terrault, N. A., & Lynch, S. V. (2018). Gut Microbial Metabolism and Nonalcoholic Fatty Liver Disease. *Hepatology communications, 3*(1), 29–43. https://doi.org/10.1002/hep4.1284(accessed on 16th July 2025).
28. Manrique, P., Montero, I., Fernández-Gosende, M., Martinez, N., Hidalgo Cantabrana, C., & Ríos-Covian, D. (2024). Past, present, and future of microbiome-based therapies. *Microbiome Research Reports, 3*. https://www.semanticscholar.org/paper/ad880e7a8180095214017f78a13315cc659791d3 (accessed on 16th July 2025).
29. Morar, N., & Skorburg, J. A. (2018). Bioethics and the Hypothesis of Extended Health. *Kennedy Institute of Ethics journal, 28*(3), 341–376. https://doi.org/10.1353/ken.2018.0020(accessed on 16th July 2025).
30. Focal Spot, Fall/Winter 2010/2011. Bernard Becker Medical Library Archives. Washington University School of Medicine, Saint Louis, Missouri(accessed on 16th July 2025).
31. Oliai, S. (2005). *Economic Environment and Applications of Telemedicine.* https://core.ac.uk/download/10685681.pdf (accessed on 16th July 2025).
32. Pei, X., Liu, L., & Han, Y. (2025). Advances in human microbiome and prostate cancer research. *Frontiers in Immunology, 16*. https://www.semanticscholar.org/paper/452c7a139e8d93f761c5699146ab2227398c3947 (accessed on 16th July 2025).
33. Pennazio, M., Rondonotti, E., Despott, E. J., Dray, X., Keuchel, M., Moreels, T. G., Sanders, D. S., et al. (2022). Small-bowel capsule endoscopy and device-assisted enteroscopy for diagnosis and treatment of small-bowel disorders: European Society of Gastrointestinal Endoscopy (ESGE) Guideline – Update 2022. *Endoscopy, 55*, 58–95. https://doi.org/10.1055/a-1973-3796 (accessed on 16th July 2025).
34. Rubino, F., Puhl, R. M., Cummings, D. E., Eckel, R. H., Ryan, D. H., Mechanick, J. I., Nadglowski, J., et al. (2020). Joint international consensus statement for ending stigma of obesity. *Nature Medicine, 26*, 485–497. https://doi.org/10.1038/s41591-020-0803-x (accessed on 16th July 2025).
35. Sadowska, M., Sarecka-Hujar, B., & Kopyta, I. (2020). Cerebral palsy: Current opinions on definition, epidemiology, risk factors, classification and treatment options. *Neuropsychiatric Disease and Treatment, 16*, 1505–1518. https://doi.org/10.2147/ndt.s235165 (accessed on 16th July 2025).
36. Sarkar, C., Das, B., Rawat, V. S., Wahlang, J. B., Nongpiur, A., Tiewsoh, I., Lyngdoh, N. M., et al. (2023). Artificial intelligence and machine learning technology driven modern drug discovery and development. *International Journal of Molecular Sciences, 24*, 2026–2026. https://doi.org/10.3390/ijms24032026 (accessed on 16th July 2025).
37. Wiita, A. P., & Schrijver, I. (2011). Clinical application of high throughput molecular screening techniques for pharmacogenomics. *Pharmacogenomics and personalized medicine, 4*, 109–121. https://doi.org/10.2147/PGPM.S15302 (accessed on 16th July 2025).
38. Seyhan, A. A., & Carini, C. (2019). Are innovation and new technologies in precision medicine paving a new era in patient-centric care? *Journal of Translational Medicine, 17*. https://doi.org/10.1186/s12967-019-1864-9 (accessed on 16th July 2025).

39. Tripathi, D., Stanley, A. J., Hayes, P., Travis, S. J., Armstrong, M. J., Tsochatzis, E., Rowe, I., et al. (2020). Transjugular intrahepatic portosystemic stent-shunt in the management of portal hypertension. *Gut, 69*, 1173–1192. https://doi.org/10.1136/gutjnl-2019-320221 (accessed on 16th July 2025).

40. Ullah, A., Kim, D. Y., Lim, S. I., & Lim, H. R. (2025). Hydrogel-based biointerfaces: Recent advances, challenges, and future directions in human–machine integration. *Gels, 11*. https://www.semanticscholar.org/paper/e13f6aa43866f58a534a2f45d8dbea024b565217 (accessed on 16th July 2025).

41. Utami, A. N. F., Baharuddin, Tawakkal, Fariaty, C. N., & Khaerah, N. (2022). *Public health services: Makassar government's response in the early phase of the COVID-19.* https://core.ac.uk/download/544196338.pdf (accessed on 16th July 2025).

42. Velikova, T. (2018). *Problems and Perspectives of Immunodiagnostics in Bulgaria* (*Vol. 3).* https://www.semanticscholar.org/paper/c6d396eb74e9533ac4e872028b8013d6d000dba0 (accessed on 16th July 2025).

43. Woo, V. L. (2015). *Oral Manifestations of Crohn's Disease: A Case Report and Review of the Literature.* https://core.ac.uk/download/85003680.pdf (accessed on 16th July 2025).

44. Yang, V. (2007). The challenges facing GI investigators today and what (more) the GI societies can do to help. *Gastroenterology, 133(6),* 1761, 1762. https://www.semanticscholar.org/paper/7733a5f8d5b3f7332865d43e30959253e3f0a1c7 (accessed on 16th July 2025).

45. Yu, P., Xu, H., Hu, X., & Deng, C. (2023). Leveraging generative AI and large language models: A comprehensive roadmap for healthcare integration. *Healthcare, 11*, 2776–2776. https://doi.org/10.3390/healthcare11202776 (accessed on 16th July 2025).

INDEX

D

G

H

I

J

L

M

Q

R

S

T

U

V

W

X

Z